General Surgery
Examination and
Board Review

NOTICE

Medicine is an ever-changing science. As new research and clinical experience broaden our knowledge, changes in treatment and drug therapy are required. The authors and the publisher of this work have checked with sources believed to be reliable in their efforts to provide information that is complete and generally in accord with the standards accepted at the time of publication. However, in view of the possibility of human error or changes in medical sciences, neither the authors nor the publisher nor any other party who has been involved in the preparation or publication of this work warrants that the information contained herein is in every respect accurate or complete, and they disclaim all responsibility for any errors or omissions or for the results obtained from the use of the information contained in this work. Readers are encouraged to confirm the information contained herein with other sources. For example, and in particular, readers are advised to check the product information sheet included in the package of each drug they plan to administer to be certain that the information contained in this work is accurate and that changes have not been made in the recommended dose or in the contraindications for administration. This recommendation is of particular importance in connection with new or infrequently used drugs.

General Surgery Examination and Board Review

Second Edition

Editors

Robert B. Lim, MD

George Kaiser Family Foundation Chair in Surgery
Vice-Chair of Education
Residency Program Director
Professor, Department of Surgery
School of Community Medicine
University of Oklahoma at Tulsa
Tulsa, Oklahoma

Daniel B. Jones, MD, MS

Professor and Chair of Surgery
New Jersey Medical School
Rutgers, The State University of New Jersey
Newark, New Jersey

New York   Chicago   San Francisco   Lisbon   London   Madrid   Mexico City
New Delhi   San Juan   Seoul   Singapore   Sydney   Toronto

1 2 3 4 5 6 7 8 9 DSS 27 26 25 24 23 22

ISBN: 978-1-260-46808-3
MHID: 1-260-46808-9

This book was set in Minion Pro by MPS Limited.
The editors were Jason Malley and Peter J. Boyle.
The production supervisor was Richard Ruzycka.
Production management was provided by Anamika Singh and Rishabh Gupta, MPS Limited.

This book is printed on acid-free paper.

Cataloging-in-publication date for this book is on file at the Library of Congress.

Disclaimer

The views expressed herein are those of the authors and do not necessarily reflect the official policy or position of the Department of the Army, the Department of the Air Force, the Department of the Navy, Department of Defense, or the U.S. Government.

*The second edition of this textbook is dedicated to my wonderful wife, Lisa,
and our children Grace, Alec, Viktoria, and Luke. Thanks for always being there.*
—RBL

*We would also like to dedicate this book to the surgeon volunteers who selflessly offer
their skills and expertise, often in harm's way, to provide care in places like Ukraine,
Nigeria, and Haiti.*

*If you are interested in learning more about surgical mission work
or in donating, please consider the following entities:*
Global Surgical and Medical Support Group at www.gsmsg.org.
International Medical Corps at www.internationalmedicalcorps.org
Doctors without borders at www.msf.org

Contents

Section 3: Surgical Subspecialties

Bariatric Surgery 253

Pediatric Surgery 283

Contributors

Alexandra Adams, MD
Department of Surgery
Brooke Army Medical Center
San Antonio, Texas
Chapter 9

Harry T. Aubin, MD
General Surgeon
Tripler Army Medical Center
Honolulu, Hawaii
Chapter 17

Eric Balent, MD
General Surgeon
Tripler Army Medical Center
Honolulu, Hawaii
Chapter 18

David W. Barham, MD
Department of Urology
University of California, Irvine, California
Chapters 93 and 97

Elise Barker, MD
OB/GYN
University of Kentucky College of Medicine
Lexington, Kentucky
Chapter 65

Ahmed B. Bayoumi, MD, MSc, MBA
Division of Neurosurgery
McMaster University
Toronto, Canada
Chapter 82

Allyson L. Berglund, DPM
Podiatric Surgeon
Department of Podiatric Surgery
Harvard Vanguard Medical Associates
Boston, Massachusetts
Chapter 90

Kenneth J. Bogenberger, MD
General Surgeon
Tripler Army Medical Center
Honolulu, Hawaii
Chapter 52

Naseem Bou-Ayash, MD
General Surgery Resident
Tufts Medical Center
Boston, Massachusetts
Chapter 8

Ryan Bram, MD
General Surgery Resident
Tripler Army Medical Center
Honolulu, Hawaii
Chapters 44, 54, and 60

Leah Brazer, MD
General Surgery Resident
Tripler Army Medical Center
Honolulu, Hawaii
Chapter 47

Danielle E. Smith, DO, MPH
Clinical Associate
Department of Surgery
Duke University School of Medicine
Durham, North Carolina
Chapter 38

Terri L. Carlson, DO
Plastics Surgeon
Tripler Army Medical Center
Honolulu, Hawaii
Chapter 15

Samantha Carson, MD
General Surgery Resident
Tripler Army Medical Center
Honolulu, Hawaii
Chapter 65

Michael Charles
Chief, Trauma Surgery
St John Medical Center
Tulsa, Oklahoma
Chapter 90

Robert C. Chick, MD
General Surgeon
Brooke Army Medical Center
Fort Sam Houston, Texas
Chapter 11

Ashley Chinn
General Surgery Resident
Tripler Army Medical Center
Honolulu, Hawaii
Chapter 46

Lindsey A. Choi, DO
Obstetrician-Gynecologist
Tripler Army Medical Center
Honolulu, Hawaii
Chapter 68

Yong Choi, MD
Assistant Professor
Baylor St. Luke's Medical Group
Baylor College of Medicine
Houston, Texas
Chapter 49

Geoffrey S. Chow
Associate Professor
Department of Surgery
School of Community Medicine
University of Oklahoma-Tulsa
Tulsa, Oklahoma
Chapter 19

William Cole, MD
General Surgeon
Tripler Army Medical Center
Honolulu, Hawaii
Chapter 22

Freeman Condon, MD
General Surgery Resident
Tripler Army Medical Center
Honolulu, Hawaii
Chapters 26 and 28

Rob Conrad, MD
General Surgeon
Wilcox Medical Center
Lihue, Hawaii
Chapters 76, 77, and 79

Erik Criman, MD
Plastic Surgery fellow
Vanderbilt University School of Medicine
Nashville, Tennessee
Chapters 39 and 78

Rachel Cuenca, MD
Orthopedic Surgeon
San Antonio Military Medical Center
San Antonio, Texas
Chapters 69, 70, 71, 72, and 73

Mia DeBarros, MD
Cardiothoracic Surgeon
Madigan Army Medical Center
Tacoma, Washington
Chapters 14 and 85

Mary Decoteau, MD
Division of Traumatology, Surgical Critical Care, and
    Emergency Surgery
Penn Surgery, University of Pennsylvania
Philadelphia, Pennsylvania
Chapter 7

Raffaella DeRosa, MD
Urologist
Womack Army Medical Center
Fort Bragg, North Carolina
Chapter 97

Charles S. Dietrich III, MD
Associate Professor
Department of Obstetrics and Gynecology
University of Kentucky College of Medicine
Lexington, Kentucky
Chapters 65 and 66

Matthew Eckert, MD
Assistant Professor
Department of Surgery
UNC School of Medicine
University of North Carolina
Chapel Hill, North Carolina
Chapter 86

Roger Eduardo, MD
Beltline Bariatric and Surgical Group
Piedmont Hospitals
Atlanta, Georgia
Chapter 4

Timiyin M. E-Nunu, MD
Urologist
Tripler Army Medical Center
Honolulu, Hawaii
Chapter 94

Jill Findlay, MD
General Surgery Resident
Tripler Army Medical Center
Honoulu, Hawaii
Chapter 50

Meaghan J. Flatley
General Surgery Resident
San Antonio Military Medical Center
San Antonio, Texas
Chapter 12

Jace J. P. Franko, MD
General Surgeon
Madigan Army Medical Center
Tacoma, Washington
Chapter 41

Matthew R. Fusco, MD
Assistant Professor of Neurosurgery
Department of Neurological Surgery
Vanderbilt University
Nashville, Tennessee
Chapters 79 and 80

Margaret E. Gallagher, MD
Pediatric Surgeon
Department of Pediatric Surgery
Vanderbilt University Medical Center
Nashville, Tennessee
Chapters 61 and 62

Alan P. Gehrich, MD
OB/GYN
Tripler Army Medical Center
Honolulu, Hawaii
Chapters 29, 66, 67, and 68

Suzanne Gillern, MD
Colorectal Surgeon
Department of Surgery
Tripler Army Medical Center
Honolulu, Hawaii
Chapter 40

John M. Giurani, DPM
Associate Professor in Surgery
Harvard Medical School
Beth Israel Deaconess Medical Center
Boston, Massachusetts
Chapter 90

Patrick Golden, DO
Staff Surgeon
Blanchfield Army Community Hospital
Fort Campbell, Kentucky
Chapter 35

C.T. Grayson, MD
General Surgeon
Landstuhl Regional Medical Center, US Army
Landstuhl, Germany
Chapter 34

Julia B. Greer, MD, MPH
Assistant Professor, Medicine
Division of Gastroenterology, Hepatology and
    Nutrition
University of Pittsburgh School of Medicine
Pittsburgh, Pennsylvania
Chapter 88

Mark A. Gromski, MD
Assistant Professor of Medicine
Indiana University School of Medicine
Indianapolis, Indiana
Chapter 6

Aditya Gutta, MD
Assistant Professor of Clinical Medicine
Indiana University School of Medicine
Indianapolis, Indiana
Chapter 6

Ally Ha, MD
General Surgery Resident
Tripler Army Medical Center
Honolulu, Hawaii
Chapter 48

Kristopher G. Hooten, MD
Neurosurgeon
Tripler Army Medical Center
Honolulu, Hawaii
Chapters 80, 82, and 83

Christopher B. Horn, MD
Surgical Critical Care Fellow
University of Cincinnati Medical Center
Cincinnati, Ohio
Chapters 86 and 89

Vernon Horst, MD
Vascular Surgeon
Shelby Baptist Medical Center
Alabaster, Alabama
Chapters 99 and 102

Bonnie B. Hunt, DO
General Surgeon
Tripler Army Medical Center
Honolulu, Hawaii
Chapter 36

Farah A. Husain, MD
Associate Professor of Surgery
Division of Bariatric Surgery
School of Medicine
Oregon Health and Science University
Portland, Oregon
Chapter 21

Theresa Jackson, MD
General Surgery Resident
Department of Surgery
University of Oklahoma-Tulsa
Tulsa, Oklahoma
Chapter 55

William J. Jordan, MD
Staff Surgeon
Sterling Ridge Orthopedics and Sports Medicine
The Woodlands, Texas
Chapter 81

Tovy Haber Kamine, MD
Assistant Professor
Division of Trauma, Acute Care Surgery, and Surgical
    Critical Care
Baystate Medical Center
University of Massachusetts
Springfield, Massachusetts
Chapter 87

Ekkehard M. Kasper, MD, PhD
Department of Neurosurgery
St. Elizabeth's Medical Center
Brighton, Massachusetts
Chapter 82

Dwight C. Kellicut, MD
Deputy Commander
Directorate of Academics, Research, and Training
Tripler Army Medical Center
Honolulu, Hawaii
Chapter 100

Kelly Kempe, MD
Associate Professor
Department of Surgery
Vascular Fellowship Program Director
School of Community Medicine
University of Oklahoma-Tulsa
Tulsa, Oklahoma
Chapters 99 and 102

Phillip M. Kemp Bohan, MD
Surgeon
Brooke Army Medical Center
Fort Sam Houston, Texas
Chapters 23 and 33

Zhamak Khorgami, MD
Assistant Professor
Department of Surgery
School of Community Medicine
University of Oklahoma-Tulsa
Tulsa, Oklahoma
Chapter 1

Hyein Kim
Vascular Surgeon
Department of Surgery
School of Community Medicine
University of Oklahoma-Tulsa
Tulsa, Oklahoma
Chapters 103 and 104

Booker T. King, MD
Chief and Professor, Division of Burn Surgery
Director, North Carolina Jaycee Burn Center
University of North Carolina
Chapel Hill, North Carolina
Chapters 87 and 101

Jordan Kopf, DO
OB/GYN Resident
Tripler Army Medical Center
Honolulu, Hawaii
Chapter 66

Omar Yusef Kudsi, MD
Chair, Department of Surgery
Good Samaritan Medical Center
Brockton, Massachusetts
Chapters 8 and 52

Kiran Lagisetty, MD
Assistant Professor of Surgery
Section of Thoracic Surgery
University of Michigan
Ann Arbor, Michigan
Chapter 32

Justin LaRocque, MD
General Surgery Resident
Tripler Army Medical Center
Honolulu, Hawaii
Chapter 17

Henry Lin, MD
Assistant Professor
Uniformed Services University of the Health
    Sciences
Captain, Medical Corps, United States Navy
Department Head of General Surgery and Urology
Naval Hospital Camp LeJeune
Camp LeJeune, North Carolina
Chapter 25

Kevin M. Lin-Hurtubise, MD
Staff Surgical Oncologist
Department of Surgery
Tripler Army Medical Center
Honolulu, Hawaii
Chapter 30

Alexander Malloy, DO
Harborview Medical Center
UW Medicine
Seattle, Washington
Chapter 102

Anita Mamtani, MD
Surgeon
Memorial Sloan Kettering Cancer Center
New York, New York
Chapter 45

Matthew J. Martin, MD
Associate Professor of Surgery
Uniformed Services University of the
    Health Sciences
Associate Professor of Surgery
University of Washington School of Medicine
Trauma Medical Director and Chief of Surgical
    Research
Madigan Army Medical Center
Tacoma, Washington
Chapters 78, 86, and 89

Pamela C. Masella, DO
Minimally Invasive Surgeon
San Antonio Military Medical Center
San Antonio, Texas
Chapter 12

Travis Mason, MD
Surgical Oncologist
Tripler Army Medical Center
Honolulu, Hawaii
Chapters 30 and 31

Kai Matthes, MD, PhD
Chief Executive Officer
Endosim, LLC
Bolton, Massachusetts
Chapter 6

Victoria Maxon, DO
Urology Resident
Tripler Army Medical Center
Honolulu, Hawaii
Chapters 91 and 92

John S. Mayo, MD
General Surgery Resident
Tripler Army Medical Center
Honolulu, Hawaii
Chapters 81 and 88

Robert A. Mazzoli, MD
Ophthalmology Surgeon
Madigan Army Medical Center
Tacoma, Washington
Chapter 84

Patrick M. McCarthy, MD
General Surgery Resident
Brooke Army Medical Center
San Antonio, Texas
Chapter 24

James McClintic
General Surgery Resident,
Department of Surgery
School of Community Medicine
University of Oklahoma-Tulsa
Tulsa, Oklahoma
Chapter 20

Robert McMurray, MD
General Surgeon
Department of General Surgery
Tripler Army Medical Center
Honolulu, Hawaii
Chapter 105

Andrea Moon, MD
General Surgery Resident
Tripler Army Medical Center
Honolulu, Hawaii
Chapter 5

Lauren P. K. Muramoto, MD
Urology Resident
Tripler Army Medical Center
Honolulu, Hawaii
Chapters 4 and 98

John E. Musser
Urologist
Tripler Army Medical Center
Honolulu, Hawaii
Chapters 94 and 98

Peter R. Nelson, MD
Professor of Surgery
Vascular Surgery Section Chief
Director of Surgical Research
School of Community Medicine
University of Oklahoma-Tulsa
Tulsa, Oklahoma
Chapter 101

Scott Nguyen, MD
General Surgery Resident
Tripler Army Medical Center
Honolulu, Hawaii
Chapters 16 and 17

Fares Nigim, MD
Clinical Fellow in Neurology
Harvard Medical School
Boston, Massachusetts
Chapter 82

Rabia Nazimani, MD
Assistant Professor, Division of Burn Surgery
North Carolina Jaycee Burn Center
University of North Carolina
Chapel Hill, North Carolina
Chapter 87

Stephen R. Odom, MD
Assistant Professor, Surgery
Harvard Medical School
Beth Israel Deaconess Medical Center
Boston, Massachusetts
Chapters 87 and 89

Mary T. O'Donnell, MD
Chief, Colon and Rectal Surgery
Walter Reed National Military Medical Center
Bethesda, Maryland
Chapter 20

Emily Ofstun, MD
General Surgery Resident
William Beaumont Army Medical Center
El Paso, Texas
Chapter 35

Christopher S. Ogilvy, MD
Director, BIDMC Brain Aneurysm Institute
Director, Endovascular and Operative Neurosurgery
Beth Israel Deaconess Medical Center
Boston, Massachusetts
Chapters 79 and 80

Morohunranti O. Oguntoye, MD
Comprehensive Ophthalmologist
Department of Ophthalmology
Madigan Army Medical Center
Tacoma, Washington
Chapter 84

Anne O'Shea, MD
General Surgery Resident
San Antonio Military Medical Center
San Antonio, Texas
Chapters 10 and 27

Chan W. Park, MD
Minimally Invasive Surgeon
Tripler Army Medical Center
Honolulu, Hawaii
Chapters 54 and 60

Brooke Pati, MD
General Surgery Resident
Tripler Army Medical Center
Honolulu, Hawaii
Chapters 56 and 58

Aaron Paul, MD
Anesthesiology Resident
Department of Surgery
School of Community Medicine
University of Oklahoma-Tulsa
Tulsa, Oklahoma
Chapter 2

Brian J. Pottorf, MD
General Surgeon
Washington Regional General Surgery Clinic
Fayetteville, Arkansas
Chapter 21

Nicholas S. Pyskir, MD
Obstetrician-Gynecologist
Program Director, Urology Residency
Tripler Army Medical Center
Honolulu, Hawaii
Chapter 67

Stuart Reynolds, MD
General Surgery Resident
Department of Surgery
School of Community Medicine
University of Oklahoma-Tulsa
Tulsa, Oklahoma
Chapter 36

William V. Rice, MD
Bariatric Center
Presbyterian Rust Medical Center
Rio Rancho, New Mexico
Chapter 53

E. Matthew Ritter, MD
Professor of Surgery
Indiana University School of Medicine
Indianapolis, Indiana
Chapter 20

Erik Roedel, MD
Chief, Department of Surgery
Madigan Army Medical Center
Tacoma, Washington
Chapter 42

Dylan Russell, MD
General Surgery Resident
Tripler Army Medical Center
Honolulu, Hawaii
Chapter 29

Joy Sarkar, MD
Surgical Oncology Fellow
Roswell Park Comprehensive Cancer Center
Buffalo, New York
Chapters 11, 13, 32, 51, 74, and 75

Justin C. Scheidt, MD
Pediatric Surgeon
Brooke Army Medical Center
Fort Sam Houston, Texas
Chapters 61 and 62

Andrew T. Schlussel, DO
Colorectal Surgeon
Department of General Surgery
Madigan Army Medical Center
Tacoma, Washington
Chapter 41

Albert Jesse Schuette, MD
Neurosurgeon
Piedmont Atlanta Hospital
Atlanta, Georgia
Chapter 83

Jigesh A. Shah, MD
Assistant Professor
Department of Surgery
UT Southwestern Medical Center
University of Texas
Dallas, Texas
Chapter 52

Zakiya Shakir, MD
General Surgery Resident
Department of Surgery
School of Community Medicine
University of Oklahoma-Tulsa
Tulsa, Oklahoma
Chapter 45

Ranjna Sharma, MD
Associate Professor of Surgery
Center for Breast, Endocrine, and Plastic Surgery
SUNY Upstate Medical University
Syracuse, New York
Chapter 47

Robert Shawhan, MD
General Surgery Resident
Madigan Army Medical Center
Tacoma, Washington
Chapter 86

Robert L. Sheffler, MD
Staff Medical Oncologist
Department of Medicine
Tripler Army Medical Center
Honolulu, Hawaii
Chapter 30

Maxwell Sirkin, MD
Critical Care Fellow
Department of Surgery
University of North Carolina
Chapel Hill, North Carolina
Chapter 53

Danielle E. Smith, DO
Vascular Surgeon
Womack Army Medical Center
Fort Bragg, North Carolina
Chapter 38

Peter L. Steinberg, MD
Urologist, Beth Israel Deaconess Medical Center
Assistant Professor of Surgery
Harvard Medical School
Boston, Massachusetts
Chapter 93

Joseph R. Sterbis
Program Director, Urology Residency
Tripler Army Medical Center
Honolulu, Hawaii
Chapters 93, 94, 95, 96, 97, and 98

Jayne Stevens, MD
Otolaryngologist, Head and Neck Surgeon
Carl R. Darnall Army Medical Center
Fort Hood, Texas
Chapter 53

Erin Swan, MD
Orthopedic Surgeon
San Antonio Military Medical Center
San Antonio, Texas
Chapter 69, 70, 71, 72, and 73

Benjamin D. Tabak, MD
Pediatric Surgeon
Tripler Army Medical Center
Honolulu, Hawaii
Chapters 63 and 64

Kelli Tavares, MD
General Surgery Resident
Tripler Army Medical Center
Honolulu, Hawaii
Chapter 42

Ajith J. Thomas, MD
Chair, Department of Neurosurgery
Professor of Neurological Surgery
Cooper Medical School of Rowan University
Camden, New Jersey
Chapters 79 and 80

Steven Vang, DO
Senior Vascular Surgery Fellow
School of Community Medicine
University of Oklahoma-Tulsa
Tulsa, Oklahoma
Chapter 101

Timothy J. Vreeland, MD
Department of Surgery
Uniformed Services University of Health Sciences
Bethesda, Maryland
Department of Surgical Oncology
Brooke Army Medical Center
San Antonio, Texas
Chapters 9, 10, 11, 23, 24, 27, and 33

Hussna Wakily, MD
Minimally Invasive Surgeon
Tri-City Medical Center
San Diego, California
Chapter 59

Paul Wetstein, MD
Ryder Trauma Center
Jackson Memorial Medical Center
University of Miami
Miami, Florida
Chapter 3

Tiffany P. Wheeler
General Surgery Resident
Department of Surgery
School of Community Medicine
University of Oklahoma-Tulsa
Tulsa, Oklahoma
Chapter 43

Bradford P. Whitcomb, MD
Associate Professor of Obstetrics and Gynecology
Division Chief, Gynecologic Oncology
UConn Health
University of Connecticut
Farmington, Connecticut
Chapter 66

Felicia N. Williams, MD
Associate Professor and Associate Division Chief
Division of Burn Surgery
North Carolina Jaycee Burn Center
University of North Carolina
Chapel Hill, North Carolina
Chapter 87

Ashley D. Willoughby, DO
General Surgery Resident
Department of General Surgery
Tripler Army Medical Center
Honolulu, Hawaii
Chapter 1

Gordon Wisbach, MD, MBA
Assistant Professor of Surgery
Uniformed Services University of the Health Sciences
F. Edward Hebert School of Medicine Bethesda,
    Maryland
Department of General Surgery
Naval Medical Center San Diego
San Diego, California
Chapter 7

Christopher G. Yheulon, MD
Assistant Professor of Surgery
Department of Surgery
Tripler Army Medical Center
Honolulu, Hawaii
Chapters 37 and 57

Preface

The first edition of *General Surgery Examination and Board Review* was a great success. Five years later, the second edition is updated with new questions, as knowledge required for general surgery certification expands. All the classic concepts of surgery are included, but so are new ideas that form the basis of management today. The reader will benefit from the knowledge of the book's many authors, most of whom are recognized experts in their field. This textbook will help the recent graduate to become board certified as he or she enters the competent phase of their career. It will also help the proficient surgeon recertify and keep abreast of the best surgical management using high-quality literature. However, many of the answers in this textbook will become obsolete someday. When I graduated from residency, it was very common to treat diverticulitis with an urgent colonic resection when on call. Later, many of those episodes were treated with antibiotics only, and now in some instances, antibiotics are not required at all. The responsible surgeon will never stop learning, and this textbook will help general surgeons continue to do so. It is a true honor to be one of its editors.

Acknowledgments

We would like to thank Cierra Gleason for her tireless work in bringing this textbook to completion

SECTION 1

Perioperative

1

Obstructive Sleep Apnea

Ashley D. Willoughby and Zhamak Khorgami

A 54-year-old male presents to his perioperative appointment to undergo elective inguinal hernia repair. The patient has a body mass index (BMI) of 38 with a height of 72 in. (1.83 m) and a weight of 127 kg (280 lb). He has a history of hypertension currently being managed with a calcium channel blocker. His wife reports increasing snoring at night with noticeable gasps for air when lying supine. The patient denies increasing daytime drowsiness. He has no history of prior surgeries and no family history of complications with anesthesia.

On physical exam, he has a neck circumference of 44 cm and a Mallampati score of 3. No cardiovascular or respiratory abnormalities are observed. His abdomen is obese with no evidence of caput medusa. Right inguinal ring weakness palpated on exam.

1. **Which of the following is NOT a criterion for obesity hypoventilation syndrome (OHS)?**

   A. Obesity (BMI >30 kg/m^2)
   B. Neck circumference of >48 cm
   C. Daytime hypoventilation
   D. Hypercapnia with $PaCO_2$ >45 mmHg
   E. Hypoxia with PaO_2 <70 mmHg

2. **Which of the following is true regarding obstructive sleep apnea (OSA) in the perioperative and intraoperative evaluation and management of this patient?**

   A. This patient has two out of three risk factors for OSA and therefore does not require polysomnography.
   B. Face mask pre-oxygenation will create a higher tidal volume than nasal prongs.

   C. The Mallampati score of 3 is not a risk for a difficult intubation.
   D. The critical closing pressure of this patient's airway is higher than non-OSA patients.
   E. The patient should be placed in the Trendelenburg position.

3. **What is the patient's ideal body weight based on the JD Robinson formula?**

   A. 75 kg
   B. 98 kg
   C. 64 kg
   D. 106 kg
   E. 86 kg

4. **Which of the following would be the best option for a paralytic agent in this patient?**

   A. Vecuronium
   B. Cistaracurium
   C. Rocuronium
   D. Pancuronium
   E. Atracurium

5. **Which of the following is true regarding the postoperative management of patients with suspected OSA?**

   A. The patient should be placed in the supine position while recovering to protect the surgical site.
   B. Continuous positive airway pressure (CPAP) should be immediately available for use in postoperative patients with known or suspected OSA.

C. Opioid dosing should be based on total body weight (TBW) rather than ideal body weight (IBW).

D. The use of thoracic epidural postoperatively is contraindicated in patients with OSA.

E. The use of CPAP postoperatively could increase the risk of complications.

A 42-year-old female with a BMI of 44 kg/m^2, along with type 2 diabetes mellitus, hypertension, and hyperlipidemia, is undergoing her preoperative evaluation for surgical management of her obesity and weight-related comorbidities. She is felt to be a good candidate for surgery, and she opted for a sleeve gastrectomy. She snores loudly with daytime sleepiness but has never been evaluated for OSA.

1. What is the average prevalence of OSA in those evaluated for bariatric surgery?

A. 5–15%

B. 20-30%

C. 30–50%

D. 60–80%

2. Which of the following is the best screen for OSA?

A. STOP-Bang score

B. Epworth sleepiness scale

C. Venous HCO$_3$$^-$

D. PaCO$_2$

3. Which is the gold standard test for the diagnosis of OSA?

A. Overnight in-laboratory polysomnography

B. Multiple sleep latency test

C. Home sleep apnea testing

D. Neck computed tomography (CT) scan

4. Based on the screening questionnaire, this patient was at risk of having OSA. You will send the patient for further evaluation. Which is compatible with the diagnosis of moderate to severe OSA?

A. Respiratory effort–related arousals >10 per hour

B. Respiratory event index ≥8 per hour

C. Apnea-Hypopnea Index ≥15 per hour

D. Respiratory Disturbance Index ≥30 per hour

5. After the appropriate test, it was confirmed that this patient has OSA. Which is the correct precaution in the perioperative period of sleeve gastrectomy for this patient?

A. Preoxygenation, induction, and intubation in a flat position

B. Continuous positive airway and positive end-expiratory pressure during induction

C. Maintenance of normal tidal volumes during surgery

D. Extubation when patients are appropriately relaxed with neuromuscular blockage

6. Which of the following would be the best option for a paralytic agent in this patient?

A. Vecuronium

B. Cistaracurium

C. Rocuronium

D. Pancuronium

ANSWERS

Scenario 1:

1. **B.** Patients with a neck circumference of >48 cm have a high probability of developing obstructive sleep apnea (OSA); however, it is not a criterion for OHS. OHS results in hypoventilation and hypoxemia due to obesity, whereas OSA is a blockage of the airway that occurs during sleep. Many obese patients have both. Patients with OHS are at a higher risk for perioperative morbidity and mortality. These patients are at a higher risk of airway collapse, blunted central respiratory stimulation, and pulmonary hypertension, therefore placing these patients at a higher surgical risk.

Criteria for OHS:

a. Obesity (BMI >30 kg/m^2)

b. Serum bicarbonate >27 mEq/L

c. SpO$_2$ <93%

d. ABG demonstrating hypercapnia PaCO$_2$> 45 mmHg and hypoxemia PaO$_2$ <70 mmHg

e. An alternative cause of hypoventilation cannot be identified

2. **D.** If the surgery is elective, if surgery is likely to require large doses of anesthetic agent or opioids intraoperatively, and if there is a high suspicion of undiagnosed OSA in the perioperative period, it should be postponed with imminent evaluation and treatment as needed preoperatively. Evidence has shown that pre-oxygenation via nasal CPAP mask is superior to face-mask oxygenation, despite potential

air leaks if the mouth is allowed to be open. Nasal CPAP increases the pressure gradient between the nasopharyngeal and oropharyngeal cavities pushing the soft palate and tongue forward and therefore opening the airway, whereas the positive pressure through the face mask will induce an obstruction. Mallampati score of 3 includes visualization of the soft palate and base of the uvula. Mallampati scores of 3 and 4 demonstrate difficulty intubation; however, they cannot predict the difficulty of bag-valve-mask ventilation.

The upstream pressure of the pharynx at which air entry/flow ceases is considered the critical closing pressure. This pressure can be increased by adding lateral pillar fat pads to compress the airway, sleep resulting in muscle relaxation, or can be induced by anesthesia. The ideal positioning for a patient with OSA is the ramped position of intubation or the lateral recumbent, if possible and in reverse Trendelenburg position to ease ventilation, increase total lung capacity, and decrease the longitudinal tension on the upper airway.

3. A. The JD Robinson formula states:

Man: 52 kg (115 lb) + 1.9 kg (4.2 lb) per in. over 60 in.

Woman: 49 kg (108 lb) + 1.7 kg (3.7 lb) per in. over 60 in.

This calculation is useful in this patient to determine optimal paralytic, anesthetic, and opioid dosing as well as mechanical ventilation control intraoperatively and postoperatively as needed.

4. C. All non-depolarizing neuromuscular blockers act by antagonizing the acetylcholine receptor in a reversible/competitive manor. A rapid-onset, short-acting non-depolarizing agent would be the best option for this patient. Out of the options listed, Rocuronium has an onset of 45 to 60 seconds and a duration of 30 to 60 minutes and would be the most ideal. Also obesity has not been found to alter the pharmacokinetics of Rocuronium and therefore can be dosed on IBW or actual body weight. Pancuronium is the longest acting and is used in patients that require paralysis >1 hour and in patients with normal hepatic and renal function. Cisatracurium and atracurium undergo Hoffman elimination with an onset of 1 to 2 minutes and are intermediate acting. These agents would be recommended in patients with renal or hepatic insufficiency. Vecuronium is also an intermediate-acting neuromuscular blocking agent (NMBA) and would be recommended in patients with cardiovascular disease as it has the least adverse side effect profile. A prolonged duration of paralysis can occur when using actual body weight in dosing atracurium and vecuronium. Avoiding prolonged paralysis or large doses of longer-acting NMBAs is key.

5. B. CPAP should be available for patients in the immediate postoperative period if OSA is known or suspected. If OSA is suspected, introducing CPAP

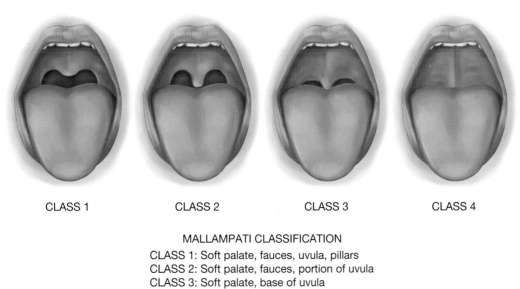

CLASS 1   CLASS 2   CLASS 3   CLASS 4

MALLAMPATI CLASSIFICATION
CLASS 1: Soft palate, fauces, uvula, pillars
CLASS 2: Soft palate, fauces, portion of uvula
CLASS 3: Soft palate, base of uvula
CLASS 4: Hard palate only

in the immediate postoperative period can induce anxiety due to the discomfort of the mask and confusion from the remaining sedatives on board. The proper positioning for optimal airway patency is in the upright and lateral decubitus position if possible. Opioid dosing should be based on IBW rather than TBW due to the potential for a prolonged duration of action with TBW in obese patients resulting in suppression of respiratory drive and decrease pharyngeal muscle stimulation. The use of a postoperative epidural can be beneficial in patients undergoing a large abdominal operation at risk for requiring large doses of opioids for pain control. The use of CPAP in the postoperative period has not been shown to increase complications; specifically, positive pressure ventilation has not been proved to increase leak rates in bariatric surgery patients.

Scenario 2:

1. D. OSA is the most common sleep-related breathing disorder. OSA is more prevalent in males, those who are older, and obese individuals. It has also been reported to be more prevalent in young African Americans compared with Caucasians of the same age.[1] The prevalence of OSA varies based on the diagnostic criteria, testing methodology, and the study population. Scoring criteria and apnea-hypopnea index (AHI) threshold vary in different studies. Peppard et al. estimated the prevalence of moderate to severe OSA (AHI ≥ 15 events per hour) to be 10% to 17% in men and 3% to 9% in women, higher in older ages, and with a significant increase in the last two decades. When AHI ≥ 5 events per hour with symptoms is considered as the diagnostic criteria (which includes mild OSA), the estimated prevalence is approximately 24% in males and 10% in females. National and international trend studies show that the prevalence of OSA is increasing which can be due to population aging, increasing obesity, and increased detection rate.

The prevalence of OSA is significantly higher in obese patients and is one of the most common comorbidities in morbidly obese patients. De Raaff et al. evaluated 14 prospective studies that investigated the prevalence of OSA before bariatric surgery using sleep studies. In their study, the prevalence of OSA was 35% to 94% (higher than 60% in 11 studies). Screening of OSA is recommended in all bariatric surgery candidates because of

- the high prevalence of OSA in morbidly obese patients,
- a significant proportion of undiagnosed OSA, and
- the increased perioperative risks in this group of patients.

Patients with mild OSA may be asymptomatic or to be noticed to have daytime sleepiness by others as the only presentation. When more severe, they will complain of daytime sleepiness with difficulty concentrating, and the bed partner will notice loud snoring, gasping, choking, or stop breathing during the sleep. Other manifestations of OSA can be sleep maintenance insomnia (repetitive awakenings), cardiovascular events during sleep (chest pain or palpitations), nighttime sweating, morning headaches, mood changes, and nocturia.

2. A. Several questionnaires have been developed to assess and screen for OSA. STOP-Bang questionnaire is a scoring model based on loud snoring, feeling tired and sleepy during the daytime, observed stop breathing in sleep, being treated for high blood pressure, body mass index, age, and neck circumference (Table 1-1). Based on 10 studies (mostly on middle-aged obese males) this questionnaire has high sensitivity (suitable for screening) but low specificity

Table 1-1   STOP-BANG QUESTIONNAIRE

Question	Answer
Do you **S**nore loudly (loud enough to be heard through closed doors)?	Yes/No
Do you often feel **T**ired, fatigued, or sleepy during daytime?	Yes/No
Has anyone **O**bserved you stop breathing during your sleep?	Yes/No
Do you have or are you being treated for high blood **P**ressure?	Yes/No
BMI more than 35 kg m²?	Yes/No
Age over 50 yr old?	Yes/No
Neck circumference: Neck circumference >40 cm?	Yes/No
Gender: Male?	Yes/No

High risk of OSA: Yes to ≥ 3 questions
Low risk of OSA: Yes to <3 questions
BMI, body mass index; OSA, obstructive sleep apnea.

Source: Reproduced, with permission, from Chung F, Subramanyam R, Liao P, Sasaki E, Shapiro C, Sun Y. High STOP-Bang score indicates a high probability of obstructive sleep apnoea. *Br J Anaesth.* 2012;108(5):768–775. doi:10.1093/bja/aes022

in detecting OSA. Although questionnaires can be used as a screening tool to stratify high-risk patients for OSA, the American Academy of Sleep Medicine (AASM) recommends that the suspicion of OSA in adults must be confirmed by polysomnography (PSG) or home sleep apnea testing (HSAT) in order to make the diagnosis. The Epworth Sleepiness Scale (ESS) is a symptom severity score assessment based on subjective daytime sleepiness. The ESS has a poor correlation in the bariatric population for the detection of OSA and is not recommended in this setting. Although ESS may have high levels of specificity, it has low sensitivity and is not appropriate for screening.

PaCO$_2$ and venous HCO$_3^-$ are not indicators of OSA but are used to diagnose OHS, which is a triad of obesity, daytime hypoxemia, and CO$_2$ elevation. Obese patients with OHS fail to maintain appropriate levels of ventilation and may face oxygen desaturation and elevated CO$_2$ levels. It is recommended to screen for OHS in bariatric surgery candidates with OSA because it can present in up to 20% of these patients, is often unrecognized, and its coexistence will increase the surgical morbidity and mortality rate.[7]

3. A. Based on the AASM practice guideline, PSG is the standard test for the diagnosis of OSA. PSG is in-laboratory, attended test and can be either a full-night or split-night test. This study can also diagnose other sleep-related breathing disorders. The key items studied and reported by PSG are data from sleep, electrocardiography, respiratory, and periodic leg movement.

In patients with suspected uncomplicated OSA who are estimated to have moderate or severe OSA, unattended HSAT with a type 3 device can be considered as an alternative to PSG (Figure 1-1). HSAT should be performed under appropriate supervision and interpreted by a clinician knowledgeable in sleep medicine. Type 3 HSAT devices measure cardiopulmonary parameters, oxygen saturation, two respiratory variables (e.g., airflow, effort to breath), and a cardiac variable (e.g., heart rate or electrocardiogram). PSG is preferred for patients with suspected mild OSA; however, some payers prefer HSAT first and proceed to PSG if HSAT is negative and OSA is still suspected.

Questionnaires, clinical tools, and algorithms are not recommended to diagnose OSA in adults. A PSG

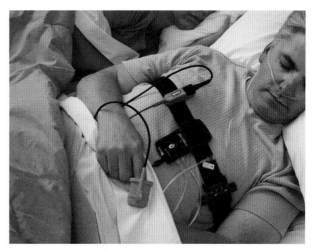

Figure 1-1 Home sleep apnea testing
Source: Sleep Insights, Rochester, NY.

or the HSAT with the appropriate device should be used to confirm the diagnosis. The HSAT can be used in uncomplicated adult patients who have signs and symptoms of moderate to severe OSA; however, if a single HSAT test is nondiagnostic, inconclusive, or technically inadequate, then a PSG is recommended to confirm or rule out OSA.

PSG is recommended to be considered in the following patients rather than HSAT:

- Complicated OSA, which refers to the presence of medical conditions that could potentially affect respiration (e.g., respiratory muscle weakness, significant cardiorespiratory disease, awake or sleep-related hypoventilation, chronic opioid use, history of stroke, severe insomnia)
- Mission-critical workers with a job in which falling asleep has a potential danger or negative consequences (e.g., airline pilots, drivers, police, military posts, astronauts)
- Suspicion of a nonrespiratory sleep disorder or coexistence of a nonrespiratory sleep disorder

4. C. The diagnostic criteria for OSA depends on the diagnostic test. If PSG is used, the diagnosis of OSA is confirmed if either (1) ≥15 predominantly obstructive respiratory events per hour of sleep are recorded, even with no documented comorbidities or associated symptom, or (2) ≥5 predominantly obstructive respiratory events per hour of sleep are recorded and the patient has typical associated symptoms of OSA or comorbidities. These can be sleepiness, fatigue, waking up with gasping or choking, loud snoring, witnessed breathing interruptions, hypertension, type 2 diabetes mellitus, coronary artery disease, cerebrovascular accident, congestive heart failure, atrial fibrillation, mood disorder, or cognitive dysfunction.

Obstructive respiratory events can be apneas (obstructive and mixed), hypopneas, or respiratory effort–related arousals (RERAs). PSG provides two quantitative indices: (1) The AHI, which is apneas + hypopneas/total sleep time in hours, and (2) the respiratory disturbance index (RDI), which is apneas + hypopneas + RERAs/total sleep time in hours. Using the RDI will confirm more patients with OSA with the same threshold values since it includes RERAs. Either the AHI or the RDI may be used for diagnosis, and it may vary based on the payor and insurance.

Most HSAT devices cannot identify RERAs and hypopneas characterized by arousals due to a lack of electroencephalogram (EEG) monitoring. Also, HSATs record the number of respiratory events per hour of recording time (should be at least 4 hours) rather than total sleep time, which is called the respiratory event index (REI). Using validated devices, the REI correlates with RDI and AHI, and the results of an HSAT in appropriately selected patients (high risk for OSA) are similar to an in-laboratory PSG. Therefore, diagnostic values for the REI to confirm OSA are the same as an in-laboratory PSG (REI ≥15 events per hour, or REI = 5–14.9 with OSA symptoms).

Patients with a diagnosis of OSA are classified as mild, moderate, or severe disease based on consensus:

- Mild OSA: patients with AHI/RDI/REI of 5 to 14.9 respiratory events per hour. These patients can be asymptomatic or may report daytime sleepiness when unstimulated (noticed by family members). Mild OSA does not impair daily life and activities.
- Moderate OSA: AHI/RDI/REI of 15 to 29.9 respiratory events per hour of sleep. Patients with moderate OSA are normally aware of their symptoms. They try to avoid falling asleep by taking a nap and avoid long activities. There is an increased risk of motor vehicle accidents, and these patients may try to avoid long driving.
- Severe OSA: AHI/RDI/REI ≥30 respiratory events per hour of sleep. Normal daily activities are impaired in this situation. These patients are at risk for injury due to falling asleep even in a sitting posture. All-cause mortality and cardiovascular comorbidities are increased in this group.

5. **B.** Anesthetic care is important in the perioperative management of bariatric surgery patients with OSA. OSA and OHS both increase perioperative complications. Table 1-2 shows recommendations on anesthetic care in this group of patients based on a consensus guideline. Appropriate anesthetic care in the preoperative, operative, and postoperative phases is critical in these patients. There is an increased risk of difficult intubation, and a ramped position is preferred for intubation. The ramped position will help with oxygenation and will facilitate the laryngoscopy for intubation (Figure 1-2). The flat supine position is not recommended due to the risk of desaturation, difficult mask ventilation, and more challenges in intubation.

In patients with moderately severe and severe OSA, CPAP, and PEEP at induction can maintain lung capacity and prevent oxygen desaturation. High-flow oxygen is also helpful in maintaining oxygenation during intubation. Video laryngoscopy needs to be considered selectively in patients with possible difficult intubation. In the immediate postoperative period, physicians should not be hesitant to place CPAP on a patient who requires it. There is no evidence that CPAP increases the risk of a sleeve gastrectomy or Roux-en-Y gastric bypass leak.

There are also considerations for anesthetic medications. Sedatives as premedication should not be used, and opioid medications should be titrated slowly with careful monitoring. At the time of extubation, the patient needs to be close to fully awake, able to open their eyes and cough well, and neuromuscular blockade needs to be fully reversed, with restored muscle function.

In the postoperative setting, opioids should be used with caution, and with the lowest dose possible. A multimodal analgesic model should be planned to decrease the use of opioids for pain control. Immediately after surgery, CPAP is beneficial especially in patients with severe OSA. Oxygen therapy

Table 1-2 RECOMMENDATIONS FOR ANESTHETIC CARE OF PATIENTS WITH OBSTRUCTIVE SLEEP APNEA IN BARIATRIC SURGERY

Recommendation	Strength of recommendation
The ramped position is preferred for induction and intubation; avoid the flat supine position	Strong
Avoid sedatives as premedication; opioid analgesia, if used at all, should be titrated slow and the patient should be monitored carefully	Strong
Video laryngoscopy is available when there are concerns for difficult intubation; routine usage may not be necessary	Weak
High-flow oxygenation could be considered in patients with predicted potential for airway difficulties during induction	Weak
Postoperative use of opioids should be minimized and, if needed, used with caution	Strong
Alternatives for opioids are paracetamol, NSAIDs, local anesthetics for incisional infiltration, epidural analgesia, and peripheral nerve blocks	Strong
Ketamine, magnesium, lidocaine, and alpha 2-agonists seem promising, yet high-quality supportive evidence regarding their use in this setting is lacking	Weak
At the end of the surgical procedure, patients should be as fully awake as soon as possible, without sedative effects, opioids, and neuromuscular weakness	Strong
CPAP is strongly recommended at induction in the diagnosed moderately severe OSA patient to maintain lung capacity and reduce time to oxygen desaturation	Strong
ERABS principles should be a standard of practice in the morbidly obese patient	Strong
The patient should only be extubated when close to fully awake, i.e., opening their eyes and coughing well, with neuromuscular blockade fully reversed and muscle function restored	Strong
In the immediate postoperative period, CPAP treatment may be beneficial, particularly in the patient with severe OSA; when needed, CPAP could be supported by increasing oxygen therapy	Strong
Instead of CPAP, noninvasive ventilation should be considered if there is persistent CO_2 retention postoperatively	Strong
When practical and as an adjunct for postoperative pain management, regional anesthesia should be considered as part of multimodal analgesia in open weight-loss surgery	Weak

Source: Reproduced, with permission, from de Raaff CAL et al. Perioperative management of obstructive sleep apnea in bariatric surgery: a consensus guideline. *Surg Obes Relat Dis.* 2017;13(7):1095–1109. doi:10.1016/j.soard.2017.03.022

NSAIDs: non-steroidal anti-inflammatory drugs; CPAP: continuous positive airway pressure; OSA: obstructive sleep apnea; ERABS: enhanced recovery after bariatric surgery

can be added for more support. In case of persistent CO_2 retention, noninvasive ventilation can be considered (Figure 1-3).

6. C. All non-depolarizing neuromuscular blockers (NDNMs) act by antagonizing the acetylcholine receptor in a reversible/competitive manner. A rapid-onset, short-acting non-depolarizing agent would be the best option in this patient. Out of the options listed, Rocuronium has an onset of 45 to 60 seconds and duration of 30 to 60 minutes and would be the most ideal. Obesity has not been found to alter

the pharmacokinetics of Rocuronium and therefore can be dosed on IBW or actual body weight. Pancuronium is the longest acting and is used in patients that require paralysis for more than 1 hour and in patients with normal hepatic and renal function. Cisatracurium and atracurium undergo Hoffman elimination in the blood plasma, with an onset of 1 to 2 minutes and are intermediate acting. These agents would be recommended in patients with renal or hepatic insufficiency. Vecuronium is also an intermediate-acting NMBA and would be recommended in patients with cardiovascular disease as

Patient positioning
- Adequate immobilization (wide hook and loop fastener strapping)
- Arms and feet supported
- Protection of pressure areas (gel pads and padding)
- Prevention of neural injury

Ramped position
- Using ramping device/pillows and/or blankets under a patient's head and shoulders
- Configuring the operating table into a back-up position

Reverse Trendelenburg position
Ear to sternal notch in the same horizontal plane

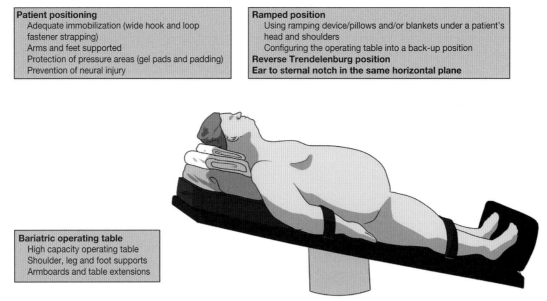

Bariatric operating table
- High capacity operating table
- Shoulder, leg and foot supports
- Armboards and table extensions

Figure 1-2 Ramped position for obese patients in the operating room
Source: Reproduced, with permission, from Carron M, Safaee Fakhr B, Ieppariello G, Foletto M. Perioperative care of the obese patient. *Br J Surg.* 2020;107(2):e39–e55. doi:10.1002/bjs.11447

it has the least adverse side effect profile. Prolonged duration of paralysis can occur when using actual body weight in dosing atracurium and vecuronium, making it less ideal as avoidance of prolonged paralysis or large doses of longer-acting neuromuscular blockers is key.

REFERENCES

Carron M, Safaee Fakhr B, Ieppariello G, Foletto M. Perioperative care of the obese patient. *Br J Surg.* 2020;107(2): e39–e55. doi:10.1002/bjs.11447.

Chung F, Subramanyam R, Liao P, Sasaki E, Shapiro C, Sun Y. High STOP-Bang score indicates a high probability of obstructive sleep apnoea. *Br J Anaesth.* 2012;108(5): 768–775.

De Raaff CAL, Gorter-Stam MAW, de Vries N, et al. Perioperative management of obstructive sleep apnea in bariatric surgery: a consensus guideline. *Surg Obes Relat Dis.* 2017;13(7):1095–1109.

Kapur VK, Auckley DH, Chowdhuri S, et al. Clinical practice guideline for diagnostic testing for adult obstructive sleep apnea: an American Academy of Sleep Medicine Clinical Practice Guideline. *J Clin Sleep Med.* 2017;13(3):479–504.

Kaw R, Bhateja P, Paz YMH, et al. Postoperative complications in patients with unrecognized obesity hypoventilation syndrome undergoing elective noncardiac surgery. *Chest.* 2016;149(1):84–91. doi:10.1378/chest.14-3216.

Kline LR, Collop N, Finlay G. Clinical presentation and diagnosis of obstructive sleep apnea in adults. In: Chervin RD, Hoppin AG, eds, *UpToDate Nederland.* Wolters Kluwer NV; 2017. https://www.uptodate.com/contents/clinical-presentation-and-diagnosis-of-obstructive-sleep-apnea-in-adults

Miller JN, Kupzyk KA, Zimmerman L, et al. Comparisons of measures used to screen for obstructive sleep apnea in patients referred to a sleep clinic. *Sleep Med.* 2018;51:15–21.

Peppard PE, Young T, Barnet JH, Palta M, Hagen EW, Hla KM. Increased prevalence of sleep-disordered breathing in adults. *Am J Epidemiol.* 2013;177(9):1006–1014.

Puhringer FK, et al. Pharmacokinetics of rocuronium bromide in obese female patients. *Eur J Anaesthesiol.* 1999;16(8):507.

Schumann R. Anaesthesia for bariatric surgery. *Best Prac Res Clin Anaesthesiol.* 2011;25:83–93.

Tietze K. Use of neuromuscular blocking medications in critically ill patients. *J Pharm D.* 2013. http://www.uptodate.com/contents/use-of-neuromuscular-blocking-medications-in-critically-ill-patients

Young T, Palta M, Dempsey J, Peppard PE, Nieto FJ, Hla KM. Burden of sleep apnea: rationale, design, and major findings of the Wisconsin Sleep Cohort study. *WMJ.* 2009;108(5): 246–249.

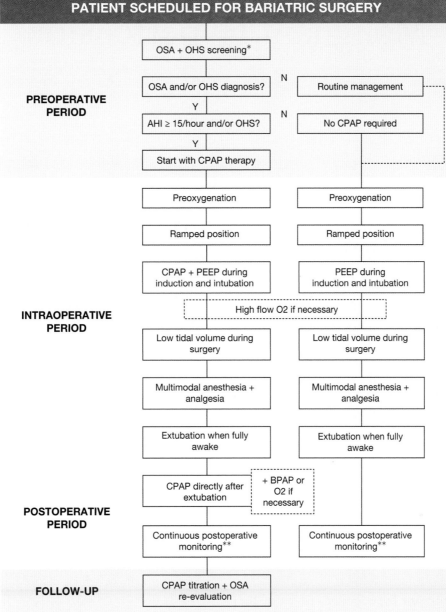

Figure 1-3 Perioperative management of the bariatric patients with and without obstructive sleep apnea

OSA: obstructive sleep apnea; OHS: obesity hypoventilation syndrome; CPAP: continuous positive airway pressure; BPAP: bilevel positive airway pressure; PEEP: positive end-expiratory pressure; AHI: Apnea-Hypopnea Index

Source: Reproduced, with permission, from De Raaff CAL, Gorter-Stam MAW, de Vries N, et al. Perioperative management of obstructive sleep apnea in bariatric surgery: a consensus guideline. *Surg Obes Relat Dis.* 2017;13(7):1095-1109. doi:10.1016/j.soard.2017.03.022

2

Malignant Hypertension

Aaron Paul

MALIGNANT HYPERTENSION AND HYPERTHERMIA

A 59-year-old female with poorly controlled hypertension on three antihypertensive medications, including a beta-blocker, an angiotensin-converting-enzyme (ACE) inhibitor, and a calcium channel blocker, presents for a routine surgery. At her preoperative visit, she is instructed to hold her home ACE inhibitor the day of surgery. She then undergoes an otherwise uncomplicated cholecystectomy with intraoperative cholangiogram. However, in the postoperative care unit, she develops hypertension with readings of 200/140. Her other vital signs are within the normal range. The anesthesia provider performs an eye exam and notes papilledema. IV nitroprusside is administered for treatment.

1. **Regarding the immediate management of this patient's malignant hypertension, which of the following is correct?**

   A. Goal blood pressure is a reduction to a normal range of systolic blood pressure (SBP) <120, diastolic blood pressure (DBP) <80 as soon as possible to prevent stroke.

   B. Reduction of DBP to 100–105 over 3 hours with maximum fall in blood pressure by 25% over 24 hours is needed to prevent stroke.

   C. Heart rate control is acutely needed to prevent worsening cerebral edema.

   D. Blood pressure should be maintained at about 150–160 SBP for at least 8 hours during the initial treatment.

2. **Regarding malignant hypertension, which of the following is a clinical sign of this diagnosis?**

   A. Blood pressure >150/110
   B. Papilledema
   C. Temperature >38.5°C
   D. Pulmonary edema
   E. Tachycardia >100

3. **Regarding the medication nitroprusside, which of the following is a feared side effect?**

   A. Cyanide toxicity
   B. Tremor
   C. Stroke
   D. Myocardial infarction
   E. Angina pectoris

4. **Regarding medications to treat malignant hypertension acutely, which of the following is most likely to cause reflexive tachycardia?**

   A. Labetalol
   B. Hydralazine
   C. Metoprolol
   D. Clevidipine
   E. Fenoldopam

5. **Regarding underlying causes of poorly controlled hypertension, which of the following is the most likely cause in this patient?**

   A. Pheochromocytoma
   B. Cushing's syndrome
   C. Renal artery stenosis
   D. Thyroid storm
   E. Glomerulonephritis

A 47-year-old male with hypertension controlled on lisinopril and amlodipine presents with a painful bulge in the right groin and no previous surgical history. He is diagnosed with an inguinal hernia and is scheduled for elective repair. Thirty minutes into the surgery, his end-tidal CO_2 begins to rise, with a blood pressure of 160/95 mmHg, a heart rate 110 beats/minute, and a temperature of 39.1°C.

6. **What is the most likely cause of the change in vitals?**

    A. Undiagnosed renal artery stenosis
    B. Catecholamine release from an adrenal tumor
    C. Non-depolarizing skeletal muscle blockade
    D. Depolarizing skeletal muscle blockade
    E. Thyroid storm

7. **What is the underlying pathophysiology of this patient's condition?**

    A. Fibromuscular dysplasia
    B. Increased skeletal muscle metabolism
    C. Overgrowth of neural crest cells
    D. Autonomic instability
    E. Transient hyperkalemia

8. **What is the best initial treatment for this patient?**

    A. Metoprolol
    B. Phenoxybenzamine
    C. Dantrolene
    D. Balloon dilation of the renal arteries
    E. High-dose propylthiouracil

9. **What information in the preoperative assessment may have helped avoid this outcome?**

    A. Family history of problems with anesthesia
    B. Personal history of frequent palpitations and diaphoresis
    C. Elevated creatinine on preoperative lab work
    D. Recent upper respiratory infection

10. **The patient is stabilized and admitted to the intensive care unit (ICU) for 24 hours of observation. Which of the following would you expect to see?**

    A. Heart block
    B. Myoglobinuria
    C. Respiratory alkalosis
    D. Hyperreflexia of proximal muscle groups

ANSWERS

1. **B.** The goal in malignant hypertension is a reduction in DBP to 100–105 with maximum fall in DBP by 25% of highest blood pressure value over 24 hours. This slow decrease prevents reflexive vasoconstriction via normal body autoregulatory mechanisms leading to stroke. A reduction of blood pressure to the normal range increases the risk of stroke and is not recommended. There are no data that suggest SBP should be kept at a certain elevated level to prevent a stroke.

    Heart rate control is not a main goal of care in malignant hypertension. The mechanism of cerebral edema is felt to be overcoming the body's autoregulatory mechanism of vasoconstriction with an increase in the mean arterial pressure (MAP), allowing for a relatively constant end organ perfusion pressure. When MAP increases above 150 mmHg, autoregulatory vasoconstriction fails, and vasodilation is seen leading to an increase in blood flow to the brain. Blood pressure control, not heart rate, prevents cerebral edema by reducing cerebral perfusion pressure (cerebral perfusion pressure = intracranial pressure – mean diastolic pressure) and permitting autoregulation, thus reducing end organ damage.

2. **B.** Malignant hypertension is defined by MAP >150 mmHg with signs of cerebral edema and/or end organ damage. Cerebral edema is characterized by clinical signs of brain swelling. Papilledema is the most worrisome sign. However, retinal hemorrhages and retinal exudates are indicative of hypertension causing damage to arterioles and capillary beds. Other end organ findings include acute kidney injury, myocardial infarction, aortic dissection, or bowel ischemia.

    Tachycardia is not a criterion for diagnosing malignant hypertension. Tachycardia is commonly seen in postoperative patients and could be attributed to catecholamine release from the stressors of surgery, pain, intravascular depletion, medications, arrhythmias, and/or atelectasis. Its presence necessitates close observation and a thorough workup.

3. **A.** Nitroprusside is an arteriovenous dilator that has rapid onset and short half-life. It, as well as fast-acting medications such as clevidipine, nicardipine,

labetalol, and fenoldopam, is used for acute treatment of hypertension. With over-administration of nitroprusside, cyanide toxicity can develop as this medication contains cyanide groups (carbon triple-bonded with nitrogen). Cyanide toxicity is detrimental to aerobic metabolism at the cellular level by inhibiting the last enzyme in oxidative phosphorylation, cytochrome oxidase (a3). Cyanide toxicity can present with headache, nausea, emesis, and flushing and hepatic and/or renal failure. The treatment of cyanide toxicity is multimodal and includes sodium nitrite, hyperbaric oxygen, and sodium thiosulfate.

Tremor is not a known side effect of nitroprusside, but hyperreflexia is commonly seen in toxic levels of this drug, leading to cyanide toxicity. Stroke, myocardial infarction, and angina pectoris are not published side effects of nitroprusside. These are more characteristic of malignant hypertension itself due to end organ damage from capillary and arteriole damage to the heart.

4. **B.** Hydralazine is a direct arteriolar vasodilator. It has rapid onset and short half-life when administered by IV. It can commonly cause reflexive tachycardia by two mechanisms. Reflexive catecholamine release in response to vasodilation and decreased vascular resistance directly stimulates the cardiac myocytes by beta-1 adrenergic receptors leading to tachycardia. Additionally, due to the decrease in renal blood flow, the juxtaglomerular apparatus secretes renin leading to increased aldosterone secretion. Aldosterone is a potent vasoconstrictor that decreases venous return. As a compensatory mechanism, heart rate increases to compensate and keep cardiac output constant ($CO = HR \times SV$). Reflexive tachycardia is commonly seen in patients who are not concomitantly on beta-blockers and ACE inhibitors.

Labetalol is both an alpha-1 and beta-1 antagonist. It has rapid onset and is ideal for patients with tachycardia and some hypertension. It does not cause reflex tachycardia due to inhibition of beta-1 receptors.

Metoprolol is a beta-blocker and will decrease heart rate. It is ideal in atrial fibrillation, with little efficacy in malignant hypertension.

Clevidipine is a dihydropyridine calcium channel blocker. It has rapid onset, has a very short half-life, and is administered intravenously. Because

it works peripherally, it does not cause reflexive tachycardia.

Fenoldopam is a dopamine-1 receptor agonist. It commonly causes flushing and hypotension. It does not cause tachycardia because it works peripherally.

5. **C.** Renal artery stenosis is a common underlying cause of malignant hypertension and is frequently seen in Caucasians who have poor blood pressure control despite multimodal therapy. Renal artery stenosis can present as worsening azotemia in relatively young individuals, poorly controlled hypertension, and/or malignant hypertension. It is diagnosed noninvasively via renal artery duplex and can be treated with renal artery stenting. However, this treatment is becoming more controversial given the recent publication of the Cardiovascular Outcomes in Renal Atherosclerotic Lesions (CORAL) trial by Hermann et al. (2013) arguing for medical management alone.

Pheochromocytoma is a catecholamine-releasing tumor that can cause hypertension. It is usually episodic and can present with flushing, palpitations, diaphoresis, and other signs of catecholamine release. It is diagnosed clinically by history and urine vanillylmandelic acid tests.

Cushing's syndrome can cause hypertension due to cortisol excess but is not as common as renal artery stenosis in malignant hypertension. Conn's syndrome, or hyperaldosteronism, is the overproduction of aldosterone by the adrenal gland and can also cause hypertension.

Thyroid storm typically presents with tachycardia. It is treated typically with nonselective beta-blockade and propylthiouracil.

Glomerulonephritis (GN) seen in nephritic syndrome can cause hypertension and renal failure. Additionally, both renal artery stenosis and malignant hypertension alone can cause renal failure. However, renal artery stenosis and not GN is associated with malignant hypertension.

6. **D.** Malignant hyperthermia (MH) is a pharmacogenetic disorder of a hypermetabolic state. The first sign is often increased end-tidal CO_2 that is resistant to increased ventilation, followed by tachycardia, acidosis, and hyperthermia. Is there a temperature that defines malignant hyperthermia? The most

common cause of a rapid onset of MH is succinylcholine, a depolarizing skeletal muscle blocker. Other potential offenders include halothane, sevofluorane, desfluorane, and isofluorane, although these have a slower onset of MH than succinylcholine. Nondepolarizing skeletal muscle blockers do not cause MH. Renal artery stenosis presenting with malignant hypertension is often associated with severe hypertension (>200 mmHg systolic or >130 mmHg diastolic blood pressure) that is resistant to outpatient medical therapy (>3 hypertensive medications) and is not associated with hypercarbia, tachycardia, or hyperthermia. Catecholamine release from a pheochromocytoma can cause tachycardia and severe hypertension; however, hyperthermia is unlikely. Thyroid storm can have significant associated tachycardia and hyperpyrexia but is not commonly associated with increased end-tidal CO_2, especially in a patient without a history of existing hyperthyroidism.

7. **B.** MH is caused by activation of a mutated Ca^{2+} channel, the ryanodine receptor, in the skeletal muscle sarcoplasmic reticulum. This leads to an uncontrolled release of intracellular Ca^{2+}-causing activation of skeletal muscle contraction and increased oxygen consumption, CO_2 production, and adenosine triphosphate consumption, which leads to continual heat production. Although there can be an associated transient hyperkalemia due to eventual rhabdomyolysis, this does not cause the symptoms seen in MH. Fibromuscular dysplasia is the most common cause of renal artery stenosis in patients <50 years old. Overgrowth of neural crest cells is seen in pheochromocytoma. Thyroid storm causes autonomic instability.

8. **C.** Dantrolene is the first-line therapy for MH, in addition to discontinuing the offending agent. Dantrolene inhibits the MH response by directly binding to the ryanodine receptor. Treatment also consists of symptomatic treatment including cooling measures, hyperventilation, and treatment of hyperkalemia and acidosis. Metoprolol would not treat the underlying problem. Phenoxybenzamine should be given preoperatively for pheochromocytoma. Balloon dilation of the renal arteries would treat renal artery stenosis. High-dose propylthiouracil is given for the treatment of thyroid storm.

9. **A.** MH is most commonly seen as an autosomal dominant mutation of the *RYR1* gene that codes the ryanodine calcium channel receptor. A personal history of palpitations and diaphoresis is a common complaint of patients with a pheochromocytoma or uncontrolled hyperthyroidism. Elevated creatinine can be seen in patients with renal artery stenosis. Recent upper respiratory infections can increase the risk for developing thyroid storm but do not commonly affect the development of MH.

10. **B.** MH causes rhabdomyolysis, which can develop up to 24 hours post-anesthesia. Patients are admitted to the ICU for observation after any MH event to monitor for recurrence as well as the development of rhabdomyolysis and any sequelae that may result, including cardiac arrhythmias secondary to hyperkalemia. Myoglobinuria is seen after rhabdomyolysis due to the breakdown of skeletal muscle membranes and the release of intracellular myoglobin that is later eliminated through the urine. EKG changes that may be seen include peaked T-waves and premature ventricular contractions, but a new heart block is not seen. Respiratory acidosis, not alkalosis, is seen in 99% of MH patients. Muscle rigidity can be seen due to MH in the acute setting, and muscle weakness is an expected side effect of dantrolene treatment; however, proximal muscle hyperreflexia is not commonly seen.

BIBLIOGRAPHY

Armario P, Dernandez del Rey R, Pardell H. Adverse effects of direct-acting vasodilators. *Drug Saf.* 1994;11(2):80–85.

Chiha M, Samarasinghe S, Kabaker AS. Thyroid storm: an updated review. *J Intensive Care Med.* 2015;30(3):131–140. doi:10.1177/0885066613498053.

Davis B, Crook J, Vestal R, Oates J. Prevalence of renovascular hypertension in patients with grade III or IV hypertensive retinopathy. *N Engl J Med.* 1979;301(23):1273.

Hermann S, Saad A, Textor S. Management of atherosclerotic renovascular disease after Cardiovascular Outcomes in Renal Atherosclerotic Lesions (CORAL). *Nephrol Dial Transplant.* Published online April 9, 2014.

Januszewicz A, Guzik, T, Prejbisz A, et al. Malignant hypertension: new aspects of an old clinical entity. *Pol Arch Med Wewn.* 2016;126(1–2):86–93.

Kaplan NM. Management of hypertensive emergencies. *Lancet.* 1994;344(8933):1335.

Marik PE, Varon J. Hypertensive crises: challenges and management. *Chest*. 2007;131(6):1949. doi:10.1378/chest.06-2490.

Mullins MF. Malignant hyperthermia: a review. *J Perianesth Nurs*. 2018;33(5):582–589.

Naranjo J, Dodd S, Martin, YN. Perioperative management of pheochromocytoma. *J Cardiothorac Vasc Anesth*. 2017;31(4):1427–1439.

Pasch T, Schulz V, Hoppelshauser G. Nitroprusside-induced formation of cyanide and its detoxification with thiosulphate during deliberate hypotension. *J Cardiovasc Pharmacol*. 1983;5(5):77–85.

Rosenberg H, Pollock N, Schiemann A, Bulger T, Stowell K. Malignant hyperthermia: a review. *Orphanet J Rare Dis*. 2015;10:93.

3

Fundamentals for Use of Surgical Energy and OR Fires

Paul Wetstein

A 74-year-old female with chronic obstructive pulmonary disease (COPD) and a baseline oxygen requirement presented to the emergency department with subjective fevers, headache, and jaw claudication. Laboratory evaluation was notable for an erythrocyte sedimentation rate (ESR) of 56 mm/hr. A noncontrast computed tomography (CT) scan of the head was obtained, which revealed no acute pathology. The patient was admitted to the internal medicine service and started on high-dose prednisone with a working diagnosis of giant cell (temporal) arteritis. During a temporal artery biopsy, an operating room fire occurs.

1. Which of the following is correct regarding operating room fires?

A. Two of the three components of the classically described "fire triad" must be present for an OR fire to occur.

B. The most common OR fire fuel is the monopolar electrosurgical energy "Bovie."

C. An oxidizer-enriched atmosphere often exists in the entire operating room.

D. Alcohol-containing prep solutions need to be completely dry before starting a procedure.

E. Fiberoptic light sources for endoscopic surgery do not serve as an ignition source.

2. Which of the following is correct regarding this scenario?

A. Surgery on the head and neck should be identified as "low risk."

B. Intraoperative communication between the surgeon and anesthesiologist is not needed.

C. Sedation with open gas delivery device would be preferred to general endotracheal anesthesia in this patient to prevent an OR fire.

D. Surgical drapes should be configured in a manner to minimize the accumulation of oxidizers.

E. Moistening surgical sponges has no impact in preventing an OR fire.

3. In the event of fire involvement of the airway or breathing circuit, the best first step is to

A. stop the flow of all gases to the airway.

B. remove all fuels from the airway.

C. activate the fire alarm.

D. perform fiberoptic bronchoscopy with the endotracheal tube in place.

E. pour saline into the airway.

4. During the preoperative huddle, the certified registered nurse anesthetist (CRNA) asks from a fire safety standpoint which situation is optimal:

A. Monitored anesthesia care only

B. Monitored anesthesia care with local

C. Local anesthesia only

D. General anesthesia via laryngeal mask airways

E. General anesthesia via endotracheal intubation

5. In deciding which form of surgical energy to perform this dissection with, which of the following is true?

A. The direct current polarization or galvanic effect of electrosurgery at the cellular level is responsible for tissue destruction.

B. Metal-to-metal arcing with monopolar energy can generate temperatures of 1000°F.

C. Ultrasonic shears have a low risk of injury from residual heat.

D. Ultrasonic electrosurgical devices generate similar amounts of current that travel through the patient.

ANSWERS

1. **D.** For a fire to occur, all three components of the "fire triad" must be present. These include fuel, an oxidizer, and an ignition source. Fuel for fire is plentiful in the operating room. Some examples include drapes, the patient's hair, surgical gowns, blankets, endotracheal tubes, laryngeal mask airways, and volatile surgical compounds (e.g., alcohol-containing prep solutions, acetone, etc.). It has been shown that alcohol-containing prep solutions with as little as 20% alcohol can ignite with diathermy or hot wire cautery, so they must be allowed to dry before surgical electricity is used. Oxidizers in the OR are generally either oxygen or nitrous oxide. These oxidizers can accumulate and form an oxidizer-enriched atmosphere in closed or semiclosed breathing systems and from tenting of surgical drapes. Ignition sources in the OR are equally as plentiful. Some common examples include electrosurgical devices, heated probes, lasers, fiberoptic light cables, argon beam coagulators, drills, and defibrillator pads.

2. **D.** According to the American Society of Anesthesiologists 2013 Task Force on OR fires, an endotracheal tube or laryngeal mask airways (LMAs) should be considered in patients undergoing moderate to deep sedation or that have a baseline oxygen requirement. Head and neck surgery should be considered "high risk" for an OR fire and, as such, communication between the surgeon and the anesthesiologist is mandatory regardless of the length of the procedure. Surgical drapes should be arranged to prevent an accumulation of oxidized air. Moistened surgical sponges can help prevent OR fires.

3. **A.** Immediate actions to be performed in the event of an airway fire include, first, removing the endotracheal tube or LMAs, then stopping the flow of *all* gases, removing fuel sources away from the airway, and pouring saline into the airway. Once the fire has been extinguished, actions should include ventilation of the patient while avoiding oxidizer-enriched environments, inspection of the tracheal tube or LMA to ensure no fragments remain in the patient's airway, and consideration of bronchoscopy. Bronchoscopy is a relatively safe procedure in experienced hands in diagnosing inhalational injury but is not part of the immediate management of an airway fire.

4. **D.** The majority of operating room fires happen during monitored anesthesia care (MAC) due to the open-source oxidizer (oxygen). One review of operating room fire claims revealed 81% happen during conscious sedation, also known as monitored anesthesia care. This patient has a baseline oxygen requirement, which makes local anesthesia only an incorrect answer. LMAs are considered closed systems and would be preferred to endotracheal intubation.

5. **B.** The galvanic effect is not used in electrosurgery. Mechanical energy is created by alternating current by oscillating proteins rapidly and is responsible for the thermal energy created at the cellular level. With monopolar energy, electrical current travels to the tip of the instrument, to the contacted tissue, and through the patient to the dispersion pad. Metal to metal arcing can generate enough heat to melt a staple or staple line or cause tissue damage. With bipolar energy, electrical energy travels to one point of the instrument and then to the other tip of the instrument. Thus, energy passes only to the tissue between the two points of the instrument. Current, therefore, does not travel through the patient to a dispersion pad.

With ultrasonic energy, electrical energy is converted to mechanical energy in the handpiece of the ultrasonic devices, and no current travels through the patient. The shaft or blade of ultrasonic shears can retain a temperature of >60°C for approximately 45 seconds and thus are not good instruments for dissecting.

BIBLIOGRAPHY

Apfelbaum JL, Caplan RA, Barker SJ, et al. Practice advisory for the prevention and management of operating room fires: an updated report by the American Society of Anesthesiologists Task Force on Operating Room Fires. *Anesthesiology*. 2013;118(2):271–290.

Bai C, Huang H, Yao X, et al. Application of flexible bronchoscopy in inhalation lung injury. *Diagnostic Pathology*. 2013;21(8):174.

Briscoe CE, Hill DW, Payne JP. Inflammable antiseptics and theatre fires. *Br J Surg*. 1976;63(12):981–983.

DeMaria S, Schwartz AD, Narine V, et al. Management of intra-operative airway fire. *Simul Healthc*. 2011;Dec(6):360–363.

Jones TS, Black IH, Robinson TN, Jones EL. Operating room fires. *Anesthesiology*. 2019;130(3):492–501.

Mehta SP, Bhananker SM, Posner KL, Domino KB. Operating room fires: A closed claims analysis. *Anesthesiology*. 2013; 118:1133–1139.

SAGES FUSE program. Society of American Gastrointestinal and Endoscopic Surgeons. Accessed March 2020. www.fusedidactic.org.

Surgical fire prevention. ECRI. https://www.ecri.org/Accident_Investigation/Pages/Surgical-Fire-Prevention.aspx.

4

Argon Gas Embolism

Lauren P. Kecskes and Roger Eduardo

The patient is a 37-year-old female without any significant past medical history undergoing a laparoscopic partial right hepatic lobectomy for a large symptomatic hepatic adenoma in segment VI of the liver. Endotracheal intubation is performed without complication and the abdomen is entered via the Hassan technique. The lesion is identified on the inferomedial aspect of segment VI. To dissect the lesion away from the liver parenchyma, an argon beam coagulator is used. Two hours after the start of the procedure, there is an abrupt decrease in the patient's $ETCO_2$ from 30 to 10 mmHg and spO_2 from 100% to 40%. This is rapidly followed by a decrease in arterial blood pressure to 60/25 mmHg and heart rate from 80 to less than 20.

1. **Why is the argon beam coagulator used over other types of electrosurgical energy?**
   - A. The flow of gas clears the site of fluids and blood, enhancing visibility.
   - B. Rapid noncontact uniform tissue coagulation over a finite area, decreasing the collateral damage.
   - C. Better hemostasis through increased depth of penetration.
   - D. There is less dense surgical smoke.
   - E. There is less of a chance of indirect coupling.

2. **What was the most likely cause of this patient's decrease in end-tidal CO_2 ($ETCO_2$) and arterial blood pressure?**
   - A. Acute myocardial infarct
   - B. Decreased venous return secondary to pneumoperitoneum
   - C. Aspiration
   - D. Gas embolism
   - E. Severe cerebral vascular accident

3. **What is the most important factor associated with an increased risk of a venous gas embolism when using argon beam coagulation?**
   - A. Use under pneumoperitoneum
   - B. High flow rate of argon gas
   - C. Holding the tip of the electrode at a right angle to the tissue
   - D. Placing tip of argon beam electrode in direct contact with the tissue surface

4. **What would be your next step in the management of this patient?**
   - A. Continue the surgery.
   - B. Administer atropine and initiate vasopressors.
   - C. Discontinue pneumoperitoneum and place patient in Durant's position.
   - D. Perform an emergent transesophageal echocardiography (TEE) to diagnose a gas embolism.
   - E. Begin immediate volume resuscitation.

A 77-year-old Caucasian male with a history of hereditary hemorrhagic telangiectasia with recurrent epistaxis and recurrent gastrointestinal (GI) bleeding undergoes an esophagogagastroduodenoscopy (EGD) with argon beam coagulation. He fails to awake from anesthesia post-procedure. The patient is transported to the intensive care unit, and an emergent head computed tomography (CT) scan is obtained, showing air within the right frontal lobe.

5. What would be the next step in management?

A. Start tissue plasminogen activator (TPA).

B. Administer naloxone.

C. Administer 100% O_2.

D. Perform a bedside transthoracic echocardiogram (TTE).

6. What additional treatment could you consider?

A. Placing the patient in the Trendelenberg position

B. Administering corticosteroids

C. Performing endovascular aspiration

D. Using hyperbaric oxygen therapy

ANSWERS

1. E. Argon beam coagulation has gained popularity among surgeons as a useful tool to achieve hemostasis in bleeding surfaces of highly vascularized organs, such as the liver and spleen. It utilizes a monopolar electrode to partially ionize a stream of argon gas that is directed toward the tissue for coagulation. The ionized argon beam acts as an efficient pathway, conducting a high-frequency electric current from the electrode to the target tissue resulting in a fine spray of electrical sparks.

As the electrical beams directed from the electrode to the target tissue causes desiccation, the electrical conductivity of the targets tissue is lost. If continually applied, the beams automatically move to nearby nondesiccated and still electrically conductive tissue, allowing for rapid uniform coagulation over a large area without any tissue contact. Furthermore, as a result of the loss of electric conductivity at a treated site, the depth of penetration of the electrical energy is reduced. This, coupled with the fact that the use of argon gas, due to its inert nature, neither carbonizes nor vaporizes biologic tissue so that the thermal effects are limited, resulting in less adjacent tissue damage and less generation of surgical smoke. Indirect coupling is not a phenomenon of this type of surgical energy.

2. D. With the use of the argon beam coagulation system in laparoscopic procedures, the argon system acts as a secondary source of pressurized gas, and argon can accumulate in the closed peritoneal cavity. With damage to any significant blood vessels, the gas under pressure can enter the vasculature, posing a risk of embolism that could be a mixture of both argon and carbon dioxide. Moreover, the argon gas stream that flows between the electrode and the tissue can cross any disrupted mucosal membrane surface and be flushed directly into the microvasculature.

Although argon is physiologically inert, it is 17 times less soluble than carbon dioxide (0.029 vs. 0.495 ml gas ml^{-1} blood) and, as such, argon-rich emboli are not as readily absorbed from the bloodstream as CO_2 and may pass into the systemic circulation. At the standard flow setting of 4 L/min used typically for hemostasis in highly vascularized organs, the argon beam electrode can produce 67 ml of gas in only 1 second, which, if embolized, can lead to significant cardiopulmonary dysfunction and be potentially lethal in an average-sized adult. Furthermore, at such a high flow rate, argon gas clearly exceeds the pressure in the venous system and can embolize not only through major veins but also through small peripheral veins.

3. D. The first few cases of venous embolism with the use of the argon beam were reported during a laparoscopic procedures and therefore, the theory of over-insufflation and over-pressurization of the abdominal cavity caused by the accumulation of argon gas under pneumoperitoneum was thought to lead to these embolic events. However, given that venous emboli have occurred in several cases of patients undergoing procedures without pneumoperitoneum, this theory cannot fully explain the incidence of these events. Ikegami et al. compared seven reported cases of venous embolism using argon beam coagulation and identified the following risk factors:

1. Using the argon gas under pneumoperitoneum
2. Puncturing the liver parenchyma (hepatic needle biopsy)
3. Possible injury to the hepatic venous system
4. Placing the tip of argon beam electrode in direct contact with the tissue surface

On review of the literature, it appears that more important than the issue of use under pneumoperitoneum is that of placing the tip of the argon beam electrode in close or direct contact with the tissue that is being treated. Multiple cases have been described without the use of penumoperitoneum, in which this is clearly the issue, and in the series described earlier, although only three cases described this, it is possible that more might have had this condition and simply not reported it.

When used at flow rates of 0.2 to 2 L/min and a power of 20 to 80 W as described in the field of interventional pulmonology for ablation of small lesions, the argon beam system can penetrate the tissue up to 5 mm in depth. However, when used for the purpose of hemostasis in highly vascularized tissues such as the spleen or hepatic parenchyma, a flow rate of 4 L/min and power of 150 W is typical. This allows for even further penetration and when coupled with direct surface contact could allow for vessel damage and for the argon gas to be flushed directly into the venous system.

To mitigate the risk of causing an air embolism, the following can be done:

1. Never place the electrode tip less than several millimeters from the surgical site.
2. Limit argon flow settings to the lowest level that will provide the desired clinical effect.
3. Hold the tip of the electrode at an oblique angle.
4. Move the handpiece away from the tissue after each activation.
5. Flush abdominal cavity with CO_2 between extended activation periods.
6. Always leave one instrument cannula open to the atmosphere during laparoscopic procedure. Alternatively, one could use a venting port at all times when operating laparoscopically and using surgical energy. This will allow gas to escape but maintain a pneumoperitoneum.

4. **C.** In conjunction with appropriate cardiac resuscitation according to Advanced Cardiovascular Life Support guidelines if indicated, the treatment of a patient suspected of having a CO_2 or any gas embolism should include immediate discontinuation of CO_2 insufflation. The patient should be placed in Durant's position (left lateral decubitus with steep head down). This allows the gas to rise into the apex of the right heart, preventing entry into the pulmonary artery and keeping it there until it slowly absorbs. The use of a nitrous oxide inhalant should be discontinued to allow for hyperventilation with 100% oxygen to increase the clearance of CO_2 or any other gas and to relieve hypoxemia. Volume expansion with bolus crystalloid may reduce further gas entry by elevating the central venous pressure. And finally, the placement of a central venous catheter for attempted aspiration of the gas from the right heart may also be performed. While a TEE may be diagnostic in the event of a venous gas embolism, it is not a priority in the unstable patient with suspected gas embolism.

5. **C.** The patient is suffering from an embolic stroke, which explains his persistent coma after general anesthesia has been withdrawn. His CT scan is concerning for the presence of an air embolus within the right frontal lobe. It is a rare but potentially devastating complication of argon plasma coagulation that has been reported during endoscopic surgery. Initial steps would include vital signs monitoring, maintaining IV access, and activating the stroke team, as well as checking labs. Placing the patient on 100% oxygen is an important first step to help accelerate the absorption of the air embolus. Because the CT scan shows an air embolism, there is no role for TPA in this setting. Finally, bedside TTE would not be useful in addressing the immediate complication at hand. Once the patient is stabilized, an echocardiogram with bubble study could be performed to evaluate for an intracardiac shunt.

6. **D.** Cerebral emboli associated with the use of argon plasma coagulation is a very rare complication. Although the first major steps in managing argon gas emboli include placing the patient in the Trendelenberg position, many authors have noted in the case of cerebral emboli that placing the head down could carry the risk of increasing cerebral edema and further compromising neurologic recovery. There has been no reported benefit to administering corticosteroids in this setting, and therefore, this treatment is not currently recommended. Endovascular aspiration has not been described in the literature in the setting of cerebral emboli. Only hyperbaric oxygen has been shown to have some benefit in neurologic recovery. Please describe the mechanism for why this should work. Does it help absorb the argon? Also are the outcomes from this stroke any different from the recovery from other causes of a cerebrovascular accident?

BIBLIOGRAPHY

Cornejo A, Liao L, Kenneth W. Argon gas embolism with the use of argon beam coagulation during open hepatic resection. *Internet J Surg.* 2009;22(2). http://ispub.com/IJS/22/2/7972.
Croce E, Azzola M, Russo R, Golia M, Angelini S, Olmi S. Laparoscopic liver tumour resection with the argon beam. *Endosc Surg Allied Technol.* 1994;2(3–4):186–188.

Economic Cycle Research Institute. Fatal gas embolism caused by overpressurization during laparoscopic use of argon enhanced coagulation. *Health Devices*. 1994;23(6): 257–259.

Farin G, Grund KE. Technology of argon plasma coagulation with particular regard to endoscopic applications. *Endosc Surg Allied Technol*. 1994;2:71–77.

Feldman L, Fuchshuber P, Jones DB. *The SAGES Manual on the Fundamental Use of Surgical Energy*. Springer-Verlag; 2012.

Ikegami T, Shimada M, Imura S, et al. Argon gas embolism in the application of laparoscopic microwave coagulation therapy. *J Hepatobiliary Pancreat Surg*. 2009;16(3): 394–398.

Kono M, Yahagi N, Kitahara M, Fujiwara Y, Sha M, Ohmura A. Cardiac arrest associated with use of an argon beam coagulator during laparoscopic cholecystectomy. *Br J Anaesth*. 2001;87(4):644–646.

Mann C, Boccara G, Grevy V, Navarro F, Fabre JM, Colson P. Argon pneumoperitoneum is more dangerous than CO2 pneumoperitoneum during venous gas embolism. *Anesth Analg*. 1997;85:1367–1371.

Min SK, Kim JH, Lee SY. Carbon dioxide and argon gas embolism during laparoscopic hepatic resection. *Acta Anaesthesiol Scand*. 2007;51(7):949–953.

Park EY, Kwon JY, Kim KJ. Carbon dioxide embolism during laparoscopic surgery. *Yonsei Med J*. 2012;53:459–466.

Reddy C, Majid A, Michaud G, Feller-Kopman D, Eberhardt R, Herth F, et al. Gas embolism following bronchoscopic argon plasma coagulation: a case series. *Chest*. 2008;134(5):1066–1069.

Shaw Y, Yoneda KY, Chan AL. Cerebral gas embolism from bronchoscopic argon plasma coagulation: a case report. *Respiration*. 2012;83:267–270.

Veyckemans F, Michel I. Venous gas embolism from an argon coagulator. *Anesthesiology*. 1996;85(2):443–444.

Wiesen J, Wiesen A, Tsuang W. All the bubbles "are-gone": an unusual cause of stroke post argon plasma coagulation in patient with hereditary hemorrhagic telangiectasia (HHT). *Chest*. 2014;146(4):255A.

5

Laparoscopic Access and the Pneumoperitoneum

Andrea Moon

A 32-year-old woman, with a body mass index of 25 kg/m^2, was admitted to the hospital with acute cholecystitis. She has been given consent for a laparoscopic cholecystectomy. She had a previous surgical history of cesarean section.

Following the administration of general anesthesia, a curvilinear infra-umbilical skin incision was made. Blunt dissection was carried down to the fascia, and the fascia was elevated and incised. Entry into the peritoneal cavity was confirmed visually, and a Hasson trocar was inserted into the peritoneal cavity.

1. **What is the safest technique to gain access to the peritoneum for laparoscopic surgery?**

   A. Open technique (Hasson)
   B. Veress needle
   C. Optical trocar technique
   D. Veress needle insufflation combined with the optical trocar technique
   E. None of the above

2. **Following insufflation, a 30° laparoscope was inserted. Upon general laparoscopic examination of the peritoneal cavity, it was apparent that a retroperitoneal hematoma was forming. What is the most commonly injured vessel during trocar placement?**

   A. Iliac artery
   B. Inferior vena cava
   C. Aorta
   D. Lumbar veins
   E. Superior mesenteric vessels

3. **Injury to a major vessel after trocar placement is usually signified by what?**

   A. Visible bleeding
   B. Retroperitoneal hematoma
   C. Bradycardia
   D. Hypoxia

4. **The distance between the abdominal wall and the aortic bifurcation in normal-weight women (BMI <25 kg/m^2) is**

   A. 1.5 cm
   B. 2.4 cm
   C. 3.5 cm
   D. 0.4 cm

5. **A Veress needle is used to gain access at the umbilicus. Anesthesia notes that the end-tidal carbon dioxide and oxygen saturation have both decreased, and the patient has become tachycardic. You note that pneumoperitoneum has not been appropriately established. What is the next most appropriate step?**

   A. Place the patient in Trendelenburg position.
   B. Place the patient in a left lateral recumbent position.
   C. Remove the Veress needle.
   D. Increase FiO$_2$ to 100%.

6. **In patients who are not obese, at what angle should the instrument be inserted to minimize the risk of major vessel injury?**

   A. 45-degree angle from the plane of the patient's spine
   B. 90-degree angle directly perpendicular to the site of insertion

C. 60 to 90 degrees from the plane of the patient's spine

D. Less than 45-degree angle from the plane of the patient's spine

ANSWERS

1. **E.** There have been many studies done comparing the safety of the open technique to the closed and direct entry techniques. There has been no obvious advantage of one technique over another. One large meta-analysis showed an incidence of vascular injury to be 0.44% with the closed technique compared to 0% in the open ones. Another large study compared the Veress, open, and direct trocar techniques and found a rate of vascular injury of 0.04%, 0.01%, and 0%, respectively. There are no data showing that an optical viewing technique is superior even when combined with a Veress needle to establish the pneumoperitoneum. Overall, one technique is not superior to the others, and surgeons should be familiar with each of them.

2. **A.** Vascular injuries may involve retroperitoneal, intraperitoneal, or abdominal wall vessels. Rates of major vascular injury during initial trocar entry are between 0.05% and 0.5%. According to limited studies, the sites of injury from most common to least common are iliac vessels, greater omental vessels, inferior vena cava, aorta, pelvic and superior mesenteric veins, and lumbar veins. Injury to a major vessel is usually signified by visible bleeding and hemodynamic instability. If an injury is confirmed or highly suspected, especially in the retroperitoneum, convert to an open procedure, ensure adequate access, initiate Massive Transfusion protocol, promptly call for surgical assistance, and explore the area in question.

3. **A.** Vascular injury is usually diagnosed by direct view of bleeding in the abdominal cavity. The absence of free intraperitoneal blood caused by retroperitoneal bleeding may delay the diagnosis because blood is not observed through the laparoscope. Clinical signs of hemodynamic instability (tachycardia, hypotension), shortly after a needle or trocar insertion, suggest a vascular injury. High intra-abdominal pressure secondary to pneumoperitoneum is associated with a decrease in venous return, which, in turn, can reduce arterial bleeding. Furthermore, a retroperitoneal hematoma can decrease a vessel leak, restraining the bleeding.

Unfortunately, 15% to 50% of the vascular injuries are not diagnosed at the time of injury. This delay has contributed to mortality rates of 13% to 30% for vascular injuries.

4. **D.** A study by Hurd et al. found that the distance between the umbilicus and the aortic bifurcation was 0.4 cm in normal-weight women (BMI <25 kg/m), 2.4 cm in overweight patients (BMI 25–30 kg/m), and 2.9 cm in obese patients (BMI >30 kg/m). Lifting the abdominal wall may improve safety by increasing the distance between the abdominal wall and the viscera. Lifting the abdominal wall by placing clamps to elevate the umbilicus has been shown to provide significant elevation of the peritoneum (6.8 cm above the viscera) that was maintained during insertion.

5. **C.** A decrease in end-tidal CO_2, oxygen saturation, tachycardia/tachyarrhythmias, a "mill wheel" murmur detected using the precordial or esophageal stethoscope, or ECG evidence of right heart strain are early clinical signs of intravascular insufflation. If there is concern for intravascular insufflation, the first step in management is to remove the Veress needle to stop insufflation. Anesthesiology and nursing should be alerted. The patient can be placed on 100% oxygen; however, this is not the first step. The literature recommends placing the patient in Trendelenburg position so that the head is lower than the heart to maximize cerebral blood flow and avoid a cerebrovascular accident with air embolism; however, this is not the first step.

6. **A.** In the nonobese patient, an important variable when inserting periumbilical instruments is the angle of insertion. It appears that the risk of major vessel injury can be minimized in most patients by inserting instruments at a 45-degree angle from the plane of the patient's spine. Increasing the angle to greater than 45 degrees is likely to increase the risk of injury to major vessels. However, in obese patients, the angle must be increased up to 90 degrees to be able to enter the peritoneal cavity; the increased subcutaneous tissue increases the distance from the skin to the major vessels that makes this approach reasonably safe when performed in a controlled manner.

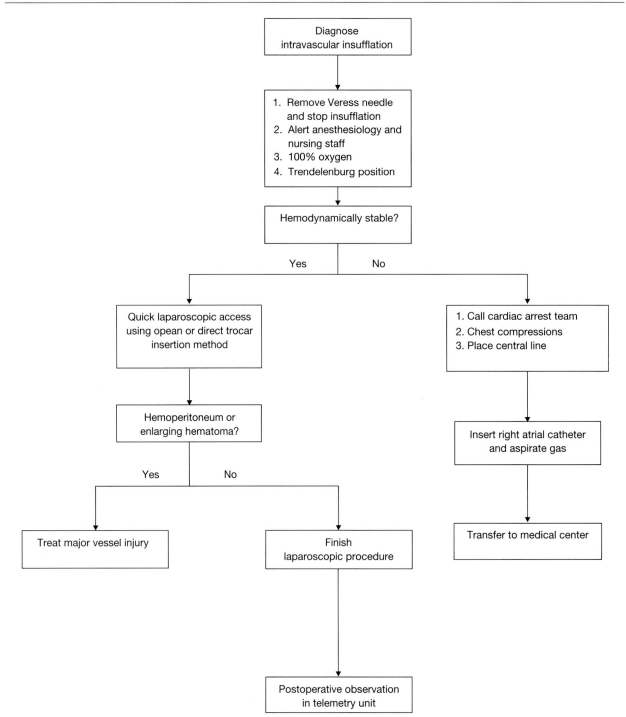

Figure 5-1 Proposed Treatment Algorithm for Intravascular Insufflation Reproduced, with permission, from Sandadi S, Johannigman JA, Wong VL, Blebea J, Altose MD, Hurd WW. Recognition and management of major vessel injury during laparoscopy. *J Minim Invasive Gynecol.* 2010;17.

BIBLIOGRAPHY

Fuller J, Ashar BS, Carey-Corrado J. Trocar-associated injuries and fatalities: an analysis of 1399 reports to the FDA. *J Minim Invasive Gynecol.* 2005;12(4):302–307.

Hurd WW, Bude RO, DeLancey JO, Pearl ML. The relationship of the umbilicus to the aortic bifurcation: implications for laparoscopic technique. *Obstet Gynecol.* 1992;80(1):48–51.

Mechchat A, Bagan P. Management of major vascular complications of laparoscopic surgery. *J Visc Surg.* 2010;147(3): e145–e153.

Pemberton RJ, Tolley DA, van Velthoven RF. Prevention and Management of Complications in Urological Laparoscopic Port Site Placement. *European Urology.* 2006;50: 958–968.

Sandadi S, Johannigman JA, Wong VL, Blebea J, Altose MD, Hurd WW. Recognition and management of major vessel injury during laparoscopy. *J Minim Invasive Gynecol.* 2010;17.

Seidman DS, Nasserbakht F, Nezhat F, et al. Delayed recognition of iliac artery injury during laparoscopic surgery. *Surg Endosc.* 1996;10:1099–101.

Shirk GJ, Johns A., Redwine DB. Complications of laparoscopic surgery: how to avoid them and how to repair them. *J Minim Invasive Gynecol.* 2006;13(4):352–359; quiz 360–361.

Vilos GA, Ternamian A, Dempter J, Laberge PY. Laparoscopic Entry: A Review of Techniques, Technologies, and Complications. *J Obstet Gynaecol Can.* 2007;29(5):433–447.

Vilos GA, Vilos AG, Abu-Rafea B, Hollett-Caines J, Nikkhah-Abyaneh Z, Edris F. Three simple steps during closed laparoscopic entry may minimize major injuries. *Surg Endosc.* 2009;23(4):758–764.

6

NOTES, Novel Endoscopy, and Advanced Laparoscopy

Aditya Gutta, Kai Matthes, and Mark A. Gromski

Ms. L is a 36-year-old female with no major medical problems who presents to the surgery clinic after a recent hospitalization for symptomatic acute blood loss manifesting as multiple episodes of melena and one episode of syncope. No associated symptoms of weight loss, nausea, emesis, dysphagia, or odynophagia are present. She has no recent nonsteroidal anti-inflammatory drug use, tobacco use, or alcohol consumption. During her hospitalization, she was initially hypotensive and required a transfusion of 4 units packed red blood cells. An upper endoscopy showed a submucosal mass in the gastric cardia with ulceration and stigmata of recent bleeding. The remainder of mucosa overlying the mass appeared normal. The margin of the ulcer was biopsied with pathology showing gastric intestinal metaplasia. Gastric antral and body biopsies were negative for *Helicobacter pylori*. CT abdomen/pelvis with IV contrast showed a mass at the gastroesophageal junction extending to the gastric cardia with smooth margins. Upper endoscopic ultrasound (EUS) showed a 39-mm × 34-mm hypoechoic mass originating from the muscularis propria layer. Her hemoglobin remained stable for the rest of her hospitalization and required no further blood transfusions.

1. **Which of the following is the appropriate management for this gastric lesion?**

   A. Endoscopic full thickness resection (EFTR)
   B. Submucosal tunneling endoscopic resection (STER)
   C. Surgical resection
   D. Surveillance upper endoscopy in 1 year

Ms. H is a 76-year-old female with a past history of Stage IV lung cancer on active chemotherapy treatment, who was hospitalized for an episode of acute cholecystitis. WBC is elevated to 16 k/mm^3. There were mild elevations in the liver tests, including total bilirubin 1.9 mg/dL. CT abdomen/pelvis with IV contrast showed a main bile duct mildly dilated to 8 mm with no intra-hepatic dilation and no filling defects. A distended gall bladder with wall thickening and pericholecystic fluid was also noted. On exam, tenderness to palpation in her right upper quadrant was elicited. She reports she has had two episodes of acute cholecystitis in the past and was managed with antibiotics. Cholecystectomy had been deferred on each occasion due to her poor performance status and her elevated surgical risk. She was started on IV antibiotics and an endoscopic retrograde cholangiopancreatography was performed. The exam showed no filling defects in the main bile duct and no contrast filled the cystic duct or the gall bladder. Attempts to cannulate the cystic duct failed. The patient would like to pursue treatment that will reduce the likelihood of future episodes of acute cholecystitis. Surgery was consulted for consideration of cholecystectomy for management of acute cholecystitis.

2. **In addition to cholecystostomy tube placement, which of the following is a reasonable alternative to surgical cholecystectomy in this patient?**

   A. No alternatives for cholecystectomy
   B. Natural orifice transluminal endoscopic surgery (NOTES) transvaginal cholecystectomy
   C. Endoscopic ultrasound (EUS)–guided transmural drainage of the gall bladder
   D. Pancreaticoduodenectomy (Whipple)

Ms. B is a 33 year-old female presenting to a general surgery clinic for a history of periodic symptomatic biliary colic over the past 9 months. A right upper quadrant ultrasound showed no evidence of cholecystitis but did show multiple small (<1-cm) stones in the gallbladder. She is an otherwise healthy individual, only taking oral birth control medications and a multivitamin daily. Her body mass index is 22 kg/m^2. She has had no previous abdominal operations.

Her main concern is scarring that may result from a potential gallbladder operation, and she comes to you to discuss this.

3. What is the most appropriate intervention to recommend at this time?

A. Standard laparoscopic cholecystectomy

B. Single-incision laparoscopic (SIL) cholecystectomy

C. Referral for transvaginal NOTES cholecystectomy

D. Ursodiol 8 to 10 mg/kg/day (in 2 divided doses daily)

4. This same patient was referred to a surgeon within the same institution who is well experienced in SIL cholecystectomy. When discussing the single-incision approach with the patient, attention should be brought to which potential complication?

A. Significant bleeding complications

B. Herniation

C. Pain

D. Surgical site infections

A 73-year-old male with a history of dysphagia and weight loss recently had a high-resolution esophageal manometry that was consistent with Type 1 achalasia. The patient has lost 10 lb recently, has a BMI of 18.5 kg/m^2, and has poor nutritional status. He is nervous about undergoing a surgical procedure.

5. Which minimally invasive technique is considered an acceptable alternative to a multiport laparoscopic Heller myotomy?

A. Per-oral endoscopic myotomy (POEM)

B. Single-port laparoscopic Heller myotomy

C. Bougie dilation of the esophagus

D. Endoscopic injection of botulinum toxin to the gastroesophageal junction

ANSWERS

1. C. This is most likely a gastrointestinal stromal tumor (GIST), and the current guidelines recommend a surgical resection of a gastric GIST (gGIST) ≥2 cm in size and endoscopic surveillance for gGIST <2 cm in size. Furthermore, a GIST that is ulcerated and bleeding is an indication for surgical resection. The nonanatomic resection (wedge/disk) of tumors in the stomach is feasible when located in the gastric body. However, for tumors extending to the esophagogastric junction (EGJ) or the pylorus, a partial gastrectomy may be required to avoid narrowing gastric inflow tract or outflow tract. For subepithelial lesions located in the stomach, two novel NOTES resection techniques have been developed: EFTR and STER. Both of these techniques appear to be equally effective and safe with the benefits of organ-sparing, fewer postoperative complications, and shorter length of hospital stay. They have also been shown to obtain en bloc resection, clear margins of resection, and low rates of recurrence on long-term follow-up. There is no data to suggest a superiority of one technique over the other. These techniques are currently limited to lesions ≤5 cm in size. However, there are no prospective randomized studies comparing these endoscopic resection techniques to surgical resection in survival and morbidity. Due to the involvement of the EGJ and cardia, these would be difficult locations to undergo endoscopic resection techniques. Thus, guideline-based management for these lesions is currently surgical in nature.

2. C. A novel endoscopic technique of transluminal drainage of the gallbladder into the gastrointestinal tract using an EUS-guided approach has recently evolved. It involves most often the placement of a lumen-apposing metal stent (LAMS) between the gall bladder and the stomach/duodenum under EUS direction and has the benefits of being minimally invasive with no external drains. A multicenter, prospective study in high-risk surgical patients with acute cholecystitis (n = 30) showed a technical success of 90% and a clinical success of 96%. Two patients (7%) developed recurrent cholecystitis due to LAMS obstruction. No LAMS-related complications were observed during a mean indwelling stent time of 364 days. Another established and accepted alternative is a percutaneous cholecystostomy tube. This, however, requires consistent nursing care and the discomfort of an external drainage catheter. The other endoscopic alternative of transpapillary gallbladder stenting was attempted but failed in this patient. NOTES for endoscopic gallbladder removal is not the standard of care and should not be considered for this patient unless part of a research protocol. A Whipple operation is not appropriate here.

3. **A.** Multiport laparoscopic is considered the gold standard approach to cholecystectomy, compared to the open approach, given equivalent serious complications, improved cosmesis, less pain, and decreased length of stay. Particularly considering the patient's concerns regarding cosmesis, an open approach would not be appropriate in this case. Ursodiol does not exert an influence on symptomatic gallstones that is nearly as efficacious or durable compared to cholecystectomy. Particularly considering this patient is a very low-risk surgical candidate, cholecystectomy is the correct approach.

Although there have been a number of series published regarding intra-abdominal NOTES (the majority of which are transvaginal cholecystectomy), NOTES procedures require highly specialized training, specialized technology, and a mastery of the flexible endoscope. Furthermore, the vast majority of clinical NOTES transvaginal cholecystectomy cases reported were hybrid cases, with at least one laparoscopic port. NOTES for endoscopic gallbladder removal is not the standard of care and should not be considered for this patient unless as part of a research protocol.

There is a definite learning curve to single-incision cholecystectomy. One particular study demonstrated a learning curve of about 25 cases, with the majority of major complications, including conversion to standard or open cholecystectomy, to occur in the first 10 cases. Given this, despite the patient's concerns regarding cosmesis, the safest and most appropriate option presented would not be a single-incision cholecystectomy unless that surgeon had adequate experience with a low complication rate.

4. **B.** A meta-analysis performed demonstrated that there were no clinically significant differences in bleeding or pain between single-incision and standard multiport cholecystectomy. Another meta-analysis also demonstrated no difference in surgical site infections. There is no high-quality data demonstrating that there is a comparative mortality difference with either procedure.

There is, however, a significant difference in postoperative incisional hernia, with more occurring in the single-incision group. This should be explained to the patient in the clinic, particularly if she is planning to become pregnant in the future. This increase in postoperative hernia is likely secondary to the length of the fascial incision required by whichever single-incision platform is chosen. The fascial incision can be up to 7 cm with some devices.

Furthermore, there are data showing that the rate of procedural failure is higher in the single-incision group (mainly relating to conversion to multiport laparoscopic), and the time of procedure is longer in the single-incision group. Finally, relative to this patient, there are data supporting that single-incision laparoscopic cholecystectomy fares better than multiport cholecystectomies on postoperative cosmesis scores.

5. **A.** Multiport laparoscopic Heller myotomy is the current gold standard operative approach for the treatment of achalasia. A SIL approach has been described in the literature, but sufficient comparative data do not exist for this approach to be considered an acceptable alternative. The anatomical location of the repair makes a single-incision approach difficult, and this technique has not been widely adopted.

Peroral endoscopic myotomy (POEM) is an endoscopic surgical approach that has gained increasing attention and adoption by surgeons and gastrointestinal endoscopists alike. The procedure consists of endoscopically creating a submucosal tunnel in the distal esophagus and gastroesophageal junction, followed by creating an endoscopic myotomy, then retraction of the endoscope and closing the submucosal tunnel with endoscopic clips or endoscopic suturing. There are no external scars involved in this procedure and it does not require laparoscopic equipment or ports. A recent comparative study of POEM and laparoscopic Heller myotomy demonstrated equal resolution of symptoms in both groups, equal esophageal acid exposure in both groups, and shorter hospitalization for the POEM group. Another prospective randomized controlled trial comparing POEM to laparoscopic Heller myotomy with Dor fundoplication demonstrated noninferiority of the POEM intervention in terms of dysphagia, but there may be some increased recurrent regurgitation. The POEM procedure should be performed in an experienced center by an expert endoscopist.

Bougie dilation of the esophagus generally does not provide durable relief in patients with achalasia.

Furthermore, botulinum toxin injection of the GE junction may modestly improve symptoms in the short term, but results are not durable.

BIBLIOGRAPHY

Aslanian HR, Sethi A, Bhutani MS, et al. ASGE guideline for endoscopic full-thickness resection and submucosal tunnel endoscopic resection. *VideoGIE*. 2019;4:343–350.

Bhayani NH, Kurian AA, Dunst CM, Sharata AM, Rieder E, Swanstrom LL. A comparative study on comprehensive, objective outcomes of laparoscopic Heller myotomy with per-oral endoscopic myotomy (POEM) for achalasia. *Ann Surg*. 2014;259(6):1098–1103.

Chukwumah C, Zorron R, Marks JM, Ponsky JL. Current status of natural orifice translumenal endoscopic surgery (NOTES). *Curr Probl Surg*. 2010;47(8):630–668.

Elmunzer, BJ, Noureldin M, Morgan KA, Adams DB, Cote GA, Waljee AK. The impact of cholecystectomy after endoscopic sphincterotomy for complicated gallstone disease. *Am J Gastroenterol*. 2017;112(10):1596–1602.

Faulx AL, Kothari S, Acosta RD, et al. The role of endoscopy in subepithelial lesions of the GI tract. *Gastrointest Endosc*. 2017;85(6):1117–1132.

Feinberg EJ, Agaba E, Feinberg ML, Camacho D, Vemulapalli P. Single-incision laparoscopic cholecystectomy learning curve experience seen in a single institution. *Surg Laparosc Endosc Percutan Tech*. 2012;22(2):114–1117.

Gill IS, Advincula AP, Aron M, et al. Consensus statement of the consortium for laparoendoscopic single-site surgery. *Surg Endosc*. 2010;24:762–768.

Huang RJ, Barakat MT, Girotra M, Banerjee S. Practice patterns for cholecystectomy after endoscopic retrograde cholangiopancreatography for patients with choledocholithiasis. *Gastroenterology*. 2017;153(3):762–71.e2.

Inoue H, Minami H, Kobayashi Y, et al. Peroral endoscopic myotomy (POEM) for esophageal achalasia. *Endoscopy*. 2010;42:265–271.

Irani S, Baron TH, Grimm IS, Khashab MA. EUS-guided gallbladder drainage with a lumen-apposing metal stent (with video). *Gastrointest Endosc*. 2015;82(6):1110–1115.

Khan MA, Khan Z, Tombazzi CR, Gadiparthi C, Lee W, Wilcox CM. Role of cholecystectomy after endoscopic sphincterotomy in the management of choledocholithiasis in high-risk patients: a systematic review and meta-analysis. *J Clin Gastroenterol*. 2018;52(7):579–589.

Kobayashi M, Mizuno M, Sasaki A, Arisue A, Akiyama S, Wakabayashi G. Single-port laparoscopic Heller myotomy and Dor fundoplication: initial experience with a new approach for the treatment of pediatric achalasia. *J Pediatr Surg*. 2011;46:2200–2203.

Lehmann KS, Ritz JP, Wibmer A, et al. The German registry for natural orifice translumenal endoscopic surgery: report of the first 551 patients. *Ann Surg*. 2010;252(2):263–270.

Liu L, Chiu PW, Reddy N, et al. Natural orifice transluminal endoscopic surgery (NOTES) for clinical management of intra-abdominal diseases. *Dig Endosc*. 2013;25(6):565–577.

Marcella C, Sarwar S, Ye H, Shi RH. Efficacy and safety of endoscopic treatment for gastrointestinal stromal tumors in the upper gastrointestinal tract. *Clin Endosc*. March 17, 2020.

Marks JM, Phillips MS, Tacchino R, et al. Single-incision laparoscopic cholecystectomy is associated with improved cosmesis scoring at the cost of significantly higher hernia rates: 1-year results of a prospective randomized, multi-center, single-blinded trial of traditional multiport laparoscopic cholecystectomy vs single-incision laparoscopic cholecystectomy. *J Am Coll Surg*. 2013;216:1037–1047; discussion 1047–1048.

Mazer L, Worth P, Visser B. Minimally invasive options for gastrointestinal stromal tumors of the stomach. *Surg Endosc*. March 27, 2020.

Milas M, Devedija S, Trkulja V. Single incision versus standard multiport laparoscopic cholecystectomy: updated systematic review and meta-analysis of randomized trials. *Surgeon*. 2014;12(5):271–289.

Omar MA, Redwan AA, Mahmoud AG. Single-incision versus 3-port laparoscopic cholecystectomy in symptomatic gallstones: A prospective randomized study. *Surgery*. 2017;162(1):96–103.

Pang T, Zhao Y, Fan T, et al. Comparison of safety and outcomes between endoscopic and surgical resections of small (≤ 5 cm) primary gastric gastrointestinal stromal tumors. *J Cancer*. 2019;10(17):4132–4141.

Pavurala RB, Li D, Porter K, Mansfield SA, Conwell DL, Krishna SG. Percutaneous cholecystostomy-tube for high-risk patients with acute cholecystitis: current practice and implications for future research. *Surg Endosc*. 2019;33(10):3396–3403.

Rajravelu RK, Ginsberg GG. Management of gastric GI stromal tumors: getting the GIST of it. *Gastrointest Endosc*. 2020;91:823–825.

Rattner D. Introduction to NOTES white paper. *Surg Endosc*. 2006;20(2):185.

Siddiqui A, Kunda R, Tyberg A, et al. Three-way comparative study of endoscopic ultrasound-guided transmural gallbladder drainage using lumen-apposing metal stents versus endoscopic transpapillary drainage versus percutaneous cholecystostomy for gallbladder drainage in high-risk surgical patients with acute cholecystitis: clinical outcomes and success in an International, Multicenter Study. *Surg Endosc*. 2019;33:1260–1270.

Song T, Liao B, Liu J, Yin Y, Luo Q, Cheng N. Single-incision versus conventional laparoscopic cholecystectomy: a systematic review of available data. *Surg Laparosc Endosc Percutan Tech*. 2012;22(4):e190–e196.

Trastulli S, Cirocchi R, Desiderio J, et al. Systematic review and meta-analysis of randomized clinical trials comparing single-incision versus conventional laparoscopic cholecystectomy. *Br J Surg*. 2013;100(2):191–208. doi:10.1002/bjs.8937

Venneman NG, Besselink MG, Keulemans YC, et al. Ursodeoxycholic acid exerts no beneficial effect in patients with symptomatic gallstones awaiting cholecystectomy. *Hepatology*. 2006;43(6):1276–1283.

Walter D, Teoh AY, Itoi T, et al. EUS-guided gall bladder drainage with a lumen-apposing metal stent: a prospective long-term evaluation. *Gut*. 2016;65(1):6–8.

Werner YB, Hakanson B, Martinek J, et al. Endoscopic or surgical myotomy in patients with idiopathic achalasia. *N Engl J Med*. 2019;381:2219–2229.

Yamada H, Yano T. Single incision laparoscopic approach for esophageal achalasia: A case report. *Int J Surg Case Rep*. 2013;4(1):1–4.

Zhang Y, Mao XL, Zhou XB, et al. Long-term outcomes of endoscopic resection for small (≤4.0 cm) gastric gastrointestinal stromal tumors originating from the muscularis propria layer. *World J Gastroenterol*. 2018;24(27):3030–3037.

Zhao Y, Pang T, Zhang B, et al. Retrospective J Gastrointest Surg 2020 Dec; 24 (12): 2714-2721.

Zorron R, Palanivelu C, Galvao Neto MP, et al. International multicenter trial on clinical natural orifice surgery—NOTES IMTN study: preliminary results of 362 patients. *Surg Innov*. 2010;17:142–158.

Robotic-Assisted Surgery

Mary Decoteau and Gordon Wisbach

A 65-year-old man with a medical history of hypertension presents to the emergency room complaining of rectal bleeding for 3 months. On physical exam, a rectal mass and scant gross blood are discovered during a digital rectal exam. A proctoscopic evaluation localizes the mass in the anterior rectum only 4 cm from the dentate line. A colonoscopy does not reveal any concomitant lesions, and a biopsy of the lesion confirms the mass is adenocarcinoma. On endoscopic ultrasound, the mass extends through the muscularis propria with one abnormal lymph node. There is no involvement with the sphincter muscles. His workup includes a computed tomography scan of the abdomen and pelvis, with no signs of metastasis. He completes neoadjuvant chemotherapy and returns to the clinic to discuss surgical treatment. Based on the location of the tumor, you recommend a robotic-assisted laparoscopic low anterior resection with a diverting loop ileostomy.

1. **Which of the following is true regarding the differences between robotic and laparoscopic resection of rectal cancer?**

   A. There is improved oncologic resection, lymph node sampling and resection of margins.
   B. There is a decreased incidence of bladder and erectile dysfunction in men undergoing robotic-assisted low anterior resection.
   C. The robotic approach has decreased conversion to open rates compared to the laparoscopic one.
   D. The increased cost of the robotic approach is offset by the significantly decreased hospital length of stay and complication rate.

2. **Of the following surgeries, which has been shown to benefit from the robotic approach?**

   A. Cholecystectomy
   B. Nissen fundoplication
   C. Colorectal resection
   D. Adrenalectomy
   E. Pancreatectomy

3. **Which of the following patients would most likely benefit from a robotic-assisted versus traditional laparoscopic surgery for colorectal cancer?**

   A. 75-year-old admitted with a lower gastrointestinal bleed, found to have a bleeding cecal tumor on colonoscopy
   B. 60-year-old man with a low rectal cancer that is abutting the prostate on endoscopic ultrasound
   C. 64-year-old man with no significant medical history with a descending colon mass
   D. 55-year-old man admitted with obstipation found to have an obstructing sigmoid tumor

4. **Of the following, which is considered to be one of the advantages of robotic surgery?**

   A. Decreased overall cost
   B. Motion scaling
   C. Improved ergonomics for the operating surgeon
   D. The ability to perform multi-quadrant procedures with ease
   E. EndoWrist (TM) technology, which allows for better tacline sensation and haptic feedback

5. **Which of the following is true regarding the training required to perform robotic-assisted laparoscopic surgery?**

    A. As part of the learning curve for robotic-assisted laparoscopic colorectal surgery, surgical efficiency is best determined by operative time.

    B. The learning curve for robotic-assisted laparoscopic colorectal surgery is well defined.

    C. Simulation for robotic surgery is undeveloped and, therefore, not useful in honing these skills.

    D. There are no regulated, standardized training programs for surgeons interested in performing robotic-assisted laparoscopic surgery.

6. **When preparing for surgery on the morbidly obese patient, which of the following considerations is most accurate when offering the robotic approach over standard laparoscopy?**

    A. The rates conversion to open when using the robot versus standard laparoscopic approach secondary to body habitus are higher.

    B. There is decreased visualization given increased intra-abdominal fat content.

    C. The hemodynamic effects of robotic surgery are more favorable over standard laparoscopy.

    D. Increased weight of organs and intra-abdominal fat can lead to higher torque requirements on surgical instruments, which can be transferred to the robot and thus decrease the physical demand on the surgeon.

7. **Regarding robotic versus laparoscopic inguinal hernia repair, which of the following is correct?**

    A. Robotic repair is associated with longer operative times.

    B. Lower complication rates occur with the robotic approach.

    C. There is a longer length of stay associated with the robot approach.

    D. Recurrence rates are less with the robot approach.

ANSWERS

1. **C.** A systematic review and meta-analysis of seven randomized clinical trials by Li et al. in 2019 identified a significantly lower conversion rate to open laparotomy in the robotic rectal surgery group (OR 0.29). However, there were no significant differences in perioperative complications, harvested lymph nodes, positive circumferential resection margins, complete total mesorectal excision, first flatus, or length of stay between the groups. One potential advantage of robotic surgery is a more accurate pelvic dissection, which could facilitate identification and preservation of autonomic nerves, leading to less postoperative bladder and sexual dysfunction. However, these advantages have not been well elucidated in the literature, with a recent comprehensive review in 2018 by Luca et al. suggesting no evidence of the superiority of robotic surgery over laparoscopy for performing nerve-sparing rectal cancer surgery.

2. **C.** The use of robotic surgery has increased precipitously over the last several years, including a widened breadth of surgical specialties and type of operations performed. The most consistent benefit of robotic surgery is decreasing operative conversions, specifically in rectal cancer, as indicated in a study by Mushtaq et al. In partial colectomies, there is evidence to support quicker return to bowel function. Oncologic outcomes compared to the laparoscopic approach are equivalent. Robotic surgery provides solutions to the challenges posed by laparoscopy, including wristed instruments, ease of intracorporeal suturing, and ergonomic advantages, which are particularly prudent to the technical challenges of colonic resections.

3. **B.** Robotic-assisted laparoscopic surgery is rarely applied to emergent operations. Also, a laparoscopic approach is rarely preferred in an urgent colorectal operation, including obstipation due to obstructing colon cancer. A randomized trial of robotic-assisted versus laparoscopic colectomy for right colon cancer showed that hospital stay, surgical complications, postoperative pain score, resection margin clearance, and number of lymph nodes harvested were similar in both groups, but the costs associated with the robotic-assisted right colectomy were higher. A nationwide analysis of robotic colorectal surgery revealed anterior resections for rectal cancers were the most common robotic-assisted colorectal surgery performed in the United States, accounting for 40% of all robotic cases. A larger percentage of all rectal cancers are being performed robotically compared to colon resections, with a tendency toward higher use of robotic-assisted techniques in males undergoing anterior resection for rectal cancer. This study suggests robotic assistance may be of no

added benefit in routine colon resections, but selective application in complex rectal cancer procedures may prove to have long-term benefits. Of the choices listed, the patient with the low rectal cancer abutting the prostate is most likely to benefit from robotic-assisted surgery.

4. **C.** There are many advantages of robotic-assisted laparoscopic surgery, including three-dimensional (3D) high-definition vision, visual magnification up to 15 times normal, motion scaling that will eliminate a natural hand tremor as motions are de-amplified up to a scale of 5 to 1, improved ergonomics for the operating surgeon, and EndoWrist technology, which allows the instrument to imitate normal wrist and elbow motions. However, there are many disadvantages, including increased operative time and cost, the loss of tactile sensation, and an evolving learning curve. It should be noted that while multiple studies report higher operative costs for robotic procedures, the overall costs for select procedures may be equivalent or lower when accounting for surgical outcomes and can reduce over time as the robot becomes more mainstream.

5. **D.** Operative time is an inadequate surrogate to determine learning curve for robotic surgery for many reasons; most important, shorter operative times are not reflected in patient outcomes. A systematic review of trials examining learning curve in robotic-assisted surgeries from multiple specialties suggests that using operative time is too simplistic and an assessment of surgical outcomes more accurately reflective of robotic expertise. Because the learning curve has been studied in multiple ways with differing numbers of parameters, the learning curve is not well defined. Simulation for robotic surgery is available and shown to be useful in attaining competency prior to performing surgeries on patients. For instance, an inexpensive and synthetic pelvic training model has been developed to teach the complex skills needed for a successful completion of robotic rectal dissection. There is no one standardized competency-based training program required prior to integrating robotic-assisted surgery into one's surgical practice. A recent literature review out of the University of Illinois[8] details the many different types of training programs described and provides guidelines for the development of a structured training program.

6. **D.** Surgery on the morbidly obese patient is technically more demanding secondary to the body habitus, increased subcutaneous adipose tissue, heavier organs, and increased intra-abdominal fat content. These factors create difficulty with instrument reach and added strain on not only the surgeon but also the laparoscopic instruments. A distinct advantage of the robot is the ability to displace this torque and physical demand onto the robot, thereby lessening the force demands of the operator. The unique placement of trocars for the robot also allows those forces to be splayed across the patient, eliminating the physical strain of reaching across a larger patient in poor ergonomic fashion. Although visualization can be a significant issue in the morbidly obese, the robot affords excellent visualization and precise dissection in small spaces given its superior up-close, 3D optics. Robotic surgeries, particularly low pelvic procedures, often require significant steep head-down positioning, which can have important hemodynamic effects on any patient but is especially important in the morbidly obese. And finally, just as robotic surgery has been found to have lower conversion rates to open surgery, lower conversion rates occur in operations involving morbidly obese patients. A retrospective review of the NSQIP database in 2018 by Harr et al.[9] comparing obese to nonobese patients undergoing colorectal surgery revealed robotic-assisted colorectal surgery was associated with fewer conversions to laparotomy, and the risk of prolonged ileus was significantly reduced in obese patients undergoing robotic surgery.

7. **A.** Utilization of robotic-assisted inguinal hernia repair (IHR) has increased dramatically in recent years, but randomized or prospective studies comparing outcomes and cost of laparoscopic and robotic-IHR are still limited. Recent studies conclude that robotic-IHR encompass a higher added cost, largely in the form of increased operative time and non-consumable instrumentation. A recent 2019 retrospective review by Khoraki et al. suggested that robotic-IHR was associated with higher perioperative complications, including higher reoperation rates and readmissions Similarly, a current ongoing clinical trial out of the University of Texas at Houston by Olavarria et al. comparing robotic versus laparoscopic ventral hernia repairs also is reporting similar perioperative outcomes with higher costs,

increased operative time, and increased enterotomies. More research will be needed to ascertain if the robotic approach truly offers any benefit in the repair of inguinal hernias. Some of these findings may be reflective of the early learning curve with the robot and as more surgeons become increasingly familiar with this surgical modality, robotic outcomes may improve.

BIBLIOGRAPHY

Al-Mazrou AM, Baser OKR. Propensity score-matched analysis of clinical and financial outcomes after robotic and laparoscopic colorectal resection. *J Gastrointest Surg.* 2018;22(6):1043–1051.

Dwyer A, Crawford DL, Michael A. Evolution and literature review of robotic general surgery resident training 2002–2018. *Updates Surg.* 2018;70(3):363–368.

Halabi WJ, Kang CY, Jafari MD, et al. Robotic-assisted colorectal surgery in the United States: a nationwide analysis of trends and outcomes. *World J Surg.* 2013;37:2782–2790.

Harr JN, Haskins IN, Amdur RL, et al. The effect of obesity on laparoscopic and robotic-assisted colorectal surgery outcomes: an ACS NSQIP database analysis. *J Robot Surg.* 2018;12(2):317–323.

Khoraki J, Gomez PP, Mazzini GS, et al. Perioperative outcomes and cost of robotic-assisted versus laparoscopic inguinal hernia repair. *Surg Endosc.* September 30, 2019.

Li L, Zhang W, Guo Y, Wang X, Yu H, Du B, et al. Robotic versus laparoscopic rectal surgery for rectal cancer: a meta-analysis of 7 randomized controlled trials. *Surg Innov.* 2019;26(4):497–504.

Luca F, Craigg DK, Senthil M, Selleck MJ, Babcock BD, Reeves ME Garberoglio, CA. Sexual and urinary outcomes in robotic rectal surgery: review of the literature and technical considerations. *Updates Surg.* 2018;70(3):415–421.

Mushtaq, HH, Shah, SK, Agarwal AK. The current role of robotics in colorectal surgery. *Curr Gastroenterol Rep.* 2019;21(11). https://doi.org/10.1007/s11894-019-0676-7

Olavarria O, Bernardi K, Shinil K, et al. Robotic versus laparoscopic ventral hernia repair: a multicenter, blinded randomized controlled Trial (09/13/2019). https://ssrn.com/abstract=3453330 or http://dx.doi.org/10.2139/ssrn.3453330

Park JS, Choi GS, Park SY, et al. Randomized clinical trial of robot-assisted versus standard laparoscopic right colectomy. *Br J Surg.* 2012;99(9):1219–1226.

Pernar, LIM, Robertson, FC, Tavakkoli A, et al. An appraisal of the learning curve in robotic general surgery. *Surg Endosc.* 2017;31:4583–4596.

Tam V, Rogers DE, Al-Abbas A, et al. Robotic inguinal hernia repair: a large health system's experience with the first 300 cases and review of the literature. *J Surg Res.* 2019;235:98–104.

8

Troubleshooting Robotic Surgery

Omar Yusef Kudsi and Naseem Bou-Ayash

You are asked to start a minimally invasive surgical (MIS) program at a new community hospital. The chief of staff has asked you to evaluate all the new minimally invasive techniques and equipment, specifically regarding patient safety, so that the hospital can purchase the proper equipment for your program.

1. **Regarding carbon dioxide (CO_2) insufflation in laparoscopic surgery, which of the following statements is true?**

   A. An average laparoscopic colectomy requires approximately 200 to 280 liters of CO_2.

   B. Insufflation filters composed of mesh with 0.1- to 0.3-micron pores have been developed to exclude the possibility of peritoneal contamination or disease transmission.

   C. Randomized controlled trials have demonstrated a clinical benefit as well as a decrease in lens fogging with the use of warmed and humidified air.

   D. Touching the laparoscope tip to the viscera should be performed cautiously as the laparoscope tip temperature can commonly exceed 200°F.

   E. If the surgeon experiences difficulty with pneumoperitoneum, inadequate relaxation of the abdominal wall is rarely a cause.

2. **Regarding the safe use of energy devices, such as monopolar instruments, in laparoscopic surgery, which of the following is true?**

   A. Thermal injury cannot occur from another instrument if the electrically active instrument is not touching it.

   B. Disruptions in the insulation of an active instrument may discharge energy to surrounding structures or tissues leading to inadvertent thermal injury.

   C. Using monopolar devices on the coagulation mode creates less lateral energy spread than the cut mode.

   D. Capacitive coupling cannot occur when a nonconductor separates two conductors.

   E. If the active electrode of a robotic instrument is inserted through a nonmetal trocar, the nonmetal trocar acts can function as a capacitor, causing potential injury.

3. **Regarding robotic-assisted laparoscopic surgery, which of the following is correct?**

   A. The current robotic surgery system has four degrees of freedom with its instruments.

   B. The current robotic surgery system has afforded the surgeon the ability to perform laparoscopic surgery with full control of up to two surgical instruments and the camera.

   C. Potential advantages of the robotic surgery system include tremor reduction, three-dimensional (3D) visualization, and increased wrist action at the surgical site compared with traditional laparoscopic instruments.

   D. Industry representatives can be present to ensure that the equipment is functional and are trained to influence surgical decisions.

   E. An intraoperative cholangiogram is not possible during a robotic-assisted laparoscopic cholecystectomy.

4. **While performing robotic-assisted or traditional laparoscopic surgery, which of the following is true regarding the management of an intraoperative complication?**

    A. While performing a robotic-assisted Nissen fundoplication, the surgeon encounters an isolated iatrogenic distal esophageal perforation. The next step would include primary single-layer repair without the planned fundoplication.

    B. While performing a laparoscopic Nissen fundoplication, the surgeon accidently entered the pleural cavity. The appropriate next step would be immediate placement of a chest tube and discontinuation of the procedure.

    C. During a robotic-assisted laparoscopic incisional hernia repair, the surgeon encounters an enterotomy while performing enterolysis on the anterior abdominal wall. The next step in management should include primary repair with permanent sutures and intraperitoneal onlay mesh placement (IPOM) with a preference of polyester mesh as it is proven to have a lower risk of mesh infection.

    D. Crepitus observed in the chest or the neck during robotic-assisted or laparoscopic Nissen fundoplication is a potential side effect and will most likely improve without any intervention.

    E. After completing a difficult laparoscopic bilateral inguinal hernia repair, the surgeon notices that the insufflation pressure was set at 40 mmHg during the case. The next step includes explaining the technical error to the patient in the recovery room and scheduling a follow-up in the office one week later.

A 76-year-old female (body mass index [BMI] = 29 kg/m^2; ASA = II), with a history of hyperlipidemia, sigmoid colectomy, and open incisional hernia repair, presents with a recurrent incisional hernia (15 × 12 cm). A robotic totally extraperitoneal retromuscular repair (TEP-RM) with posterior component separation is done and a 30 × 35-cm synthetic uncoated mesh was placed in the retrorectus space.

Insufflation settings: 15 mmHg
Ventilator settings: Assist-control mode
  - Tidal volume (V$_T$) = 460 ml
  - Respiratory rate (RR) = 14 bpm
  - Peak inspiratory pressure (PIP) = 32 cm H$_2$O
  - Positive end-expiratory pressure (PEEP) = 5 cm H$_2$O

5. **While performing the posterior component separation with monopolar scissors, what is an** appropriate precaution for avoiding thermal injury to the small bowel behind the posterior layer?

    A. Using a metal cannula with a plastic anchor (hybrid cannula system) to avoid capacitive coupling

    B. Using another instrument to push the posterior layer away from the dissection plane to avoid direct coupling

    C. Using the "coagulation" mode to divide the muscle fibers due to the decreased voltage and lateral spread of energy associated with this mode

    D. Using the monopolar device with continuous activation in order to decrease the risk of injury to adjacent tissues

    E. Using the lowest possible power setting

6. **While dissecting the retromuscular space, a tear was created in the posterior layer, causing a loss of working domain. Which of the following should be avoided?**

    A. Closing the tear using absorbable suture

    B. Inserting a Veress needle into the peritoneal cavity to help decompress intra-abdominal pressure

    C. Creating a larger retromuscular flap

    D. Converting to open surgery

    E. Communicating with the anesthesiologist to ensure the patient is adequately relaxed

7. **Toward the end of the operation, both end-tidal carbon dioxide (Pet$_{CO2}$ = 54) and blood pressure (BP = 175/95) were found to be elevated. Which of the following is the most appropriate next step in management?**

    A. Decrease the abdominal insufflation pressure, complete the operation, keep the patient intubated and mechanically ventilated until parameters normalize, and extubate intraoperatively.

    B. Decrease abdominal insufflation pressure, complete the operation, and extubate immediately.

    C. Complete the operation, keep the patient intubated, and administer narcotics to address pain-induced hypertension.

    D. Obtain an arterial blood gas sample, complete the operation, extubate immediately, and monitor.

    E. Complete the operation, check for a cuff leak, and keep the patient intubated.

ANSWERS

1. D. To maintain pneumoperitoneum throughout a case, a significant amount of CO_2 is frequently required. The duties of the surgical team include monitoring the intra-abdominal pressure during the case, identifying the amount of CO_2 remaining prior to the start of the surgical procedure, and having a replacement tank in reach if needed, especially for long or difficult cases. One report estimated that an average laparoscopic colectomy requires approximately 110 to 180 L of carbon dioxide. The surgeon should be aware of that fact, making sure to check CO_2 pressure in the tank prior to the start of he surgery and clarify that a replacement tank is available, if needed.

The possibility of peritoneal contamination or disease transmission through the flow of intraperitoneal fluid or particulate matter from the patient to the insufflator (and then to the next patient) has been a concern since the early days of laparoscopy. To address this concern, insufflation filters composed of mesh with 0.1- to 0.3-micron pores have been developed that limit, but do not exclude, the possibility of disease transmission.

Warmed, humidified gas is sent directly from the insufflator (or gas is sent from the insufflator through a warming and humidification system prior to patient delivery) in order to enter the peritoneal cavity at body temperature. In addition to the theoretical benefit of improved visualization attributable to condensation prevention, there is some evidence that warm, humidified gas can also reduce hypothermia and pain; however, several randomized controlled trials have failed to show either a clinical benefit or a decrease in lens fogging with the use of warmed, humidified air.

Wiping the laparoscope tip on the viscera, often the liver or small bowel, is another maneuver commonly used and is often effective. However, this should be performed with extreme caution as the laparoscope tip temperature can often exceed 200°F.

An inadequate pneumoperitoneum can also be due to incomplete muscle relaxation. Whenever the intra-abdominal pressure is 15 mmHg or greater and there is inadequate visualization, then the patient's muscles may not be completely relaxed. As such it is always a good idea to check with the anesthesia provider.

Inadequate pneumoperitoneum may be secondary to incomplete muscular relaxation. This often manifests as poor visualization with a simultaneous intra-abdominal pressure of 15 mmHg or greater.

Communicating such concerns with the anesthesia provider is warranted.

2. B. Current concepts in electrosurgery are based on the idea of monopolar and bipolar instrumentation. Monopolar instruments are an "active" electrode, deliver concentrated energy, and require a second "dispersive" electrode, placed on the patient to complete the circuit. Often, the size of the dispersive electrode is much larger than the active electrode to decrease the delivered energy and prevent thermal injury. Bipolar instruments in comparison contain both the "active" and "dispersive" electrodes in a single-hand instrument, thereby delivering concentrated and focused energy to a particular location. Additionally, two modes of energy delivery are used in modern-day electrosurgical units. The "cut" mode delivers a low-voltage, continuous output, while the "coagulation" mode delivers a high-voltage, interrupted output. These modes reflect the energy waveforms and not their designated labels. For further information, please refer to the *SAGES FUSE* (Fundamental Use of Surgical Energy) Handbook.

Metallic trocars are often utilized in both laparoscopic and robotic surgery for cost reduction with current robotic surgery instrumentation requiring the use of metal trocars. It is important to understand the associated possible injuries if these trocars are placed beyond the suggested fascial point and/or come in touch with intra-abdominal organs. With direct coupling, the capacitor generates an electrostatic field between the active electrode and the metal trocar, and as electricity passes through the active electrode, the electrostatic field can transfer energy to the metal trocar, which will then discharge the energy in the form of heat, leading to burns of the skin and abdominal wall, which is common in robotic-assisted surgery performed using metal trocars. The use of nonconductive plastic trocars can avoid this phenomenon.

The use of monopolar instruments possesses an additional risk, known as capacitive coupling, whereby electrical energy is stored in a capacitor (instrument) and then discharged when the circuit is completed. Often, injuries of this type occur with accidental contact of a recently used instrument, which retains stored energy, with nearby tissue causing accidental thermal injuries. Thus, whenever monopolar electrical energy is being utilized, it is important to ensure that there is a safe distance between the active instrument and all other metallic objects.

3. C. Robotic surgery has up to 7 degrees of freedom with its instruments and provides the ability to perform laparoscopic surgery with full control of up to three different surgical instruments as well as the camera by a single operator. The potential advantages of robotic-assisted laparoscopic surgery include tremor reduction, 3D visualization, and increased wrist action at the surgical site.

An intraoperative cholangiogram is possible during robotic cholecystectomy and, if needed, any of the robotic arms can be undocked and moved away for cholangiography and/or placement of assistant ports. The application of surgical safety standards to robotic surgery includes credentialing, mentorship, knowledge of laparoscopic physiology, case selection appropriateness to skill levels, conversion to an open procedure when needed, and industry representatives can be present to ensure that the equipment is functional; however, they are not trained or credentialed to influence any surgical decision-making.

4. D. Given that safely performing minimally invasive surgery requires an advanced set of skills, the American Board of Surgery adapted the Fundamentals of Laparoscopic Surgery (FLS) course prior to being eligible to sit for board examination. Surgeons performing minimally invasive surgery should be prepared to deal with potential complications that could arise, as well as be comfortable with the open technique, if needed.

Possible complications of both robotic-assisted and laparoscopic Nissen fundoplication include entering the pleural cavity, which is often managed by decreasing the insufflation pressure and good communication with the anesthesiologist. As long as the patient remains stable and there is no difficulty in ventilation, the procedure can continue as planned and postoperative chest x-rays can be obtained to confirm the resolution of CO_2. Chest tube placement is not immediately required unless the patient becomes symptomatic.

Iatrogenic injury to the esophagus is a potential complication during Nissen fundoplication and can be avoided by handling the esophagus with umbilical tape (the no-touch technique). It is recommended to repair an iatrogenic injury with a primary, two-layer closure, with the planned portion of the Nissen wrap covering the primary repair site. An enterotomy is a contraindication for synthetic mesh placement irrespective of the amount of spillage or contamination.

Is this still true? Some studies have shown it is okay to place mesh if there is a little spillage.

Crepitus is often seen after mediastinal dissection and usually resolves spontaneously without any additional treatment. Monitoring insufflation pressures during surgery is important throughout the duration of a case since high insufflation pressures can lead to serious complications, such as difficulty with extubation due to CO_2 retention and end-organ ischemia (e.g., acute renal failure). For these reasons, patients that undergo procedures with high insufflation pressures should be admitted to the hospital for observation and closely followed clinically.

5. E. Using the lowest possible power setting minimizes the risk of thermal injury. The power setting used should cater to the resistance of the target tissue. Edematous tissues may necessitate a higher power setting in order to vaporize the water present. Regardless of tissue type, the lowest power setting needed to achieve the desired effect should be used.

Capacitance is stored energy created by an electrostatic field whenever a non-conductor separates two conductors. An example of such is a hybrid cannula system (A), whereby the active electrode is surrounded by an insulator. This, in turn, is surrounded by a metal cannula that is held in place with a nonconductive plastic anchor. The plastic anchor prevents current dissipation through the abdominal wall, which may result in the discharge of this current from the cannula to surrounding tissues (capacitive coupling). In order to minimize this risk, an all-metal cannula system is recommended.

When an active electrode comes in contact with a conductive instrument, a process known as direct coupling may occur (B). Although this process may be intentional, such as with the use of a monopolar device and forceps for coagulation, inadvertent coupling of secondary instruments may lead to serious injury to surrounding tissues in both laparoscopic and robotic procedures.

Two modes of energy delivery are used in modern-day electrosurgical units. The "cut" mode delivers a continuous low-voltage output, while the "coagulation" mode delivers an interrupted high-voltage output. Either mode may be used to cut or coagulate. When using the "coagulation" mode, holding the electrode slightly away from the tissue results in a process called fulguration, which coagulates the tissue over a wide area. By holding the electrode in direct contact with tissue, a higher concentration of current is delivered, resulting in a cutting action. However, due to the "coagulation" mode's higher voltage, direct contact with tissues may result in excessive energy dispersion and thermal injury (C).

Using brief, intermittent activation of energy devices helps maintain better control while coagulating or cutting the target tissue. It also reduces the risk of inadvertent injury to surrounding structures (D).

6. **D.** A peritoneal breach during robotic TEP hernia repair may have several consequences. Insufflated gas quickly enters the peritoneal cavity, causing a loss of working domain and hinders further dissection. Peritoneal or posterior layer tears, if left unclosed, may potentially lead to incarceration, strangulation, and/or bowel obstruction. Therefore, it is good practice to close any tears using absorbable sutures (A).

Inserting a Veress needle into the peritoneal cavity helps release the pneumoperitoneum and restore the working domain (B). This has shown to be effective in laparoscopic inguinal TEP repair as well.

Other troubleshooting options include creating a larger retromuscular flap in order to increase the working space available and reduce the effect of the pneumoperitoneum (C). Increased muscular tone due to insufficient relaxation could also further limit the working domain. Clear and structured communication with the anesthesiologist and operating room team members about such issues is essential (E).

If all the preceding measures fail, converting to a transabdominal preperitoneal approach is an available option. However, converting to an open repair is unnecessary in such situations and may compound the risks of minimally invasive surgery with that of open surgery.

7. **A.** The most widely adopted form of abdominal insufflation for minimally invasive procedures involves the use of CO_2 gas. Its high solubility decreases the risk of accidental venous embolism as compared to other gases used for insufflation. However, this same property may also have several adverse sequelae. The effect of hypercarbia on the cardiovascular system may include tachycardia and increased systemic vascular resistance secondary to activation of neurohumoral mechanisms. Another consequence is the development of subcutaneous emphysema, which can be recognized by the presence of crepitus in the subcutaneous tissue as well as an elevation in end-tidal CO_2. The extent of the subcutaneous emphysema and the ability of the patient to clear excess CO_2 are what determine whether significant physiologic perturbances occur. Although arterial CO_2 also mirrors these disturbances, obtaining an arterial blood gas sample intraoperatively may not provide significant value because arterial CO_2 is almost always elevated as a consequence of abdominal insufflation (D). Relying on early indicators such as end-tidal CO_2 can help address these issues promptly.

In such cases, it is recommended that insufflation pressure be decreased to the lowest level necessary for adequate exposure and completion of the operation. Minute ventilation should also be elevated by increasing the tidal volume or respiratory rate in order to help clear excess CO_2. When these complications are noted toward the end of a case, it is important to ensure end-tidal CO_2 returns to normal limits prior to extubation (B). Only patients with severe chronic obstructive pulmonary disease or those with compromised ventilatory function should be mechanically ventilated postoperatively.

Complications, such as subcutaneous emphysema, may also result in airway compression. Therefore, prior to extubation, a "cuff-leak" test can be performed, whereby deflation of the endotracheal balloon can assess the presence or absence of an air leak around the tube, indirectly screening for airway compression (E). This minimizes the need for reintubation and its associated risks.

Although postoperative hypertension, secondary to increased pain, is a common occurrence with these procedures, treating patients with narcotics may fail to address the actual underlying cause of hypertension. It may also further compromise the patient's ability to expel CO_2, ultimately worsening outcomes (C).

BIBLIOGRAPHY

Ahmad A, Schirmer BD. Summary of intraoperative physiologic alterations associated with laparoscopic surgery. In: Whelan RL, ed. *The SAGES Manual: Perioperative Care in Minimally Invasive Surgery.* Springer; 2006: 56–62.

Alkatout I, Schollmeyer T, Hawaldar NA, Sharma N, Mettler L. Principles and safety measures of electrosurgery in laparoscopy. *JSLS.* 2012;16(1):130–139.

Bittner R, Arregui ME, Bisgaard T, et al. Guidelines for laparoscopic (TAPP) and endoscopic (TEP) treatment of inguinal hernia [International Endohernia Society (IEHS)]. *Surg Endosc.* 2011;25(9):2773–2843.

Brunt LM. Fundamentals of electrosurgery part II: Thermal injury mechanisms and prevention. In: Feldman LS, Fuchshuber PR, Jones DB, eds. *The SAGES Manual on the Fundamental Use of Surgery Energy (FUSE)*. Springer-Verlag; 2012; 61–79.

Fundamentals of electrosurgery part II: thermal injury mechanisms and prevention. In: Feldman L, Fuchshuber P, Jones DB, eds. *The SAGES Manual on the Fundamental Use of Surgical Energy (FUSE)*. Springer; 2012: 61–79.

De Backer D. The cuff-leak test: what are we measuring? *Crit Care*. 2004;9(1):31.

Diamantis T, Kontos M, Arvelakis A, et al. Comparison of monopolar electrocoagulation, bipolar electrocoagulation, ultracision, and ligasure. *Surg Today*. 2006;36:908–913.

Farley DR, Greenlee SM, larson DR, Harrington JR. Double-blind, prospective, randomized study of warmed, humidified carbon dioxide insufflation vs standard carbon dioxide for patients undergoing laparoscopic cholecystectomy. *Arch Surg*. 2004;139:739–743; discussion 743–744.

Funk LM, Greenberg JA. Minimally invasive surgery: equipment and troubleshooting. In: Souba WW, Fink MD, Jurkovich GJ, Pearce WH, Pemberton JH, Soper NJ, eds. *ACS Surgery: Principles and Practice*. Marcel Dekker; 2011: 1–10.

Larson JA, Johnson MH, Bhayani SB. Application of surgical safety standards to robotic surgery: five principles of ethics for nonmaleficence. *J Am Coll Surg*. 2014 Feb;218(2): 290–293.

Lomanto D, Katara AN. Managing intra-operative complications during totally extraperitoneal repair of inguinal hernia. *J Minim Access Surg*. 2006;2(3):165–170.

Ludwig KA. Implications of subcutaneous emphysema and how to avoid and/or limit its development. In: Whelan RL, ed. *The SAGES Manual: Perioperative Care in Minimally Invasive Surgery*. Springer; 2006: 273–280.

Randles VC. The art and science of monopolar electrosurgery. In: Feldman LS, Fuchshuber PR, Jones DB, eds. *The SAGES Manual on the Fundamental Use of Surgery Energy (FUSE)*. Springer-Verlag; 2012: 81–91.

Sammour T, Kahokehr A, Hayes J, et al. Warming and humidification of insufflation carbon dioxide in laparoscopic colonic surgery: a double-blinded randomized controlled trial. *Ann Surg*. 2010;251:1024–1033.

Trastulli S, Cirocchi R, Desiderio J, et al. Robotic versus laparoscopic approach in colonic resections for cancer and benign disease: systematic review and meta-analysis. *PLoS One*. 2015;10(7):1–26.

Tyler JA, Fox JP, Desai MM, et al. Outcomes and costs associated with robotic colectomy in the minimally invasive era. *Dis Colon Rectum*. 2013 Apr;56(4):458–466.

9

Ethics/Legal Issues—Decision-Making

Alexandra Adams and Timothy J. Vreeland

A 70-year-old woman from a nursing facility with mild dementia is admitted with a high-grade small bowel obstruction. She is admitted to the floor for bowel rest and resuscitation. Over the next 24 hours, her nasogastric (NG) output remains bilious, her abdominal pain worsens, and her lactate rises. You determine she urgently needs to go to the operating room (OR), but when you discuss surgery she states, "I don't want surgery, I want to go home and cook dinner with my husband," and she states she will just get better on her own without surgery. She is insistent that she leave the hospital and continues speaking to her husband as if he is in the room. When you call the nursing home, they state that her husband died decades ago, she has no advance directives on file, her siblings have all died, and she has no children. They state she normally lives in an independent unit.

1. **What is the next best step in her management?**
   A. Obtain a court order to proceed with surgery.
   B. Respect the patient's verbal wishes and do not perform surgery, but continue medical management.
   C. Obtain a second physician's opinion, and proceed with surgery if they agree with your assessment.
   D. Respect the patient's verbal wishes and discharge her back to the nursing facility with hospice.
   E. Proceed with surgery as she is unable to refuse at this time, and it is an emergency.

2. **Which principle(s) can be used to justify this decision?**
   A. Autonomy
   B. Beneficence
   C. Nonmaleficence
   D. Justice

3. **You decide to go to the OR, and you call your partner to assist in the case. He informs you that he was diagnosed with HIV today. Which of the following statements are true?**
   A. If the surgeon knows their viral load is $>5 \times 10^2$ copies, the surgeon should refrain from operating until the viral burden is better controlled.
   B. The surgeon needs to disclose their status to the patient.
   C. The surgeon should not be allowed to operate due to this diagnosis.
   D. Due to recent diagnosis, the risk of healthcare worker–to–patient transmission is high ($>33\%$).
   E. The patient should have an HIV test prior to discharge from the hospital.

4. **The patient improves during her hospitalization, but during her care, a nurse accidentally gives her a double dose of narcotic, causing her to sleep for a whole day and require some supplemental oxygen. What should you tell the patient, if anything?**
   A. Do not disclose the medication error as the outcome was not too bad.
   B. Tell the patient she should file an allergy to that medication.
   C. Make the nurse disclose the error and call risk management.
   D. Apologize to the patient and assure her that a patient safety report was filed.
   E. Inform the patient, and tell them that the nurse will be losing her job.

5. **The patient makes a full recovery and is discharged to her prior living arrangement. She returns to the emergency room 6 months later and is diagnosed with acute cholecystitis. She desires for you to remove her gallbladder. However, in the last 6 months, she established a living will and has a do not resuscitate (DNR) order. What is true of her DNR status in this current clinical situation?**

   A. She must revoke her DNR status prior to proceeding to the operating room.
   B. She cannot have a conditional DNR order in place prior to the operation (i.e., medications are allowed, but compressions are not).
   C. Her DNR is invalid due to her mild dementia.
   D. Assume surgical consent implicitly revokes her DNR order in the OR; resume DNR status postoperatively.
   E. She can proceed to the OR with a DNR order in place after a discussion among the patient, the surgeon, and the anesthetist to define the goals of care.

ANSWERS

1. **C.** Obtain a second physician's opinion, and proceed with surgery if they agree with your assessment.

   This patient lacks decisional capacity, likely secondary to delirium. There are five elements that must be present for informed consent: disclosure of relevant medical and procedural details, decisional capacity, the patient understanding the information, voluntariness, and consent. A patient must have decisional capacity to participate in this process, without factors such as neurological impairment to include delirium or sedation. If this patient was alert and oriented, and she was able to voice the benefits and risks of the procedure and the consequences of not operating, it would be her right to refuse surgery even in the setting of mild dementia, as she is still living independently and making everyday decisions on her own (B, D). The surgeon can continue the discussion to understand her reasoning but cannot force the patient to undergo surgery if she refuses.

   In the case of an urgent or emergent operation, two physicians can agree that a patient lacks competence and that a procedure is in their best interest. In this case, the patient has a high probability of recovery and meaningful quality of life after surgery given her reported prior independent status. If her prognosis was poor with projected low quality of life, two physicians could also agree on the futility of surgery and forego aggressive treatment. A second physician's opinion is required in an emergency situation to determine if a patient does not have the capacity to refuse treatment (E). Every effort to find a surrogate decision-maker or advanced directive should be made. In the case of a nonurgent procedure, an ethics committee can be consulted or a court order can be obtained, but this is not appropriate in this scenario given the time limitations of an urgent procedure (A).

2. **B.** The four principles of autonomy, beneficence, nonmaleficence, and justice are the foundations for medical ethics, and the basis for physicians to make moral decisions in clinical dilemmas. Beneficence would be the justification in this scenario, as the surgeon would be balancing the potential benefits and risks of surgery versus nonoperative management, and taking necessary action to mitigate harm to the patient. The decision to operate is believed to be in the best interest of the patient, as not operating will likely result in deterioration and death.

   Autonomy (A) refers to respecting an individual's decisions, allowing them to make their own informed choices based on their own values and beliefs. If the patient was not delirious and was able to understand the benefits and risks of the procedure, the surgeon should not operate and honor the patient's wishes based on the principle of autonomy. This principle does not apply to children, as parents have the right to accept or decline treatment on their behalf. However, some state laws allow adolescents to make their own healthcare decisions independently of their parents.

   Nonmaleficence (C) refers to avoidance or mitigation of harm or injury, which can be active or inactive. It is rooted in the Hippocratic adage "to do no harm." In the realm of surgery, it must be considered that the treatment itself does not cause more harm than benefit; because one can operate does not mean one should.

   Justice (D) is the fourth principle, establishing that benefits, risks, costs, and resources of health care are distributed fairly or equitably. It does not apply in this case.

3. **A.** If the surgeon knows their viral load is $>5 \times 10^2$ copies, the surgeon should refrain from operating until the viral burden is better controlled.

The Society for Healthcare Epidemiology of America (SHEA) provides specific guidelines for healthcare providers infected by hepatitis B, hepatitis C, and HIV. This includes the recommendation that providers with an HIV viral load of $>5 \times 10^2$ copies not participate in Category III procedures, which include general surgery procedures, due to the definite risk of virus transmission (A). This risk is exceedingly low at a reported 0.32% when exposed to HIV-blood contaminated objects (D). Under SHEA guidelines, providers with a viral load of $>5 \times 10^2$ copies can participate without restriction in Category I or II procedures, such as endoscopy, percutaneous procedures, and minor superficial surgical procedures, but do recommend double gloving.

The SHEA guidelines state that providers are ethically bound to report their status to their institution, undergo at least twice yearly testing to ensure maintenance of low viral burden, and seek treatment for their diagnosis. However, providers' duties should not be limited based on HIV diagnosis if the viral burden is acceptably low ($<5 \times 10^2$ copies; C). Some state laws require HIV-positive providers to notify their patients of their status prior to treatment; in most states, this requirement is determined on a case-by-case basis by an expert panel or advisory committee (B). Otherwise, the patient does not require an HIV test prior to discharge unless otherwise clinically indicated (E).

4. **D.** Apologize to the patient and assure her that a patient safety report was filed.

This is an adverse event, and a patient safety report should be filed. Medical errors should be disclosed to the patient, even if the consequences were relatively minor (A). As the physician, you should honestly inform them of what happened, the consequences of the event, and sincerely apologize for the error (D). This conversation is ideally held sitting down, with no distractions, jargon, euphemism, or blaming of other individuals (C, E). Multiple studies have shown that open conversation and apologies lead to fewer lawsuits and lower litigation costs. Many states have apology laws, which prohibit statements of sympathy from being admissible in court as admissions of fault.

5. **E.** She can proceed to the OR with a DNR in place, after a discussion among the patient, surgeon, and anesthesiologist defining goals of care.

Despite mild dementia, the patient would have the capacity to decide her own DNR status if she can demonstrate that she understands the consequences (C). Although she may desire "do not resuscitate," this does not equate to "do not treat." Patients with DNR orders may still benefit from a surgical procedure, although it may not change the course of their underlying disease; this patient would benefit from cholecystectomy if deemed fit for surgery, or a patient with a malignant bowel obstruction may benefit from a palliative bypass. A frank conversation should be held again among the surgeon, anesthesiologist and the patient (or surrogate) to revisit her DNR status and modify her wishes as appropriate, as the consequences of her health have now changed, following the American College of Surgeons recommendation of "required reconsideration" (E). By shared decision-making with the team, she can clarify what interventions are acceptable to her, such as permission to treat easily remediated issues such as pressors for hypotension or blood transfusion, but her desire for no compressions or defibrillation (B). It would violate her right to self-determination to mandate that she must revoke her DNR status to visit the OR, if that is not what she desires (A, D). Based on the principle of autonomy, the patient has the right to maintain her DNR status but proceed with surgery after revisiting the conversation with the medical team.

BIBLIOGRAPHY

American College of Surgery. Statement on advance directives by patients: "do not resuscitate" in the operating room. *Bull Am Coll Surg.* 2014;99(1):42–43.

Chan DK, Gallagher TH, Reznick R, Levinson W. How surgeons disclose medical errors to patients: a study using standardized patients. *Surgery.* 2005;138(5):851–858.

Convie LJ, Carson E, McCusker D, et al. The patient and clinician experience of informed consent for surgery: a systematic review of the qualitative evidence. *BMC Med Ethics.* 2020;21(1):58.

Gallagher TH, Waterman AD, Ebers AG, Fraser VJ, Levinson W. Patients' and physicians' attitudes regarding the disclosure of medical errors. *JAMA.* 2003;289(8):1001–1007.

Henderson DK, Dembry L, Fishman NO, et al. SHEA guideline for management of healthcare workers who are infected with hepatitis B virus, hepatitis C virus, and/or human immunodeficiency virus. *Infect Control Hosp Epidemiol.* 2010;31(3):203–232.

Herron PD. Clinical ethics and professionalism. In: Swartz, MH, ed. *Textbook of Physical Diagnosis: History and Examination*. 8th ed. Elsevier; 2021: 664–664.

Moye J, Marson DC. Assessment of decision-making capacity in older adults: an emerging area of practice and research. *J Gerontol B Psychol Sci Soc Sci*. 2007;62(1):P3–P11.

Robbennolt JK. Apologies and medical error. *Clin Orthop Relat Res*. 2009;467(2):376–382.

Shapiro ME, Singer EA. Perioperative advance directives: do not resuscitate in the operating room. *Surg Clin North Am*. 2019;99(5):859–865.

Turkel S, Henderson DK. Current strategies for managing providers infected with bloodborne pathogens. *Infect Control Hosp Epidemiol*. 2011;32(5):428–434.

Wall A, Angelos P, Brown D, Kodner IJ, Keune JD. Ethics in surgery. *Curr Probl Surg*. 2013;50(3):99–134.

10

End-of-Life Care

Anne O'Shea and Timothy J. Vreeland

SCENARIO 1

An 85-year-old female presents to the hospital with nausea, vomiting, abdominal pain, and distension for the past two days. The pain rapidly worsens over the next hour, and the patient is taken to the operating room (OR) with the diagnosis of mesenteric ischemia. The patient has a past medical history of coronary artery disease, chronic obstructive pulmonary disease, and osteoporosis. She currently lives in a nursing home and is able to perform activities of daily living with assistance. Before taking the patient to the OR, you confirm that the patient has no living will or durable power of attorney but does state that she "wouldn't want to be a vegetable on a machine." During the surgery, the patient is found to have extensive necrotic bowel from the ligament of Treitz to the transverse colon. The patient is closed without resection. After surgery, the patient rapidly deteriorates and develops severe septic shock. A discussion occurs with the patient's family about the poor prognosis of this illness. The patient's daughter, the next of kin, states that she wants everything to be done for her mother and threatens legal action if her wishes are not granted.

1. **What is the next appropriate step in managing this patient?**

    A. Take the patient back to the OR to perform a subtotal colectomy as per the daughter's wishes.
    B. Inform the daughter that she has no decision-making capabilities and proceed with palliative care.
    C. Remove the patient from nutritional support and hydration.
    D. Consult the hospital's ethics committee.

    E. Continue to discuss options with the family.

2. **Regarding advance directives, which statement is correct?**

    A. Advanced directives are not transferable between states.
    B. Oral advance directives are legally valid.
    C. A living will takes precedence over appointed surrogate decision-making.
    D. Advance directives are always followed verbatim.

3. **Regarding life-sustaining medical treatment, which statement is correct?**

    A. There is no ethical difference between withdrawing and withholding treatments.
    B. Risk management personnel must be consulted before life-sustaining medical treatment may be terminated.
    C. A patient has to be terminally ill for life support to be stopped.
    D. It is permissive to withhold "extraordinary" care but not "ordinary" care.
    E. It is illegal to provide palliative care to a terminally ill patient if there is a possibility that this may hasten the patient's death.

SCENARIO 2

A 68-year-old female with a history of poorly differentiated colorectal cancer who previously underwent a right hemicolectomy presents to the emergency department with complaints of abdominal pain, bloating, nausea, vomiting, and anorexia for the last 2 weeks. She notes an approximately 20-lb weight loss with associated fatigue over the last 6 months. The computed tomography (CT) scan demonstrates dilated fluid-filled loops of small bowel with air-fluid levels and multiple transition points, numerous peritoneal masses concerning for peritoneal carcinomatosis, and a new mass in the lower lobe of the patient's right lung, which is concerning for extra-abdominal metastases. You admit the patient, begin IV fluids, and place a nasogastric (NG) tube for abdominal decompression. On admission you note that she has a current living will that states that she would like to be full code. She has not named a durable power of attorney for health care at this time. Her husband died a few years ago following a heart attack, but she does have an adult daughter who lives on the other side of the country.

4. **Despite 48 hours of decompression and bowel rest, the patient remains obstipated with large amounts of bilious NG tube output. What is the next best step in the management of this patient?**

   A. Proceed immediately to the OR for laparotomy with bowel resection and possible colostomy.
   B. Refer the patient for cytoreductive surgery (CRS) with hyperthermic intraperitoneal chemotherapy (HIPEC).
   C. Contact the patient's daughter, present her with the treatment options, and ask her to make a decision regarding her mother's care as she is the next of kin.
   D. Initiate a goals-of-care discussion with the patient and outline palliative options.

5. **In discussing the patient's options for treatment, you mention that the goals of treatment would be palliative and not curative. Which of the following is correct regarding palliative care?**

   A. Life-prolonging treatments are not a component of palliative care
   B. Surgeons may be prone to selecting more aggressive treatment interventions secondary to a paucity of palliative care training and education.
   C. Palliative care encompasses only the medical/surgical treatments provided at the end of life, not psychological or spiritual support.
   D. The majority of patients who qualify for palliative care receive it.

6. **Following your discussion on prognosis, the patient states that she would like to have a do not resuscitate (DNR) order despite what her living will currently states. Which of the following is correct regarding advance directives?**

   A. Patients with advance directives are likely to receive care that is consistent with their preferences.
   B. A living will cannot be superseded by the orally conveyed interests of the patient.
   C. In the presence of a DNR order, medical staff will make every effort to restore cardiac function in the event of cardiac arrest or non-perfusing cardiac rhythms.
   D. In order to remain valid, advance directives must be reviewed and renewed every year.

7. **The patient elects to forego any surgical palliation, and despite attentive supportive care, she progresses quickly, continuing to have significant amounts of abdominal pain. You recommend that the patient consider hospice care. Which of the following is true regarding hospice?**

   A. Hospice care can only be provided in a medical treatment facility (i.e., hospital, nursing home, or assisted living center.
   B. Patients are eligible for hospice when they have 6 months or less to live.
   C. Treatments or medications with curative intent are covered by hospice.
   D. Only adults suffering from cancer are eligible for hospice.

ANSWERS

1. **E.** When making decisions about end-of-life care it is important for all involved parties to have a consensus about care. Emotions and psychological strain can heavily influence decision-making, but it is important to remind involved parties that the most important decision-making factor is what the patient would have wanted. If the patient is no longer competent to make decisions, it is reasonable to ascertain what they would have wanted from previous comments about similar situations. Advanced directives, living wills, or appointed surrogates are commonly used to make decisions, but in their absence, informal advanced directives or next of kin is implicated. In this case, the patient has stated she would not want any heroic lifesaving measures to be taken. Oral advance directives are legally valid and should be documented in the patient's medical records. The

next of kin has rights regarding making decisions about a patient's care as long as these decisions are consistent with the patient's autonomous wishes. Further discussion with the family may make this clear and avoid unwanted court intervention.

2. **B.** Advance directives provide information about a patient's wishes regarding their health care when they are no longer competent to make decisions. Many advance directives contain provisions allowing the directive to be enforceable in whichever state they are currently residing in. Even without such a provision, oral "informal" advance directives made about treatment preferences are legally valid and are upheld in court as a sworn testimony about statements the patient made prior to their illness. Living wills often lack the specific details to direct care in unforeseen circumstances. A surrogate can be appointed to make real-time decisions on behalf of the patient, removing the responsibility of a provider to attempt to interpret a patient's wishes. When a durable power of attorney is appointed, they become an extension of the patient and may make decisions that conflict with a written advance directive so long as they promote the best interest of the patient. Regardless of the preparation a patient takes in preparing an advanced directive, their wishes cannot always be carried out. A recent study showed that a large portion of patients that requested aggressive care did not receive it as either such care was not an option or the patient had appointed a surrogate that overrode the previous preference.

3. **A.** There is no difference between withdrawing and withholding care, such that one action is not more ethically sound than the other. It is not more unethical to stop life-sustaining therapy versus never having started in the first place. However, physicians are less likely to withdraw care once it has been initiated.

Risk management personnel are consulted to limit legal risk regarding patient care. Some hospital policies may require a consult before terminating life-sustaining treatment, but there is no law that indicates this as a prerequisite.

There is a very fine line that marks the distinction between "extraordinary" care and "ordinary" care. Extraordinary care or heroic measures are ones that take over normal physiologic function of the body in end-organ failure. Examples would include the use of ventilators for pulmonary failure or hemodialysis for kidney failure. Ordinary care helps the body sustain itself, with treatment such as IV fluids, tube feeds, or antibiotics. In a Supreme Court ruling in 1983, it was found that any treatment could be declined under the Fourteenth Amendment of the U.S. Constitution, be it extraordinary or ordinary, as long as this is in the best interests in the patient and the burden of medical care outweighs the benefits.

The principle of "double effect" states that it is ethical to initiate a treatment that is intended to benefit a patient even if there is an unintended negative consequence. The benefit must be sufficiently substantial to outweigh the risk. The act must also directly cause the benefit and not be intrinsically harmful. An example would be giving a patient high-dose opiates to relieve pain but then unintentionally hastening the patient's demise by way of respiratory depression.

4. **D.** This patient is presenting with a malignant bowel obstruction secondary to peritoneal carcinomatosis. Her peritoneal carcinomatosis is coupled with the extraperitoneal metastasis, which bars any curative therapies. A frank discussion should be had with the patient clarifying her prognosis. It is important to be as unambivalent as possible, as terminal patients who are not fully aware of prognosis tend to overestimate their survival, which can influence their decisions regarding treatment. At this point, the goals of care should be directed towards symptom control. Options for this include surgical debulking, surgical decompression through bypass or diversion (ostomy), endoscopic interventions (stenting), palliative G tube, and conservative therapy with continued NG tube decompression, or medicinal palliation.

Given that curative intervention is not a realistic option for this patient, any surgical intervention must be carefully considered. CRS with HIPEC is a treatment option for patients with peritoneal carcinomatosis secondary to CRC shown to improve overall survival in some studies; however, the patient's concomitant extraperitoneal metastasis eliminates this as a therapeutic option (B). Surgical decompression via bypass or ostomy is a palliative option but should not be done until the risks and benefits of such an operation have been discussed and weighed. Anywhere from 32% to 100% of patients with malignant bowel obstructions obtain some symptomatic relief following surgery; however, this comes at the cost of significantly increased perioperative morbidity and mortality secondary to malnourishment and high disease burden. In addition, surgical decompression will likely prove futile in patients with multilevel obstruction, as the patient may require multiple bowel resections and the likelihood of re-obstruction is high. Surgical decompression is most effective when there is clearly one or two sites of obstruction located distal in the gastrointestinal tract. Given that this patient has a multilevel obstruction, moving to the OR early (A) would likely be detrimental. Finally, palliative surgery for malignant bowel obstruction has been shown to increase a patient's hospitalization time relative to their survival time, meaning that a majority of their remaining life may be spent in the hospital. Overall, it is important to have an evidence-based discussion with the patient regarding her prognosis and the risks and benefits of the palliative treatment options available to her.

These discussions should include both the patient and family members if possible. However, because this patient maintains her decision-making capacity and therefore her autonomy, decisions regarding care are to be made by the patient, not the daughter (C).

5. **B.** Palliative care was defined in 1990 by the World Health Organization (WHO) as "the active and total care of patients whose disease is not responsive to curative treatment. Control of pain and other distressing symptoms and of psychological, social, and spiritual problems, is paramount." In 2005, the Task Force on Surgical Palliative Care and the Committee on Ethics of the American College of Surgeons published a statement of 10 principles of palliative care echoing this. In summary, these principles are aimed at respecting the dignity of patients by honoring their autonomy to decide what treatments they undergo, if any. Ultimately the patient's goals should be elicited based on the importance they place on longevity, comfort, and function. A care plan should be developed that strikes a balance suitable to patients and their families and can include anything from life-prolonging treatments all the way through hospice (A). It is also important to recognize and address the psychological, social, and spiritual issues that arise after an incurable, life-limiting diagnosis (C). A patient should be provided with the support necessary to alleviate both physical and nonphysical symptoms.

The American College of Surgeons has been an advocate for palliative care since the late 1990s. However, studies published as recently as 2019 have demonstrated that deficiencies in palliative care education in surgical training affect care recommendations. Bateni et al. determined that a lack of training was associated with advocating for major operative interventions in clinical vignettes regarding treatment in patients with advanced cancer when compared with physicians with >40 hours of palliative care training. As mentioned earlier, this could lead to increased morbidity and mortality, a need for reoperation, and longer hospital stays. Determining what is important to the patient and what would improve their perceived quality of life is imperative.

Although each year approximately 40 million people qualify, according to the WHO, approximately only 14% receive palliative care (D). Financial constraints, restrictive regulations, and misconceptions regarding palliative medicine and when and how it should be practiced limit access. Policies, programs, resources, and training on palliative care for healthcare professionals are necessary in order to integrate palliative care into the health system and promote its full potential in the care of patients, not only at the end of life but also in chronic disease states. Ultimately, when employed early, palliative care has the ability to increase quality of life and decrease healthcare costs by reducing unnecessary hospitalizations and the use of other healthcare resources.

6. **A.** Advance directives are legal documents created and signed by competent individuals that provide guidance for healthcare decisions in the event that an individual is incapacitated and unable to make them for themselves. The most common types of advance directives are the living will and the durable power of attorney for health care. A living will is a document outlining the types of life-sustaining treatment a person would want to receive in certain situations, namely, in terminal illness or in cases of prolonged unconsciousness. A durable power of attorney for health care (also known as a medical power of attorney) is a legal document naming a surrogate decision-maker responsible for making healthcare decisions on behalf of a patient if the individual becomes unable to do so. The purpose of advance directives is to protect a patient's autonomy. A retrospective analysis of patients who died between 2000 and 2006 and their advance directives or lack thereof determined that patients who had prepared advance directives were more likely to receive care that was congruent

with their preferences (A). Therefore, inquiring about and encouraging patients to prepare advance directives can help direct end-of-life care and prevent potentially unwanted invasive interventions.

However, advance directives are subject to change as a person ages, is diagnosed with new illnesses, or if their condition changes. Our goals are dynamic. Orally stated interests of a competent patient supersede any prior living wills and are legally valid (B). In this case, our patient's stated desire to change her code status to DNR renders her previous living will null and void. These statements, when and if made, should be thoroughly documented in the medical record.

A DNR order conveys to healthcare workers that a patient does not wish to undergo cardiopulmonary resuscitation, defibrillation, or other life-sustaining measures in the event of cardiac arrest or development of a non-perfusing cardiac arrhythmia. Without a DNR order in your medical file, hospital staff will make every attempt to restore cardiac function. In the presence of a DNR order, medical staff should not make such efforts, but instead follows the wishes of the patient. (C).

Advance directives do not require yearly renewal to remain valid (D). However, it is recommended that they be reviewed every few years in order to ensure wishes regarding treatment or healthcare proxies have not changed.

7. **B.** Hospice is medical care provided to those with terminal illnesses at the end of life with the sole objective of improving quality of life. Hospice care is multidisciplinary and addresses the physical, psychosocial, and spiritual needs of both the patient and their families. Hospice care differs from palliative care in that all treatments with curative intent are stopped (C). A patient becomes eligible for hospice once they have 6 months or less to live according to a physician. Although most often associated with malignancy, hospice is not only for adults with cancer. A significant number of patients on hospice today have other terminal illnesses, such as late-stage pulmonary, cardiac, or renal disease. In addition, infants, children, and adolescents with terminal illness at the end of life also qualify for hospice (D). Hospice care can be provided anywhere—at home, a skilled nursing facility, an assisted living facility, or in the hospital (A).

BIBLIOGRAPHY

Annas GJ. Nancy Cruzan and the right to die. *N Engl J Med.* 1990;323(10):670–673. doi:10.1056/NEJM199009063231010

Balaban RB. A physician's guide to talking about end-of-life care. *J Gen Intern Med.* 2000;15(3):195–200.

Bateni SB, Canter RJ, Meyers FJ, Galante JM, Bold RJ. Palliative care training and decision-making for patients with advanced cancer: a comparison of surgeons and medical physicians. Bateni SB, Canter RJ, Meyers FJ, Galante JM, Bold RJ. Palliative care training and decision-making for patients with advanced cancer: a comparison of surgeons and medical physicians. *Surgery* 2018. DOI: 10.1016/j.surg.2018.01.021.

Dunn GP. Surgery, palliative care, and the American College of Surgeons. *Ann Palliat Med.* 2015;4(1):5–9. doi:10.3978/j.issn.2224-5820.2015.01.03

Dunn GP, Milch RA, Mosenthal AC, Lee KF, Easson AM, Huffman JL. Palliative care by the surgeon: how to do it. *J Am Coll Surg.* 2002;194(4):509–537.

Emanuel EJ. Palliative and end-of-life care. In: Longo DL, Fauci AS, Kasper DL, et al. eds. *Harrison's Principles of Internal Medicine.* 18th ed. McGraw Hill; 2012. Available from http://www.accessmedicine.mhmedical.com

Hall DE, Angelos P, Dunn GP, et al. Ethics, palliative care, and care at the end of life. In: Brunicardi F, Andersen DK, Billiar TR, et al. eds. *Schwartz's Principles of Surgery.* 9th ed. McGraw Hill; 2010. http://www.accessmedicinemhmedical.com

Lo B. Surrogate decision making. In: Lo B., ed. *Resolving Ethical Dilemmas: A Guide For Clinicians.* 4th ed. Lippincott Williams & Wilkins; 2009:101–106.

Meisel A, Synder L, Quill T. Seven legal barriers to end-of-life care: myths, realities, and grains of truth. *JAMA.* 2000;284(19):2495–2501.

Meisel A, Snyder L, Quill T, American College of Physicians–American Society of Internal Medicine End-of-Life Care Consensus P. Seven legal barriers to end-of-life care: myths, realities, and grains of truth. *JAMA.* 2000;284(19):2495–2501.

National Comprehensive Cancer Network Clinical Practice Guidelines in Oncology: Colon Cancer. National Comprehensive Cancer Network. June 15, 2020. https://www.nccn.org/professionals/physician_gls/pdf/colon.pdf

National Institute on Aging: End of Life — What are Palliative Care and Hospice Care? National Institute of Health National Institute on Aging. May 17, 2017. https://www.nia.nih.gov/health/what-are-palliative-care-and-hospice-care#palliative

Paul Olson TJ, Pinkerton C, Brasel KJ, Schwarze ML. Palliative surgery for malignant bowel obstruction from carcinomatosis: a systematic review. *JAMA Surg.* 2014;149(4):383–392.

Pawlik TM. Withholding and withdrawing life-sustaining treatment: a surgeon's perspective. *J Am Coll Surg.* 2006;202(6):990–994.

Sabatino C. Top ten myths and facts about health care advance directives. *Bifocal.* 2015;37(1):6–9.

Silveira MJ, Kim SY, Langa KM. Advance directives and outcomes of surrogate decision making before death. *N Engl J Med.* 2010;362(13):1211–1218.

World Health Organization Palliative Care. World Health Organization. August 5, 2020. who.int/en/news-room/fact-sheets/detail/palliative-care

SECTION 2

General Surgery

11

Skin Cancer and Melanoma

Joy Sarkar, Robert C. Chick, and Timothy J. Vreeland

1. **A 70-year-old male presents to your office with a concerning 2-cm painless lump on his left hip that he noticed over the last year, which is firm and dome-shaped. An excisional biopsy is performed, demonstrating a Merkel cell carcinoma (MCC) with negative margins. Regarding MCC, which of the following is true?**

   A. The Merkel cell polyomavirus likely contributes to the development of most MCC.
   B. A sentinel lymph node biopsy is required only for tumors >2 cm in size.
   C. Risk factors for MCC include having dark skin, a weakened immune system, and overexposure to ultraviolet (UV) radiation.
   D. Merkel cell dense-core granules stain positively for the neuroendocrine marker neuron-specific enolase.
   E. Current recommendations for tumor excision are with a 0.5-cm margin for tumors <2 cm in size and 2-cm margins for those >2 cm in size.

2. **An 86-year-old female presents to your office with a 1.5-cm lesion on her forehead (refer to photo) which has been gradually enlarging over the past year. Which of the following would be the best option in her management?**

   A. Surgical excision with 4-mm margins
   B. Cryotherapy
   C. Mohs microsurgery
   D. Radiation therapy
   E. Topical imiquimod

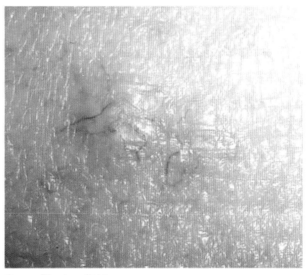

Source: Usatine, 2009.

3. **A 61-year-old male presents to your office with a lesion on his lower lip. Biopsy confirms a squamous cell carcinoma, 2 cm in diameter. Which of the following is true?**

   A. Squamous cell carcinoma of the lip most often presents on the upper lip.
   B. Squamous cell carcinoma is the second-most common cutaneous cancer in patients who have had a kidney transplant.
   C. Actinic keratosis is not a risk factor for the development of squamous cell carcinoma.
   D. Lip defects involving at least one-third of the lip require regional flaps such as an Abbe flap.
   E. Margins for low-risk squamous cell carcinoma range from 1.0 to 2.0 cm.

4. A 41-year-old female patient presents with an 8-mm, flat pigmented skin lesion with irregular borders on her right posterior lower leg. There is no regional lymphadenopathy on exam. An excisional biopsy is performed, and results show superficial spreading melanoma with Breslow thickness 0.9 mm and no ulceration; microsatellitosis is present. Which of the following is true regarding the staging of this tumor?

   A. The T category of this tumor is T1b.
   B. Information about the tumor mitotic rate is needed to determine the T category.
   C. Evaluation of the lymph node status to determine the N category requires dissection of the inguinofemoral and iliac lymph nodes.
   D. Determination of the M category is based on the site of metastasis and serum lactate level.
   E. The most significant prognostic factor for melanomas of this stage is tumor thickness.

5. A 38-year-old male presents for evaluation of a changing mole on his left dorsal upper arm. He endorses a history of severe, blistering sunburns in his teens and is noted to have several moles on his body. He does not have clinically appreciable regional lymphadenopathy. The lesion is biopsied and found to be consistent with superficial spreading melanoma, with a Breslow depth of 2.3 mm, present ulceration, tumor mitotic rate of 1 mitosis/mm², and no evidence of microsatellitosis. He undergoes wide local excision and sentinel lymph node biopsy, and final pathology returns with negative margins and no evidence of metastases in the sentinel lymph nodes. The most appropriate next step in his treatment is:

   A. a serum lactate dehydrogenase level (LDH) test.
   B. a whole-body fluorodeoxyglucose (FDG) positron emission tomography (PET)/computed tomography (CT) scan.
   C. an axillary lymphadenectomy.
   D. a skin exam every 3 to 6 months for 2 years.
   E. adjuvant nivolumab treatment.

A 50-year-old Caucasian female was referred by her primary care provider for evaluation of a mole to her left medial calf. On examination of her left medial calf, she has a 9 mm-diameter pigmented lesion with irregular borders and color variation. Excisional biopsy is performed.

6. Pathology will most likely show which histologic subtype of melanoma?

   A. Acral lentiginous
   B. Desmoplastic
   C. Lentigo maligna
   D. Nodular
   E. Superficial spreading

7. Which of the following is a poor prognostic indicator in melanoma patients?

   A. Extremity location
   B. Low Breslow depth
   C. Female gender
   D. Elevated LDH
   E. Younger age

8. If the patient above is diagnosed with a 2.2-mm-thick melanoma, the radial margin for a wide local excision of the primary lesion should be at least:

   A. 0.5 cm.
   B. 1 cm.
   C. 2 cm.
   D. 3 cm.
   E. 4 cm.

9. Regarding sentinel lymph node biopsy in patients with melanoma, which of the following is TRUE?

   A. Sentinel lymph node biopsy has been shown to improve disease-free survival in patients with intermediate thickness melanomas.
   B. Sentinel lymph node biopsy is indicated for all thin melanomas with ulceration.
   C. Sentinel lymph node biopsy is not indicated in patients with thick melanomas.
   D. In patients with clinically localized melanoma, thickness is the most important prognostic indicator.
   E. Sentinel lymph node biopsy is recommended in patients with T1a melanomas.

10. If the patient above with a 2.2-mm-thick melanoma had a positive sentinel lymph node biopsy (inguinal node), what is the next best step in management?

   A. Superficial groin dissection
   B. Superficial and deep groin dissection
   C. Superficial groin dissection, with deep groin dissection only if Cloquet's node was positive
   D. Ultrasound surveillance of the nodal basin

11. Regarding metastatic melanoma disease, which of the following is TRUE?

A. The primary objective of metastasectomy for stage IV melanoma is relief of the tumor burden.

B. Recurrent stage IV disease is a contraindication to surgery for metastatic melanoma.

C. In-transit metastases occur <2 cm from the primary melanoma.

D. Fifty percent of patients with stage IV melanoma will develop brain metastases.

12. A 50-year-old fair-skinned, blue-eyed male presents to your office with a skin lesion on the pinna of his right ear concerning for a melanoma. Biopsy determines a superficial spreading melanoma with a depth of 1.1 mm. What is the next step in the management of this patient?

A. Wide local excision and sentinel lymph node biopsy

B. High-dose interferon alpha-2b

C. Radiation therapy

D. Excisional biopsy and a total parotidectomy

E. Complete surgical excision with a 0.5-cm clinical margin

ANSWERS

1. A. The mainstay of therapy for patients newly diagnosed with primary MCC remains surgical. Current recommendations are based on the clinical size of the primary tumor and call for tumor excision with 1-cm margins for tumors up to 2 cm in size and 2-cm margins for those that are greater than 2 cm in size. Radiotherapy has been used as monotherapy for primary tumors with reported success, but until more data become available, surgery remains the mainstay of therapy for primary MCC tumors. Furthermore, Feng et al. characterized a novel polyomavirus, the MCPyV, and suggested an association between it and the pathogenesis of MCC. Baseline MCPyV antibody determination can identify patients at higher risk of recurrence requiring closer surveillance, and rising titers may be an early indicator of recurrence. However, there are no data confirming a polyomavirus is responsible for the development of MCC.

The role of chemotherapy in the treatment of MCC remains unclear. Because nearly one-third of clinically node-negative patients harbor microscopic nodal disease, sentinel lymph node (SLN) biopsy is currently recommended for MCC at the time of wide local excision. SLN biopsy has been shown to be important in the staging and prognosis of MCC, and SLN status is included in the most recent American Joint Committee on Cancer (AJCC) staging guidelines. SLN biopsies should be examined by both hematoxyin and eosin (H&E) and immunoperoxidase staining, including CK20. If sentinel nodes are positive, completion lymph node dissection of the nodal basin followed by radiotherapy of the basin is recommended. In cases in which SLN positivity is found on immunostaining but not H&E staining of the lymph node, radiotherapy without complete lymph node dissection has been suggested as sole regional therapy. Dark skin is not a risk factor; fair skin is. The other two are risk factors.

2. C. Basal cell carcinoma (BCC) is the most common form of skin cancer, followed by squamous cell carcinoma (SCC). Multiple subtypes of BCC exist, including nodular, superficial, and morpheaform. Nodular BCC often presents as pearly nodules with telangiectasias and may bleed occasionally, while superficial BCCs may appear as scaly patches, and morpheaform BCC tends to have a scar-like appearance.

The principles of treatment of basal cell carcinoma are based on the risk of tumor recurrence, which in turn is determined by histologic subtype, tumor size, and location (see Table 11-1). This patient's BCC, which is located on the forehead and >1.0 cm in size, is categorized as high risk. Surgical treatment options for high-risk BCCs include Mohs microsurgery or surgical excision with wider surgical margins

Table 11-1 BASAL CELL

	Low Risk	High Risk
Histology	Nodular or superficial	Aggressive pattern
Perineural invasion	Absent	Present
Size	<2cm	2cm or greater
Location	Trunk, extremities if <2cm	Head/neck, hands, feet, pretibial, anogenital (any size)

(as opposed to standard 4-mm margins). Surgical treatment options for low-risk BCCs would include standard excision with 4-mm clinical margins or curettage and electrodessication. Nonsurgical treatments, typically reserved for nonsurgical candidates include radiotherapy and topical and photodynamic therapy. Topical therapy includes 5-fluorouracil and imiquimod. Imiquimod, a nonspecific immune-response modifier, has been approved for the treatment of superficial BCC smaller than 2 cm for five times per week for the duration of 6 weeks, with a clearance rate more than 80%.

On the other hand, SCCs, rather than basal cell carcinomas, most often arise in chronically damaged skin or within actinic keratosis, in burn scars, and in chronic inflammatory wounds. Margins for low-risk SCC range from 0.5–1.0 cm. Mohs microsurgery is indicated for high-risk nonmelanoma skin cancers, tumors >2.0 cm, tumors with indistinct margins or with positive margins identified after excisional biopsy, or tumors in cosmetically sensitive areas.

3. D. In immunosuppressed transplant patients, SCC is the most common skin cancer, and it tends to have a more aggressive behavior. Lip carcinoma is the most common oral cavity cancer, with a majority of these lesions occurring on the lower lip. A majority of patients with oral cavity carcinomas have a history of either excessive alcohol intake or tobacco use. Lip carcinoma most likely presents as an exophytic mass, and diagnosis is obtained by biopsy. Risk factors for SCC include actinic keratosis, burn wound scars, and chronic inflammatory wounds. Large defects that involve up to two-thirds of the lip require local flaps such as Abbe or Estlander. What margins are recommended for lesions <1/3 of the lip? Please explain why answer E is wrong.

4. A. The 8th edition of the AJCC guidelines for melanoma staging has been modified from the 7th edition to remove the tumor mitotic rate as a T1 staging criterion. T1b tumors are now defined as either with ulceration (≤1.0 mm in depth), or 0.8–1.0 mm in depth regardless of ulceration. The presence of microsatellitosis in the excised biopsy specimen upstages the tumor to stage III, and evaluation of the nodal status is indicated. For patients without microsatellitosis or clinically positive nodes, sentinel lymph node biopsy is indicated for melanomas that are at least Stage IB (T2a) or Stage II or selected

Stage IA tumors with high-risk features. The management of clinically negative regional lymph nodes in melanoma remains controversial, but the basic National Comprehensive Cancer Network (NCCN) algorithm for a positive groin sentinel node involves an inguinofemoral lymph node dissection, with the iliac and obturator lymphadenectomy only performed for ≥3 positive nodes within the specimen, positive Cloquet's node, or positive pelvic CT scan. In patients with Stage IV disease, the M designation is categorized by site of metastases and LDH level, not serum lactate level. The most important prognostic factor in patients with localized melanoma is tumor thickness, while the most important prognostic factor in patients with node-positive disease is the number of positive nodes.

5. D. This patient has a T3bN0M0 (Stage IIB) melanoma. After a sentinel lymph node biopsy is negative for metastasis in patients with clinical Stage I or II disease, no completion lymphadenectomy is recommended. Routine laboratory tests such as serum LDH are not recommended, nor is imaging such as CT, PET, or MRI scans unless clinically directed by patient symptoms. Baseline serum LDH would be appropriate for a patient with Stage IV disease, and baseline imaging for staging would be appropriate in a patient with at least clinical Stage III disease. Reasonable follow-up for a patient with Stage II disease that has been fully resected, and with risk factors such as multiple nevi and history of blistering sunburn, would include a history and physical (H&P) every 3–6 months for the first 2 years, every 3–12 months for the following 3 years, and then annually thereafter. Nivolumab is an immune checkpoint inhibitor that is used as adjuvant therapy in resected Stage III melanoma, recurrent disease, or primary systemic therapy in unresectable/metastatic disease.

6. E. Seventy-five percent of all malignant melanomas are superficial spreading melanomas(E). Most arise *de novo*, but they may be associated with a preexisting nevus. They grow radially before growing vertically and thus are usually more superficial when diagnosed. This means they have a relatively good prognosis because the depth of the tumor is the most important prognostic factor. Typical locations are in sun-exposed areas, namely, the back in men and the legs in women. Nodular melanomas (D) comprise 15–30% of melanomas and are often dome-shaped and dark. They quickly develop a vertical growth phase, which then means that they are generally deeper (higher T stage) at the time of diagnosis and have a worse prognosis. Lentigo maligna melanoma (also called Hutchinson's Freckle; C) typically develops as a brown macule in sun-damaged skin of older individuals and may grow radially for years before vertical growth develops. Classically these will be on the head/neck. These will often present as a wide lesion but only as melanoma in situ; thus, these generally have a good prognosis. Acral lentiginous melanoma (A) is the rarest melanoma in Caucasians but is the most common type in Asians and dark-skinned people. They are aggressive and commonly arise on palmar, plantar, subungual, and mucosal surfaces. Desmoplastic melanoma (B) is a rare variant that may be mistaken for a scar, fibroma, or other benign lesion and should be referred to an experienced dermatopathologist for evaluation. Desmoplastic melanoma has a higher risk of local recurrence and is treated with radiation therapy in addition to wide local excision with sentinel lymph node biopsy.

7. **D.** Evidence-based prognostic indicators are integrated into the current AJCC staging system to provide staging that reflects disease biology. An earlier version of the AJCC staging system relied upon a prospective study of 17,600 melanoma patients to determine factors predictive of melanoma-specific survival. The investigators determined that patients with melanomas of the head, neck, or trunk had a significantly worse survival rate than patients with melanomas of the extremities (A). Males had a poorer prognosis than females (C). Increasing Breslow thickness was predictive of lower survival rates (B).

The presence of ulceration was more frequent among patients with thick melanomas (63% ulceration for Breslow thickness >4 mm) than among patients with thin melanomas (6% ulceration for Breslow thickness <1 mm). At all thickness levels, patients with ulcerated melanomas were found to have survival curves similar to patients with melanomas of the next-higher Breslow thickness. The investigators found a significant stepwise decrease in survival based on increasing age (E). Patients with a higher number of nodal metastases and patients with clinically palpable nodal metastases had poorer survival. Pretreatment LDH has been found to correlate with poorer 2-year survival in stage IV melanoma (D) and is often used as a tumor marker in metastatic

disease. More recent data in the era of BRAF/MEK inhibitors and checkpoint inhibitors have revealed factors in the tumor microenvironment that influence survival by changing the way the immune system interacts with the tumor. The most important of these to date, at least in terms of response to immunotherapy, is BRAF mutation (patients with BRAF mutations have a worse prognosis).

8. **C.** Wide local excision is the standard treatment for melanoma. Excision should be carried through skin and subcutaneous tissue down to muscular fascia. Current recommendations are as follows.

Breslow depth	Margins
Melanoma in situ	0.5–1 cm
Up to 1 mm	1 cm
≥1.01	2 cm

The data supporting these recommendations is somewhat heterogeneous, but importantly, it was shown in a randomized controlled trial that there was no benefit in local recurrence or overall survival of 4-cm margins compared to 2-cm margins in patients with melanomas >2 mm thick.

9. **A.** The Multicenter Selective Lymphadenectomy Trial I (MSLT-I) enrolled patients with cutaneous melanoma and randomized to two arms: (1) sentinel lymph node biopsy followed by lymphadenectomy for patients with positive sentinel node(s) and (2) nodal observation with lymphadenectomy for nodal relapse. The major findings of this trial included no difference in melanoma-specific survival in the overall study population but improved disease-free survival in patients with an intermediate thickness (1.2–3.5 mm) or thick (>3.5 mm) melanomas (A). Additionally, 10-year melanoma-specific survival was improved for patients with intermediate-thickness melanoma and nodal metastases (it was better in these patients to know those nodes were positive up front than to wait for clinical recurrence). Finally, the prognostic significance of sentinel lymph node was confirmed as 10-year melanoma-specific survival was 20.8% among node-positive versus 79.2% in node-negative patients (D). This prognostic and staging information is probably even more important in the current era of effective adjuvant therapy for patients with stage III (node-positive) disease.

The most recent NCCN guidelines recommend offering sentinel lymph node biopsy for all T2 or greater melanomas (≥1 mm thick) in the absence of clinically positive lymph nodes (B, C). The guidelines recommend consideration of sentinel lymph node biopsy for T1b melanomas (<0.8 mm with ulceration or 0.8–1 mm). The NCCN recommends against sentinel lymph node biopsy for T1a melanomas (E), as the rate of node positivity in these patients is <5%.

10. **D.** The recent MSLT-II trial enrolled patients with a positive sentinel lymph node biopsy and compared completion lymph node dissection to observation with ultrasound of the nodal basin. It found no difference in melanoma-specific survival between groups, but completion lymphadenectomy did improve locoregional disease control while also increasing lymphedema considerably (24.1% vs 6.3%). Based on the lack of survival benefit and considerable morbidity of completion lymph node dissection, completion lymphadenectomy is currently not recommended for patients with clinically negative lymph nodes who have a positive sentinel lymph node biopsy and can undergo observation with serial ultrasound and physical exam. This patient meets criteria for this trial and therefore should undergo ultrasound surveillance of the nodal basin (D), as opposed to any form of completion lymphadenectomy (A–C). The positive sentinel lymph node biopsy does, however, mean stage III disease, so this patient would be offered adjuvant therapy with either a checkpoint inhibitor (nivolumab ± ipilimumab or pembrolizumab) or a BRAF/MEK inhibitor, depending on BRAF-mutation status.

11. **D.** In-transit metastasis is defined as intralymphatic tumor in skin or subcutaneous tissue more than 2 cm from the primary tumor but not beyond the nearest regional lymph node basin. Satellite lesions refer to lesions within 2 cm of the primary tumor (C). Regarding metastasectomy, a subgroup analysis from MSLT-I demonstrated improved survival with surgery with or without systemic therapy compared to systemic therapy alone, but systemic therapy has evolved since that time. More recently, metastasectomy in combination with systemic immunotherapy was found to improve survival compared to systemic immunotherapy alone. In practice and in multiple ongoing trials, many such patients receive neoadjuvant immunotherapy followed by surgical resection of residual disease when it can all be resected. Multiple sites of disease and even recurrent stage IV

disease are not contraindications to resection (B). The goal of metastasectomy is the removal of all known disease (A) and not just relief of the tumor burden. The most important preoperative considerations include the resectability of all known disease, tumor biology such as tumor volume doubling time, and patient comorbidities. The most common metastatic sites for melanoma are skin, lung, lymph nodes, brain, liver, and gastrointestinal tract. More than 50% of patients with stage IV melanoma will develop brain metastasis, but surveillance imaging for patients with no prior brain metastasis is not well defined (D). Currently, NCCN guidelines recommend consideration of brain MRI every 3–12 months for 2 years and then every 6–12 months for another 3 years in patients without central nervous system symptoms.

12. **A.** Tumor thickness is critical for establishing the prognosis in melanoma, and regional metastases indicates poor prognosis even on difficult anatomic places like the ear. Frozen sections have no role in the diagnosis or treatment of melanoma. Once the dermis is invaded, the probability of regional or distant metastases increases substantially. Lymphoscintigraphy and sentinel lymph node biopsy became the primary method of identifying nodal drainage patterns replacing the prior suggested nodal drainage based on location. Tragus and anterior pinna lesions were thought to metastasize to the parotid gland and anterior cervical lymph nodes, whereas posterior pinna lesions were thought to spread to the mastoid bone and occipital and posterior cervical nodes. Complete surgical excision with 1- to 2-cm margin is the treatment of choice. Elective neck dissection is generally not recommended for lesions less than 1 mm in thickness, whereas lymphadenectomy may offer a survival advantage and better local control for lesions >1 mm in depth and positive sentinel lymph node biopsy (see Table 11-2). Interferon

Table 11-2 EXCISION MARGIN OF MELANOMAS

T Stage	Depth of Invasion (mm)	Suggestion Margin (cm)
T1	<1	1
T2	1–2	1
T3	2.01–4	2
T4	>4	2

Table 11-3 TYPES OF MELANOMA

Type	Characteristics
Superficial spreading	Most common, associated with congenital nevi/dysplastic nevi. Prominent radial growth
Nodular	Prominent vertical growth, dark pigmentation
Lentigo maligna	Arise in sun-exposed areas, occur at dermal–epidermal junction
Acral lentiginous	Least common, arise on palmar, plantar, mucosal, and subungual regions. Common in dark-skinned and Asian patients

alpha-2b has previously been widely used in node-positive melanoma but has now been supplanted by immune checkpoint inhibitors and BRAF-targeted therapy. Different types of melanoma are described in Table 11-3.

BIBLIOGRAPHY

Allen PJ, Bowne WB, Jaques DP, et al. Merkel cell carcinoma: Prognosis and treatment of patients from a single institution. *J Clin Oncol.* 2005;23(10):2300–2309.

Amaria RN, Prieto PA, Tetzlaff MT, et al. Neoadjuvant plus adjuvant dabrafenib and trametinib versus standard of care in patients with high risk, surgically resectable melanoma: a single centre, open-label, randomized, phase 2 trial. *Lancet Oncol.* 2018;19(2):181–193.

Balch CM, Soong SJ, Gershenwald JE, et al. Prognostic factors analysis of 17,600 melanoma patients: validation of the American Joint Committee on Cancer melanoma staging system. *J Clin Oncol.* 2001;19(16):3622–3634.

Balch CM, Soong SJ, Smith T, et al. Long-term results of a prospective surgical trial comparing 2 cm vs. 4 cm excision margins for 740 patients with 1-4 mm melanomas. *Ann Surg Oncol.* 2001;8(2):101–108.

Bartlett EK, Gupta M, Datta J, et al. Prognosis of patients with melanoma and microsatellitosis undergoing sentinel lymph node biopsy. *Ann Surg Oncol.* 2014;21(3):1016–1023.

Bartlett EK, Karakousis GC. Current staging and prognostic factors in melanoma. *Surg Oncol Clin N Am.* 2015; 24:215–217.

Campbell JP. Surgical management of lip carcinoma. *J Oral Maxillofac Surg.* 1998;56(8):955.

Coe MD, Jakowatz J, Evans GR. Evaluation of nodal patterns for melanoma of the ear. *Plast Reconstr Surg.* 2003;112(1):50–56.

Diepgen TL, Mahler V. The epidemiology of skin cancer. *Br J Dermatol.* 2002;146 (Suppl 61):1–6.

Feng H, Shuda M, Chang Y, Moore PS. Clonal integration of a polyomavirus in human Merkel cell carcinoma. *Science.* 2008;319(5866):1096–1100.

Funk GF, Hynds K, Arnell L, Robinson RA, et al. Presentation, treatment, and outcome of oral cavity cancer: a National Cancer Data Base Report. *Head Neck.* 2002;24(2):165.

Gershenwald, JE. "8th Edition AJCC Melanoma Staging System." AJCC Physician to Physician. 2 February 2018.

Howard JH, Thompson JF, Mozzillo N, et al. Metastasectomy for distant metastatic melanoma: analysis of data from the first Multicenter Selective Lymphadenectomy Trial (MSLT-I). *Ann Surg Oncol.* 2012;19(8):2547–2555.

Jemal A, Siegel R, Ward E, et al. Cancer statistics, 2008. *CA Cancer J Clin.* 2008;58(2):71–96. https://www.nccn.org/professionals/physician_gls/pdf/nmsc.pdf

National Comprehensive Cancer Network. Cutaneous Melanoma Version 2.2019. 2019. Accessed October 1, 2019. https://www.nccn.org/professionals/physician_gls/pdf/cutaneous_melanoma_blocks.pdf

National Comprehensive Cancer Network. National Comprehensive Cancer Network Guidelines Version 1.2020: Cutaneous Melanoma. December 19, 2019. Accessed March 1, 2020. https://www.nccn.org/professionals/physician_gls/pdf/cutaneous_melanoma.pdf

National Comprehensive Cancer Network. National Comprehensive Cancer Network Guidelines Version 1.2020: Squamous Cell Skin Cancer. October 2, 2019. Accessed March 1, 2020. https://www.nccn.org/professionals/physician_gls/pdf/squamous.pdf

National Comprehensive Cancer Network Guidelines Version 1.2020: Basal Cell Skin Cancer. October 24, 2019. Accessed March 1, 2020.

Nelson DW, Fischer TD, Graff-Baker AN, et al. Impact of effective systemic therapy on metastasectomy in stage IV melanoma: a matched-pair analysis. *Ann Surg Oncol.* 2019;26(13):4610–4618.

Odgson NC. Merkel cell carcinoma: Changing incidence trends. *J Surg Oncol.* 2005;89(1):1–4.

Pockaj BA, Jaroszewski DR, DiCaudo DJ, et al. Changing surgical therapy for melanoma of the external ear. *Ann Surg Oncol.* 2003;10(6):689–696.

Rubin AI, Chen EH, Ratner D. Basal cell carcinoma. *N Engl J Med.* 2005;353:2262–2269.

Shinkai K, Fox LP. Dermatologic disorders. In: Papadakis MA, McPhee SJ, Rabow MW, eds., *Current Medical Diagnosis and Treatment 2020.* 59th ed. McGraw Hill Education; 2020:106–173.

Usam KJ, Jungbluth AA, Rekthman N, et al. Merkel cell polyomavirus expression in Merkel cell carcinomas and its absence in combined tumors and pulmonary neuroendocrine carcinomas. *Am J Surg Pathol.* 2009;3(9):1378–1385.

Usatine RP, Smith MA, Mayeaux EJ Jr, Chumley H, Tysinger J. *The Color Atlas of Family Medicine.* McGraw Hill; 2009.

Weber J, Mandala M, Del Vecchio M, et al. Adjuvant nivolumab versus ipilimumab in resected stage III or IV melanoma. *N Engl J Med.* 2017;377(19):1824–1835.

Wolchok JD, Chiarion-Sileni V, Gonzalez R, et al. Overall survival with combined nivolumab and ipilimumab in advanced melanoma. *New Engl J Med.* 2017;377(14):1345–1356.

12

Decubitus Ulcers

Meaghan J. Flatley and Pamela C. Masella

You are consulted on a previously healthy 35-year-old male, who was initially admitted 26 days ago in septic shock secondary to a necrotizing soft tissue infection of the right lower extremity. He required high-dose vasopressors for several days following emergent operative debridement and institution of broad-spectrum antibiotics. He was recovering well in the ICU and was recently extubated. However, he developed tachycardia, fever, and leukocytosis. The ICU team calls you to evaluate because the team is unable to identify a source of infection. You examine him and find a black eschar with surrounding cellulitis overlying his right ischial tuberosity approximately 4 × 5 cm in size with a black eschar overlying, expressible malodorous fluid, and surrounding cellulitis.

1. What is the stage of this pressure ulcer?

   A. Stage I
   B. Stage II
   C. Stage III
   D. Stage IV
   E. Unstageable

2. Surgery is performed and when the black eschar is removed, purulent fluid is expressed. On continued debridement, you find that the wound extends to bone. Which is the most appropriate next step?

   A. Debride to healthy, bleeding tissue, and utilize the least invasive, most beneficial musculocutaneous flap reconstruction option.
   B. Debride to healthy, bleeding tissue, and employ temporary coverage with negative pressure wound therapy (NPWT).

   C. Debride to healthy, bleeding tissue, obtain bone biopsy, and employ temporary coverage with NPWT.
   D. Halt surgical debridement until magnetic resonance imaging (MRI) is obtained to rule out osteomyelitis.
   E. Halt surgical debridement until X-ray, Erythrocyte Sedimentation Rate (ESR), and C-Reactive Protein (CRP) are obtained to rule out osteomyelitis.

3. Which of the following would preclude use of NPWT?

   A. Chronic wounds
   B. Diabetic wounds
   C. Wound location
   D. Meshed skin grafts
   E. Wounds that require hemostasis

4. Six days after initial debridement, the patient develops profuse, watery diarrhea and tests positive for *C. diff.* infection. Despite multiple attempts at reinforcement by the nursing staff and the intern, the wound vacuum could not hold a seal due to continued exposure to fecal matter. Which is the best next step?

   A. Bedside wound wash out and wound vacuum replacement
   B. Repeat of operative debridement and replacement of the wound vac
   C. Placement of a fecal management system
   D. Fecal diversion with loop colostomy
   E. Fecal diversion with loop ileostomy

5. **Which of the following patients would be the best candidate for flap reconstruction?**

    A. A 48-year-old male with Stage I sacral ulcer and has no medical comorbidities

    B. A 34-year-old male recovering from brain injury with a Stage IV ischial ulcer that recently underwent treatment for osteomyelitis

    C. A 74-year-old homeless male with Stage III sacral ulcer

    D. A 48-year-old poorly controlled diabetic male with Stage III pressure sore overlying the right greater trochanter

    E. A 56-year-old male with Stage III chronic sacral ulcer who refuses to stop smoking despite hospitalization

6. **Multiple options for treatment of pressure sores exist. Which of the following options offers the best coverage with the least amount of functional deformity?**

    A. Primary closure
    B. Local wound care
    C. Skin grafts
    D. Musculocutaneous reconstruction
    E. Fasciocutaneous reconstruction

ANSWERS

1. **E.** Accurate staging of pressure wounds is important because it guides management. Staging is as follows:

    Stage I: Non-blanchable erythema of intact skin; impending skin ulceration.

    Stage II: Partial-thickness skin loss involving epidermis or dermis; ulcer is superficial and presents clinically as an abrasion, blister, or shallow crater.

    Stage III: Full-thickness skin loss involving damage or necrosis of subcutaneous tissue that may extend down to, but not through, underlying fascia; ulcer presents clinically as a deep crater with or without undermining of adjacent tissue.

    Stage IV: Full-thickness skin loss with extensive destruction, tissue necrosis, or damage to muscle, bone, or supporting structures.

    Unstageable/Unclassified: There are also "unstageable" pressure sores that are commonly incorrectly staged. These are pressure sores with slough/eschar that need to be debrided before one can see how deep they truly are, and can then be accurately staged.

    Suspected Deep Tissue Injury: Purple or maroon localized area of discolored intact skin or blood-filled blister due to damage of underlying soft tissue from pressure and/or shear.

2. **C.** It is true that laboratory tests and imaging can be useful in the workup of osteomyelitis (OM). In a patient who presents with concern for OM, positive X-ray findings combined with elevated ESR or CRP, or positive MRI findings would suggest a diagnosis of OM. However, a bone biopsy and culture are needed to confirm the diagnosis. Specimens should be obtained after debridement of overlying tissue to decrease the risk of contamination. If bone biopsy is positive, broad-spectrum antibiotic therapy should be initiated in addition to serial debridement and temporary coverage/NPWT. Permanent wound coverage should not be considered until CRP levels trend down and granulation tissue is present.

3. **E.** NPWT is becoming a valuable resource used by surgeons to manage difficult wounds. NPWT devices consist of an adhesive semi-occlusive dressing, tubing connected to a collection canister and a vacuum source, and an interface material to distribute the vacuum (open-pore polyurethane hydrophobic foam).

    Negative pressure on the sealed, airtight wound results in:

    - Increased blood flow to the wound
    - Removal of excess fluid that may retard cell growth and proliferation
    - Micro- and macro-deformation of the wound:
        - Macro-deformation is the visible stretch that occurs when the sponge contracts. It serves to draw the wound edges together, provide direct and complete wound bed contact, distribute negative pressure, and remove exudate and infectious materials.
        - Micro-deformation occurs at the cellular level and leads to cell stretch. It reduces edema, promotes perfusion, and promotes granulation tissue formation by facilitating cell migration and proliferation.
        - Maintenance of wound homeostasis: The semi-occlusive dressing and foam with insulation qualities minimizes evaporation, desiccation, and heat loss.

    The following are common indications for NPWT:

    - Chronic, diabetic wounds or pressure ulcers
    - Meshed grafts (before and after)
    - Flaps
    - Chronic and acute wounds
    - Subacute wounds (dehisced incisions)

The following are contraindications to NPWT:

- Fistulae to organs/body cavities
- Necrotic tissue that has not been debrided or eschar
- Untreated osteomyelitis
- Wounds that require hemostasis
- Placing dressing on exposed blood vessels (including anastomotic sites) or organs
- Wound malignancy

Caring for the pressure sore patients involves more than addressing the wound. Healing in chronic wounds requires a systemic strategy, including nutritional assessment and maintenance, control of both systemic and local infection, avoidance of excessive moisture/incontinence, pressure and muscle spasm relief, surgical debridement, and wound closure.

4. C. Temporary non-surgical fecal diversion with a fecal management system can be used for approximately 1 month. Surgical fecal diversion should be considered in patients with long-standing, medically intractable sacral or ischial pressure injuries. The type of surgical diversion performed should take into consideration patient factors and the probability for temporary vs. permanent diversion. Temporary diversion options include loop colostomy or loop ileostomy. Advantages of loop ileostomy include technical ease of reversal and lower morbidity. Loop colostomy results in less dehydration and electrolyte abnormalities and may be preferred in older patients. Permanent diversion with end colostomy should be considered in patients with perianal sepsis or fecal incontinence related to spinal cord injury, paraplegia or those unable to perform adequte toileting. It is important to prevent wound contamination, particularly if it is in close proximity to the fecal stream as in ischial or sacral pressure injuries. In addition to leading to infection of the wound itself, stool and urine can be irritating to the surrounding skin, causing further skin breakdown and extension of the existing ulcer. Rectal tubes and fecal management systems are a viable option for fecal diversion, especially if the patient is having liquid stools. These fecal management systems are not without their own risks/complications, including pressure ulcers from the device itself. However, this is often a reasonable first step before considering surgical diversion.

5. B. Most commonly, Stage III/IV pressure sores are referred for soft tissue reconstruction. Unfortunately, some of these patients are not suitable candidates for medical or social reasons. Since these surgeries are frequently fraught with complications, there are multiple patient characteristics to optimize before coverage can be considered:

- Nutritional status
- Control of medical comorbidities
- Presence of muscle spasticity
- Tobacco use
- Social situation (assess for presence of a responsible caretaker at home—and subsequent appropriate residence at own home vs facility), appropriate specialty mattress at residence, strict regimen of frequent turning to prevent flap necrosis/failure, appropriately padded wheelchair
- In case of osteomyelitis, patient requiring bony debridement and tailored IV antibiotic therapy (typically for 6 weeks) before soft tissue reconstruction are attempted
- Consideration of adverse drug factors like use of steroids or immunosuppressants
- Control of different causes of maceration like fecal or urine incontinence
- Medical noncompliance

Once these medical/social issues are addressed, the wound can then be optimized with thorough debridement and dressing care, in preparation for flap reconstruction.

6. E. When planning therapeutic treatment of pressure sores, the choice of closure strategy depends not only on the location, size, and depth of the ulcer but also on the previous management strategies employed. Primary closure should be avoided. These wounds tend to have an absence of adequate tissue and primary closure leads to tension, scarring over the original bony prominence, and dehiscence. Skin grafting has a limited success rate, as grafting tends to provide unstable coverage. Musculocutaneous flaps provide adequate blood supply, bulky padding, and are effective in treating infected wounds. Fasciocutaneous flaps offer an adequate blood supply, durable coverage, and low rates of functional deformity.

BIBLIOGRAPHY

Bauer JD, Mancoll JS, Phillips LG. Pressure sores. In: Thome CH, ed. *Grabb and Smith's Plastic Surgery*. 5th ed. Lippincott Williams & Wilkins; 2007;722–729.

Boyko TV, Longaker MT, Yang GP. Review of the current management of pressure ulcers. *Adv Wound Care.* 2018;7(2):57–67.

Eray IC, Alabaz O, Akcam AT, et al. Comparison of diverting colostomy and bowel management catheter applications in fournier gangrene cases requiring fecal diversion. *Indian J Surg.* 2015;77(2):438–441.

European Pressure Ulcer Advisory Panel and National Pressure Ulcer Advisory Panel. *Prevention and Treatment of Pressure Ulcers: Quick Reference Guide.* National Pressure Ulcer Advisory Panel; 2009.

de la Fuente SG, Levin LS, Reynolds JD, et al. Elective stoma construction improves outcomes in medically intractable pressure ulcers. *Dis Colon Rectum.* 2003;46(11): 1525.

Nicksic PJ, Sasor SE, Tholpady SS, Wooden WA, Gutwein LG, Peter J. Management of the pressure injury patient with osteomyelitis: an algorithm. *J Am Coll Surg.* 2017;225(6):817–822.

Ohjimi H, Ogata K, Setsu Y. Modification of the gluteus maximus V-Y advancement flap for sacral ulcers: the gluteal fasciocutaneous flap method. *Plast Reconstr Surg.* 1996;98(7):1247–1252.

13

Sarcoma and Lymphoma

Joy Sarkar

SCENARIO 1

A 47-year-old female presents with a several months history of a slowly growing painless mass in her right thigh. On physical exam, she is noted to have a 5-cm firm, nontender mass in the right lateral mid-thigh.

1. Which of the following is true?

A. Routine imaging of the mass should include a positron emission tomography (PET) scan.

B. Incisional biopsy should be routinely performed to confirm the diagnosis and identify the histological subtype.

C. The most common histologic subtypes for extremity sarcomas include liposarcoma and malignant fibrous histiocytoma.

D. Staging includes an abdominal and pelvic computed tomography (CT) scan to evaluate for metastatic disease in this lesion.

E. Multidisciplinary evaluation is not needed for simple early-stage sarcomas.

2. Regarding surgical management of this patient, which of the following is true?

A. A functional outcome is the highest priority.

B. Surgical margin of 1 to 2 cm should be sought whenever possible.

C. Regional lymph node dissection is also required.

D. Amputation should be strongly considered as the primary therapy for most extremity sarcomas.

E. Histologic subtype has little impact on surgical planning.

3. Regarding neoadjuvant and adjuvant therapies for soft tissue sarcoma, which of the following is true?

A. Chemotherapy is the most important therapeutic intervention for outcomes from sarcoma.

B. Metastatectomy has no role in the management of sarcomas.

C. Radiation therapy has been shown to be of benefit in the treatment of sarcomas.

D. Local recurrence is rare after appropriate therapy.

E. Gastrointestinal stromal tumors (GIST) are treated similarly to other sarcomas.

SCENARIO 2

A 26-year-old male presents with a painless mass in his left axilla that has been present for several months. Upon questioning, he endorses unexplained low-grade fevers, night sweats, and an unplanned weight loss of 10 lb over the previous 3 months. On physical exam, he is noted to have a 2-cm firm, rubbery, nontender mass in the left axilla.

4. Which of the following considerations is true for this patient?

A. Observation is warranted.

B. History of fever, chills, night sweats, and weight loss are considered A-level symptoms.

C. Physical examination should include a thorough exam of all accessible lymph node basins as well as potential sites of a primary malignancy.

D. Sexually transmitted diseases can be ruled out by physical exam in younger patients.

E. Fine-needle aspiration (FNA) biopsy of suspicious lymph nodes in this patient is usually adequate for diagnosis.

5. Regarding lymphoma, which of the following is true?

A. Surgeons play a major role in the treatment of lymphoma.

B. The hallmark of treatment is surgery and chemotherapy.

C. Staging for Hodgkin's lymphoma is based upon a different staging system than is non-Hodgkin's lymphoma.

D. Of the immunosuppressive states, only HIV infection has been shown to increase the incidence of lymphoma.

E. Mucosa-associated lymphoid tissue (MALT) lymphoma may be definitively treated with *Helicobacter pylori* eradication in its early stages.

SCENARIO 3

A 61-year-old male presents with a 6-month history of early satiety, nausea, and vague abdominal pain. On physical exam, his abdomen is soft and nondistended, with no palpable mass. Laboratory examination is only notable for a mild anemia. A contrast-enhanced CT scan of the abdomen and pelvis demonstrates an exophytic 4- × 4.5-cm mass arising from the posterior aspect of the fundus along the greater curvature. There is no evidence of metastasis or invasion into adjacent organs or vasculature. The patient undergoes upper endoscopy, which demonstrates a subtle submucosal bulge in the posterior fundus, without overlying mucosal changes. An endoscopic biopsy is taken and returns as normal gastric mucosa.

6. What is the next best step in the diagnosis of this patient?

A. Percutaneous biopsy

B. Endoscopic ultrasound

C. Repeat EGD with four-quadrant biopsies of the mass

D. Contrast-enhanced MRI scan

E. Diagnostic laparoscopy

7. Biopsy of the mass is successfully performed and shows spindle cells with eosinophilic cytoplasm, which stains strongly and diffusely positive for KIT. The mitotic rate is 2 mitoses/50 HPFs. The tumor tests positive for an exon 11 mutation in KIT. What is the next best step in treatment?

A. Neoadjuvant imatinib followed by surgery

B. Wedge resection followed by close surveillance

C. Wedge resection with adjuvant imatinib

D. Subtotal gastrectomy with adjuvant imatinib

E. Total gastrectomy with D1 resection

ANSWERS

Answers to Scenario 1

1. C. Regarding preoperative imaging of the tumor, an MRI scan is generally preferred for extremity sarcomas, while a CT scan tends to be preferable for abdominal and retroperitoneal sarcomas. However, there has not been demonstrated a statistically significant difference between the two modalities. High-quality cross-sectional imaging is nevertheless critical for preoperative evaluation and planning. A PET scan can give information regarding the grade, prognostication, and response to chemotherapy in select high-grade, large, deep sarcomas and can be considered for use but does not have a role in the routine evaluation of all sarcomas.

Incisional biopsy may be required, but generally, for both extremity and retroperitoneal sarcomas, needle core biopsy (with or without image guidance) provides adequate tissue sampling with good diagnostic correlation to final pathology. However, when unavailable or inadequate, incisional biopsy for extremity sarcomas remains a reasonable diagnostic option. Care should be taken if an incisional biopsy is necessary. Incisions should be oriented longitudinally and thoughtfully, as reexcision of biopsy site will be necessary with definitive operation. In some selected institutions with clinical and pathologic expertise, FNA may be adequate but should probably not be considered adequate at low-volume centers.

There are more than 50 histologic subtypes of soft tissue sarcoma recognized. Overall, the most common subtypes are liposarcoma, malignant fibrous histiocytoma (MFH), and leiomyosarcoma; however, the prevalence is site-specific. The most common types of extremity sarcomas are liposarcoma and MFH, while retroperitoneal sarcomas are more commonly liposarcoma and leiomyosarcoma. GIST and leiomyosarcoma are the histological types found in visceral tumors.

Overall, the lung is the most common site of metastasis for extremity sarcomas. For visceral tumors, the liver is more common. A chest CT scan is generally advocated for extremity sarcomas to rule out metastatic disease.

Due to the complexity, rarity, and histology-based therapy for soft tissue sarcomas, prior to initiating therapy, all patients should be evaluated by a multi-disciplinary team with expertise in sarcoma therapy.

2. **B.** Until the early 1980s, amputation remained a primary therapy for most extremity sarcomas. In 1982, Rosenberg and colleagues at the National Cancer Institute published a randomized trial of amputation versus limb-sparing surgery plus radiation and demonstrated equivalent overall survival and acceptable local recurrence rate of 15% with limb-salvage versus 0% with amputation. Currently, limb salvage surgery can be safely performed in over 90% of patients with extremity sarcoma with excellent local recurrence rates. The proximity of critical structures (bone, nerves, blood vessels, etc.) should be considered carefully during preoperative planning and the expected functional outcome assessed to assist in making the decision for limb salvage versus amputation.

Careful preoperative planning is imperative for a successful resection of these tumors. Failure to obtain a negative surgical margin is the most important risk factor for local recurrence. Careful scrutiny of preoperative imaging can result in improved outcomes by allowing the surgeon to have a thorough understanding of the extent of the tumor and relationship to local structures. Functional outcomes are also improved by careful consideration of the extent of resection required. Similarly, this allows for appropriate consultation with subspecialists, including plastic or vascular surgeons preoperatively when anticipated being necessary.

Wide margins should be the goal of therapy. A margin of 1 to 2 cm of normal tissue can help to minimize the risk of local recurrence. However, strong tissues such as fascia can severely limit the spread of most types of sarcoma into adjacent structures. Therefore, a narrow fascial margin may be acceptable where such a narrow margin of muscle or fat would likely result in an increased risk of recurrent disease. In some cases, such as retroperitoneal sarcomas, wide margins may not be feasible.

The resection of nerves and blood vessels is occasionally unavoidable but can often be avoided by careful skeletonization of blood vessels and resection of the perineurium along with the tumor. The concept of "planned positive margin" is feasible in many cases with the use of adjuvant radiation therapy. As long as the structure of concern is not fixed to the tumor, this carefully planned positive margin provides similar outcomes to controls with negative margins. Neoadjuvant radiation has been advocated in this setting for "marginally resectable" tumors in order to allow a negative margin functional resection.

Histologic subtype does play an important factor in planning surgical intervention. Well-differentiated liposarcoma (formerly called atypical lipomas) have a similar recurrence rate to other types of sarcoma, but metastatic disease is rare, so surgical resection can be less aggressive when necessary. Dermatofibrosarcoma protuberans (DFSP) and myxofibrosarcoma are particularly difficult due to the common finding of microscopic tentacles that extend laterally from these lesions. DFSP has a tendency to respect fascial borders, whereas myxofibrosarcoma often penetrates fascia and can have multifocal skip lesions, so these factors must be considered. Lymph node metastasis is rare in soft tissue sarcomas (STS) in general but can be seen more commonly with epithelioid or clear cell variants. For this reason, sentinel lymph node biopsy can give prognostic information, so although no clear therapeutic benefit has been shown, it may be considered in this setting.

3. **C.** Radiation therapy has been repeatedly demonstrated to be of benefit in disease-free survival, although not significantly different overall survival. There remains some controversy regarding the optimal timing of the radiation therapy. When comparing neoadjuvant versus adjuvant therapy, the local control rate is similar. However, preoperative radiation has been found to double wound complications in the months following surgery compared to increased rates of long-term complications such as fibrosis, edema, and joint stiffness with postoperative radiation. External beam, brachytherapy, and intraoperative radiotherapy have all been used with some success. Patients at low risk for recurrence (i.e., small [<5-cm] superficial tumors, low-grade tumors, wide surgical margins) may not derive a significant benefit from radiation and may be treated with surgery alone.

Surgery is the dominant therapeutic modality for extremity, retroperitoneal, and visceral sarcomas. Complete surgical resection is the primary factor in outcomes. Only a few clinical trials have demonstrated a statistically significant improvement in outcomes with adjuvant chemotherapy. Specific histology-directed regimens have shown the most promise and have achieved excellent and sustained results in specific subtypes to include GIST, rhabdomyosarcoma, Ewing sarcoma, and osteosarcoma.

Patients with an isolated metastasis can be considered for metastatectomy if resection with or without chemotherapy or radiation may result in a cure. This may include the removal of limited disease in a single organ or regional node dissection if nodal metastasis is isolated. Specifically in the setting of isolated lung metastasis, median survival is lengthened from 11 to 33 months compared to observation. Patients with widely metastatic disease may be considered for palliation using a variety of modalities including surgery, chemotherapy, radiation, embolization, and ablation procedures.

Local recurrence rate varies with the site of the initial tumor and the adequacy of surgical resection. Local recurrence after treatment for extremity soft tissue sarcoma approaches one out of three patients. The median disease-free interval is 18 months but can be quite remote. Considerations for treatment of recurrent disease are similar to primary disease and can include reexcision, chemotherapy, and radiation, often with similar success to the primary tumors for extremity sarcomas. Recurrence of visceral and retroperitoneal sarcomas often is unable to be completely reexcised.

GIST is the most common mesenchymal tumor of the GI tract and has gained significant interest in recent years. The discovery of the KIT proto-oncogene mutation present in the majority of GIST tumors led to the ability to specifically target GIST tumors at a molecular level with the tyrosine kinase inhibitor (TKI) imatinib mesylate (Gleevec; Novartis Pharmaceutical, Basel, Switzerland). This advancement marks a new era in treating solid tumors with specific molecular targeting. Surgery remains of vital importance, but several studies have demonstrated improved disease-free and overall survival for patients at significant risk for recurrence who are treated adjuvantly with TKIs, so this has become an important, disease-specific therapy for these rare tumors. In general, enucleation of the tumor represents an adequate surgical resection.

The staging of soft tissue extremity sarcomas is determined by tumor size, grade, and presence or absence of nodal and distant metastases. The tumor grade, in turn, is determined by three parameters: mitotic rate, tumor differentiation, and tumor necrosis. Tumor grade is the most important prognostic factor determining the pattern of recurrence, disease-free survival, and overall survival. Because sarcoma spreads predominantly by hematogenous rather than lymphatic routes, the specific number of affected lymph nodes is not factored into sarcoma staging.

Answers to Scenario 2

4. **C.** In patients without a tissue diagnosis of malignancy, but concern for lymphoma, FNA is generally not considered to be adequate for diagnosis. FNA may be able to identify some cases of metastatic carcinoma (i.e., breast, lung, etc.) but is limited in hematologic malignancies (especially lymphoma) as lymph node architecture is a critical pathologic component of making these diagnoses. FNA may be useful in searching for recurrent disease. As knowledge and the use of molecular markers are expanded in the future, FNA may become a viable alternative to open biopsy of suspicious nodes. When lymphadenopathy is generalized the largest, most suspicious, and accessible note is selected for biopsy. The diagnostic yield does vary by site with inguinal nodes having the lowest yield and supraclavicular nodes the highest. Careful and appropriate handling of tissue specimens is critical to allow pathologic diagnosis. Adequate tissue sampling is critical to allow an assessment of nodal architecture. Specimens should be submitted to pathology dry or in saline, not formalin or another preservative, to allow flow cytometric and immunohistochemical studies to supplement traditional pathology.

The differential diagnosis for lymphadenopathy is extremely broad and includes malignancy (lymphoma, metastatic disease), infections (cat-scratch disease, HIV, mononucleosis, tuberculosis, etc.), autoimmune disorders, iatrogenic causes such as medications, and unusual causes including sarcoidosis and Kawasaki's disease. A thorough history and physical (H&P) can be used to help narrow this broad differential. In patients without concerning signs or symptoms suggestive of malignancy or other severe disease (e.g., B symptoms, etc.), a period of observation of 4 to 6 weeks is appropriate. If the lymphadenopathy persists beyond this period of observation, further evaluation to include complete blood count (CBC) and chest x-ray should be pursued. Other testing to include serology for cytomegalovirus (CMV), heterophile testing (monospot), purified protein derivative (PPD) testing, HIV testing, rapid plasma reagin (RPR) testing, and so on may be utilized based on the H&P and specific concerns. Several nonspecific laboratory tests reflecting inflammation, including electrolyte sedimentation, C-reaction protein, and fibrinogen, may be used but do not typically help narrow the differential diagnosis. Lactate dehydrogenase is often similarly nonspecific, although very high levels may suggest a lymphoid neoplasm. Ultimately, persistent lymphadenopathy without an obvious etiology warrants lymph node biopsy as discussed earlier.

Fever, chills, night sweats, and weight loss >10% over 6 months are the classically described "B" symptoms associated with lymphoma and the presence of these findings should increase the suspicion of this diagnosis and prompt a more aggressive approach to diagnosis.

A careful physical exam should be an important part of the evaluation of every patient with lymphadenopathy. The differential diagnosis is highly dependent upon the presence of generalized versus isolated lymphadenopathy and the lymph node basin involved when localized. Examining sites of possible metastatic spread, for example, breast, skin, oropharynx, and so on, is important in narrowing the differential.

5. **E.** *Lymphoma* refers to a spectrum of diseases, including Hodgkin's and non-Hodgkin's lymphomas (NHL) with multiple subtypes within each group. The role of the surgeon in patients with lymphoma is limited. By far, the most important role of the surgeon is in assisting with the diagnosis by means of lymph node biopsy. Once the diagnosis has been made, the treatment of lymphoma is overwhelmingly the role of chemotherapy and radiation. Historically, surgery was more involved through the use of staging laparotomy, but this is now rarely indicated with the availability and use of PET/CT scans for staging purposes. Surgical intervention to include splenectomy is limited to significantly symptomatic situations such as anemia, thrombocytopenia, neutropenia, and massive splenomegaly, and should be done only in close consultation with oncology.

Staging for lymphoma is based on modifications of the original Ann Arbor classification, initially described for Hodgkin's lymphoma but now also used for NHL. Staging is based on the number and location of lymph node groups and extra-nodal involvement and has modifiers to signify presence or absence of B symptoms.

Several risk factors for lymphoma have been identified. There has been a significant increase in incidence since the 1970s, which has been partially explained by the HIV epidemic. Other contributors to the increase include other infections (i.e., *H. pylori*-induced MALT lymphoma), autoimmune diseases, immunosuppression (as with organ transplant), environmental factors including pesticides, and aging of the population (NHL increases in incidence with age and peaks during the fifth through seventh decades). Hodgkin's lymphoma is more common in higher socioeconomic groups and less common in Asian populations.

MALT lymphoma has been shown to be dependent on *H. pylori* infection. Gastric inflammatory response to this infection stimulates the acquisition of genetic abnormalities and malignant transformation of B cells. In the early stages of this disease, *H. pylori* eradication can reverse the disease process in as many as 77% of patients. However, in later stages of the disease, further genetic injury to these malignant cells makes the tumor resistant to bacterial eradication, so more aggressive therapy, including chemotherapy and radiation, is indicated. Like other forms of lymphoma, surgery is generally reserved for rare situations with complications, such as life-threatening hemorrhage.

Answers to Scenario 3

6. **B.** The presentation of an exophytic gastric mass appearing as a submucosal/subepithelial mass suggests a GIST, which accounts for 5% of all sarcomas. The differential diagnosis is wide and includes gastric schwannoma, desmoid fibromatosis, carcinoma, melanoma, and other types of sarcomas. As GISTs arise from the mesenchymal stem cells which differentiate into interstitial cells of Cajal in the intramuscular layer, they often appear as a submucosal bulge on endoscopy (with or without mucosal ulceration) rather than an intraluminal mass, and endoscopic biopsy is often nondiagnostic. In patients with gastric carcinoma presenting as an ulcer on endoscopy, the diagnostic accuracy does increase with the number of mucosal biopsies taken (up to 4–5 specimens); however, this is unlikely to be high yield for a mesenchymal tumor such as a GIST. As GISTs are fragile, endoscopic

ultrasound-guided FNA is preferable to percutaneous biopsy, due to the risk of intra-abdominal tumor dissemination with percutaneous biopsy. Similarly, a diagnosis should be confirmed prior to proceeding with surgery, as neoadjuvant therapy may be indicated. MRI scans may be helpful for clarifying the extent of metastases if present or for surveillance of treatment but will not provide a definitive diagnosis.

7. B. For resectable gastric GISTs with an activating mutation in the KIT tyrosine kinase gene, the standard of care is surgical resection, with or without an adjuvant TKI, such as imatinib. GISTs are stratified based on their predicted risk of recurrence, from very low to high. The classification is based on tumor size, mitotic rate, site, and presence/absence of rupture. Gastric GISTs have a lower rate of recurrence than nongastric GISTs. Multiple classification systems exist, including the National Institutes of Health (NIH) classification, Armed Forces Institute of Pathology (AFIP) classification, and revised NIH classification, but in general, nonperforated gastric GISTs, which are ≤5 cm in size with a mitotic rate <5 per 50 HPFs, are considered to be at a low risk of recurrence. Gastric GISTs should be excised by wedge resection, either laparoscopic or open. There is generally no indication to perform an extended anatomic resection such as subtotal or total gastrectomy, as there is limited intramural extension and low incidence of metastasis to regional lymph nodes, unlike as seen in gastric adenocarcinoma. In this patient with a resectable, nonperforated gastric GIST, which is 4.5 cm in size and a low mitotic rate of 2 per 50 HPFs, the risk of recurrence is considered to be low, and wedge resection followed by close surveillance (H&P, CT/MRI) is the most appropriate.

BIBLIOGRAPHY

Bazemore AW, Smucker DR. Lymphadenopathy and malignancy. *Am Fam Physician.* 2002;66(11):2103–2110.

Billingsley KG, Burt ME, Jara E, et al. Pulmonary metastases from soft tissue sarcoma: analysis of patterns of diseases and post-metastasis survival. *Ann Surg.* 1999;229(5):602–610.

Du MQ, Isaccson PG. Gastric MALT lymphoma: from aetiology to treatment. *Lancet Oncol.* 2002;3(2):97–104.

Ferrone ML, Raut CP. Modern surgical therapy: limb salvage and the role of amputation for extremity soft-tissue sarcomas. *Surg Oncol Clin N Am.* 2012;21(2):201–213.

Fong Y, Coit DG, Woodruff JM, Brennan MF. Lymph node metastasis from soft tissue sarcoma in adults. Analysis of data from a prospective database of 1772 sarcoma patients. *Ann Surg.* 1993;217(1):72–77.

Heslin MJ, Lewis JJ, Woodruff JM, Brennan MF. Core needle biopsy for diagnosis of extremity soft tissue sarcoma. *Ann Surg Oncol.* 1997;4(5):425–431.

Hueman MT, Thornton K, Herman J, Ahuja N. Management of extremity soft tissue sarcomas. *Surg Clin N Am.* 2008;88(3):539–557.

Kaushal A, Citrin D. The role of radiation therapy in the management of sarcomas. *Surg Clin North Am.* 2008;88(3):629–646.

Kingham TP, DeMatteo RP. Multidisciplinary treatment of gastrointestinal stromal tumors. *Surg Clin North Am.* 2009;89(1):217–233.

Larrier NA, Kirsch DG, Riedel RF, et al. Practical radiation oncology for extremity sarcomas. *Surg Oncol Clin N Am.* 2013;22(3):433–443.

Motyckova G, Steensma DP. Why does my patient have lymphadenopathy or splenomegaly? *Hematol Oncol Clin North Am.* 2012;26(2):395–408.

National Comprehensive Cancer Network Clinical Practice Guidelines in Oncology: soft tissue sarcoma. Accessed May 15, 2014. Available at https://www.nccn.org/professionals/physician_gls/pdf/sarcoma.pdf

National Comprehensive Cancer Network Clinical Practice Guidelines in Oncology: Hodgkin Lymphoma. Accessed May 15, 2014. Available at https://www.nccn.org/professionals/physician_gls/pdf/hodgkins.pdf

National Comprehensive Cancer Network Clinical Practice Guidelines in Oncology: Non-Hodgkin's Lymphomas. Accessed May 15, 2014. Available at https://www.nccn.org/professionals/physician_gls/pdf/nhl.pdf

Nayak LM, Deschler DG. Lymphomas. *Otolaryngol Clin N Am.* 2003;36(4):625–646.

Nishida T. The role of endoscopy in the diagnosis of gastric gastrointestinal stromal tumors. *Ann Surg Oncol.* 2015;22:2810–2811.

O'Sullivan B, Davis AM, Turcotte R, et al. Preoperative versus postoperative radiotherapy in soft-tissue sarcoma of the limbs: a randomized trial. *Lancet.* 2002;359(9325):2235–2241. doi:10.1016/S0140-6736(02)09292-9

Panicek DM, Gatsonis C, Rosenthal DI, et al. CT and MR imaging in the local staging of primary malignant musculoskeletal neoplasms: Report of the Radiology Diagnostic Oncology Group. *Radiology.* 1997;202(1):237–246. Doi:10.1148/radiology.202.1.8988217

Ravi V, Patel S. Adjuvant chemotherapy for soft tissue sarcomas. *Surg Oncol Clin N Am.* 2012;21(2):243–253.

Rosenberg SA, Tepper J, Glatstein E, et al. The treatment of soft-tissue sarcomas of the extremities: prospective randomized evaluations of (1) limb-sparing surgery plus radiation therapy compared with amputation and (2) the role of adjuvant chemotherapy. *Ann Surg.* 1982;196(3):305–315.

Schuetze SM, Rubin BP, Vernon C, et al. Use of positron emission tomography in localized extremity soft tissue sarcoma treated with neoadjuvant chemotherapy. *Cancer.* 2005;103(2):339–348.

Singer S. Soft tissue sarcomas. In: Townsend DM, Beauchamp RD, Evers BM, et al. eds. *Sabiston Textbook of Surgery.* 18th ed. Saunders Elsevier; 2008: 786–799.

Taghizadeh M, Muscarella P. Splenectomy for hematologic disorders. In: Cameron JL, Cameron AM, eds. *Current Surgical Therapy*. 10th ed. Elsevier Saunders; 2011: 473–479.

Twist CJ, Link MP. Assessment of lymphadenopathy in children. *Pediatr Clin N Am*. 2002;49(5):1009–1025.

Wong SL. Sarcomas of soft tissue and bone. In: Mulholland MW, Lillemoe KD, Doherty GM, et al. eds. *Greenfield's Surgery: Scientific Principles and Practice*. 5th ed. Lippincott Williams & Wilkins; 2010.

Zhao X, Yue C. Gastrointestinal stromal tumor. *J Gastrointest Oncol*. 2012;3(3):189–208.

14

Lung Cancer—Cough

Mia DeBarros

A 65-year-old male who is a former smoker (quit 10 years ago; smoked 1 pack per day for 50 years) with chronic obstructive pulmonary disease (COPD), type 2 diabetes mellitus, and coronary artery disease (CAD) status post–coronary artery bypass graft (CABG) for three diseased vessels 5 years ago, is referred to surgery after presenting to his primary care physician with a 4-month history of a nonproductive cough and 10-lb weight loss in the past 3 months. Given his past medical history and risk factors, a low-dose screening computed tomography (CT) chest scan was obtained that demonstrated a 2- × 1.5-cm solid-appearing mass in his right upper lobe (RUL) that was not present on a prior CT chest scan from 5 years ago.

1. **Which of the following patients should be screened for lung cancer?**
   1. 65-year-old male who is an active smoker with a 30-pack-year history.
   2. 50-year-old female with pulmonary fibrosis and 25-pack-year history.
   3. 77-year-old male with a 15-pack-a-year history who quit smoking 30 years ago.
   4. 55-year-old female with a 20-pack-year history who quit 20 years ago and worked for 30 years in the electronics industry.
   A. 1, 2, 3
   B. 1, 2, 4
   C. 1, 2
   D. 1, 3, 4
   E. 2, 3, 4

2. **What is the best appropriate next step in the management of this patient?**

A. Positron emission tomography (PET) CT scan
B. Cervical mediastinoscopy
C. Right upper lobectomy
D. Right upper lobectomy with mediastinal lymph node sampling
E. Endobronchial ultrasound-guided biopsy (EBUS)

3. **After a complete staging workup, a tissue diagnosis is obtained of the RUL mass demonstrating adenocarcinoma. Which of the following patients is a candidate for upfront surgical resection?**

A. RUL tumor measuring 7 cm with likely invasion into the esophagus but no hilar lymph nodes found on preoperative PET CT.
B. RUL tumor measuring 3 cm and palpable fixed mass in the right supraclavicular fossa
C. RUL peripherally located tumor measuring 2 cm extending into the parietal pleura but not the chest wall with no fluorodeoxyglucose (FDG) avid lymph nodes
D. RUL tumor measuring 2 cm and patient symptoms of shoulder and arm pain, hand numbness/weakness in the ulnar nerve distribution, and miosis and ptosis on the right side
E. RUL tumor measuring 1 cm and positive left paratracheal lymph node (4L) on cervical mediastinoscopy

4. **The patient described earlier has been clinically staged as T1bN0M0, stage IA2. He has been evaluated by cardiology and deemed optimized for surgery. In addition to labs, he also undergoes pulmonary function tests (PFTs) as part of his preoperative workup. He is consented for a video-assisted**

thoracoscopic surgery (VATS) RUL lobectomy. Which of the following PFTs results is a contraindication to surgery without further workup?

A. A preoperative forced expiratory volume in 1 second (FEV1) of 84%, diffusing capacity of the lung for carbon monoxide (DLCO) of 80%

B. A preoperative FEV1 of 1.0 L, a DLCO of 50%, and is able to climb three flights of stairs

C. A predicted postoperative FEV1 of 45%

D. A predicted postoperative FEV1 of 60% and predicted postoperative DLCO of 40%

E. A preoperative FEV1 of 0.8 L and a DLCO of 65%

5. **The patient is consented for a VATS RUL. In the operating room, there is no evidence of pleural disease; the lymph nodes are sampled and negative for N2 disease on the frozen section. The anterior hilum is exposed. What is the order of division of the hilar structures?**

A. Superior pulmonary vein/upper lobe bronchus/recurrent ascending arterial branch/truncus anterior

B. Truncus anterior/superior pulmonary vein/recurrent ascending arterial branch/upper lobe bronchus

C. Superior pulmonary vein/truncus anterior/recurrent ascending arterial branch/upper lobe bronchus

D. Recurrent ascending arterial branch/upper lobe bronchus/truncus anterior/superior pulmonary vein

E. Truncus anterior/upper lobe bronchus/superior pulmonary vein/recurrent ascending arterial branch

6. **The patient undergoes successful VATS RUL lobectomy. The final pathology is well-differentiated adenocarcinoma with negative margins, pT2aN0, stage IB. Which of the following is correct?**

A. He will need surveillance with a CT chest scan every 6 months for the first 2 years and then annually for the next 3 years.

B. Patients with T3 tumors or N1 disease do not need adjuvant chemotherapy if they have an R0 resection.

C. Adjuvant radiation therapy can be used in lieu of chemotherapy for systemic control.

D. An R1 resection for a stage I tumor can be observed or treated with chemotherapy.

E. Radiation therapy is only useful in the preoperative setting.

7. **The same patient presents to thoracic surgery with the same imaging and clinical staging. Preoperative tissue diagnosis is obtained and is small cell carcinoma. Mediastinal staging is undertaken with EBUS and cervical mediastinoscopy and is negative. A brain MRI scan is negative. His clinical stage is T1bN0. Which of the following is correct?**

A. He should be referred for definitive chemotherapy alone.

B. He should undergo RUL lobectomy with mediastinal lymph node sampling followed by adjuvant chemotherapy.

C. He should be referred for definitive radiation therapy alone.

D. He should be referred for definitive chemotherapy and radiation therapy.

E. He should undergo RUL lobectomy, and if he does not have lymph node disease on final pathology, he should undergo observation only.

ANSWERS

1. **B.** Although lung cancer represents 13% of all cancer cases in the United States, it is often diagnosed in advanced stage, resulting in a dismal 5-year survival of 19%. Currently, lung cancer represents 25% of all cancer deaths in the United States. The purpose of cancer screening is to identify and diagnose cancer in earlier stages and increase the chance of curative treatment. The National Lung Screening Trial (NSLT) randomized 55,454 patients at high risk for lung cancer to annual low-dose CT chest (LDCT) scan or chest x-ray. High-risk factors considered were those ages 55 to 74 years, history of cigarette smoking for at least 30 pack years, and former smokers who quit in the last 15 years. The group who underwent LDCT saw a 20% reduction in lung cancer–specific mortality. The trial investigators determined the number needed to screen to prevent one lung cancer death was 320. This was the first randomized control trial to demonstrate a reduction in mortality. Another study, the Nederlands–Leuvens Longkanker Screenings On-derzoek, or NELSON trial (also randomized control trial), recently published results confirming the findings of NLST with a 26% reduction in mortality. This mortality benefit was even higher in women on post hoc analysis.

Based on the results of NSLT, the U.S. Preventive Task Force issued screening guidelines for lung cancer. Currently, multiple societies, including the National

Comprehensive Cancer Network (NCCN), the Centers for Medicare and Medicaid Services (CMS), CHEST, and the American Association of Thoracic Surgery (AATS) recommend lung cancer screening with slight variations in inclusion criteria on who should be screened. The majority recommend screening starting at age 55 years with at least a 30-pack-year history and less than 15 years from smoking cessation. Most recommend stopping screening at the age of 74–77 years.

The NCCN splits patients into two groups. Group 1 recommends screening in ages 55–74 years with a greater than 30-pack-year history and smoking cessation less than 15 years. Group 2 recommends screening in patients older than 50 years, greater than 20-pack-year history, and one other risk factor (personal cancer history, positive family history, exposure to radon, asbestos, arsenic, cadmium, beryllium, silica, diesel fumes, coal smoke, soot, or chronic lung disease—those with COPD or pulmonary fibrosis). The AATS has recommended three groups for screening. Group 1 recommends screening in ages 55–79 years with a a greater than 30-pack-year history and less than 15 years from smoking cessation. Group 2 consists of lung cancer survivors who have completed greater than 4 years of surveillance without recurrence. Group 3 consists of patients ages 50–79 years with greater than 20-pack-year history and additional comorbidities that produce 5% risk of lung cancer in 5 years. The patients in the question all meet screening criteria with the exception of patient 3, who is 77 years old but with a pack-year history of only 15 years and quit 30 years ago.

Despite these robust recommendations, lung cancer screening in the United States continues to be low, with some studies reporting only 1–4% of all eligible patients being screened. The lack of screening is likely multifactorial including the patient population itself, which tends to be less educated, less likely to have primary care access, and less likely to agree to screening or treatment of cancer found on screening compared to nonsmokers. Furthermore, many primary care providers are un aware of the new screening guidelines for lung cancer highlight the importance of continued outreach and education to both health care providers and patients.

2. **A.** In order to determine if a patient has a resectable lung cancer, staging of tumor, lymph nodes, and metastatic disease must be completed. A PET CT scan combines the anatomic data of CT with the functional and metabolic information of PET. This study allows for noninvasive assessment of metastatic or mediastinal lymph node disease, which would preclude up-front surgical resection of a suspected lung cancer. In a meta-analysis of 56 studies, PET CT scans showed a pooled sensitivity and specificity of 72–91%, respectively, in mediastinal lymph node staging. Another meta-analysis reported pooled sensitivity and specificity of 77–95% for all extrathoracic metastatic disease. Current NCCN guidelines recommend the use of PET CT scans in staging with mandatory histopathological tissue diagnosis for any evidence of suspicious mediastinal or metastatic FDG avid lesions prior to surgical resection. Cervical mediastinoscopy and EBUS-guided biopsy are both options to obtain tissue diagnosis in patients with T2 tumors and those with FDG avid lesions present in the mediastinum. It is important to remember that a negative tissue diagnosis with EBUS biopsy in a suspicious lesion on a PET CT scan is a discordant finding, and tissue diagnosis should be obtained via cervical mediastinoscopy as confirmation before proceeding with surgery. PET CT has replaced abdominal CT and bone scan. Surgical resection of any kind should not proceed until staging workup is completed.

3. **C.** The current NCCN guidelines recommend upfront surgical resection for early-stage lung cancers assuming no other contraindication for surgery (i.e., cardiopulmonary comorbidities). Accurate preoperative staging is important to prevent unnecessary surgery in non-resectable tumors or provide neoadjuvant therapy to downstage an unresectable tumor to a resectable one. The current TNM staging is the AJCC 8th edition. The patient in choice A has 7-cm tumor with possible invasion of the esophagus. This is a T4 tumor that is unresectable and definitive chemoradiation therapy is recommended. The patient in choice B has 3-cm tumor (T2) and fixed palpable mass in the right supraclavicular fossa, which represents N3 disease. The stage for this patient is T2N3M0, stage IIIB. Tissue diagnosis of the lymph node should be obtained and if this is positive, and definitive chemoradiation is recommended. The patient in C has RUL mass measuring 2 cm with parietal pleural involvement and no lymph nodes positive. This is a T3N0, stage IIB and should

undergo up-front surgical resection. The patient in choice D has a superior sulcus tumor or Pancoast tumor (automatically at least a T3 tumor regardless of size) with signs and symptoms of Pancoast syndrome (a superior sulcus tumor with the triad of shoulder and arm pain, wasting of the hand muscles and ipsilateral Horner's syndrome). A trial of chemoradiation is mandatory followed by restaging with CT chest scan and PET CT scan to determine resectability. The patient in choice E has a 1-cm tumor T1b and a positive 4L (left or contralateral paratracheal lymph node), which is N2 disease, which makes this patient stage IIIA. Patients with N2 disease should undergo induction chemoradiation therapy followed by restaging or definitive chemoradiation therapy.

4. **E.** Postoperative pulmonary complications continue to be one of the most common complications in thoracic surgery. There is a significant impact on respiratory physiology from the resection of lung parenchyma, single-lung ventilation, and proximity to the diaphragm. Many patients with lung cancer have underlying chronic lung disease and abnormal lung function. It is important to determine their baseline and expected postoperative pulmonary function prior to a planned resection that could result in lifelong supplemental oxygen, need for lung transplant, or death. Pulmonary function tests use spirometry to determine pulmonary function prior to surgery and help the surgeon determine if the planned resection is appropriate for the patient. The FEV1 and the DLCO are considered to be the two most important predictive values for postoperative pulmonary complications. Either value is useful in predictions and they are also used in the calculation of predicted postoperative values for FEV1 and DLCO (ppo FEV1 and ppo DLCO).

Prediction of postoperative lung function is based off a "simple calculation" which assumes that all lung function is evenly distributed among the 19 segments of the lungs. In order to complete the calculation, the number of resected segments and preoperative FEV1 and DLCO must be known.

The right lung contains 10 segments broken down into three in the upper lobe, two in the middle lobe, and five in the lower lobe. The left lung contains nine segments broken down into the five in the upper lobe and four in the lower lobe.

$$\text{ppo FEV1} = \text{preop FEV1} \times (\text{\# of segments remaining/total number of segments})$$

$$\text{ppo DLCO} = \text{preop DLCO} \times (\text{\# of segments remaining/total number of segments})$$

In general, patients with FEV1>2L can tolerate a pneumonectomy, FEV1 > 1L can tolerate a lobectomy and >0.6L can tolerate a segmentectomy or wedge resection. Patients with postoperative predicted FEV1 of 30–40% and a DLCO of >40% are considered low risk for a minimally invasive lobectomy. If preoperative FEV1 or DLCO is less than 80%, further workup to determine functional capacity is warranted. A simple test for functional capacity is the stair-climbing test. Patients who can climb three flights of stairs can tolerate a lobectomy and do not need further workup.

5. **C.** Structures in the hilum are typically divided in an anterior to posterior fashion. The superior pulmonary vein is the most anterior structure. Division of this structure exposes the truncus anterior and its branches. These can be divided individually or as one trunk depending on the situation. The interlobar pulmonary artery is next to be dissected out for the purpose of finding and dividing the recurrent ascending arterial branch which supplies the posterior segment of the upper lobe. Finally, the bronchus is the last structure to be dissected and divided. This represents normal anatomy, but it is vital to review preoperative imaging for aberrant anatomy.

6. **A.** Adenocarcinoma of the lung is most likely to recur in the first 2 years following curative resection. NCCN guidelines recommend surveillance with a history and physical and CT chest scan every 6 months for the first 2–3 years and then annually for up to 5 years following surgery. Following 5 years of surveillance with no evidence of recurrence, a patient is considered cured.

Patients with T3 or N1 disease are considered to have stage IIB and adjuvant chemotherapy is recommended if the patient is able to tolerate it. Patients with high-risk tumors, such as those that are poorly differentiated, >4 cm, visceral pleural involvement, lymphovascular invasion, and non-anatomic wedge resections, should also be considered for adjuvant chemotherapy.

Radiation is used for locoregional control and has no role in the systemic control of cancer. In lung cancer, it can be useful in both the pre- and postoperative periods.

Patients who have R1 resection, even in early stage tumors, should either undergo re-resection to obtain clear margins or be referred for adjuvant radiation therapy.

7. B. Small cell carcinoma represents 10–15% of all lung cancers. Unfortunately, most patients present with metastatic or extensive disease, with only 4–12% presenting with limited disease. Patients who present with T1 or T2 disease and no lymph node involvement should undergo surgery followed by platinum-based chemotherapy. Patients with more extensive disease (stage IV, T3 and T4 tumors or multiple nodules that cannot be treated by radiation therapy alone) should be referred for definitive chemoradiation therapy. All patients with small cell carcinoma should all receive a brain MRI scan for evaluation of brain metastases, which are more common prior to undergoing any surgical resection as this would be a contraindication for resection. Additionally, the history and physical should focus on signs and symptoms of paraneoplastic syndromes such as syndrome of inappropriate antidiuretic hormone secretion (SIADH). In addition to hyponatremia, the diagnosis of SIADH is confirmed by demonstrating a serum osmolarity <275 mOsm/kg, urine osmolarity > serum osmolarity, and urine sodium >25 meq/L. Associated symptoms may include lethargy, nausea, vomiting, altered mental status, and seizure.

BIBLIOGRAPHY

Aberle DR, DeMello S, Berg CD, et al. Results of the two incidence screenings in the National Lung Screening Trial. *N Engl J Med.* 2013;369:920–931.

De Koning HJ, van der Aalst CM, de Jong PA, et al. Reduced lung cancer mortality with volume CT screening in a randomized control trial. *N Engl J Med.* 2020;382:503–513.

International Association for the Study of Lung Cancer. TNM Classification for Lung Cancer. 8th edition. January 2018. Accessed February 19, 2020. https://www.iaslc.org

Kandathil A, Kay FU, Butt YM. Role of FDG PET CT in the Eighth Edition of TNM Staging of non-small cell lung cancer. *Radiographics.* 2018 Nov–Dec;38(7):2134–2149.

Low M, Ben-Or S. Thoracic surgery in early stage small cell lung cancer. *Thorac Surg Clin.* Feb 2018;28(1):9–14.

National Comprehensive Cancer Network. NCCN Clinical Practice Guidelines in Oncology Non-Small Cell Lung Cancer (version 1.2022). January 10, 2022. Accessed January 10, 2022. https://www.nccn.org/professionals/physician_gls/pdf/nscl.pdf

National Comprehensive Cancer Network. NCCN Clinical Practice Guidelines in Oncology Small Cell Lung Cancer (version 2.2022). January 10, 2022. Accessed January 10, 2022. https://www.nccn.org/professionals/physician_gls/pdf/sclc.pdf

Nicastri DG, Swanson SJ. VATS lobectomy. In: Sugarbaker DJ, Bueno R, Colson YL et al. eds. *Adult Chest Surgery.* 2nd ed. McGraw Hill Education.

Fuhlbrigge A. Preoperative Evaluation of the Thoracic Surgery Patient. In: Sugarbaker DJ, Bueno R, Burt BM, Groth SS, Loor G and Wolf AS, Adult Chest Surgery 3rd Edition, 2020 McGraw Hill Education.

Thomas NA, Tanner NT. Lung cancer screening: patient selection and implementation. *Clin Chest Med.* 2020 Mar;41(1):87–97.

15

Abdominal Wall Reconstruction

Terri L. Carlson

A 53-year-old female presents to your clinic with complaint of an abdominal bulge and occasional discomfort. She tells you that the bulge is worse when she stands and causes pain throughout the day when she is active and that it seems to be getting bigger over the past year. She has no obstructive symptoms at this time. She has a history of a midline laparotomy for trauma 10 years ago and a ventral hernia repair 6 years ago with synthetic mesh. She did have an episode of cellulitis postoperatively that was treated with oral antibiotics. She has diabetes, which is controlled by oral medications, and otherwise is healthy. On exam, she has a large palpable defect and computed tomography (CT) scan revealed a 6-cm midline defect containing omentum and small bowel, as well as two additional 1-cm defects superiorly without evidence of obstruction.

1. **According to the Ventral Hernia Work Group (VHWG) classification system, what grade would this hernia be considered?**

   A. Grade 1
   B. Grade 2
   C. Grade 3
   D. Grade 4

2. **Regarding ventral hernias which of the following is correct?**

   A. Primary suture repair and mesh repair have similar recurrence rates.
   B. Suture type for midline closure has been shown to affect the risk of a postoperative hernia.

   C. Secondary ventral hernias are thought to be related to an abnormal ratio of types I and III collagen.
   D. Ventral hernia repair is the most common procedure performed by general surgeons.

3. **Which of the following mesh placement locations has the highest rate of recurrence?**

   A. Underlay
   B. Onlay
   C. Retro-rectus inlay
   D. Interpositional

4. **Regarding complications of hernia repair, which of the following is true?**

   A. Surgical site infection rates range from 0–12% for clean cases and up to 34% for clean-contaminated and contaminated cases.
   B. The Centers for Disease Control and Prevention (CDC) define mesh infections as occurring up to 6 months after implantation of prosthetic mesh.
   C. Seroma formation is common postoperatively despite drain placement and therefore drains should be removed within 1–2 weeks to prevent retrograde infection.
   D. The most common organisms identified in mesh infections are gram-negative organisms such as *Klebsiella* and *Proteus* species.

5. **Which of the following is true with respect to mesh?**

   A. The use of biologic mesh material in a contaminated field has about a 30% surgical site infection rate.
   B. Recurrence rates after biologic mesh can be as high as 30% in contaminated fields.

C. Advanced age does not increase the risk of complications after abdominal wall reconstruction.

D. Synthetic mesh infections have been successfully treated using a vacuum-assisted closure (VAC) technique without the need for mesh explantation.

6. What avascular layer is developed during an anterior component separation technique?

A. Between internal oblique and transverse abdominis muscles

B. Between anterior rectus fascia and rectus muscle

C. Between internal and external oblique muscles

D. Between posterior rectus fascia and rectus muscle

ANSWERS

1. C. A grading system was created to help identify the risk of morbidity from a ventral hernia repair and to help decide which type of mesh to utilize. This patient would be considered a grade 3 because of her history of previous infection despite not requiring mesh removal. If there was no previous infection then she would be considered a grade 2 because of her history of diabetes.

Grade 1 (low risk): No comorbidities (i.e., a young healthy individual).

Grade 2 (comorbid): Comorbidities (i.e., smoking, diabetes, immunosuppression, chronic obstructive pulmonary disease, obesity, etc.) that increase the risk of surgical site infections (SSIs). There is no evidence of wound contamination or active infection.

Grade 3 (potentially contaminated): Evidence of wound contamination (i.e., stoma, violation of the GI tract, or history of wound infection). This includes patients with active or suspected wound contamination.

Grade 4 (infected): Active infection such as infected synthetic mesh or septic wound dehiscence.

2. C. It has long been established that direct suture repair for ventral hernia has an unacceptably high recurrence rate with the exception of small 1–2-cm primary hernias. There has been speculation that at the time of primary operation the type of suture used for closure correlates with the rate of incisional hernia formation; however, there is no conclusive evidence to support this notion. Primary ventral hernias are thought to have a genetic predisposition, which secondary or incisional hernias are likely related to abnormal ratios of types I and III collagen, as well as the amount of metalloprotease expression. An average of 150,000 to 250,000 ventral hernias are performed each year, making it the fifth-most common procedure performed by general surgeons.

3. D. Interpositional repair or "bridge" repair in which the mesh is sutured directly to the fascial edge has been largely abandoned due to the extremely high recurrence rates. Onlay mesh repair places the mesh above the rectus sheath. There are several types of inlay repair. In the retro-rectus repair, the mesh is placed between the rectus abdominis muscle and the posterior rectus sheath. Alternatively, the mesh can be placed preperitoneal between the posterior rectus sheath and the preperitoneal fat. An intraperitoneal or underlay type repair places the mesh underneath the peritoneum. This type of repair is used for laparoscopic repairs. Because the mesh is placed under the peritoneum, intraperitoneal repair is thought to have higher rates of adhesions and erosion of the mesh into the bowel. In general, the type of repair is surgeon preference.

Advances in mesh products such as composite mesh with anti-adhesive barriers have been developed to decrease complications. Onlay-type mesh repair has more potential for seroma formation because large subcutaneous dissection is required and is also more susceptible to contamination from infection because of the superficial location. Inlay mesh repairs are generally preferred because of their ability to distribute the intra-abdominal wall pressure and decrease overall tension. Underlay and inlay repairs have been shown to have the lowest recurrence rates of all types of mesh repair.

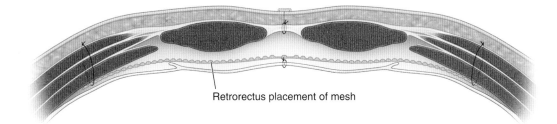

Retrorectus placement of mesh

4. A Surgical site infections are common after ventral hernia repair and are defined as superficial, deep, and organ space infections. The intraoperative level of wound contamination based on CDC criteria includes clean, clean-contaminated, contaminated, and dirty correlates with the rate of surgical site infections. Clean cases have an infection rate of 0–12%; whereas clean-contaminated and contaminated have infection rates as high as 34%. The CDC defines mesh infections as occurring up to 1 year after mesh implantation. The most common organism cultured from infected mesh is *Staphylococcus aureus* and is seen in up to 81% of cases. This suggests a possible skin flora contamination at the time of mesh implantation. While gram-negative organisms are present in mesh infection, they occur only 17% of the time. Seromas are common after ventral hernia, and drains are recommended to decrease the dead space. While they can cause retrograde bacterial contamination, there is no definitive recommendation of time for removal and are often necessary for up to 4–6 weeks.

5. D. Prolonged operative time and American Society of Anesthesiologists (ASA) >2 have been associated with major operative complications; however, advanced as has not been shown to be a predictor of morbidity. Particular comorbidities identified were obesity, smoking, hypertension, diabetes, and anemia. The use of VAC techniques can be successful in treating surgical site infections, including mesh infections leading to mesh salvage. A meta-analysis including 60 studies by Bellows et al. showed a 17% surgical site infection and 15% recurrent rate in grade 3 contaminated fields after biologic mesh repair.

6. C. The incision for an anterior component separation is made 1–2 cm lateral to the rectus sheath or linea semilunaris, and the external oblique fascia is incised.

After dividing 1–2 cm lateral to the linea semilunaris, the external oblique fibers are released, and a plane is developed between the internal and external oblique muscles (avascular). Full release can allow medial fascial advancement of 3–5 cm in the upper abdomen, 7–10 cm at the umbilicus, and 1–3 cm in the suprapubic region for each side.

BIBLIOGRAPHY

Albino FP, Patel KM, Nahabedian MY, Sosin M, Attinger CE, Bhanot P. Does mesh location matter in abdominal wall reconstruction? A systematic review of the literature and a summary of recommendations. *Plast Reconstr Surg.* 2013;132(5):1295–1304.

Bellows CF, Smith A, Malsbury J, Helton WS. Repair of incisional hernias with biological prosthesis: a systematic review of current evidence. *Am J Surg.* 2013;205(1): 85–101.

Butler CE, Baumann DP, Janis JE, Rosen MJ. Abdominal wall reconstruction. *Curr Probl Surg.* 2013;50(12):557–586.

Fischer JP, Wink JD, Nelson JA, Kovach SJ. Among 1,706 cases of abdominal wall reconstruction, what factors influence the occurrence of major operative complications? *Surgery.* 2014;155(2):311–319.

Montgomery A. The battle between biological and synthetic meshes in ventral hernia repair. *Hernia.* 2013;17: 3–11.

Rosen, MJ. Chapter 1. Abdominal wall anatomy and vascular supply In: *Atlas of abdominal wall reconstruction.* 2nd edition. Philadelphia, PA: Elsevier, Inc.; 2017

Tamhankar AP, Raki K, Everitt NJ. Vacuum-assisted closure therapy in the treatment of mesh infection after hernia repair. *Surgeon.* 2009;7(5):316–318.

16

Hernia - Umbilical/Ventral with Cirrhosis

Scott H. Nguyen

A 44-year-old male presents to the emergency department. He has had complaints of abdominal pain over the last several days. Today, he was bending over to pick up something off the floor and felt a sudden sharp pain at his belly button. He states the area is now very tender and achy. He has felt some nausea for the last hour or two. There has been no change in bowel habits prior to this episode. His past medical history is significant for an umbilical hernia, hypertension, and cirrhosis. Past surgical history is for an appendectomy when he was 27. He smokes a half pack per day and has 2–3 drinks per day. He denies any drug use. When pressed, he states that his doctors told him his liver problems are because he "drinks too much."

Vital signs are heart rate 105, blood pressure 140/91, respiratory rate 18, and pulse Ox 98% on the radial artery. On exam, there is no evidence of jaundice. He is noted to have tenderness directly at the umbilicus with a protuberant abdomen. It is dull to percussion. There are skin changes noted at the umbilicus, specifically an area of ulceration, and a nonreducible hernia is noted.

Labs:

WBC: 13.1; Hgb/Hct: 13.5/40; Platelets: 202
Na: 138; K: 3.7; BUN/Cr: 23/1.4; TBili: 1.7; INR: 1.6

1. **Regarding cirrhosis, which of the following negatively affects the patient's perioperative mortality risk?**
   A. White blood cell count of 13.1
   B. Hypertension
   C. Alcohol consumption
   D. Smoking
   E. International normalized ratio (INR)

2. **Which of the following factors is associated with increased incidence of abdominal wall hernias in patients with cirrhosis?**
   A. Increased clotting time
   B. Single episode of ascites formation
   C. Rising creatinine
   D. Recanalized umbilical vein
   E. Decreased mobility

3. **Which of the following relates to worse outcomes in the setting of emergent repair of an umbilical hernia in the cirrhotic patient?**
   A. Mesh insertion
   B. Smoking
   C. Omentectomy
   D. Small bowel resection
   E. Anemia

4. **Best management of an umbilical/ventral hernia in a patient with cirrhosis and ascites would include which of the following?**
   A. Elective repair rather than emergent management
   B. Preoperative ascites control only
   C. Postoperative ascites control only
   D. Primary repair of the hernia
   E. Intraoperative drain placement only

5. **The described patient, while waiting in the emergency department, tells a nurse that his umbilical bulge just started seeping clear fluid. He asks if he should be concerned and what should be the immediate next steps in management.**

A. Applying an absorbent sterile dressing only as this is self-limiting
B. Emergent surgical repair
C. Antibiotics, fluid resuscitation, and sterile dressing
D. Intra-abdominal drain placement
E. Urgent paracentesis

6. **What is the definitive management of the patient's umbilical hernia pathology described in question 5?**

A. Nonoperative management because it is self-limiting and an intervention that has high morbidity and mortality
B. Urgent surgical repair
C. Transjugular intrahepatic portosystemic shunt (TIPS)
D. Urgent paracentesis
E. Elective surgical repair on an outpatient basis

ANSWERS

1. **E.** In a cirrhotic patient, the extent of the cirrhosis affects the perioperative mortality; but the etiology of cirrhosis does not have to be taken into consideration. To determine the patient's 90-day mortality, the model for end-stage liver disease (MELD) score can be used. The MELD score is calculated by the equation:

$$MELD = 3.78 \times \ln[\text{serum bilirubin (mg/dL)}] + 11.2 \\ \times \ln[\text{INR}] + 9.57 \times \ln[\text{serum creatinine} \\ \text{(mg/dL)}] + 6.43$$

As such, the patient's bilirubin, INR, and creatinine affect his survival chances. This system was developed to determine outcomes for patients having undergone transjugular intrahepatic portosystemic shunt (TIPS) procedures. It has now become the standard for determining the severity of liver disease (having replaced the Childs Classification), and in the criteria outlined by the United Network for Organ Sharing (UNOS), the frequency of dialysis was applied to the formula. The etiology of the cirrhosis (or end-stage liver disease) was not found to be a significant prognostic indicator and was removed from the original MELD score. In our particular patient, the MELD score is 17, which correlates with a 6% 3-month mortality.

MELD Scores	
40 or more	71.3% mortality
30–39	52.6% mortality
20–29	19.6% mortality
10–19	6.0% mortality
<9	1.9% mortality

2. **D.** Patients with liver cirrhosis and ascites have a risk of developing an umbilical hernia that approaches 20%. A single episode of ascites is not highly associated with abdominal wall hernia formation. However, as the number of episodes of ascites increases, so does the incidence of hernia formation such that by the third episode, about 70% of patients will have developed an umbilical hernia. The other factors, which include increased intra-abdominal pressure, muscle wasting and weakening of the abdominal fascia related to malnutrition, and recanalization of the umbilical vein, are all contributing factors to the development of umbilical hernias in the cirrhotic patient. The decreased functional status, rising creatinine from kidney dysfunction, and the increased platelet dysfunction due to uremia do not influence the development of a hernia.

3. **E.** In the setting of emergent repair of the abdominal wall/umbilical hernia in the cirrhotic patient, preoperative anemia was the only preoperative predictor of complicated outcome. The other factors found to be statistically significant and related to major complications were age older than 65 and a higher MELD score. Additionally, the authors in this study noted that small bowel obstruction, but not resection, in this setting had a 9-fold increase in risk for postoperative complications. Additionally, smoking, omentectomy, and mesh insertion were not significant factors in the development of postoperative complications.

4. **A.** In a randomized controlled trial of 80 patients having repair with or without mesh by Ammar, the author found that primary repair of an umbilical/ventral hernia in the setting of cirrhosis and ascites has a significantly higher recurrence rate than when a mesh repair is performed (14.2% vs. 2.7%, p < 0.05). Most authors now advocate for more aggressive elective repair of hernias in patients with cirrhosis and

ascites even in the setting of Class B and C cirrhosis. In their study, Carbonell et al. found that elective surgical morbidity in patients with cirrhosis was no different from those without cirrhosis (15.6% vs. 13.5%; p = 0.18). Emergent surgery morbidity was statistically significant between the two groups (17.3% vs. 14.5%; p = 0.04). While differences in elective surgical mortality in cirrhotics approached significance (0.6% vs. 0.1%; p = 0.06), mortality was sevenfold higher in emergency surgery (3.8% vs. 0.5%; p < 0.0001). In addition, the opportunity to utilize laparoscopy in the elective setting in this patient population has the ability to mitigate postoperative complications and decrease the length of hospitalization. Medical diuresis, postoperative paracentesis, and drain placement at time of surgery are all factors that improve the postoperative course after hernia repair in these patients. Odom et al. noted a significant increase in major complications when no invasive measure was used to control the ascites.

5. **C.** The patient is experiencing "Flood syndrome," first named by Frank B. Flood in 1961, is described as spontaneous perforation or rupture of the umbilicus. This complication is rare and associated with high morbidity and mortality. In Flood's case report, all five patients reported on had died. These patients can have large fluid and electrolyte shifts due to ascites loss; therefore, early and aggressive fluid resuscitation is recommended in addition to antibiotics to mitigate the risk of infection and subsequent peritonitis. Finally, sterile dressing should be applied to additionally help prevent infection risks and further spillage of ascites that may lead to fluid shifts.

6. **B.** Definitive management is urgent surgical intervention and repair of the hernia after initial fluid resuscitation, hemodynamic stabilization, and antibiotic administration. Primary repair versus the use of mesh are still controversial topics are this time.

If the patient were to undergo liver transplant surgery, an umbilical hernia repair is recommended at the time of the transplant operation. Nonoperative management of complicated hernias in the cirrhotic patient can be associated with mortality ranging from 60–80% versus 6–20% with urgent surgical intervention as described by Coelho et al. Large-volume paracentesis has been associated with large fluid shifts and electrolyte abnormalities in an already possibly hemodynamically unstable patient.

BIBLIOGRAPHY

Ammar SA. Management of complicated umbilical hernias in cirrhotic patients using permanent mesh: randomized clinical trial. *Hernia.* 2010;14(1):35–38.

Belli G, D'Agostino A, Fantini C, et al. Laparoscopic incisional and umbilical hernia repair in cirrhotic patients. *Surg Laparosc Endosc Percutan Tech.* 2006;16:330–333.

Carbonell AM, Wolfe LG, DeMaria EJ. Poor outcomes in cirrhosis-associated hernia repair: a nationwide cohort study of 32,033 patients. *Hernia.* 2005;9:353–357.

Choi SB, Hong KD, Lee JS, et al. Management of umbilical hernia complicated with liver cirrhosis: an advocate of early and elective herniorrhaphy. *Dig Liver Dis.* 2011;43: 991–995.

Coelho JC, Claus CM, Campos AC, Costa MA, Blum C. Umbilical hernia in patients with liver cirrhosis: a surgical challenge. *World J Gastrointest Surg.* 2016;8(7): 476–482.

Eker HH, van Ramshorst GH, de Goede B, et al. Prospective study on elective umbilical hernia repair in patients with liver cirrhosis and ascites. *Surgery.* 2011;150:542–546.

Flood FB. Spontaneous perforation of the umbilicus in Laennec's cirrhosis with massive ascites. *N Engl J Med.* 1961;264:72–74.

Kamath PS, Kim WR. The model for end-stage liver disease (MELD). *Hepatology.* 2007;45(3):797–805.

Odom SR, Gupta A, Talmor D, et al. Emergency hernia repair in cirrhotic patients with ascites. *J Trauma Acute Care Surg.* 2013;75:404–409.

Online MELD calculator: http://www.mayoclinic.org/ medical-professionals/model-end-stage-liver-disease/ meld-model-unos-modification

17

Inguinal and Femoral Hernias

Justin LaRocque, Harry T. Aubin, and Scott Nguyen

An otherwise healthy 31-year-old male presents with a painless bulge in his right groin. Although it does not bother him or limit his daily activities, he notices fluctuation in its size, from being absent when he lies flat for a few minutes to a golf-ball-sized mass upon coughing or strenuous exercises. Physical examination confirms the presence of a right inguinal hernia. No abnormalities were noted on the contralateral side.

1. **Regarding the management and indications for surgical intervention of asymptomatic inguinal hernias, which of the following is correct?**
   A. The incidence of inguinal hernia strangulation is greater than 10% after 5 years.
   B. Elective surgical repair is advised for all otherwise healthy patients.
   C. Most patients will develop symptoms over time and require an operation.
   D. Incarceration is much more likely with direct hernias.
   E. Emergency and elective inguinal hernia repairs share similar morbidity and mortality rates.

2. **Which of the following is considered the most common early complication after open inguinal hernia repair?**
   A. Surgical site infection
   B. Hematoma/seroma
   C. Urinary tract infection
   D. Small bowel obstruction
   E. Recurrence

3. **Which of the following is true regarding laparoscopic inguinal hernia repair?**
   A. It is generally less expensive than the open repair.
   B. Potential complications are similar, or less severe, to those seen with open repair.
   C. The procedure is limited to the repair of only one defect in the inguinal region.
   D. They are associated with greater chronic pain and numbness compared to the open approach.
   E. It is used only for recurrent or bilateral inguinal hernias.

4. **After an open inguinal hernia repair, which symptom is most likely to appear?**
   A. Numbness on ipsilateral upper lateral thigh
   B. Numbness on ipsilateral medial thigh
   C. Hyperreflexia of the cremasteric muscles
   D. Hypersthesia of the ipsilateral hemiscrotum
   E. Numbness of the suprapubic region

A 55-year-old Caucasian male with a history of hypertension and tobacco use disorder presents to a clinic for follow-up after a two-column hemorrhoidectomy. He states that he is doing well overall, with good pain control after his procedure 3 weeks ago. He has increased his fiber intake and has been drinking more water in order to keep his stools soft. The patient inquires about a small round mass he has noticed for the past 6 months in his inguinal region. He denies significant pain and states he is unsure if the mass changes size throughout the day or when he is lying down.

5. **The patient notices more pain in the area when he strains himself. On physical exam, no mass is palpable even with Valsalva. Which of the following is more likely the cause of his pain?**

    A. Fat-containing hernia on CT scan
    B. Varicocele
    C. Intermittent testicular torsion
    D. Athletic pubalgia
    E. Hydrocele

6. **In all patients, which side is most common for an inguinal hernia to occur, and why?**

    A. The most common side is the left side because the sigmoid colon puts pressure on the inguinal canal, making it weaker over time.
    B. This patient's history of constipation leading to need for hemorrhoidectomy makes it likely he has bilateral disease.
    C. The most common side is the right side because the right testicle descends into the scrotum later, which delays closure of the processes vaginalis.
    D. The most common side is the left side because the testicular vein connects to the left renal vein meaning renal development has to occur first, which delays closure of the processes vaginalis.
    E. The most common side is the right side because the cecum and appendix overlay the right hemi-pelvis and protect against hernia formation.

7. **As a hernia was not palpated on physical exam, which of the following is the next best step in management?**

    A. Consider an alternative diagnosis
    B. Ultrasound
    C. Computerized tomography (CT) scan
    D. Magnetic resonance imaging (MRI)

A 65-year-old female is seen in your clinic for a "lump" in her groin. She states the lump has been present for a few years and intermittently becomes larger in size. On exam, there is no evidence of adenopathy or venous thrombosis. A reducible hernia is palpated. You perform an uncomplicated McVay repair, and she is seen in follow-up 1 year later with a recurrence.

8. **Regarding femoral hernias, which of the following is true?**

    A. It is an acquired defect.
    B. It has a male preponderance.
    C. It is the most common of the inguinal hernias.
    D. The incidence of incarceration is lower than inguinal hernias.

9. **Regarding the recurrence of this patient's hernia, which of the following is the most likely etiology?**

    A. Congenital collagen disorder
    B. Wound infection
    C. Tension on suture line
    D. Poor tissue due to her age

10. **Regarding an open repair of groin hernias, which of the following techniques will fix a femoral hernia?**

    A. Bassini repair
    B. Marcy repair
    C. Shouldice repair
    D. Preperitoneal repair
    E. Lichtenstein tension-free with mesh repair

11. **How are femoral hernia most typically diagnosed?**

    A. History and physical exam alone
    B. With ultrasound imaging.
    C. With computed tomography
    D. With herniography
    E. With magnetic resonance imaging

12. **What is the most common type of hernia in this patient if she presented with groin pain?**

    A. Obturator hernia
    B. Direct inguinal hernia
    C. Femoral hernia
    D. Indirect inguinal hernia
    E. Spigelian hernia

ANSWERS

1. **C.** As one of the naturally weak points in the abdominal wall, the groin area is prone to the protrusion of the peritoneal sac. When this occurs in the presence of minor symptoms or in the absence of symptoms altogether, the condition is known as an asymptomatic inguinal hernia. One-third of patients with inguinal hernias fall within this category, presenting with a nontender bulge in the area.

    The inferior epigastric vessels, as well as the internal and external inguinal rings, provide anatomic landmarks that help in distinguishing direct and indirect inguinal hernias. The sac of a direct hernia protrudes outward and forward, medial to the internal inguinal ring and the inferior epigastric vessels. On the other hand, indirect hernias pass from the internal ring obliquely toward the external ring, lateral to the inferior epigastric vessels. A pantaloon-type hernia occurs when both of these features are present. Regardless, the anatomic distinction between these is of little importance given the similarities in the approach for operative repair. Moreover, there is no difference in rates of incarceration, strangulation, and need for emergent repair among the direct, indirect, and pantaloon hernias. More traditional descriptions of inguinal hernias are made on the basis of their contents (e.g., sliding, Richter's, Littre's) or the status of the contents (e.g., sliding, incarcerated, strangulated).

With more than 20 million operations performed annually around the world, inguinal hernia repair is the most common elective procedure performed in the United States and Europe. There is a well-documented debate as to what the best management is for asymptomatic inguinal hernias: operative management or the watchful waiting approach. The rationale of repairing all inguinal hernias, whether symptomatic or not, lies in their risk of incarceration and strangulation. Elective repairs are considered relatively safe with low short-term morbidity, mortality, and recurrence rates. This is different from emergent operations, which carry higher morbidity and mortality rates given the additional risks of gangrene, perforation, and infection of the peritoneal cavity. Nonetheless, watchful waiting spares the patient from the complications of elective surgery, such as surgical site infection, hematoma, and urinary retention, and may result in more long-term chronic groin pain, neuralgia, and recurrence.

Studies by Fitzgibbons et al. and O'Dwyer et al. both show no difference in terms of discomfort and pain across groups, but there is a rate of conversion driven mainly by pain of 54% and 72% after 5 and 7.5 years, respectively, in those managed nonoperatively. A more recent systematic review of the evidence by Mizrahi et al. shows that the rate of strangulation in those who do not pursue surgery is quite low at less than 1% after a 2- and a 4-year follow-up period. On the other hand, the range of operative complications in those undergoing elective surgery goes from 0%–22.3%, with a recurrence rate of 2.1%. Both treatment options are thus considered safe, although most patients will progress to develop symptoms and eventually require an operation.

2. B. The overall risk of complications following open inguinal hernia repair is low, and fortunately, these are oftentimes transient and easy to manage. Several factors play a role in the occurrence of complications, including the surgical technique, surgeon experience, and anesthetic choices. Neumayer et al. compared open mesh versus laparoscopic inguinal hernia repair and reported a combined incidence of hematoma or seroma of 13.6% in open cases and 16.4% in those performed laparoscopically. Other less common adverse events seen in the immediate postoperative period include urinary retention, orchitis, pain, and urinary tract and wound infections. As for long-term complications, chronic pain tops the list, with a reported rate of 14%–19% following open repairs with some series reporting frequencies as low as 6% or as high as 75.5%. The risk is lower following laparoscopic cases, with rates ranging between 9.8% and 13.8%. Orchitis, infection, and hernia recurrence are amongst other common late complications.

3. B. The approach and operative technique for the repair of inguinal hernias has evolved throughout the years. Repairs can be either done open or laparoscopically. The open approach can be either a tissue repair or a prosthetic (tension-free) repair. Although the former might be of historical interest, there are some situations in which these may be indicated, such as in a contaminated field, in pediatric patients, or in those places where access to prostheses is limited. By identifying increased tension as the main cause of recurrence, Lichtenstein popularized the use of a synthetic mesh to bridge the hernia defect and provide a tension-free repair. This approach is the gold standard of open hernia repairs, as it has proved to decrease the rates of postoperative discomfort, duration of hospital stay, and recurrence. The laparoscopic approach also offers a tension-free repair. Those who support this technique emphasize the quicker time to recovery, less pain, better visualization of the anatomy, and the ability to repair all the defects in the inguinal region. On the other hand, critics note the longer operative times, technical challenges, risk of recurrence, and increased costs. A meta-analysis study by Voyles et al. compared the two approaches and showed that both provide equivalent outcomes, with open repairs being lower in cost, and entailing a lower risk of severe postoperative complications. Those unique to the laparoscopic approach include small bowel obstruction, internal hernia, bladder perforation, infarcted omentum, and port-site hernia.

Special situations may favor the use of the laparoscopic approach. In the setting of bilateral inguinal hernias, the ability to use the same access sites evidently translates into faster recovery and less postoperative pain. However, whether done openly or laparoscopically, the simultaneous repair of bilateral hernias does not increase the risk of reoperation for recurrence. Another typical challenge for the surgeon is that of recurrent hernias. These may be caused by either technical problems (e.g., knot slipped, crushed suture, inadequate bites of fascia) or patient factors (e.g., malnutrition, steroid use, and smoking). A second groin exploration entails cutting through scar tissue that in itself adds a certain degree of difficulty and additional trauma with increased risk of damage to the testicular blood supply and sensory nerves. Access through virgin territories through a posterior approach explains the advantage of laparoscopic repairs in these situations.

4. **B.** Depending on the approach used, specific nerves in the area will be more prone to injury. For example, in open hernia repairs, the ilioinguinal nerve can be most commonly injured at the external ring where it runs on top of the cord. This results in loss of the cremasteric reflex and numbness to the ipsilateral penis, scrotum, and thigh. On the other hand, the posterior approach used in laparoscopic surgery can result in injuries to the lateral femoral cutaneous, femoral branch of the genitofemoral (sensory, upper lateral thigh) and, rarely, the femoral nerves. Hypersthesia of the hemiscrotum and numbness of the suprapubic region are not complications of nerve injury from inguinal hernia repairs.

5. **A.** Any of these entities are potential causes of the patient's inguinal mass. Detailed history and physical can further aid in achieving the correct diagnosis. This patient has multiple potential risk factors for inguinal hernia, including male sex, increasing age, Caucasian race, constipation, and tobacco use, leading to chronic cough. Inguinal hernias can result in groin "heaviness," are typically worse with walking/activity, and masses usually enlarge with standing or Valsalva and decrease in size with recumbency. Location of the bulge can also help narrow the differential in a patient presenting with an inguinal mass. A bulge or pain originating near the scrotum could represent varicocele, hydrocele, or testicular torsion, whereas the other answer choices are commonly located higher in the groin.

6. **C.** Right-sided inguinal hernias are more common. During fetal development, the testis descends into the scrotum following the processus vaginalis through the layers of the abdominal wall as the gubernaculum foreshortens and pulls the testis to its final location. This transit is completed between the 7th–9th months of gestation. The processus vaginalis then spontaneously underdoes obliteration. If the peritoneal defect does not fully obliterate, the individual will have an increased risk of inguinal hernia over the course of their lifetime. In the fetus, this process occurs on the left, followed by the right, increasing the chance of incomplete obliteration on the right side of the groin. Although it is true that the left testicular vein drains into the left renal vein, this has no impact on the inguinal wall's development.

Premature and low-birth-weight infants are at greatly increased risk of inguinal hernia, with increasing risk correlating with the magnitude of their prematurity. Their risk of bilateral inguinal hernia is similarly increased. It is thought that the incidence of right-sided inguinal hernia, and specifically femoral hernia, compared to the left side is a result of the sigmoid colon offering a protective effect on the left inguinal and femoral canals.

7. **B.** Ultrasound can be highly sensitive (>90%) and specific (82–86%) in identifying inguinal hernia when completed by trained practitioners. It is safe, noninvasive, relatively inexpensive, and widely available. X-rays are unable to differentiate soft tissue in a manner that would aid in diagnosing inguinal hernias. Radial imaging modalities, such as CT and MRI, tend to be more expensive and less available, and both expose the patient to ionizing radiation, in the case of CT, or are time-intensive, in the case of MRI. MRI can be useful in the workup of athletic pubalgia as it can better identify the subtle tenoperiosteal disruption and osteitis pubis typically associated with the diagnosis. If the ultrasound is nondiagnostic, then a CT scan or an MRI scan can be ordered. A CT scan in the prone position may be the most sensitive test for diagnosing an inguinal hernia.

8. **A.** Femoral hernias are acquired hernias and NOT of congenital origin. They are more common in females and more common in older women who are multiparous, as laxity of the abdominal wall

and stretching of the femoral ring with aging or pregnancy is felt to be the leading cause. Given the mostly fixed, confined spaces of the femoral canal, these hernias are notorious for incarcerating, leading to emergent/urgent hernia repair.

A study from the Swedish Hernia Register showed an incidence of 2–4% of all groin hernias over a 14-year period. Of these hernias, 35.9% of femoral hernias were found to present as incarcerated needing emergency surgery, and of these, 22.7% required bowel resection. This is compared to only 4.9% needing emergency surgery in the inguinal group.

All femoral hernias should be repaired, and in the presence of incarcerated contents, the sac should be assessed for viability, which may include a laparotomy or laparoscopic evaluation of the small bowel. Delayed diagnosis will lead to higher morbidity and mortality. Different repair techniques are available and mainly depend on the clinical presentation. Many consider mesh plug repair as the technique of choice in elective and noninfected cases. In contrast, tissue repair (i.e., McVay operation) may be preferred in strangulated cases in which severe infection is present.

The McVay repair, aka the Cooper's ligament repair, is a tissue repair that is effective in repair of all three groin hernias (indirect, direct, femoral). It is performed with nonabsorbable sutures in an interrupted fashion. Sutures are placed to sew the transversus abdominus aponeurosis to Cooper's ligament beginning at the pubic tubercle toward the femoral sheath. Once the femoral sheath is reached, place a transition stitch containing transversus abdominus, Cooper's ligament, femoral sheath medial to femoral vein, and inguinal ligament (iliopubic tract); then approximate the transversus abdominal aponeurosis to the inguinal ligament laterally to the internal ring. Exposing the Cooper's ligament is done prior to suturing. Additionally, to avoid tension, a curvilinear relaxing incision is made through the anterior rectus sheath starting 1 cm cephalad of the pubic tubercle to near its lateral border.

9. C. Tension on the suture line is felt to be the most common cause of hernia recurrence in general and especially in tissue repairs. This is why an adequate relaxing incision is necessary in the McVay repair. Most likely, there was some tension on the repair despite the relaxing incision.

A shift has been made to tension-free repairs with the usage of mesh. Tissue versus mesh repair was compared in a large meta-anaylsis including more than 11,000 patients, specifically looking at recurrence rates after hernia surgery. Findings of this study show the odds of developing a recurrent hernia with mesh repairs were reduced by about half, although recurrence rates were relatively small with each repair. Other factors can contribute to recurrence, such as wound infection, but are not the primary/most common cause. Congenital collagen disorder is a rare disorder and is not likely to be seen in this patient.

10. D. Lichtenstein tension-free hernia repair with mesh is the most common hernia repair done at most institutions. It requires little suturing, does not need a relaxing incision, and does not require general anesthesia. Unfortunately, the drawback of this repair is that it does not close, or cover, the femoral ring. Therefore, it is not used for repairing femoral hernias.

The Marcy repair only repairs the deep inguinal ring and is mostly used in pediatric patients. The Bassini and Shouldice repairs only repair the inguinal floor and will not treat a femoral hernia.

The preperitoneal repair, a variation known as the Kugel repair, involves placing mesh in the preperitoneal space and suturing the mesh from the pubic tubercle to the Cooper's ligament. Bilayer mesh repair, in theory is a combined preperitoneal and Lichtenstein repair with mesh and is used for femoral hernia repair. Plug and patch repair can be utilized to obliterate the femoral canal in femoral hernia repair. Laparoscopic repair, as with the previously mentioned repairs, is a described technique for repair of femoral hernias and utilizes the preperitoneal space.

11. A. History and physical exam alone are most often adequate for diagnosing clinically apparent femoral hernias. Features that suggest a femoral hernia include older patients, female patients, and those with a mass or bulge palpable below the level of the inguinal ligament and along the medial aspect of the ipsilateral upper leg. Femoral hernias have an increased risk of incarceration and strangulation and should be repaired regardless of symptomology.

For occult hernias with equivocal clinical exams, diagnostic imaging can aid in the diagnosis.

In Robinson et al.'s systemic review and meta-analysis of the role of radiology in the diagnosis of occult inguinal hernias, first-line radiographic modality should be the use of ultrasound imaging due to its low cost, lack of radiation exposure, and moderate sensitivity (86%) and specificity (77%). CT is less sensitive (80%) and specific (65%).

12. D. Although femoral hernias are more common in females, indirect inguinal hernias remain the most common type of groin hernia in both males and females. Femoral hernias account for 4% of all groin hernias, and they only constitute 20–30% of all female groin hernia repairs. For females older than 70 years of age, they represent approximately half of groin hernia repairs.

BIBLIOGRAPHY

Aasvang EK, Bay-Nielsen M, Kehlet H. Pain and functional impairment 6 years after inguinal herniorrhaphy. *Hernia.* 2006;10:316–321.

Alimoglu O, Alimoglu O, Kaya B, Okan I, et al. Femoral hernia: a review of 83 cases. *Hernia.* 2006;10:70–73.

Amid PK, Shulman AG, Lichtenstein IL. Open "tension-free" repair of inguinal hernias: the Lichtenstein technique. *Eur J Surg.* 1996;162:447–453.

Bittner R, Schwarz J. Inguinal hernia repair: current surgical techniques. *Langenbecks Arch Surg.* 2012;397:271–282.

Bradley M, Morgan D, Pentlow B, et al. The groin hernia—an ultrasound diagnosis? *Ann R Coll Surg Engl.* 2003;85:178–180.

Bullen NL, Massey LH, Antoniou SA, Smart NJ, Fortelny RH. Open versus laparoscopic mesh repair of primary unilateral uncomplicated inguinal hernia: a systematic review with meta-analysis and trial sequential analysis. *Hernia.* 2019;23(3);461–472.

Chung L, Norrie J, O'Dwyer PJ. Long-term follow-up of patients with a painless inguinal hernia from a randomized clinical trial. *Br J Surg.* 2011;98:596–599.

Dahlstrand U, Wollert S, Nordin P, Sandblom G, Gunnarsson U. Emergency femoral hernia repair: a study based on a national register. *Ann Surg.* 2009;249(4):672–676.

EU Hernia Trialists Collaboration. Repair of groin hernia with synthetic mesh: meta-analysis of randomized controlled trials. *Ann Surg.* 2002;235(3):322–332.

Fitzgibbons RJ, Giobbie-Hurder A, Gibbs JO, et al. Watchful waiting vs repair of inguinal hernia in minimally symptomatic men: a randomized clinical trial. *JAMA.* 2006;295:285–292.

Fitzgibbons RJ Jr, Ramanan B, Arya S, et al. Long-term results geal reflux disease. In: Townsend CM, Beauchamp RD, Evers BM, Mattox K, eds. *Sabiston Textbook of Surgery: The Biological Basis of Modern Surgical Practice.* 19th ed. Elsevier Saunders; 2012:1114–1140.

Fitzgibbons RJ Jr, Ramanan B, Arya S, et al. Long-term results of a randomized controlled trial of a nonoperative strategy (watchful waiting) for men with minimally symptomatic inguinal hernias. *Ann Surg.* 2013;258:508–515.

Hachisuka T. Femoral hernia repair. *Surg Clin North Am.* 2003;83:1189–1205.

Humes DJ, Radcliffe RS, Camm C, West J. Population-based study of presentation and adverse outcomes after femoral hernia surgery. *Br J Surg.* 2013;100:1827–1832.

Jones DB. *Master Techniques in Surgery: Hernia.* Lippincott Williams & Wilkins; 2012.

Kald A, Fridsten S, Nordin P, Nilsson E. Outcome of repair of bilateral groin hernias: a prospective evaluation of 1,487 patients. *Eur J Surg.* 2002;168;150–153.

Kark AE, Kurzer M. Groin hernias in women. *Hernia.* June 2008;12(3):267–270.

Kingsnorth A, LeBlanc K. Hernias: inguinal and incisional. *Lancet.* 2003;362;1561–1571.

Kurzer M, Belsham PA, Kark AE. Prospective study of open preperitoneal mesh repair for recurrent inguinal hernia. *Br J Surg.* 2002;89:90–93.

Lichtenstein IL, Shulman AG, Amid PK, Montllor MM. The tension-free hernioplasty. *Am J Surg.* 1989;157(2):188–193.

Malagoni MA, Rosen MJ. Hernias. In: Townsend CM, Beauchamp RD, Evers BM, Mattox K, eds. *Sabiston Textbook of Surgery: The Biological Basis of Modern Surgical Practice.* 19th ed. Elsevier Saunders; 2012:1114–1140.

Malangoni MA, Rosen MJ. Inguinal hernia. In: Townsend CM, Beauchamp RD, Evers BM, Mattox K, eds. *Sabiston Textbook of Surgery: The Biological Basis of Modern Surgical Practice.* 20th ed. Elsevier Saunders; 2016:44.

Matthews RD, Neumayer L. Inguinal hernia in the 21st century: an evidence-based review. *Curr Probl Surg.* 2008;45:261–312.

McCormack K, Scott NW, Go PM, Ross S, Grant AM. Laparoscopic techniques versus open techniques for inguinal hernia repair. *Cochrane Database Syst. Rev.* 2003;2003(1):CD001785.

McVay CB, Chapp JD. Inguinal and femoral hernioplasty: the evaluation of a basic concept. *Ann Surg.* 1958;148(4):499–510; discussion 510–512.

Miyaki A, Yamaguchi K, Kishibe S, Ida A, Miyauchi T, Naritaka Y. Diagnosis of inguinal hernia by prone- vs. supine-position computed tomography. *Hernia.* 2017;21(5):705–713.

Mizrahi H, Parker MC. Management of asymptomatic inguinal hernia: a systematic review of the evidence. *Arch Surg.* 2012;147:277–281.

Naude GP, Ocon S, Bongard F. Femoral hernia: the dire consequences of a missed diagnosis. *Am J Emerg Med.* 1997;15:680–682.

Neumayer L, Giobbie-Hurder A, Jonasson O, et al. Open mesh versus laparoscopic mesh repair of inguinal hernia. *N Engl J Med.* 2004;350:1819–1827.

O'Dwyer PJ, Norrie J, Alani A, Walker A, Duffy F, Horgan P. Observation or operation for patients with an asymptomatic inguinal hernia: a randomized clinical trial. *Ann Surg.* 2006;244:167–173.

Page B, Paterson C, Young D, O'Dwyer PJ. Pain from primary inguinal hernia and the effect of repair on pain. *Br J Surg.* 2002;89:1315–1318.

Perez AJ, Strassle PD, Sadava EE, Gaber C, Schlottmann F. Nationwide analysis of inpatient laparoscopic versus open inguinal hernia repair. *J Laparoendosc Adv Surg Tech A.* 2020;30(3):292–298.

Primatesta P, Goldacre MJ. Inguinal hernia repair: incidence of elective and emergency surgery, readmission and mortality. *Int J Epidemiol.* 1996;25:835–839.

Robinson A, Light D, Nice C. Meta-analysis of sonography in the diagnosis of inguinal hernias. *J Ultrasound Med.* 2013;32(2):339–346.

Sherman V, Macho JR, Brunicardi FC. Inguinal hernias. In: Brunicardi FC, Andersen D, Billiar T, et al., eds. *Schwartz's Principles Surgery.* 9th ed. McGraw Hill Professional; 2010:1305–1342.

van den Heuvel B, Dwars BJ, Klassen DR, Bonjer HJ. Is surgical repair of an asymptomatic groin hernia appropriate? A review. *Hernia.* 2011;15:251–259.

Voyles CR, Hamilton BJ, Johnson WD, Kano N. Meta-analysis of laparoscopic inguinal hernia trials favors open hernia repair with preperitoneal mesh prosthesis. *Am J Surg.* 2002;184:6–10.

18

Inguinal Neuralgia

Eric Balent

A 35-year-old male presents to a clinic 3 months after an uncomplicated open right inguinal hernia repair with mesh for a chronic, minimally symptomatic, indirect inguinal hernia. During the operation, the ilioinguinal nerve was intentionally divided. He reports continued right-sided sharp, episodic groin pain radiating to his testicle that is worse than the symptoms he had prior to repair. He took ibuprofen and acetaminophen for 6 weeks after the surgery with minimal relief. The pain is beginning to limit his activities at work. He now complains of worsening pain.

1. **Regarding the pathophysiology of chronic groin pain after hernia surgery, which of the following is correct?**

   A. Most commonly, it is felt to be neuropathic and due to primary nerve injury during the operation.

   B. It is felt to be due to inflammatory mechanisms from the operation and healing.

   C. It is nociceptive.

   D. Tacking mesh to nerves in a laparoscopic repair is an uncommon cause.

   E. Secondary nerve injury from nerve degeneration from mesh contact is the most common cause.

2. **Regarding the management of chronic groin pain in this patient, which of the following is the best course of action?**

   A. Imaging studies (ultrasound, CT scan, and/or MRI)

   B. Peripheral nerve block

   C. Referral to a pain management specialist

   D. Triple neurectomy

3. **Regarding nerve injuries in hernia repair, which of the following is correct?**

   A. Injury to the ilioinguinal nerve causes loss of cremasteric reflex and numbness to the ipsilateral scrotum, penis, and medial thigh.

   B. Injury to the femoral branch of the lateral femoral cutaneous nerve causes loss of sensation to the medial thigh.

   C. Tack placement inferior to the iliopubic tract and medial to the spermatic cord is avoided to minimize nerve damage in laparoscopic hernia repair.

   D. Injury to the genital branch of the genitofemoral nerve results in a loss of sensation of the entire scrotum and a lack of cremestric reflex on the contralateral side.

4. **Regarding surgical management of postherniorrhaphy neuralgia, which of the following is correct?**

   A. Tailored neurectomy is more effective than triple neurectomy at decreasing symptoms postoperatively.

   B. Triple neurectomy is effective at eliminating pain in upwards of 80% of patients.

   C. Mesh explantation alone is an effective strategy and has been shown to be superior to neurectomy with or without mesh explantation.

   D. Patients with preexisting pain hypersensitization are ideal candidates for neurectomy.

5. **Regarding the intentional division of the ilioinguinal nerve at the time of initial herniorrhaphy, which of the following is correct?**

A. There is no difference in sensory loss between division and preservation of the nerve.

B. A significant decrease in postoperative chronic pain is seen when the ilioinguinal nerve is intentionally divided during the initial surgery.

C. There is no significant difference in decreasing chronic postoperative groin pain.

D. There is less debilitating pain with routine division of the ilioinguinal nerve.

E. Energy.

6. **Regarding the evaluation of postherniorrhaphy neuralgia, which of the following is correct?**

   A. There are no preoperative risk factors to estimate the likelihood of the incidence of postherniorrhaphy neuralgia.

   B. An escalating algorithmic approach to postoperative pain should be employed to perform the least invasive to most invasive workups and treatments.

   C. A therapeutic nerve block can only be repeated once for postoperative pain.

   D. Imaging to guide nerve blocks is not needed.

7. **For postherniorrhaphy neuralgia, if an ultrasound-guided peripheral nerve block fails to achieve pain control, which is the next best course of action?**

   A. Ablation of the iliohypogastric, ilioinguinal, and genital branch of the genitofemoral nerves

   B. Peripheral nerve stimulators

   C. Dorsal root ganglion stimulators

   D. Triple neurectomy

ANSWERS

1. **A.** Chronic postoperative groin pain is felt to be secondary to neuropathic pain from aberrant nerve conduction resulting from either primary or secondary nerve injury. Typically, it is ongoing pain, which is difficult to manage. Initial postoperative pain is due to inflammatory cytokine release and nociceptive mechanisms. Nocioceptive pain is pain felt via neural pathways in which tissue damage surrounding the nerves is the stimulus. This type of pain typically resolves over 6 weeks and is amendable to anti-inflammatory medications such as nonsteroidal anti-inflammatory drugs.

   Primary nerve injury is defined as direct nerve injury and can occur during hernia repair in multiple ways. During dissection, complete or partial nerve transection can occur later, forming a neuroma. Additionally, handling of the nerve can result in crushing, stretching, or burns from surgical energy. Most commonly, the nerve is incidentally entrapped with mesh, suture, and/or staple.

   Secondary nerve injury is defined as nerve degeneration/demyelination from an inflammatory process. It is not as common as primary nerve injury in the pathogenesis of postherniorrhaphy neuralgia. Secondary nerve injury is felt to be from meshoma, excessive scar tissue, or contact with mesh not involving entrapment.

2. **B.** Chronic groin pain, or chronic postherniorrhaphy inguinal pain, after hernia surgery is diagnosed by chronic pain at site or region of prior hernia repair that persists postoperatively for more than 3 months that cannot be attributed to another cause. The prevalence of postoperative chronic groin pain varies from study to study. A large Swedish survey including 2,500 patients, noted that 14% of patients had lifestyle-limiting groin pain and 30% chronic pain that didn't hinder their lifestyle. A smaller series noted 1.5% of patients had moderate to severe pain at 5 years. Interestingly, it is more common in younger patients, with persistent pain in 58% of patients under the age of 40, and only 14% of those older than age 40.

   Upon presentation of a patient you suspect has chronic postoperative groin pain, anti-inflammatory treatment has already been attempted and, as stated, usually has little effect on neuropathic pain. In this instance, an ilioinguinal nerve block can help confirm the diagnosis and is indicated. This can be done by a surgeon or by a pain management specialist. Additionally, nerve ablation with phenol or radiofrequency ablation is used. Patients who fail less invasive means of treatment should undergo triple neurectomy.

   Nonneuropathic pain must be excluded. This is done with history, physical, and imaging studies. The ideal imaging study has not been determined by randomized trials. In general, ultrasound is the least expensive test with minimal risk to the patient. However, CT and MRI scans can provide a better representation of the location of mesh, location of neuronal structures, and presence of recurrent hernias.

3. **A.** An injury to the femoral branch of the lateral femoral cutaneous nerve causes a lack of sensation to

the lateral thigh, not the medial thigh as mentioned in the answer. This nerve is seen in laparoscopic hernia repairs and is not encountered during open inguinal hernia repair. Other nerves encountered laparoscopically include the lateral femoral cutaneous nerve, the ilioinguinal nerve lateral to the internal ring, the iliohypogastric (which cannot be seen but could be injured with mesh fixation), the genital branch of the genitofemoral nerve, and the femoral nerve. The so-called triangle of pain is defined as the iliopubic tract superiolaterally, the spermatic vessels posteriomedially, and the reflected peritoneal edge laterally. This contains the genitofemoral nerve and the lateral femoral cutaneous nerve. Minimizing nerve injuries laparoscopically is achieved by avoiding tack placement inferior to the iliopubic tract laterally beyond the external iliac artery.

For open inguinal hernia repairs, the ilioinguinal nerve is the most common cause of pain. Injury to this nerve can also cause ipsilateral scrotal, thigh, and penis numbness, as well as loss of the cremasteric reflex. Injury to the genital branch of the genitofemoral nerve can less commonly cause pain. More commonly, scrotal sensation and a lack of cremasteric reflex on the ipsilateral side are seen.

4. **B.** Given the significant morbidity and difficulty of the operation, neurectomy is reserved for patients who fail pain management strategies. Patients with preexisting pain syndromes or hypersensitization are not ideal surgical candidates. Of the operative strategies, triple neurectomy of the ilioinguinal, iliohypogastric, and genital branch of the genitofemoral nerve has been shown to be the best at a surgical cure. There have been a few small trials studying success rates for triple neurectomy, the largest looking at 225 patients. Of these, 80% reported resolution of pain, 15% had transient pain, and only 2 patients reported no improvement.

Tailored neurectomy could be beneficial as it is less morbid, leaving the patient with less sensory loss. Although tailored neurectomy has not been compared to triple neurectomy and has only been studied in small studies, it was found to provide complete pain relief in only 54% of patients, giving partial relief in 24% of patients and leaving 24% with no benefit.

Mesh explantation alone is not likely to be an effective strategy for the treatment of chronic postherniorrhaphy neuralia unless secondary nerve injury either by excessive scar formation over the mesh or nerve contact with the mesh not associated with entrapment or meshoma by imaging is suspected. No randomized controlled trials have compared triple neurectomy with and without mesh explantation, but if mesh removal alone does not relieve the pain, then proceeding with a third operation in the inguinal region may result in a very difficult dissection, an inability to identify all three nerves, and worsening pain.

5. **C.** Intentional ilioinguinal nerve division during herniorrhaphy has been postulated to decrease chronic groin pain. Its benefits have been studied in multiple randomized control trials. It is clear that operative division will decrease sensation along the distribution of the nerve (the groin and hemiscrotum). However, no statistically significant advantage at decreasing postherniorrhaphy neuralgia at 1-month, 6-month, and 1-year follow-ups has been shown in large studies and a meta-analysis of more than 1,200 patients.

6. **B.** The evaluation of postherniorrhaphy neuralgia involves a multifaceted approach. The assessment of a patient's risk of postoperative pain should be conducted during the preoperative visit. Several preoperative risk factors have been described for postherniorrhaphy neuralgia to include young age, female gender, high pain intensity level, lower preoperative optimism, impairment of everyday activities, and operation for a recurrent hernia. After the patient develops postoperative pain, a systematic approach to find the etiology of the patient's pain should be employed. This involves the characterization and localization of the pain, a physical examination for recurrence and inflammation, imaging for recurrence, imaging-guided nerve blocks, an evaluation for nerve ablation versus nerve stimulator, and, finally, neurectomy. Therapeutic nerve blocks have been repeated in multiple clinical trials with positive results in decreasing pain as well as bridging therapy to nerve ablation or neurectomy. The nerves within the region of the inguinal canal have been to found to vary significantly in course, advocating for the role of imaging for nerve blocks during the evaluation and treatment of postherniorrhaphy pain.

7. **B.** Ultrasound-guided nerve blocks, peripheral nerve stimulators, and dorsal root ganglion stimulators have all been found to improve

postherniorrhaphy neuralgia, occasionally eliminating the need for possible nerve ablation or neurectomy. Although it is generally accepted that attempted identification of nerves within the inguinal canal should be performed during inguinal herniorrhaphy in an effort to protect them, evidence has been presented by Bischoff et al. that there is no difference in the risk of pain-related impairment with identification of these nerves. There is more data on the success of peripheral nerve stimulators and thus they should be considered next in the algorithm for chronic pain management after inguinal herniorrhaphy. Dorsal root ganglion stimulators have also shown some success in pain control after surgery, but fewer data have been seen for inguinal pain. Nerve ablation and then triple neurectomy are next in the line for treatment.

BIBLIOGRAPHY

Amid PK. Causes, prevention, and surgical treatment of postherniorrhaphy neuropathic inguinodynia triple neurectomy with proximal end implantation. *Hernia*. 2004 Dec;8(4):343–349.

Beauchamp RD, Evers BM, Mattox K, eds. Sabiston Text book of Surgery: The Biological Basis of Modern Surgical Practice. 19th ed. Elsevier Saunders; 2012: 1114–1140.

Bischoff J, Aasvang E, Kehlet H, Werner M. Does nerve identification during open inguinal herniorrhaphy reduce the risk of nerve damage and persistent pain? *Hernia*. 2012;16:573–577.

Bjurstrom MF, Nicol AL, Amid PK, Chen DC. Pain control following inguinal herniorrhaphy: Current perspectives. *J Pain Res*. 2014;7:277–290.

Franneby U, Sandblom G, Nordin P, Nyren O, Gunnarsson U. Risk factors for long-term pain after hernia surgery. *Ann Surg*. 2006;244:212.

Hakeem A, Shanmugam V. Current trends in diagnosis and management of post-herniorrhaphy chronic groin pain. *World J Gast Surg*. 2011;3:73.

Hsu W, Chen CS, Lee HC, et al. Preservation versus division of ilioinguinal nerve on open mesh repair of inguinal hernia: a meta-analysis of randomized controlled trials. *World J Surg*. 2012 Oct;36(10):2311–2319.

Kehlet H, Jensen TS, Woolf CJ. Persistent postsurgical pain: risk factors and prevention. *Lancet*. 2006;367:1618.

Liem L, Mekhail N. Management of postherniorrhaphy chronic neuropathic groin pain: a role for dorsal root ganglion stimulation. *Pain Pract*. 2016;16:915–923.

Malangoni MA, Gagliani RJ. Hernias. In: Townsend CM, Beauchamp RD, Evers BM, Mattox K, eds. Sabiston Textbook of Surgery: The Biological Basis of Modern Surgical Practice. 19th ed. Philadelphia, PA: Elsevier Saunders; 2012: 1114–1140.

Picchio M, Palimento D, Attanasio U, Matarazzo PF, Bambini C, Caliendo A. Randomized controlled trial of preservation or elective division of ilioinguinal nerve on open inguinal hernia repair with polypropylene mesh. *Arch Surg*. 2004;Jul;139(7):755–758.

Poobalan AS, Bruce J, King PM, Chambers WA, Krukowski ZH, Smith WC. Chronic pain and quality of life following open inguinal hernia repair. *Br J Surg*. 2001;88:1122.

Rab M, Ebmer AJ, Deloon AL. Anatomic variability of the ilioinguinal and genitofemoral nerve: implications for the treatment of groin pain. *Plast Reconstr Surg*. 2001;108: 1618–1623.

Reinpold WM, Nehis J, Eggert A. Nerve management and chronic pain after open inguinal hernia repair: a prospective two phase study. *Ann Surg*. 2011;254:163.

Verhagen T, Loos M, Cheltinga M, et al. The GroinPain Trial: a randomized controlled trial of injection therapy versus neurectomy for postherniorrhaphy inguinal neuralgia. *Ann Surg*. 2018;267:841–845.

Voorbrood CE, Burgmans JP, Van Dalen T, et al. An algorithm for assessment and treatment of postherniorrhaphy pain. *Hernia*. 2015;19:571–577.

19

Hiatal and Paraesophageal Hernia

Geoffrey S. Chow

A 58-year-old female presents with a long-standing history of gastroesophageal reflux disease (GERD). She takes a proton pump inhibitor (PPI) twice daily and complains of increasing regurgitation over the past 6 months. She has a history of diabetes mellitus, morbid obesity, and hypertension. She denies alcohol use, currently smokes 1/2 pack of cigarettes per day, and is independent for all activities of daily living. She is otherwise in good health with no other problems. Her vitals are normal, body mass index (BMI) is 39 kg/m^2, and physical exam is normal.

1. **What is the most likely cause of her symptoms?**
   A. Gastroparesis
   B. Esophageal cancer
   C. Gastric ulcers
   D. Hiatal hernia
   E. Obesity

2. **What should be the next appropriate test?**
   A. Chest x-ray
   B. Esophageal manometry
   C. Endoscopy
   D. 24-hour pH monitoring
   E. Computed tomography (CT) scan of chest, abdomen, and pelvis

3. **What is the most common type of hiatal hernia?**
   A. Type I
   B. Type II
   C. Type III
   D. Type IV

4. **Regarding the formation of hiatal hernias, which etiology is most common?**
   A. Congenitally acquired
   B. Have no familial hereditary pattern
   C. Secondary to blunt abdominal trauma
   D. Weakening of the phrenoesophageal ligament

5. **What is the next best step in the management of this patient?**
   A. Laparoscopic Roux-en-Y-gastric bypass
   B. Smoking cessation, weight loss
   C. Laparoscopic hiatal hernia repair
   D. Increase PPI dose

6. **The patient subsequently underwent an uneventful diaphragm repair and a Nissen fundoplication. Two years' postoperative, the patient presents with recurrent heartburn and regurgitation. On evaluation, it is noted that the Nissen fundoplication is slipped. What is the best alternative at this point?**
   A. Collis gastroplasty
   B. Ivor-Lewis esophagectomy
   C. Roux-En-Y gastric bypass
   D. Esophagomyotomy

7. **After reduction of the hernia sac at the time of surgery, there is a large diaphragmatic defect with stiff musculature. The crura are unable to be approximated with suture. Which is the next best step at this point?**
   A. Collis gastroplasty
   B. Truncal vagotomy

C. Diaphragmatic relaxing incision

D. Bridged hiatal repair with permanent mesh

ANSWERS

1. D. Hiatal hernias are common, with up to 60% of the population having such hernias. Approximately 10% are truly asymptomatic. Regurgitation and heartburn may be the only presenting symptoms, although some patients will have cardiac and pulmonary symptoms. Esophageal cancer must be on the differential diagnosis with anyone presenting with regurgitation, GERD, and dysphagia or weight loss. Gastric ulcers are associated with GERD but will usually present with abdominal pain. Diabetic neuropathy can affect the intestinal tract and can cause gastroparesis. Patients with this condition can have regurgitation, abdominal fullness, and pain. This patient has no other symptoms consistent with diabetic peripheral neuropathy. Obesity is a risk factor for GERD, but the most common cause in this patient is likely a hiatal hernia.

2. C. Endoscopy is essential to the evaluation of patients presenting with GERD; to evaluate for esophagitis, Barrett's esophagus, and hiatal hernia; and to rule out maligancy. Esophageal manometry evaluates esophageal motility and is essential for the diagnosis of named esophageal motility disorders. Twenty-four-hour pH monitoring is the gold standard for diagnosing and quantifying acid reflux. Impedance pH can also be performed to discern the difference between nonacid and acidic reflux. The use of either a CT scan or a swallow study can be used for evaluation of the esophagus and stomach and may be beneficial for preoperative evaluation and planning.

3. A. Type I (sliding) hernia: Upward herniation of the cardia in the posterior mediastinum, the gastroesophageal (GE) junction migrates above the diaphragm. Type I are the most common and account for 90% of hiatal hernias.

Type II (paraesophageal) hernia: The GE junction remains in the normal anatomical position, and the fundus herniates through the hiatus.

Type III (mixed) hernia: Characterized by an upward herniation of both the GE junction and the gastric fundus.

Type IV hiatal hernia: An additional organ, most commonly the omentum or colon, herniates as well. The spleen, pancreas, and small bowel may be herniated.

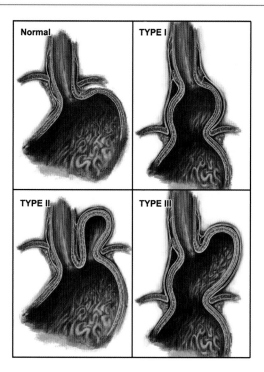

4. D. Cephalad migration of the gastroesophageal junction may result from a weakening of the phrenoesophageal ligament. A depletion of elastin fibers leads to stretching of the ligament and cephalad displacement of the gastroesophageal junction. Most cases of hiatal hernia are acquired and not congenital. A small number of cases of familial hiatal hernias have been shown. Bochdalek hernias are congenital hernias involving the right posterior diaphragm usually found in children. Morgagni hernias are also congenital and seen in the anterior portion of the diaphragm. Traumatic diaphragmatic hernias are often secondary to rupture at a site separate from the hiatus or from penetrating transdiaphragmatic injury and have a lower incidence than hiatal hernias.

5. B. Smoking cessation and weight loss should be considered as part of a quality initiative to optimize the health and outcome of surgical patients. Twice-daily PPI therapy can decrease heartburn and reflux symptoms in patients who have ongoing symptoms on once-daily therapy. In patients who have continued reflux on twice daily therapy, you should confirm that patients are taking PPI therapy on an empty stomach before meals. Trial of a dual release PPI formulation may also improve patient symptoms. Laparoscopic hiatal hernia repair concurrent with an anti-reflux procedure can alleviate reflux symptoms and critical steps of the operation include reduction of the hernia, reduction of the hernia sac, restoration of intra-abdominal esophageal length, closure of the diaphragmatic defect, and performance of an antireflux operation. Roux-en-Y gastric bypass is a surgical option for patients with morbid obesity who are interested surgical weight loss as part of a multidisciplinary program. Additionally, it is considered a better surgical option for patients with a BMI >35 kg/m^2 than a fundoplication since obesity is a risk factor for GERD.

6. **D.** A patient with morbid obesity and a failed fundoplication can benefit from a Roux-en-Y gastric bypass. Kim et al. showed that at 11 months, 93.3% of patients were symptom-free. A Collis gastroplasty is used as a lengthening procedure in patients with a short esophagus and can be performed in open, laparoscopic, or thoracosopic approach. A wedge fundectomy technique can be employed when using a minimally invasive abdominal approach. Esophagectomy has no role in the revision of slipped fundoplication. Esophagomyotomy is used to treat achalasia and are relieve the associated symptoms of chest pain and dysphagia. A slipped fundoplication occurs when there is a migration of the wrap into the chest, onto the stomach, or when the body of the stomach is used to perform the wrap. These mechanical failures can be identified on upper gastrointestinal contrast study. This is different from a recurrence where the stomach reherniates into the chest.

7. **C.** A Collis gastroplasty, as described in the previous answer, has no benefit in treating patients with a large esophageal hiatus. A truncal vagotomy can be performed in patients with refractory ulcer disease and has been done to allow great mobility of the esophagus to assist with reflux control in conjunction with a fundoplication. If this is performed with a primary anti-reflux operation, patients may present with symptoms of gastroparesis. Permanent mesh should be avoided at the esophageal hiatus due to risks of dysphagia and mesh erosion into the esophagus. Bridged repairs should be avoided due to a risk of recurrent reflux and mesh-related complications. A diaphgramatic relaxing incision can decrease the radial tension at the hiatus and allow for primary closure around the esophagus. Strong consideration Strong consideration should be given to use mesh reinforcement over both the relaxing incision and the diaphragmatic closure around the esophageal hiatus.

BIBLIOGRAPHY

Alam U, Asghar O, Malik RA. Diabetic gastroparesis: therapeutic options. *Diabetes Ther.* August 2010;1(1):32–43.

Baglaj SM, Noblett HR. Paraoesophageal hernia in children: familial occurrence and review of the literature. *Pediatr Surg Int.* 1999;15:85–87.

Curci JA, Melman LM, Thompson RW, Soper NJ, Matthews BD. Elastic fiber depletion in the supporting ligaments of the gastroesophageal junction: a structural basis for the development of hiatal hernia. *J Am Coll Surg.* 2008;207:191–196.

Hawn MT, Houston TK, Campagna EJ, Graham LA, Singh J, Bishop M, Henderson WG. The attributable risk of smoking on surgical complications. *Ann Surg.* 2011;254(6):914–920.

Kahrilas PJ, Bredenoord AJ, Fox M, Gyawali CP, Roman S, Smout AJ, Pandolfino JE. International High Resolution Manometry Working Group. The Chicago Classification of esophageal motility disorders, v3.0. *Neurogastroenterol Motil.* 2015 Feb;27(2):160–174.

Kim M, Navarro F, Eruchalu CN, Augenstein VA, Heniford BT, Stefanidis D. Minimally invasive Roux-en-Y gastric bypass for fundoplication failure offers excellent gastroesophageal reflux control. *Am Surg.* July 2014;80(7):696–703.

Kohn GP, Price RR, DeMeester SR, Zehetner J, Muensterer OJ, Awad Z, et al. Guidelines for the management of hiatal hernia. SAGES Guidelines Committee. *Surg Endosc.* Dec;2013;27(12):4409–4428.

Maish MS. Esophagus. In: Townsend CM, Beauchamp RD, Evers BM, Mattox K, eds. *Sabiston Textbook of Surgery: The Biological Basis of Modern Surgical Practice.* 19th ed. Elsevier Saunders; 2012;1012–1066.

Patti MG, Fisichella PM, Perretta S, et al. Impact of minimally invasive surgery on the treatment of esophageal achalasia: a decade of change. *J Am Coll Surg.* 2003;196:698–705.

Petersen RP, Pellegrani CA, Oelschlager BK. Hiatal hernia and gastroesophageal reflux disease. In: Townsend CM, Beauchamp RD, Evers BM, Mattox K, eds. *Sabiston Textbook of Surgery: The Biological Basis of Modern Surgical Practice.* 19th ed. Philadelphia, PA: Elsevier Saunders; 2012:1067–1086.

Stylopoulos N, Gazelle GS, Rattner DW. Paraesophageal hernias: operation or observation? *Ann Surg.* 2002;236(4),492–501.

Ward MA, DeMeester SR. Diaphragmatic Relaxing Incisions for Crural Tension During Hiatal Hernia Repair. Yeo CJ, ed. *Shackelford's Surgery of the Alimentary Tract.* 8th ed. Elsevier; 2019;301–304.

20

Achalasia

Mary T. O'Donnell, E. Matthew Ritter, and James A. McClintic

A 50-year-old female is referred to your clinic by their primary care provider with a chief complaint of progressive difficulty swallowing some solids and occasionally liquids. She reports this has been worsening for the last 5 months and is associated with chest discomfort and regurgitation of undigested food. She also notes a 10-kg weight loss over the last 2 months. She has been treated with daily omeprazole, but this does not seem to be improving her symptoms. She appears healthy and her vital signs are normal.

1. **Of the listed studies, which is the most appropriate initial study to narrow the differential diagnosis of this patient's dysphagia?**

   A. Contrast esophagram
   B. Endoscopic esophageal ultrasound
   C. Computed tomography (CT) chest scan with contrast
   D. *H. pylori* testing
   E. Chest x-ray

2. **A contrast esophagram is shown to the right. What additional study or studies should be ordered to workup this patient?**

   A. Esophageal manometry
   B. Esophagogastroduodenoscopy (EGD)
   C. 24-hour pH monitoring
   D. 24-hour pH monitoring and EGD
   E. Esophageal manometry and EGD

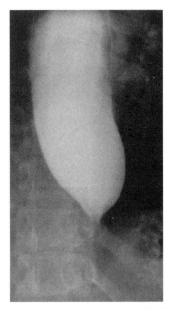

Barium esophagogram showing a markedly dilated esophagus and characteristic "bird's beak" in achalasia. (Reproduced with permission from Waters PF, DeMeester TR: Foregut motor disorders and their surgical management, Med Clin North Am. 1981 Nov;65(6):1235-1268.)

3. **Upper endoscopy reveals no evidence of esophagitis, diverticulum, or lesion. Some food is present in a dilated distal esophagus. The food is suctioned with no underlying lesion noted. Manometry shows aperistalsis and a nonrelaxing lower esophageal sphincter (LES). Which initial treatment offers the patient the most durable relief of symptoms?**

A. Pneumatic dilation of the LES
B. Calcium channel blocker therapy
C. Esophageal myotomy with fundoplication
D. Botulinum toxin injection at the LES
E. Esophagectomy

4. **Suppose in the same patient's esophageal manometry shows 10/10 normal propagated swallows with a mean distal esophageal amplitude pressure of 293 mmHg. The LES relaxes completely. The results of ambulatory pH monitoring and EGD were both normal. What is the most likely diagnosis?**

A. Achalasia
B. Pseudoachalsia
C. Diffuse esophageal spasm
D. Nutcracker esophagus
E. Esophageal stricture

5. **The patient with achalasia underwent thoracoscopic Heller myotomy and presented postoperatively with resolved dysphagia but persistent heartburn with a 24-hour pH test demonstrating a pH <4 time of 12% with 157 reflux events. What would have been the best option to prevent this while treating the patient's achalasia.**

A. Laparoscopic approach, avoiding thoracoscopy
B. Nissen fundoplication after myotomy
C. Toupet fundoplication after myotomy
D. Peroral endoscopic myotomy
E. Pyloroplasty after myotomy

6. **The patient undergoes appropriate treatment with resolution of symptoms at a 2-year follow-up. She does not follow up until 13 years later. She reports progressive dysphagia, 20-kg weight loss in the last 6 months, and appears malnourished. She reports a cough at night, and she was recently treated in the hospital for pneumonia, and hilar adenopathy was noted on a chest x-ray. What is the most appropriate next step in management of this patient?**

A. Transfer to the hospital for antibiotic therapy
B. Esophageal manometry
C. Placement of jejunostomy feeding tube
D. Esophagogastroduodenoscopy
E. CT chest scan with oral (PO) contrast

ANSWERS

1. A. Contrast esophagram is a useful initial diagnostic tool to narrow the differential diagnosis of a patient with dysphagia. The esophagram shown demonstrates the characteristic bird's beak appearance of achalasia and rules out diverticula and hiatal hernia. It may also demonstrate other pathology such as a mass or Schatzki's ring/stricture.

2. E. This esophagram is consistent with achalasia, and esophageal manometry is the gold standard to diagnose esophageal motility disorders; however, a neoplasm or stricture must be ruled out with an esophagogastroduodenoscopy (EGD). An EGD would also document any evidence of Barrett's esophagus, ulceration, or eosinophilic esophagitis. If there are sequelae of reflux seen on EGD, a 24-hour pH study could confirm the presence of functional reflux disease.

Differential Diagnosis	Confirmatory Test
Esophageal perforation	Esophagram
Diverticulae	EGD
Hiatal hernia	
Neoplasm	
Eosinophilic esophagitis	
Barrett's esophagus	
Schatzki's ring/stricture	
Esophageal ulcer	
Typical reflux	24-hr pH monitoring
Atypical reflux	Esophageal impedance
Biliary reflux	
Achalasia	Manometry
Diffuse esophageal spasm	
Nutcracker esophagus	
Connective tissue disorder	

3. C. This patient has achalasia. In the absence of an obstructing entity (neoplasm, hiatal hernia, diverticula, stricture) retained food in the esophagus is suspicious for achalasia. The diagnosis is confirmed by manometry. In patients with classic achalasia, manometry demonstrates an esophagus in which there is a complete absence of peristalsis and an LES pressure that is normal to moderately elevated but fails to completely relax. Although a hypertensive

LES and an LES that fails to completely relax are often associated with achalasia, only the complete absence of peristalsis is required for the diagnosis. The pathophysiology of achalasia is not fully understood but involves the loss of ganglion cells in the myenteric plexus and interruption of inhibitory vagal nerve innervation.

The treatment for achalasia requires relaxing the hypertensive smooth muscles of the LES. This can be done surgically by dividing the muscles of the LES and endoscopically by injecting botulinum toxin or balloon dilating the LES. Surgical treatment with myotomy (laparoscopic, thorascopic, or open) provides long-term treatment of achalasia, with a high success rate reported at 95% at 5 years and 75% at a mean of 15.8 years. This is accompanied by partial fundoplication to reduce subsequent reflux. Calcium channel blockers have shown inconsistent success and do not have a role in achalasia treatment. Botulinum toxin requires repeated interventions every 6–12 months, as does dilation. Some studies have shown similar outcomes at two years between repeated pneumatic dilation and myotomy. Repeated pneumatic dilation comes with a higher risk of perforation at 4% compared to 1% and mortality of 0.5% compared to 0.2% with myotomy. Botulinum and pneumatic dilation may be good options in persons who are poor operative candidates or in those who refuse surgery.

Esophagectomy may be required in the setting of some cancers, sigmoid esophagus, megaesophagus, or in the setting of persistent symptoms after two myotomies. The POEM, or per oral endoscopic myotomy, technique involves dividing the LES muscle endoscopically. This has the advantage of avoiding most surgical risks. The long-term success rate, however, is unknown and is not yet considered the equivalent of a surgical myotomy.

4. **D.** Manometry is used to rule out esophageal motility disorders by measuring the pressure along the esophagus and LES. The normal pressure of the LES is 10 to 15 mmHg. Patients with GERD will often have a hypotensive LES with a pressure of around 5 to 8 mmHg and normal to moderately abnormal peristalsis. The low LES pressure allows gastric contents to reflux back into the esophagus.

Twenty-four-hour ambulatory manometry can be used to diagnose spastic disorders such as diffuse esophageal spasm (DES), nutcracker esophagus,

or hypercontractile esophageal motility disorder. Nutcracker esophagus is characterized by very high LES pressures (>50 mmHg) during swallowing with otherwise normal peristalsis. DES would be characterized by high pressures throughout the esophagus (25–50 mmHg) and poor peristalsis. Psuedoachalasia would show a slightly hypertensive but relaxing LES and abnormal but not absent peristalsis. Connective tissue disorders, such as scleroderma, would demonstrate poor peristalsis and a normal LES.

5. **C.** This patient is presenting with acid reflux after myotomy without fundoplication. A laparoscopic approach over a thorascopic approach would allow for easier performance of fundoplication but would not prevent reflux by itself. Although a Nissen fundoplication has been shown to have acceptable post myotomy reflux rates, it has significantly higher rate of persistent dysphagia when compared to Dor fundoplication during a randomized trial. A recent randomized trial comparing Dor and Toupet fundoplication show similar long-term outcomes with acceptable rates of post op reflux and dysphagia. There are not long-term data for the efficacy of POEM and it does not include an antireflux procedure. There are no data to support a pyloroplasty after myotomy and it may lead to biliary reflux.

6. **D.** This patient presents with symptoms concerning for esophageal cancer. Patients with achalasia even after therapy have an 8% risk of developing cancer over a 20-year period. The most common being squamous cell carcinoma followed by adenocarcinoma. There is also concern for recurrent achalasia. The best next step would be EGD with biopsy. If cancer was found, a CT chest and abdomen scan with PO and IV contrast would be indicated for staging followed by esophageal ultrasound if no sign of M1 disease. Any metastatic disease should be biopsied. Appropriate surgical versus medical therapy would then be performed. A feeding jejunostomy would be considered in this patient after a diagnosis of cancer was confirmed.

If no sign of lesion or mass is noted on EGD, then manometry could be performed to assess for recurrent achalasia. If recurrent achalasia is found, then repeat myotomy could be performed after nutritional optimization. If the patient is a poor surgical candidate pneumatic dilation could be considered. If the patient has progressed to having a megaesophagus, then an esophagectomy could be considered if the patient could be medically optimized. There no widely accepted screening guidelines for patients with achalasia, but their increased risk for recurrence and esophageal cancer warrants consideration.

BIBLIOGRAPHY

Ajani J, D'Amico T. NCCN Guidelines Version 4.2019 Esophageal and Esophagogastric Junction Cancers. August 14, 2020. Accessed August 15, 2020. https://www.nccn.org/professionals/physician_gls/pdf/esophageal.pdf

Castell DO, Diederich L, Castell JA. *Esophageal Motility and pH Testing, Technique and Interpretation.* 3rd ed. Sandhill Scientific, Inc.; 2000.

Csendes A, Braghetto I, Burdiles P, Korn O, Csendes P, Henriquez A. Very late results of esophagomyotomy for patients with achalasia: clinical, endoscopic, histologic, manometric, and acid reflux studies in 67 patients for a mean follow-up of 190 months. *Ann Surg.* 2006;243:196–203.

Csendes A, Braghetto I, Henriquez A, Cortes C. Late results of a prospective randomised study comparing forceful dilatation and oesophagomyotomy in patients with achalasia. *Gut.* 1989;30:299–304.

O'Neill OM, Johnston, BT, Coleman HG. Achalasia: a review of clinical diagnosis, epidemiology, treatment and outcomes. *World J Gastroenterol.* 2013;19(35):5806–5812. https://doi.org/10.3748/wjg.v19.i35.5806

Society of American Gastrointestinal and Endoscopic Surgeons (SAGES). Guidelines for the Surgical Treatment of Esophageal Achalasia. May 2011. Accessed June 2014. http://www.sages.org/publications/guidelines/guidelines-for-the-surgical-treatment-of-esophageal-achalasia/

Stefanidis, D, et al. *Guidelines for the Surgical Treatment of Esophageal Achalasia.* Society of American Gastrointestinal and Endoscopic Surgeons (SAGES); May 2011.

Torres-Villalobos G, Coss-Adame E, Furuzawa-Carballeda J, et al. Dor Vs Toupet fundoplication after laparoscopic Heller myotomy: long-term randomized controlled trial evaluated by high-resolution manometry. *J Gastrointest Surg.* 2018;22(1):13–22. https://doi.org/10.1007/s11605-017-3578-8

Tutuian R, Castell DO. Review article: esophageal spasm—diagnosis and management. *Aliment Pharmacol Ther.* 2006;23(10):1393–1402.

21

Gastric Cancer

Brian J. Pottorf and Farah A. Husain

A 68-year-old male with a history of hypertension and hypercholesterolemia presents to his primary care physician's office with a chief complaint of worsening epigastric pain and weakness. The pain is improved with oral intake, especially milk-based products. The patient has been treating his pain with naproxen. In the office, the patient is nontoxic with normal vital signs. His physical examination reveals mild epigastric tenderness with deep palpation. His serum hemoglobin was 8.3 g/dL. Fecal occult blood testing was positive. The patient underwent colonoscopy, which was normal. Esophagogastroduodenoscopy (EGD) revealed a 2.5-cm ulcerated lesion with elevated, irregular borders 5 cm distal to the gastroesophageal junction.

1. **The appropriate management of the ulcer includes which of the following?**
   A. Observation
   B. Cessation of naproxen and begin sucralfate and a proton pump inhibitor with repeat EGD in 3 months
   C. Biopsy the ulcer
   D. Proximal gastrectomy
   E. Total gastrectomy

2. **Final pathology reveals a poorly differentiated adenocarcinoma. Which is the most sensitive preoperative examination to determine T and N stage?**
   A. Positron emission tomography (PET) scan
   B. Endoscopic ultrasound (EUS)
   C. Magnetic resonance imaging (MRI) with gadolinium

   D. Diagnostic laparoscopy
   E. Triple-phase helical computed tomography (CT) scan

3. **The EUS suggests a T3N0 lesion. Which would be the most appropriate next step?**
   A. Neoadjuvant therapy
   B. Proximal gastrectomy with negative margins (R0) only
   C. Total gastrectomy
   D. Total gastrectomy with splenectomy and distal pancreatectomy
   E. Esophagogastrectomy with colonic interposition graft

4. **Following neoadjuvant therapy, a total gastrectomy is performed. The final pathology revealed a T4N1 lesion with negative margins. Which should the patient next receive?**
   A. No additional therapy
   B. Imatinib
   C. External-beam radiation only
   D. Fluorouracil-based chemotherapy only
   E. External-beam radiation and fluorouracil-based chemotherapy

5. **Which of the following describes the association between Irish's node and gastric cancer?**
   A. An anterior mass palpable on digital rectal examination
   B. A metastatic left supraclavicular lymph node
   C. An ovarian mass from metastatic tumor
   D. Metastatic left axillary lymph node

E. Umbilical mass suggestive of metastatic gastric cancer

6. **As part of the workup for the same patient, imagine that the tumor was found in the midbody of the gastric antrum and that a staging CT scan was performed revealing a lesion in segment 2 of the liver without evidence of carcinomatosis. The lesion was biopsied and positive for metastatic disease of gastric origin. Which tumor marker will affect management and potentially increase patient survival?**

   A. EGFR1
   B. VEGF
   C. HER2
   D. HGF/c-Met
   E. FGFR2

7. **The patient is now diagnosed with Stage IV disease. Which is the most accurate statement regarding his treatment approach?**

   A. Palliative chemotherapy should be the only treatment offered.
   B. Cytoreductive surgery with hyperthermic intraperitoneal effusion chemotherapy is the gold standard treatment.
   C. Palliative gastrectomy alone should be offered to ameliorate symptoms.
   D. A bypass procedure is the operation of choice to avoid a gastric outlet obstruction.
   E. Chemotherapy in addition to partial gastrectomy and hepatic metastatectomy if diagnostic laparoscopy confirms no carcinomatosis.

ANSWERS

1. **C.** Historically, a biopsy of gastric ulcers was a uniform practice throughout medical and surgical disciplines because there was a 5–11% attendant risk of malignancy. However, data now suggest that the incidence of gastric cancer is decreasing, thereby rendering mandatory biopsy of all gastric ulcers unnecessary. When gastric ulcers have features suggestive of malignancy, such as elevated irregular folds, association with a polypoid or fungated mass, and abnormal adjacent mucosal folds, then a biopsy is warranted (Figure 21-1). Several biopsies, typically six or more, are necessary to minimize the false-negative risk. If benign ulcers are diagnosed, then EGD is repeated in 6 weeks to ensure resolution. All ulcers should be followed and biopsied until complete resolution occurs. If malignancy is detected, then further workup with potential operative intervention is pursued.

Ulcers with a diameter of 3 cm or greater are termed *giant gastric ulcers* (Figure 21-2). These large ulcers harbor an underlying malignancy in 30% of lesions. Given the higher incidence of malignancy, perforation, and bleeding surgical treatment is warranted.

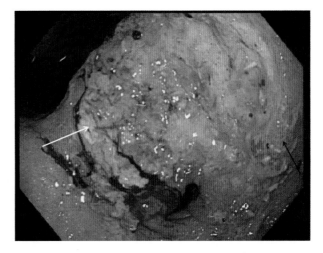

Figure 21-1 Endoscopic view of an ulcerated fungating gastric mass (white arrow) with irregular mucosal folds (black arrow).

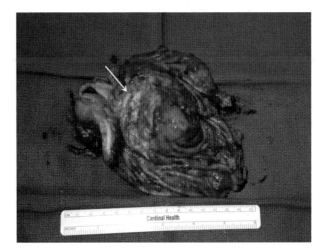

Figure 21-2 *Ex vivo* surgical specimen containing giant gastric ulcer (white arrow). Note the ulcerated, necrotic center with irregular circumferential mucosal folds. Final pathology revealed a poorly differentiated adenocarcinoma.

2. **B.** EUS is important in preoperative locoregional staging for gastric cancer. It is currently the best imaging modality for assessing both tumor depth and nodal invasion. A spatial resolution of 0.1 mm can be achieved with EUS. T-staging accuracy ranges from 60–90%, whereas N-staging accuracy ranges from 50% to 80%. EUS is better at identifying T1 (80%) and T3 (90%) lesions as opposed to T2 (38.5%). EUS is not reliable for delineating between individual benign and malignant lymph nodes. Increasing T stage directly correlates with increased risk of nodal and distant metastasis (>80% likelihood of nodal metastasis in T3 disease versus <5% in stage T1 m).

CT remains an important preoperative tool to evaluate for metastatic disease. If metastatic disease is present, an unnecessary operation can be avoided. T-staging accuracy with CT approaches 80% (66–77%). N stage determination is variable with a wide range of 25–86%. Small gastric tumors and metastases smaller than 5 mm can be missed on CT scans. CT, MRI, and PET scanning show promise for preoperative staging but have yet to become standard of care.

Routine diagnostic laparoscopy to minimize unnecessary operations has become a less popular preresection strategy. However, diagnostic laparoscopy still has a role in advanced gastric cancer. Power et al., in 2009, evaluated patients with known gastric cancer without obvious metastatic disease and stratified them into low-risk (T1–2, N0) and high-risk (T3–4, N+, or both) groups based on EUS. Both groups underwent diagnostic laparoscopy, which identified M1 disease in 20.5% of the high-risk patients and 4% of the low-risk patients. The study concluded that laparoscopy can be avoided in patients by using EUS to identify early-stage cancer, whereas more advanced gastric cancers would benefit from diagnostic laparoscopy to rule out occult metastatic disease. When diagnostic laparoscopy is performed, peritoneal lavage cytology should be obtained as positive results can alter further therapy. Diagnostic laparoscopy, however, does not address the T or N stage.

3. **A.** Although the patient will ultimately need an operation, the MAGIC trail demonstrates that the patient will benefit from neoadjuvant therapy instead of proceeding straight to the operating room, unless the patient is hemorrhaging from the mass resulting in hemodynamic instability. Neoadjuvant therapy consisting of epirubicin, cisplatin, and fluorouracil is recommended for patients with T2 lesions or higher.

The benefits of the preoperative therapy are to reduce the tumor's size and stage, eliminate micrometastases, improve tumor-related symptoms, and determine whether the tumor is sensitive to chemotherapy.

Gastric adenocarcinoma exists as two distinct entities: diffuse and intestinal types. Table 21-1 summarizes these distinct subtypes. Controversies surrounding the surgical management of gastric adenocarcinoma include the adequacy of surgical margins, the need for resection of adjacent structures (i.e., spleen and distal pancreas), and the extent of lymphadenectomy. Diffuse-type gastric adenocarcinoma spreads in the submucosa, thereby increasing the risk of microscopic residual positive margin (R1 resection). To minimize the risk of leaving microscopic disease or recurrence, a 5–6-cm margin is considered acceptable for an R0 resection. Newer studies emerging from Japan suggest that smaller proximal resection margins of 2–3 cm are adequate for T1 lesions. If the patient went straight to surgery, total gastrectomy is preferred as the tumor is within 5 cm of the gastroesophageal junction.

Table 21-1 SUMMARY COMPARING INTESTINAL AND DIFFUSE GASTRIC ADENOCARCINOMA

Characteristic	Intestinal	Diffuse
Age	Older	Younger
Gender	Male > Female	Male = Female
Metastatic route	Hematologic	Lymphatic, submucosal spread which can result in a thickened, non-distensible stomach known as linitis plasticans
Site of metastasis	Liver	Peritoneum
Risk factors	Atrophic gastritis, intestinal metaplasia, *Helicobacter pylori* infection, and diet high in salt, smoked, and preserved foods	CHD-1 mutation, obesity
Cellular etiology	Glandular gastric mucosa	Lamina propria
Prognosis	Better	Poor

Esophagogastrectomy is unnecessary when the gastroesophageal junction has no direct tumor involvement and surgical margins exceed 5 cm.

Assessing nodal disease at the time of operation can be difficult. A minimum of 15 lymph nodes is recommended for staging. Most surgeons tend to remove the perigastric lymph nodes (D1 resection). In countries such as Japan, where gastric cancer has a higher prevalence, a more aggressive D2 lymphadenectomy is frequently employed, harvesting lymph nodes along the celiac trunk and its named branches, the middle colic artery, the superior mesenteric artery, and the periaortic area. Several studies have demonstrated prolonged survival with the more aggressive (D2) lymphadenectomy. This is thought to be related to better locoregional disease control. A recent randomized trial comparing D1 versus D2 lymphadenectomy did not reveal a significant difference in long-term survival. Accordingly, more studies regarding the extent of lymphadenectomy are required before a long-term endorsement of this more aggressive strategy can be made.

Removal of adjacent structures (i.e., distal pancreas and spleen) confer no survival benefit and actually increase morbidity and mortality. Resection of these adjacent structures should be reserved for primary tumor invasion.

4. E. The final pathology revealed Stage III gastric cancer. Given the high rate of locoregional failure (40–70%) and a 5-year survival rate of 20–28%, adjuvant therapy is recommended. This recommendation originates from the Intergroup Trial 0116, which demonstrated a benefit for those patients with advanced gastric cancer undergoing curative resection combined with postoperative fluorouracil-based chemotherapy and radiation. The CLASSIC trial demonstrated survival advantages using an adjuvant chemotherapy therapy regimen of capecitabine and oxaliplatin.

Resection without adjuvant therapy resulted in decreased survival when compared with those who received postoperative chemoradiation. Palliation can be achieved with either external-beam radiation or chemotherapy, but local control and long-term survival are poor. Imatinib is a tyrosine-kinase inhibitor currently used for gastrointestinal stromal tumors and other malignancies.

5. D. In general, physical findings portend advanced disease. Patients are typically cachectic and jaundiced when nodal metastatic disease obstructs the common bile duct. *Irish's node* is an enlarged lymph node within the left axilla. A prerectal mass palpable on digital rectal examination is a Blumer's shelf suggestive of a drop metastasis. Virchow's node, also known as Troisier's sign, refers to carcinomatous involvement of the left supraclavicular lymph nodes at the junction of the thoracic duct with the subclavian vein. Krukenberg tumors are ovarian masses from metastatic gastric cancer. The Sister Mary Joseph node is a periumbilical nodule suggestive of carcinomatosis. It reflects tumor extension from the falciform ligament.

6. C. As discussed, adjuvant treatment of gastric adenocarcinoma with epirubicin-based chemotherapy regimens has increased overall survival and quality of life. Recent research has shown benefits in targeted biologic therapy. Trastuzumab is a monoclonal antibody to human epidermal growth factor receptor 2 (HER2) that confers overall survival benefit to patients with gastric tumors expressing HER2. The trastuzumab for gastric cancer (ToGA) trial demonstrated that the addition of trastuzumab to traditional chemotherapy regimens ought to be the new standard of care for patients with metastatic gastric cancer expressing HER2.

HER2 expression is often associated with a high-grade histology, tumor invasion, advanced staging, and overall poor prognosis. Expression is most commonly observed in intestinal histology (34%) as opposed to the diffuse type (6%). There is a higher incidence of HER2 expression with gastroesophageal junction tumors (32%) when compared to purely gastric cancers (18%).

Epidermal growth factor receptor 1 (EGFR) is overexpressed in of 60% of gastric cancer and is associated with advanced stage and poor prognosis. Cetuximab is a chimeric monoclonal antibody that targets EGFR and induces apoptosis. The EXPAND trial demonstrated no survival benefit when added to chemotherapy regimens. Moreover, more patients experienced adverse effects of the medication. Vascular endothelial growth factor (VEGF) is also overexpressed in 60% of gastric cancers. When present, gastric cancer is associated with an increased risk of recurrence, aggressiveness, and advanced stage at presentation. Bevacizumab is a humanized monoclonal antibody that targets VEGF receptors, which are responsible for the angioneogenesis in tumorigenesis. Although effective in the treatment of other malignancies, the AVAGAST trial failed to show any survival benefit with the addition of bevacizumab to a chemotherapy regimen. Hepatic growth factor is a ligand receptor that activates key oncogenic pathways that is encoded within the mesenchymal-epithelial transition factor (c-MET) oncogene. Overexpression is associated with poor prognosis and is seen in 4–10% of gastric cancers. Ornartuzumab is a monovalent, humanized anti-c-MET antibody. The METGastric study concluded that the addition of ornatuzumab to a chemotherapy regimen did not improve clinical benefits. Fibroblastic growth factor (FGF2) amplification has been reported in 9% of gastric cancer with a higher frequency seen in the histopathologic diffuse type. The SHINE study compared the effect of adding AZD4547, which selectively inhibits *FGF1*, *FGF2*, and *FGF3*, to paclitaxel for second-line chemotherapy. Unfortunately, no perceivable benefit was identified in the data.

Although not listed, the mammalian target of rifampin (mTOR) is an important tumorigenesis pathway that affects cell proliferation as well as apoptosis, protein translation, and angiogenesis. Everolimus is a serine-threonine kinase inhibitor that inhibits the PI3K/Akt/mTOR pathway. When studied within the GRANITE trial, its addition to chemotherapy failed to show any improvement in overall survival in patients with advanced disease.

7. **E.** Although treatment for gastric cancer has improved dramatically, early detection remains a problem. As a result, 40% of gastric cancers are diagnosed as Stage IV. Advanced uncurable disease can present as obvious metastatic disease, macroscopic peritoneal metastases, or nonvisible cytopathologic disease. In patients with obvious peritoneal carcinomatosis, gastrectomy is oftentimes avoided, and palliative chemotherapy is routinely administered. In those few patients who have cytology-positive disease, chemotherapy can be administered with repeat lavage of the abdomen to see if the patient converts to having no evidence of advanced disease on cytology. These patients may be operative candidates if testing is negative. Hyperthermic intraperitoneal chemotherapy (HIPEC) surgery is a controversial topic given the uncertainty of the data as well as

the high morbidity associated with the operation. More promising studies from a minimally invasive approach with HIPEC are underway and inconclusive currently. A bypass of a tumor can be applicable when it causes gastric outlet obstruction. However, studies have shown that palliative gastrectomy for symptomatic tumors (obstruction, hematemesis, pain, etc.) is an acceptable treatment for patients with advanced disease. Quality of life is improved, and morbidity and mortality are comparable to curative operations. Case series from multiple institutions examined combined chemotherapy, gastrectomy with hepatic metastectomy suggested improved overall survival when compared to palliative gastrectomy alone. Studies have suggested a 5-year survival rate of 25% when using a combined approach in an appropriate candidate. The Japanese Gastric Cancer Treatment Guidelines committee concluded that a solitary lesion, a lack of other non-curative markers, and favorable T and N staging from the primary tumor portend to an overall better long-term prognosis. Studies are currently looking at the role of radiofrequency ablation for patients with a "small number" of metastatic lesions and 5-year survival rates of 30% have been reported. This is an evolving area of gastric cancer management and additional studies are underway and still needed.

REFERENCES

Al-Refaie WB, Abdalla EK, Ahmad SA, Mansfield PF. Gastric Cancer. In: Fieg BW, Berger DH, Fuhrman GM, eds. *The M D Anderson Surgical Oncology Handbook*. 4th ed. Lippincott Williams & Wilkins; 2006:205–240.

Arrington AK, Nelson R, Patel SS, et al. Timing of chemotherapy and survival in patients with resectable gastric adenocarcinoma. *WJGNET*. 2013;5:321–328.

Bang YJ, Kim YW, Yang HK, et al. Adjuvant capecitabine and oxaliplatin for gastric cancer after D2 gastrectomy (CLASSIC): a phase 3 open-label, randomised controlled trial. *Lancet*. 2012;379:315–321.

Bilici A. Treatment options in patients with metastatic gastric cancer: current status and future perspectives. *World J Gastroenterol*. 2014;40(6):692–700.

Committee ASoP, Banerjee S, Cash BD, et al. The role of endoscopy in the management of patients with peptic ulcer disease. *Gastrointest Endosc*. 2010;71:663–668.

De Angelis C, Pellicano R, Manfre SF, Rizzetto M. Endoscopic ultrasound in the 2013 preoperative evaluation of gastric cancer. *Minerva Gastroenterol Dietol*. 2013;59:1–12.

Degiuli M, Sasako M, Ponti A, et al. Randomized clinical trial comparing survival after D1 or D2 gastrectomy for gastric cancer. *BJS*. 2014;101:23–31.

Joensuu H, Eriksson M, Hall KS, et al. One versus three years of adjuvant imatinib for operable gastrointestinal stromal tumor: a randomized trial. *JAMA*. 2012;307:1265–1272.

Kodera Y. Surgery with curative intent for Stage IV gastric cancer: is it a reality of illusion? *Ann Gastroenterol Surg*. 2018;2(5):339–347.

Kodera Y, Fujitani K, Fukushima N, et al. Surgical resection of liver metastasis from gastric cancer: a reviewer and new recommendation in the Japanese Gastric Cancer Treatment Guidelines. *Gastric Cancer*. 2014;17:206–212.

Lasithiotakis K, Antoniou SA, Antoniou GA, et al. Gastrectomy for Stage IV gastric cancer: a systematic review and meta-analysis. *Anticancer Res*. 2014;34(5):2079–2085.

Macdonald JS, Smalley SR, Benedetti J, et al. Chemoradiotherapy after surgery compared with surgery alone for adenocarcinoma of the stomach or gastroesophageal junction. *NEJM*. 2001;345:725–730.

McLoughlin JM. Adenocarcinoma of the stomach: a review. *Proceedings*. 2004;17:391–399.

Naeem AN, Mufeed S, Makary MA. The Stomach. In: Cameron JL, Cameron AM, eds. *Current Surgical Therapy*. 10th ed. Elsevier; 2011:63–92.

Pavlidis TE, Pavlidis ET, Sakantamis AK. The role of laparoscopic surgery in gastric cancer. *JMAS*. 2012;8:35–38.

Power DG, Schattner MA, Gerdes H, et al. Endoscopic ultrasound can improve the selection for laparoscopy in patients with localized gastric cancer. *J Am Coll of Surg*. 2009;208:173–178.

Schulte N, Ebert MP, Härtel N. Gastric cancer: new drugs – new strategies. *Gastrointest Tumors*. 2014;1(4):180–194.

Shah MA, Bang YJ, Lordick F, et al. Effect of fluorouracil, leucovorin, and oxaliplatin with or without ornartuzumab in HER2-negative MET-positive gastroesophageal adenocarcinoma. *JAMA Oncol*. 2017;3(5):620–627.

Shin D, Park SS. Clinical importance and surgical decision-making regarding proximal resection margin for gastric cancer. *WJGO*. 2013;5:4–11.

Stolte M, Seitter V, Muller H. Improvement in the quality of the endoscopic/bioptic diagnosis of gastric ulcers between 1990 and 1997—An analysis of 1,658 patients. *Zeitschrift fur Gastroenterologie*. 2001;39:349–355.

Sun J, Song Y, Wang Z, et al. Clinical significance of palliative gastrectomy on the survival of patients with incurable advanced gastric cancer: a systematic review and meta-analysis. *BMC Cancer*. 2013;13:577.

Van Cutsem E, Bang YJ, Mansoor W, et al. A randomized, open-label study of the efficacy and safety of AZD4547 monotherapy versus paclitaxel for the treatment of advanced gastric adenocarcinoma with FGFR2 polysomy or gene amplification. *Ann Oncol*. 2017;28(6)1316–1324.

Wu CW, Hsiung CA, Lo SS, et al. Nodal dissection for patients with gastric cancer: a randomised controlled trial. *The Lancet Oncology*. 2006;7:309–315.

22

Gastrointestinal Stromal Tumors

William Cole

A 62-year-old man was referred to the general surgery clinic for further evaluation of chronic abdominal pain, bloating, and early satiety, which had been worsening over several months. He was previously healthy except for mild hypertension controlled with metoprolol and a history of inguinal hernia repair. His last screening colonoscopy, performed 2 years ago, was negative. On review of systems, he endorses significant fatigue. Laboratory results are consistent with mild anemia. An abdominal CT scan was obtained by his primary physician for further evaluation and revealed a large tumor of gastric origin (pictured below).

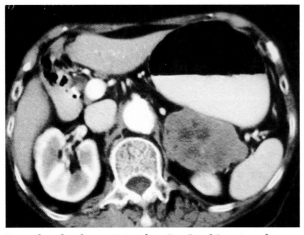

Reproduced with permission from Lua S et al. Imaging of gastrointestinal stromal tumor (GIST). *Clin Radiol.* 2004;59:487–498.

1. **Which is the best next step to definitively diagnose this lesion?**

   A. Abdominal magnetic resonance imaging (MRI)
   B. Endoscopic ultrasound with fine-needle aspiration
   C. Percutaneous image-guided biopsy
   D. Diagnostic laparoscopy with biopsy and peritoneal washings

2. **Biopsied tissue is positive for KIT (CD117) upon immunochemical staining. Which of the following is true of this type of tumor?**

   A. Gastrointestinal stromal tumor (GIST) most commonly arises from the stomach.
   B. The most common subtype is epithelioid.
   C. A positive stain for KIT (CD117) is required to make the diagnosis of GIST.
   D. The most common site of metastatic spread is the peritoneum.
   E. All tumors >1 cm should be considered potentially malignant.

3. **Which of the following is true of gastrointestinal stromal tumors in general?**

   A. Because they arise from the mucosa, GISTs are easily identified at endoscopy.
   B. Surgical resection is often appropriate for patients with recurrent or metastatic GIST.
   C. These tumors arise from the smooth-muscle cells of the intestinal wall.
   D. GIST tends to arise as a solitary lesion.
   E. Abdominal pain is the most common clinical manifestation of GIST.

4. **Further review of the computed tomography (CT) scan raises concerns that this 6-cm tumor may involve the neck of the pancreas. There is no evidence of distant metastatic disease. Further**

therapy in this case should include which of the following?

A. Surgical resection with en-bloc removal of the involved pancreas to achieve 1-cm negative margins

B. Neoadjuvant imatinib prior to surgical therapy

C. Avoidance of pancreatectomy by enucleation of the tumor

D. An open, rather than laparoscopic, approach should be used

E. An extended lymphadenectomy should be performed

5. **After appropriate therapy, the final pathology returns with a GIST of gastric origin, 6 cm at the greatest dimension, with 15 mitoses per high-power field. Which of the following is true regarding this patient?**

A. Adjuvant therapy with imatinib will increase his chance of recurrence-free and overall survival at 5 years.

B. If this lesion were in the small bowel, the prognosis would be better.

C. This patient is at low risk of tumor recurrence.

D. Five-year overall survival for all GIST patients is about 50%.

6. **A CT scan of the abdomen performed after the endoscopy reveals metastatic disease in the liver, in addition to the recurrent disease in the stomach. Which is the next best step in treating this patient?**

A. Cytoreductive surgery followed by adjuvant imatinib

B. Ifosfamide-based chemotherapy

C. At least 6 months of imatinib followed by surgery if the tumors respond

D. Medical therapy alone, with imatinib therapy until resistance develops, followed by sunitinib

7. **Another patient with suspected gastric GIST undergoes esophageal-ultrasound (EUS)–guided biopsy. The histologic appearance is consistent with GIST, but it does not stain positive for cKIT or PDGFRα. Which of the following is true of this tumor?**

A. This is not a GIST.

B. This tumor is more likely to respond to imatinib.

C. These patients often require extensive serial resections to achieve long-term survival.

D. This comprises up to 10% of all GISTs.

ANSWERS

1. **B.** The CT slice shown demonstrates a large, well-demarcated, heterogeneously enhancing mass that appears to grow outward from the wall of the stomach. These findings are characteristic of gastric GIST, although the differential diagnosis includes gastric adenocarcinoma, carcinoid, lymphoma, or leiomyosarcoma, as well as tumors of pancreatic, renal, or adrenal origin. GIST is a relatively uncommon neoplasm, with an incidence of about 7 per million population in the United States and Europe. The benefits of EUS include defining the layer of the stomach wall from which the tumor originates, delineating its relationship to surrounding structures, and obtaining a tissue diagnosis transluminally, which avoids the risk of seeding a percutaneous biopsy tract. A percutaneous image-guided biopsy may result in intraperitoneal tumor spillage or hemorrhage as a result of the friable, vascular nature of these tumors and is therefore less desirable. MRI offers no additional benefit over CT diagnostically, although it may provide more information regarding the tumor's relationship to surrounding tissues. Diagnostic laparoscopy with peritoneal washings for cytology has a prognostic role in gastric adenocarcinoma, but a similar role has not been established in GIST. Laparoscopic excision of the lesion may be performed without a tissue diagnosis for a small tumor, but the goal of surgery in this case is resection to clear margins. Endoscopic ultrasound is the best choice.

2. **A.** The presence of the KIT receptor tyrosine kinase on tumor cells, as in this case, is pathognomonic for GIST. However, it is noteworthy that only about 80% have a KIT mutation. Other useful histologic markers include PDGFRα, CD34, and smooth-muscle actin, if KIT-negative GIST is suspected. The most common histologic subtype is the spindle-cell variety (70%), followed by epithelioid (20%) and mixed subtypes (10%). All tumors greater than 2 cm in size should be considered malignant, even in the absence of metastases on initial workup. The most common site of metastatic spread of GIST is the liver, followed by the omentum and peritoneum. If present, these metastases are often identified by contrast-enhanced CT scanning. Metastasis to the lymph nodes, lung, or other distant sites may occur, but this is quite rare. Thus, extended surgical lymphadenectomy is not indicated for these tumors. Over half of all GISTs

arise from the stomach, making it the most common primary site.

3. D. Gastrointestinal stromal tumors are more likely to be solitary than multiple. This stands in contrast to carcinoid tumors, which often occur multiply. They arise from the muscular layer of the intestinal wall, but from the interstitial cells of Cajal, not the smooth-muscle cells. Their location in the muscular layer can make small GISTs somewhat difficult to detect and lead to underestimation of tumor extent by endoscopy.

At presentation, GISTs are frequently metastatic, usually to the liver or peritoneum. Presenting symptoms may include abdominal pain, dyspepsia, or early satiety. Gastrointestinal bleeding is the most common sign. Life-threatening hemorrhage from intraperitoneal rupture of these highly vascular tumors may also occur. Generally speaking, imatinib, a tyrosine kinase inhibitor (TKI), is considered first-line therapy for metastatic or recurrent GIST, and surgical resection is often inappropriate due to high rates of recurrence. However, some patients with tumors responsive to imatinib and/or lesions felt to be completely resectable may benefit.

4. B. When surgical morbidity can be reduced by its use, preoperative therapy with imatinib should be strongly considered. In this case, response to the TKI could potentially eliminate pancreatic involvement and obviate the need for pancreatectomy. For localized GIST, surgical resection is indicated and is curative for low-risk lesions. If necessary to achieve an R0 resection, en bloc removal of involved organs outside the primary site is indicated. However, there is no additional survival benefit to resection beyond microscopically negative margins. An extended lymphadenectomy also offers no benefit to the patient, as nodal metastasizes are uncommon with GIST occurring only 1% of the time.

Enucleation of the tumor risks violating its pseudocapsule, which may result in intraoperative tumor spillage, resulting in recurrence rates approaching 100%. In the past, an open approach for tumors larger than 5 cm has been recommended. Although laparoscopic surgery for GIST has not been prospectively evaluated, there is good retrospective evidence to show adequate oncologic outcomes with this approach if the surgeon is adequately skilled. Rates of R0 resection between 97% and 100% and disease-free

survival and overall survival rates of more than 90% have been reported for laparoscopy. Current guidelines indicate that laparoscopy is appropriate for larger tumors provided sound oncologic principles are maintained.

5. A. Tumor size, mitotic rate, and location are important prognostic factors in GIST. Tumors with a size <5 cm have a 5-year overall survival of about 70%. This drops to about 45% when tumor size is >10 cm.

Similarly, about 75% of patients with <5 per high-power field will survive 5 years, while only 20% of those with ≥5 per high-powered field will. Tumors of gastric origin carry a better prognosis than those originating in the small bowel, with survival rates of approximately 75% and 50%, respectively, at 5 years. Tumor rupture before or during surgery also portends a poor prognosis, as discussed earlier. Given the mitotic rate of the tumor in this case, the patient has a relatively poor prognosis. Adjuvant therapy with imatinib for 1 year has been shown to increase recurrence-free survival by 15% and, if continued for 3 years, improve 5-year overall survival by 10%. However, about half of all patients will develop resistance to the drug within 2 years of its initiation. For these patients, other TKIs (i.e., sunitinib) remain effective second-line therapy. Historically, the overall survival for all patients with GIST at 5 years has been about 50%. However, in the era of TKIs, the 5-year overall survival has improved to 84%, although survival varies markedly between patients with early-stage tumors (nearly 100%) versus more advanced tumors (22%).

6. C. As discussed previously, a trial of imatinib of at least 6 but no more than 24 months should be given prior to resection of recurrent or metastatic GISTs. There are two reasons for this. First, only about 25% of metastatic disease is resectable at presentation, and a good response to a TKI may change this. Second, response to TKI in this setting is predictive of outcomes after surgery and longer-term survival, allowing appropriate patient selection. Thus, surgery for metastatic GIST is indicated when there is resectable, responsive, or stable disease on TKIs; a limited, resectable focus of disease progression due to TKI resistance; and palliation of oncologic emergencies, including bleeding, rupture, abscess, or obstruction. Conventional chemotherapy has no role in the treatment of GIST as only 10% 5-year survival was achieved with its use. Sunitinib is used for imatinib-resistant, generally progressive disease, but surgery should not be omitted entirely from the treatment plan, as described earlier, as the combination of surgery and TKIs led to better overall survival than TKIs alone.

7. D. This scenario describes a wild-type GIST. These tumors compose as many as 10% of all GISTs. They often demonstrate mutations in SDH, NF1, or BRAF, for which the tissue should be tested, if it is negative for KIT and PDGFRα mutations. Unfortunately, these tumors are generally resistant to TKIs because they lack the gain-of-function mutation of cKIT or PDGRFα. Because of this, generalized progressive disease is common and, after primary resection, there seems to be no benefit to extensive, repeated debulking procedures as they do not lead to long-term survival.

BIBLIOGRAPHY

Dematteo RP, Gold JS, Saran L, et al. Tumor mitotic rate, size, and location independently predict recurrence after resection of primary gastrointestinal stromal tumor (GIST). *Cancer*. 2008;112:608–615.

Dematteo RP, Ballman KV, Antonescu CR, et al. Long-term results of adjuvant imatinib mesylate in localized, high-risk, primary gastrointestinal stromal tumor. *Ann Surg*. 2013;258:422–429.

Dematteo RP, Maki RG, Singer S, et al. Results of tyrosine kinase inhibitor therapy followed by surgical resection for metastatic gastrointestinal stromal tumor. *Ann Surg*. 2007;245:347–352.

Demetri GD, von Mehren M, Antonescu CR, et al. NCCN task force report: update on the management of patients with gastrointestinal stromal tumors. *J Natl Compr Canc Network*. 2010;8:S1–S41.

Eisenberg BL, Harris J, Blanke C, et al. Phase II trial of imatinib mesylate (IM) for advanced primary and metastatic/recurrent operable gastrointestinal stromal tumor (GIST)—early results of RTOG 0132. *J Surg Oncol*. 2009;99(1):42–47.

Emory TS, Sobin LH, Lukes L, Lee DH, O'Leary TJ. Prognosis of gastrointestinal smooth-muscle stromal tumors: dependence on anatomic site. *Am J Surg Pathol*. 1999;23(1):82–87.

Ford SJ, Gronchi A. Indications for surgery in advanced/metastatic GIST. *Eur J Cancer*. 2016;63:154–167.

Gervaz P, Huber O, Morel P. Surgical management of gastrointestinal stromal tumors. *Brit J Surg*. 2009;96:567–578.

Gold JS, DeMatteo RP. Combined surgical and molecular therapy: the gastrointestinal stromal tumor model. *Ann Surg*. 2006;244:176–184.

Hohenberger P, Ronellenfitsch U, Oladeji O, et al. Pattern of recurrence in patients with ruptured primary gastrointestinal stromal tumor. *Brit J Surg*. 2010;97;1854–1859.

Joensuu H, Eriksson M, Sundby Hall K, et al. One versus three years of adjuvant imatinib for operable gastrointestinal stromal tumor. *JAMA*. 2012;307(12):1265–1272.

Joensuu H, Hohenberger P, Corless C. Gastrointestinal stromal tumour. *Lancet*. 2013;382:973–983.

Kays JK, et al. Approach to wild-type gastrointestinal stromal tumors. *Transl Gastroenterol Hepatol*. 2018;3:92–99.

Lee SD, Ryu KW, Eom BW, Lee JH, Kook MC, Kim Y-W. Prognostic significance of peritoneal washing cytology in patients with gastric cancer. *Br J Surg*. 2012;99(3):397–403.

Lua S, Tam KF, Kam CK, et al. Imaging of gastrointestinal stromal tumor (GIST). *Clin Radiol*. 2004;59:487–498.

Novitsky YW, Kercher KW, Sing RF, Heniford BT. Long-term outcomes of laparoscopic resection of gastric gastrointestinal stromal tumors. *Ann Surg*. 2006;243:738–747.

Rutkowski P, Wozniak A, Dębiec-Rychter M, et al. Clinical utility of the new American Joint Committee on Cancer staging system for gastrointestinal stromal tumors. *Cancer*. 2011;117:4916–4924.

Sepe PS, Brugge WR. A guide for the diagnosis and management of gastrointestinal stromal cell tumors. *Nat Rev Gastroenterol Hepatol*. 2009;6(6):363–371.

Tabrizian P, Sweeney RE, Uhr JH, Nguyen SQ, Divino CM. Laparoscopic resection of gastric and small bowel gastrointestinal stromal tumors: 10-year experience at a single center. *J Am Coll Surg*. 2014;218:367–373.

Winer JH, Raut CP. Management of recurrent gastrointestinal stromal tumors. *J Surg Oncol*. 2011;104:915–920.

Zhaolun C, Yuan Y, Chaoyong S, et al. Role of surgical resection for patients with recurrent or metastatic gastrointestinal stromal tumors: a systematic review and meta-analysis. *Int J Surg*. 2018;56:108–114.

23

Gastric Lymphoid Tumors

Phillip M. Kemp Bohan and Timothy J. Vreeland

A 56-year-old man with a 4-month history of vague epigastric abdominal pain, decreased appetite, and weight loss presents to his local gastroenterologist for evaluation. An esophagogastroduodenoscopy (EGD) reveals non-specific gastritis and a polypoid lesion in the region of the antrum. Laboratory findings note mild anemia, elevated lactate dehydrogenase (LDH), and *Heliobacter pylori*–positive samples, and there is no t(11;18) translocation.

A follow-up endoscopic ultrasound (EUS) notes a thickened antral wall, and multiple biopsies obtained reveal an extra-nodal marginal zone B-cell lymphoma of mucosa (gut)-associated lymphoid tissue (MALT) type (MALT lymphoma). A computed tomography scan of the chest, abdomen, and pelvis reveals thickening of the distal half of the stomach with no evidence of adenopathy.

1. **After the patient has undergone a complete staging workup as noted, what stage lesion does this patient have?**

    A. Stage I
    B. Stage II
    C. Stage III
    D. Stage IV
    E. Unknown

2. **The proper surgical management of this patient with gastric lymphoma is**

    A. a total gastrectomy with D2 lymph node dissection.
    B. a total gastrectomy with D1 lymph node dissection.
    C. a partial gastrectomy with D1 lymph node dissection.
    D. a partial/total gastrectomy with no lymph node dissection.
    E. a surgical resection is not warranted in most cases.

3. **If this patient were *H. pylori*–negative, therapy would consist of which of the following?**

    A. Surgical resection
    B. Radiation therapy
    C. Chemotherapy
    D. Endoluminal resection
    E. No additional therapy

4. **What is the management for persistent, localized MALT lymphoma following repeated failed efforts at *H. pylori* eradication therapy?**

    A. Radiation therapy
    B. Surgical resection
    C. Chemotherapy
    D. Rituximab
    E. Bevacizumab

5. **What is the best treatment strategy in patients with *H. pylori*–negative high-grade gastric lymphoma (advanced MALT lymphoma or diffuse large B-cell lymphoma [DLBCL])?**

    A. Surgical resection
    B. Radiation therapy alone
    C. Chemotherapy alone
    D. *H. pylori* eradication alone
    E. Combination targeted therapy and chemotherapy with or without radiation therapy

ANSWERS

1. A. Gastrointestinal lymphomas are staged using the Lugano Staging System for Gastrointestinal Lymphomas in accordance with the latest National Comprehensive Cancer Network (NCCN) guidelines. Broadly, stage I disease is confined to the gastrointestinal (GI) tract, stage II disease involves lymph nodes in the abdomen (B), stage IIE disease denotes penetration of the serosa of adjacent organs, and stage IV disease describes disseminated extra-nodal involvement or disease on both sides of the diaphragm (D). While stage III is a category of the Ann Arbor staging system for DLBCLs, there is no category for stage III disease in the Lugano system or the modified Ann Arbor system for MALT lymphomas (C). A diagnostic workup for a gastric MALT lymphoma requires endoscopy (EGD) with biopsy. Enough tissue should be sampled during the biopsy procedure to allow for immunohistochemical characterization and *H. pylori* staining. The association of *H. pylori* and lymphomagenesis is well documented, with *H. pylori* infection reported in more than 90% of patients with MALT lymphoma. Accurate determination of *H. pylori* status is essential. A negative *H. pylori* stain should be confirmed with noninvasive stool antigen or urea breath test. A positive *H. pylori* stain should prompt polymerase chain reaction (PCR) testing for t(11;18). The presence of the t(11;18) translocation has been associated with shortened progression-free survival, higher rates of disseminated disease, and the persistence of MALT lymphoma following *H. pylori* eradication. Finally, a CT scan of the chest, abdomen, and pelvis should be obtained to evaluate for distant disease, which can be present in 10–25% of cases at initial diagnosis. Cumulatively, *H. pylori* status, the presence or absence of the t(11;18) translocation, and evidence of distant disease dictate the initial treatment course.

2. E. This patient has stage I disease and is positive for *H. pylori*. The preferred treatment for these patients is antibiotic therapy for *H. pylori* eradication followed by endoscopy to confirm disease remission. Surgical intervention should be reserved for the control of residual local disease following *H. pylori* eradication and radiation/chemotherapy or in patients who develop a complication but should not be routinely employed in the treatment of gastric MALT lymphoma (A–D) as it provides no additional survival benefit.

Lugano Staging System	Lugano Modification of Ann Arbor Staging System
Stage I: The tumor is confined to the gastrointestinal (GI) tract. I₁: invades the mucosa or submucosa I₂: invades the muscularis propria or serosa	**Stage I_E:** The tumor is confined to the GI tract (equivalent to stage I)
Stage II: The tumor extends into the abdomen. II₁: Involvement of local nodes II₂: Involvement of distant nodes	**Stage II_E:** The tumor extends into the abdomen (equivalent to stage II–stage IIE).
Stage IIE: The tumor penetrates the serosa to involve adjacent organs or tissues.	
Stage IV: There is disseminated extranodal involvement or concomitant supra-diaphragmatic nodal involvement.	**Stage IV:** There is disseminated extra-nodal involvement or concomitant supra-diaphragmatic nodal involvement (equivalent to stage IV).

3. D. For patients who also have the t(11;18) translocation, radiation therapy should accompany *H. pylori* eradication given higher rates of recurrence. Similarly, for patients with *H. pylori*–negative stage I or II₁ disease, radiation therapy is recommended (B). Radiation therapy has excellent complete response rates and a high 10-year recurrence-free survival rate. Patients with stage I disease who are positive for *H. pylori* with unknown t(11;18) status should receive *H. pylori* eradication therapy as first-line therapy. *H. pylori* eradication has been associated with lymphoma remission in 75–77% of patients. Chemotherapy (C) can also be considered in patients with low-grade MALT lymphoma if *H. pylori* eradication is ineffective, although chemotherapy appears to be less efficacious than radiation therapy. For advanced disease (II₂, IIE, IV), rituximab combined with multiagent chemotherapy is a first-line treatment (C). Surgery, including endoluminal resection, should not be pursued routinely for treatment of gastric MALT lymphoma (A). Watchful waiting is inappropriate as the patient has early-stage disease and intervention at this stage can be curative (E).

4. A. The management of persistent, localized, early-stage gastric MALT lymphoma is dependent on *H. pylori* status. If *H. pylori* has been eradicated but MALT lymphoma persists, then appropriate treatment would consist of radiation therapy. If the patient remains *H. pylori*–positive (i.e., resistant to eradication) with persistent MALT lymphoma, then a second course of antibiotic therapy with or without concurrent radiation therapy would be appropriate. In general, radiation therapy (external beam, 25–40 Gy) produces excellent rates of complete response, even when given as salvage therapy for patients who underwent *H. pylori* eradication but continued to have persistent residual lymphoma. Among a study of patients with stage I–II MALT lymphoma, *H. pylori* eradication produced complete remission in 43% of patients, and adding radiation to the treatment of these patients with residual disease after eradication increased the complete remission rate to 89%. Radiation also produces durable local control, with a separate study demonstrating 88% of patients who received radiation therapy remained free from treatment failure at 15 years. Rituximab (in combination with *H. pylori* eradication therapy) can be given to patients with stage I/stage II disease who are *H. pylori*–positive and t(11;18) positive if radiation therapy is contraindicated but should not be considered a first-line treatment in a patient who can receive radiation (D). Chemotherapy is typically reserved for stage IIE or IV disease (C). Surgery rarely is utilized in the treatment of MALT lymphoma (B). Bevacizumab has no role in the treatment of MALT lymphoma (E).

5. E. As noted earlier, surgery should not be routinely utilized in the treatment of any MALT lymphoma, including high-grade MALT lymphoma (A). The treatment of gastric DLBCL utilizes with rituximab (a monoclonal antibody against CD20) and CHOP (cyclophosphamide, doxorubicin, vincristine, prednisone), also known as R-CHOP. A study of patients with DLBCL (gastric and nongastric) that compared CHOP and R-CHOP found that 6-year event-free survival was 55.8% versus 74.3% (p<0.001; C). In gastric DLBCL specifically, a retrospective study comparing chemotherapy to chemotherapy plus rituximab found a significantly lower complete response rate (76.6% vs 100%) and significantly lower disease-free survival at 5 years (73.3% vs 100%) in the group that did not receive rituximab

(E). The addition of radiation therapy to chemotherapy is associated with improved event free survival in patients with bulky disease (≥7.5 cm). In a study of aggressive DLBCL, patients with bulky disease who did not receive radiation had worse progression-free survival rates (HR 4.4, CI 1.8–10.6) and overall survival rates (HR 4.3, CI 1.7.11.1). The role of radiation therapy in limited-stage (stage I–II) non-bulky DLBCL is more controversial. In a randomized controlled trial comparing R-CHOP with radiation to R-CHOP alone in patients with limited-stage (stage I–II) non-bulky DLBCL, the addition of radiation to R-CHOP provided no event-free survival or overall survival benefit.

An additional consideration in the treatment of DLBCL patients is the role of *H. pylori* eradication. The reported incidence of *H. pylori* infection in patients with DLBCL is relatively high (61.9%). Those with *H. pylori*–positive DLBCL tends to have a lower clinical stage, a better response to chemotherapy, and an improved 5-year event-free and an overall survival rate relative to those with *H. pylori*–negative DLBCL. Although not part of the generalized NCCN guidelines for treatment of DLBL, treatment with *H. pylori* eradication should be considered in patients with early-stage *H. pylori*–positive pure DLBCL as *H. pylori* eradication alone has been shown to produce a pathologic complete remission in 68.8% of stage IE/IIE$_1$cases. Given this patient is *H. pylori*–negative, there is no role for *H. pylori* eradication (D).

BIBLIOGRAPHY

Goda JS, Gospodarowicz M, Pintilie M, et al. Long-term outcome in localized extranodal mucosa-associated lymphoid tissue lymphomas treated with radiotherapy. *Cancer.* 2010;116(16):3815–3824.

Gong EJ, Ahn JY, Jung HY, et al. *Helicobacter pylori* eradication therapy is effective as the initial treatment for patients with *H. pylori*-negative and disseminated gastric mucosa-associated lymphoid tissue lymphoma. *Gut Liver.* 2016;10(5):706–713.

Held G, Murawski N, Ziepert M, et al. Role of radiotherapy to bulky disease in elderly patients with aggressive B-cell lymphoma. *J Clin Oncol.* 2014;32(11):1112–1118.

Koch P, del Valle F, Berdel WE, et al. Primary gastrointestinal non-Hodgkin's lymphoma: II. Combined surgical and conservative or conservative management only in localized gastric lymphoma—results of the prospective German Multicenter Study GIT NHL 01/92. *J Clin Oncol.* 2001;19(18):3874–3883.

Koch P, Probst A, Berdel WE, et al. Treatment results in localized primary gastric lymphoma: data of patients registered within the German multicenter study (GIT NHL 02/96). *J Clin Oncol.* 2005;23(28):7050–7059.

Kuo SH, Chen LT, Lin CW, et al. Expressions of the CagA protein and CagA-signaling molecules predict Helicobacter pylori dependence of early-stage gastric DLBCL. *Blood.* 2017;129(2):188–198.

Kuo SH, Yeh KH, Chen LT, et al. Helicobacter pylori-related diffuse large B-cell lymphoma of the stomach: a distinct entity with lower aggressiveness and higher chemosensitivity. *Blood Cancer J.* 2014;4(6):e220.

Kuo SH, Yeh KH, Wu MS, et al. Helicobacter pylori eradication therapy is effective in the treatment of early-stage H. pylori-positive gastric diffuse large B-cell lymphomas. *Blood.* 2012;119(21):4838–4844; quiz 5057.

Lamy T, Damaj G, Soubeyran P, et al. R-CHOP 14 with or without radiotherapy in nonbulky limited-stage diffuse large B-cell lymphoma. *Blood.* 2018;131(2):174–181.

Leopardo D, Di Lorenzo G, De Renzo A, et al. Efficacy of rituximab in gastric diffuse large B cell lymphoma patients. *World J Gastroenterol.* 2010;16(20):2526–2530.

Liu H, Ye H, Ruskone-Fourmestraux A, et al. T(11;18) is a marker for all stage gastric MALT lymphomas that will not respond to *H. pylori* eradication. *Gastroenterology.* 2002;122(5):1286–1294.

Matysiak-Budnik T, Jamet P, Ruskone-Fourmestraux A, et al. Gastric MALT lymphoma in a population-based study in France: clinical features, treatments and survival. *Aliment Pharmacol Ther.* 2019;50(6):654–663.

Nakamura S, Sugiyama T, Matsumoto T, et al. Long-term clinical outcome of gastric MALT lymphoma after eradication of *Helicobacter pylori*: a multicentre cohort follow-up study of 420 patients in Japan. *Gut.* 2012;61(4):507–513.

NCCN Clinical Practice Guidelines in Oncology: B-Cell Lymphomas. 2020. Updated January 22, 2020. Accessed March 19, 2020. https://www.nccn.org/professionals/physician_gls/pdf/b-cell.pdf

Ohkubo Y, Saito Y, Ushijima H, et al. Radiotherapy for localized gastric mucosa-associated lymphoid tissue lymphoma: long-term outcomes over 10 years. *J Radiat Res.* 2017;58(4):537–542.

Pfreundschuh M, Kuhnt E, Trümper L, et al. CHOP-like chemotherapy with or without rituximab in young patients with good-prognosis diffuse large-B-cell lymphoma: 6-year results of an open-label randomised study of the MabThera International Trial (MInT) Group. *Lancet Oncol.* 2011;12(11):1013–1022.

Schechter NR, Portlock CS, Yahalom J. Treatment of mucosa-associated lymphoid tissue lymphoma of the stomach with radiation alone. *J Clin Oncol.* 1998;16(5):1916–1921.

Schmelz R, Miehlke S, Thiede C, et al. Sequential H. pylori eradication and radiation therapy with reduced dose compared to standard dose for gastric MALT lymphoma stages IE & II1E: a prospective randomized trial. *J Gastroenterol.* 2019;54(5):388–395.

Stathis A, Chini C, Bertoni F, et al. Long-term outcome following *Helicobacter pylori* eradication in a retrospective study of 105 patients with localized gastric marginal zone B-cell lymphoma of MALT type. *Ann Oncol.* 2009;20(6):1086–1093.

Tomita N, Kodaira T, Tachibana H, Nakamura T, Mizoguchi N, Takada A. Favorable outcomes of radiotherapy for early-stage mucosa-associated lymphoid tissue lymphoma. *Radiother Oncol.* 2009;90(2):231–235.

Toyoda K, Maeshima AM, Nomoto J, et al. Mucosa-associated lymphoid tissue lymphoma with t(11;18)(q21;q21) translocation: long-term follow-up results. *Ann Hematol.* 2019;98(7):1675–1687.

Violeta Filip P, Cuciureanu D, Sorina Diaconu L, Maria Vladareanu A, Silvia Pop C. MALT lymphoma: epidemiology, clinical diagnosis and treatment. *J Med Life.* 2018;11(3):187–193.

Vrieling C, de Jong D, Boot H, de Boer JP, Wegman F, Aleman BM. Long-term results of stomach-conserving therapy in gastric MALT lymphoma. *Radiother Oncol.* 2008;87(3):405–411.

Wirth A, Gospodarowicz M, Aleman BM, et al. Long-term outcome for gastric marginal zone lymphoma treated with radiotherapy: a retrospective, multi-centre, International Extranodal Lymphoma Study Group study. *Ann Oncol.* 2013;24(5):1344–1351.

Wotherspoon AC, Ortiz-Hidalgo C, Falzon MR, Isaacson PG. *Helicobacter pylori*-associated gastritis and primary B-cell gastric lymphoma. *Lancet.* 1991;338(8776):1175–1176.

Yoon SS, Coit DG, Portlock CS, Karpeh MS. The diminishing role of surgery in the treatment of gastric lymphoma. *Ann Surg.* 2004;240(1):28–37.

Zucca E, Conconi A, Laszlo D, et al. Addition of rituximab to chlorambucil produces superior event-free survival in the treatment of patients with extranodal marginal-zone B-cell lymphoma: 5-year analysis of the IELSG-19 Randomized Study. *J Clin Oncol.* 2013;31(5):565–572.

Zucca E, Dreyling M. Gastric marginal zone lymphoma of MALT type: ESMO Clinical Practice Guidelines for diagnosis, treatment and follow-up. *Ann Oncol.* 2010;21(Suppl 5):v175–176.

Zullo A, Hassan C, Andriani A, et al. Treatment of low-grade gastric MALT-lymphoma unresponsive to *Helicobacter pylori* therapy: a pooled-data analysis. *Med Oncol.* 2010;27(2):291–295.

24

Gastroesophageal Reflux Disease

Patrick M. McCarthy and Timothy J. Vreeland

SCENARIO 1

A 49-year-old man presents to your clinic after referral from his primary care manager (PCM) for complaints of post-prandial, retrosternal burning sensation that is worse when supine. He receives some initial relief with over-the-counter (OTC) antacids and a low-dose proton pump inhibitor (PPI), but his symptoms quickly recur. His body mass index (BMI) is 33; he does not smoke and consumes one alcoholic drink per day.

1. **What is the next best step in the management of this patient?**

    A. Omeprazole 20 mg once a day
    B. Esophageal manometry
    C. Anti-reflux procedure
    D. Barium swallow
    E. Omeprazole 40 mg twice a day

2. **After 8 weeks of appropriately timed maximal PPI therapy, the patient continues to have symptoms and now reports a globus sensation and hoarseness. What preoperative tests are REQUIRED prior to surgical intervention in this patient with typical gastroesophageal reflux disease (GERD) symptoms?**

    A. Esophagogastroduodenoscopy (EGD) and pH monitoring
    B. Barium swallow, EGD, pH monitoring, and esophageal manometry
    C. pH monitoring
    D. pH monitoring, EGD, and esophageal manometry
    E. EGD and barium swallow

3. **Your preoperative evaluation reveals a DeMeester score of 15.2 as well as evidence of a Type 1 hiatal hernia with an area of esophageal mucosal erythema involving two mucosal folds measuring approximately 50% of the esophageal circumference. What class of esophagitis is this?**

    A. LA Class A
    B. LA Class B
    C. LA Class C
    D. LA Class D
    E. LA Class E

4. **The high-resolution manometry for this patient shows an incompetent lower esophageal sphincter at baseline with appropriate relaxation. Additionally, there is an absence of normal esophageal peristalsis. Given all the preceding findings, what is the optimal surgical plan for this patient?**

    A. Magnetic sphincter augmentation without crural repair
    B. Toupet fundoplication with crural repair
    C. Nissen fundoplication without crural repair
    D. Nissen fundoplication with crural repair

5. **During your procedure, you are unable to mobilize the appropriate length of the intra-abdominal esophagus. Which of the following would be the next step to obtain the required length?**

    A. Mobilize the esophagus to the level of pulmonary vein
    B. Collis gastroplasty
    C. Transthoracic mediastinal mobilization

D. Stapled wedge gastroplasty

E. Vagus nerve division

SCENARIO 2

A 64-year-old obese male smoker is referred to your clinic after finding Barrett's esophagus without dysplasia on recent EGD performed after his GERD symptoms failed to improve on adequate PPI therapy.

1. **What is the best course of action?**

    A. Observation for worsening of symptoms

    B. Repeat endoscopy in 6 months

    C. Repeat endoscopy in 1 year

    D. Repeat endoscopy in 3 years

    E. Fundoplication

2. **After a repeat endoscopy is performed for surveillance, the patient returns with biopsies showing low-grade intestinal metaplasia. What is the best next step?**

    A. Repeat surveillance in 6 months

    B. Repeat surveillance in 3 years

    C. Endoscopic mucosal resection

    D. Esophagectomy

3. **The patient returns to the clinic later after surveillance EGD with biopsy revealing high-grade dysplasia. Examination of the patient also reveals a past surgical history of two-vessel coronary artery bypass graft (CABG), ejection fraction of 42%, and 60 pack-year history. What is the best course of action for this patient?**

    A. Anti-reflux surgery

    B. Endoscopic mucosal resection

    C. Esophagectomy

    D. Chemotherapy

ANSWERS

SCENARIO 1

1. **E.** The patient has classic GERD symptoms and does not present with any alarm symptoms that warrant additional investigation. GERD should be initially managed with pharmacologic therapy and lifestyle changes. Lifestyle changes include weight loss, smoking cessation, head of bed elevation, and avoidance of large or late evening meals. Initial management is typically once a day PPI or an H2 blocker. If initially, a low-dose PPI does not manage symptoms, the next

step would be to increase the dose to twice-daily maximal dose PPIs.

2. **D.** Globus sensation and hoarseness constitute alarm symptoms in addition to the failure of improving the patient's reflex after appropriate medical therapy. Other alarm or extraesophageal symptoms include persistent coughing, asthma, or regurgitation. Prior to performing a reflux operation, malignancy must always be ruled. This is done with EGD as it allows for direct mucosal visualization and biopsy if needed. In addition, in general, pH monitoring should be performed to confirm that the patient's symptoms correlate with objective findings of reflux. Finally, prior to performing a full 360-degree wrap (Nissen), it is ideal to confirm normal peristalsis of the esophagus. Although manometry, pH monitoring, EGD, and barium swallow are all acceptable tests to order, a barium swallow is most relevant for patients where there is a concern for a large hiatal hernia. Furthermore, most hiatal hernias can be identified on EGD; thus, a barium swallow is generally not needed.

3. **C.** The classification of esophagitis is useful in cases of serial endoscopy. The presence of LA Class C or D esophagitis is considered pathognomonic for GERD. There is no LA Class E.

LA Class	Criteria
Grade A	One or more mucosal breaks no longer than 5 mm that do not extend between the tops of two mucosal folds
Grade B	One or more mucosal breaks more than 5 mm long that do not extend between the tops of two mucosal folds
Grade C	One or more mucosal breaks that are continuous between the tops of two or more mucosal folds but involve less than 75% of the circumference
Grade D	One or more mucosal breaks that involve at least 75% of the esophageal circumference

4. **B.** High-resolution manometry fails to show a competent lower esophageal sphincter (LES) at baseline with appropriate relaxation. Incompetent LES on manometry is typical in cases of significant GERD

and explains why the patient has reflux. The absence of peristalsis down the esophagus tells us that esophageal motility is compromised for some reason; this presents a relative contraindication for a 360-degree fundoplication (Nissen). Therefore, a partial wrap, such as a Toupet, is likely a better choice for this scenario. The presence of a Type 1 hiatal hernia from the prior question is an indication for crural repair. Some surgeons never do full 360-degree wraps, choosing instead to perform partial wraps (Toupet or Dor) for all patients. The data on this topic are rather mixed, so the choice of a full versus partial wrap in patients with normal peristalsis is very controversial; either choice is reasonable. In the setting of poor progression of peristalsis, however, a partial wrap is the best choice.

5. **A.** Long-standing GERD and inflammation of the esophagus can cause shortening that prevents adequate mobilization of 2–3 cm of the intra-abdominal esophagus, which is required when doing any anti-reflux surgery. If this occurs, dissection should be carried to the level of the inferior pulmonary vein within the mediastinum to obtain additional length of intra-abdominal esophagus. This should be the first maneuver before any additional maneuvers are performed. Additional steps that can be taken include division of one or both vagus nerves, stapled wedge gastroplasty, or Collis gastroplasty. Division of a single vagus nerve is reported to provide 1–2 cm of additional esophageal length per nerve. However, this maneuver can lead to delayed gastric emptying, bloating, and abdominal pain. The performance of a stapled wedge gastroplasty or Collis gastroplasty is effective in providing a replacement for the function of the LES but is rarely required and places the patient at risk of postoperative leak and/or stricture.

SCENARIO 2

1. **D.** There is a current lack of evidence to definitively recommend screening endoscopy for patient's with Barrett's esophagus without evidence of dysplasia. However, certain risk factors place a subset of patients at increased risk of esophageal adenocarcinoma and Barrett's esophagus. These risk factors include age >50, Caucasian race, central obesity, current or past smoking history, or a family history of Barrett's esophagus or esophageal adenocarcinoma. Patients with two or more of these risk factors should be most strongly considered for screening endoscopy. In patients undergoing endoscopic surveillance of Barrett's esophagus without dysplasia, the current recommendation is for an endoscopy every 3–5 years. A fundoplication at this time is not required.

2. **C.** Low-grade dysplasia represents a risk factor for progression to Barrett's esophagus. There is a growing body of literature to suggest that ablative endoscopic procedures for low-grade dysplasia provide greater risk reduction with respect to progression to high-grade dysplasia and adenocarcinoma. In fact, recent guidelines have been updated to reflect this, although for patients unwilling to undergo these procedures, endoscopic surveillance every 12 months is an acceptable alternative. Esophagectomy is unnecessarily morbid for low-grade dysplasia. Three years is too long an interval to detect a meaningful change in patients elected for surveillance of low-grade dyspasia.

3. **B.** This patient has had progression of his Barrett's esophagus to high-grade dysplasia. Evidence suggests that endoscopic mucosal resection, radiofrequency ablation, and/or photodynamic therapy are adequate therapies for the treatment of targeted dysplastic lesions. These lesions were previously treated with esophagectomy, which would also be difficult for this patient with serious comorbidities and surgical risk factors. Chemotherapy is an option for esophageal adenocarcinoma, but would NOT be appropriate for the treatment for noninvasive disease.

BIBLIOGRAPHY

American Gastroenterological A. GERD care pathway. *Gastroenterology.* 2016;150(4):1026–1030. doi:10.1053/j.gastro.2016.02.038

Epstein D, Bojke L, Sculpher MJ, Reflux Trial Group. Laparoscopic fundoplication compared with medical management for gastro-oesophageal reflux disease: cost effectiveness study. *BMJ.* 2009;339:b2576. doi:10.1136/bmj.b2576

Kahrilas PJ, Boeckxstaens G. The spectrum of achalasia: lessons from studies of pathophysiology and high-resolution manometry. *Gastroenterology.* 2013;145(5):954–965. doi:10.1053/j.gastro.2013.08.038

Katz PO, Gerson LB, Vela MF. Guidelines for the diagnosis and management of gastroesophageal reflux disease. *Am J Gastroenterol.* 2013;108(3):308–328; quiz 329. doi:10.1038/ajg.2012.444

Ness-Jensen E, Hveem K, El-Serag H, Lagergren J. Lifestyle intervention in gastroesophageal reflux disease. *Clin Gastroenterol Hepatol.* 2016;14(2):175–182.e173. doi:10.1016/j.cgh.2015.04.176

Pech O, Alqahtani SA. Update on endoscopic treatment of Barrett's oesophagus and Barrett's oesophagus–related neoplasia. *Ther Adv Gastrointest Endosc.* 2020;13: 263177452093524. doi:10.1177/2631774520935241

Qumseya B, Sultan S, Bain P, et al. ASGE guideline on screening and surveillance of Barrett's esophagus. *Gastrointest Endosc.* 2019;90(3):335–359.e332. doi:10.1016/j.gie.2019.05.012

Shaheen NJ, Falk GW, Iyer PG, Gerson LB. ACG clinical guideline: diagnosis and management of Barrett's esophagus. *Am Journal Gastroenterol.* 2016;111(1):30–50. doi:10.1038/ajg.2015.322

Stefanidis D, Hope WW, Kohn GP, Reardon PR, Richardson WS. Fanelli RD. Guidelines for surgical treatment of gastroesophageal reflux disease. *Surg Endosc.* 2010;24(11):2647–2669. doi:10.1007/s00464-010-1267-8

Townsend CM, Beauchamp RD, Evers BM, Mattox KL. *Sabiston Textbook of Surgery: The Biological Basis of Modern Surgical Practice.* 20th ed. Elsevier; 2017. https://yale.idm.oclc.org/login?URL=https://www.clinicalkey.com/dura/browse/bookChapter/3-s2.0-C20130186151

25

Perforated Peptic Ulcer Disease

Henry Lin

A 58-year-old active female with arthritis and asthma presents to the emergency department with an acute onset of epigastric pain a couple of hours ago. Her pulse is 104, her blood pressure is unchanged from her baseline of 110/74 mmHg, and her temperature is 98.2 degrees Fahrenheit. Her medications include naproxen for her arthritis & prednisone occasionally for asthma. On physical exam, her abdomen demonstrates significant epigastric tenderness with rebound. She has a mild leukocytosis of 12.5 cells/mcL. Her acute abdominal series demonstrates a small amount of free air.

1. **Which radiologic study would most expeditiously decide management in this patient?**

    A. Computed tomography (CT) abdomen and pelvis scan
    B. Upright chest x-ray
    C. Ultrasound of the abdomen
    D. Hepatobiliary iminodiacetic acid (HIDA) scan
    E. Magnetic resonance imaging (MRI) of the abdomen

2. **What is the most reasonable current treatment option for this patient as the next step?**

    A. Laparoscopic highly selective vagotomy without resuscitation
    B. Nasogastric tube insertion, cessation of all oral feeds, and intravenous fluid initiation for the next 24 hours
    C. Truncal vagotomy with pyloroplasty
    D. Open Graham patch with parietal cell vagotomy
    E. Emergent anterior seromyotomy

3. **If she does not demonstrate improvement during the 12 hours after onset of symptoms, what is the most reasonable and expedient next step?**

    A. Truncal vagotomy with antrectomy and a Bilroth II reconstruction
    B. Continued observation
    C. Selective angioembolization
    D. Laparoscopic Graham patch only and *Helicobacter pylori* testing with possible treatment
    E. Laparoscopic Graham patch with parietal cell vagotomy

4. **What testing should be done for follow-up?**

    A. Secretin stimulation test
    B. *H. pylori* stool antigen testing
    C. Emergent urea breath testing
    D. Colonoscopy

5. **What further follow-up is necessary if she has no further symptoms?**

    A. Long-term intravenous pantoprazole
    B. Close interval follow-up
    C. Chronic suppressive antibiotics
    D. Serum gastrin level
    E. Esophagogastroduodenoscopy with biopsy of ulcer if still present

6. **Which of the following factors increase the risk of mortality after surgery for perforated peptic ulcer disease?**

    A. Age < 40 years old
    B. A lack of comorbidities/comorbid cardiac disease

C. Early operative treatment, that is, treatment within 24 hours of onset of symptoms

D. Presence of septic shock

E. Size of the perforated ulcer is smaller than 9 mm/ perforations >10 mm

ANSWERS

1. **B.** An upright chest x-ray is the quickest imaging study that would increase the clinical suspicion of this patient who presented with the classic triad of perforated peptic ulcer disease: sudden severe onset of epigastric pain, tachycardia, and abdominal rigidity. Although a CT abdomen and pelvis scan may be confirmatory in equivocal cases or if a patient with high clinical suspicion has a negative chest x-ray, the length of time to obtain in most institutions far exceed the time to obtain a chest x-ray that has 60–80% sensitivity and 15% false-negative rate. An ultrasound of the abdomen for free air is user-dependent. An MRI tends to take significant time. An HIDA scan does not contribute to the workup for perforated peptic ulcer disease (PUD).

2. **B.** This patient manifests the classic triad of sudden onset of abdominal pain, abdominal rigidity, and tachycardia of perforated PUD. Of all the listed options, nasogastric tube insertion with NPO status and initiation of IV fluid is a very reasonable first step in the modern era of *H. pylori* detection and treatment, especially in a stable patient in a resource-rich environment where close monitoring and surgeon access is readily available. Approximately 40–80% of perforated PUD spontaneously seal. Graham patch with parietal cell vagotomy is also a very reasonable option, and an open approach may result in more complications if laparoscopic experience and resources are available. The verification of resuscitation is required prior to going to the operating room for patients. The verification in this patient can simply be assessing volume status (e.g., urine output of 0.5 cc/kg/hour or normal heart rate for a patient not on a beta-blocker). Truncal vagotomy with pyloroplasty is not a first-line treatment in the modern era of *H. pylori*. Anterior seromyotomy, division of the seromuscular layer of the lesser curvature in order to achieve a highly selective vagotomy effect, has been a reasonable approach but not as a first option.

3. **D.** Laparoscopic Graham patch with *H. pylori* testing and subsequent testing is the best choice of those presented. Truncal vagotomy with antrectomy is no longer a first-line option in the modern era of *H. pylori* detection and treatment. Observation is not reasonable if the patient is not improving and a more aggressive management choice is most likely necessary. Angioembolization may be considered for bleeding PUD in selective cases but not for the perforation of an ulcer. Parietal cell vagotomy is no longer considered one of the early line treatments but to be reserved as a treatment option for refractory PUD.

4. **B.** *H. pylori* stool antigen testing is a very reasonable approach and can even be ordered semi-emergently in the emergency department at some institutions to help in decisions with early treatment options. Secretin stimulation test is utilized for gastrinoma workup, which is not yet necessary during this part of the workup for this patient because recalcitrant PUD is not yet identified. Urea breath testing for *H. pylori* is reasonable but is not an emergent process as obtaining this test requires a clinic visit. Colonoscopy is reasonable in a patient older than 50 who has not had a screening process done but is not required to address the follow-up for PUD perforation.

5. **E.** Esophagogastroduodenoscopy is necessary to rule out a gastric carcinoma that caused the perforation, especially in older patients. Pantoprazole, another proton pump inhibitor, or H2 blockers are reasonable to start on admission for perforated PUD, but long-term intravenous treatment is not necessary, especially after treatment for *H. pylori*. The treatment of *H. pylori* involves a course of antibiotics, and chronic suppression should not be necessary. Serum gastrin level can be checked for a patient who is suspected of gastrinoma but is not necessary if the patient's peptic ulcer is healed.

6. **D.** Presence of septic shock at the time of surgery increases complications by 30%. A patient who is 40 years old or more increases the mortality rate postrepair; more than 60 years old increases the mortality rate 3–5 times (12–47%), and more than 65 years old increases the mortality rate to 37.7% from 1.4%. Comorbidities increase the mortality rate by 9 times. Both delay of treatment from onset of symptoms and perforated ulcer size greater than 9 millimeters also increase mortality rates.

BIBLIOGRAPHY

Baker RJ. The perforated duodenal ulcer. In: Fischer JE, Jones DB, Pomposelli FB, et al. eds. *Fischer's Masters of Surgery.* 5th ed. Lippincott Williams & Wilkins; 2007:891–901.

Bertleff MJ. Perforated peptic ulcer disease: a review of history and treatment. *Dig Surg.* 2010;27(3):161–169.

Bhogal RH. Comparison between open and laparoscopic repair of perforated peptic ulcer disease. *World J Surg.* 2008;32(11):2371–2374.

Chung KT, Shelat VG. Perforated peptic ulcer – an update. *World J GI Surgery.* 2017;9(1):1–12.

Donovan AJ, Berne TV, Donovan JA. Perforated duodenal ulcer: an alternative therapeutic plan. *Arch Surg.* 1998;133(11):1166–1171.

Gustafson J, Welling D. "No acid, no ulcer"—100 years later: a review of the history of peptic ulcer disease. *J Am Coll Surg.* 2010;210(1):110–117.

Jones DB, Mathiel SK, Schneider BE. Laparoscopic management of peptic ulcer disease. *Atlas of Minimally Invasive Surgery.* Cine-Med; 2006:196–225.

Lin H, Jones DB. Surgery for peptic ulcer disease. In: Talley et al., eds. *Practical Gastroenterology and Hepatology: Esophagus and Stomach.* Blackwell Publishing; 2010:404–411.

Napolitano L. Refractory peptic ulcer disease. *Gastroenterol Clin North Am.* 2009;38:267–288.

Stabile BE. Redefining the role of surgery for perforated duodenal ulcer in the *Helicobacter pylori* era. *Ann Surg.* 2000 Feb;231(2):159–160.

26

Gallbladder Mass

Freeman Condon

A 66-year-old Japanese female is referred by her primary physician for long-standing biliary colic symptoms. She describes 10–15 years of intermittent right upper quadrant (RUQ) pain with nausea that typically resolves after 1–2 hours. She went to the emergency department once 6 years ago and had an ultrasound that showed gallstones. Her medical history is significant for hypertension and osteoporosis. Her vitals and exam are unremarkable. A repeat RUQ ultrasound ordered by her primary care physician now shows a large 3-cm gallstone, as well as a fixed mass in the fundus, 2 cm in diameter, that appears to originate from the gallbladder wall. The immediate surrounding gallbladder wall is thickened to 8–11 mm. A complete blood count (CBC), basic chemistry, and liver function tests are all within normal limits.

1. **Which of the following is a risk factor for gallbladder carcinoma?**

   A. Hemolytic anemia
   B. Biliary dyskinesia
   C. *Clonorchis sinensis* infection
   D. Anomalous union of the pancreaticobiliary ductal system or pancreaticobiliary maljunction (PBM)
   E. Autoimmune diseases

2. **Which of the following radiographic findings is associated with the highest incidence of gallbladder carcinoma?**

   A. PBM without biliary dilatation identified on magnetic resonance cholangiopancreatography (MRCP)
   B. Strongly enhancing thick inner layer and a weakly enhancing or nonenhancing outer layer of the gallbladder wall on the portal phase of a multidetector computed tomography (MDCT) scan
   C. Gallbladder polyp 10–20 mm on ultrasound
   D. Gallbladder wall calcifications; "porcelain gallbladder"
   E. Asymptomatic gallstone greater than 3 cm in size

3. **A review of all imaging studies shows a gallbladder tumor invades the muscularis propria. There is no lymphadenopathy or distant metastases seen. What is the most appropriate next step in management?**

   A. Referral for definitive treatment with chemotherapy and radiation
   B. Referral for neoadjuvant chemotherapy and radiation
   C. Schedule for cholecystectomy
   D. Schedule for cholecystectomy with removal of regional lymph nodes and en bloc hepatic resection

4. **The same patient with the same history of present illness and past medical history instead presents to the emergency department with RUQ pain. The ultrasound in this case is read as two large gallstones with diffuse gallbladder wall thickening up to 11 mm, pericholecystic fluid, and a normal common bile duct. Labs show a white blood cell count of 13 and normal liver function. You take the patient for laparoscopic cholecystectomy.**

There was no concern for malignancy during the procedure. The gallbladder was removed without spillage and with a retrieval bag. You see her 2 weeks later in clinic, and a review of the pathology report shows T2 adenocarcinoma. All surgical margins, including cystic duct margin, are reported as clear. What is the most appropriate course of action?

A. No additional surgery, surveillance with imaging every 6 months

B. Staging with imaging followed by radical cholecystectomy to include liver resection with at least 3 cm of margin around gallbladder bed and regional lymphadenectomy

C. Staging with imaging followed by radical cholecystectomy and excision of the previous laparoscopic port sites

D. Staging with imaging followed by radical cholecystectomy and excision of the common bile duct

E. Staging with imaging followed by radical cholecystectomy and excision of both the common bile duct and the laparoscopic port sites

5. **Which of the following is true regarding the surgical management for T2 or T3 gallbladder cancers?**

A. Formal segmentectomy (4b + 5) improves overall survival over wedge resection.

B. Formal segmentectomy reduces local recurrence rates compared to wedge resection, but overall survival is the same.

C. Formal segmentectomy improves disease-free survival but not overall survival.

D. A clear survival benefit for formal segmentectomy over wedge resection has not been demonstrated.

6. **Which of the following is true regarding gallbladder adenomyomatosis?**

A. Adenomyomatosis is a premalignant condition, and all patients with adenomyomatosis found on imaging should be offered cholecystectomy.

B. Adenomyomatosis has no relationship to gallbladder malignancy and should be treated as an incidental finding.

C. There is an unclear relationship between adenomyomatosis and gallbladder cancer, but the presence of adenomyomatosis may obscure

the finding of a synchronous malignant lesion on sonography. Symptomatic patients with adenomyomatosis should therefore be offered cholecystectomy.

D. The presence of adenomyomatosis on imaging is usually a harbinger of locally advanced malignancy and should be treated with up-front radical cholecystectomy.

7. **The patient described earlier presents complaining of the same symptoms, but her ultrasound demonstrates a 9-mm polyp in the gallbladder fundus without wall thickening. A previous ultrasound from 1 year prior demonstrated a 4-mm polyp in the same location. The patient would prefer to avoid surgery. Which is true regarding the lesion's malignant potential and the appropriate next steps?**

A. Polyps smaller than 10 mm are seldom malignant. It would be reasonable to repeat an ultrasound in 12 months and recommend cholecystectomy only if the lesion is >10 mm in size.

B. Despite the polyp's size of less than 10 mm, its growth is concerning, and the patient should be counseled to undergo cholecystectomy.

C. The lesion likely represents a cholesterol polyp given its size. Treatment should be initiated with ursodeoxycholic acid and the lesion assessed for regression with sonography at 1 year.

D. Positron emission tomography (PET) may be pursued as it is helpful for excluding malignancy from polyps discovered on ultrasound.

ANSWERS

1. D. A history of gallstones is common, and 65–90% of those with biliary carcinoma, have a history of gallstones. The relation of gallstones to gallbladder cancer (GBC) is thought to be mediated by chronic inflammation. There is a relatively well-defined sequence of flat-epithelial premalignant changes leading to GBC. Chronic inflammation leads to intermediate low-grade dysplastic changes. Dysplastic progression over time leads to carcinoma in situ and finally invasive carcinoma. An anomalous union of the pancreaticobiliary ductal system, where the pancreatic duct and common bile duct merge outside the wall of the duodenum and form a long common channel, is also associated with an increased risk of

GBC. This PBM leads to chronic reflux of pancreatic enzymes.

The progression to GBC is likely mediated through an epithelial hyperplasia, with resultant papillary or villous epithelial changes progressing to GBC. Further evidence that this is a distinct pathway from chronic inflammation is that the gene alterations of cancers arising in the setting of cholelithiasis differ from anomalies of the duct system–associated cancers. Adenomas do occur in the gallbladder and can progress to cancer. However, this is less common than the other two pathways, given a lack of cancer-related molecular changes in most of these lesions. Inflammatory bowel disease is also associated with increased risk for gallbladder carcinoma. Clonorchis infection is associated with risk for cholangiocarcinoma, but it has not been linked to carcinoma of the gallbladder. Chronic *Salmonella typhi* or *paratyphi* infection is, however, associated with increased risk for gallbladder cancer. Hemolytic anemia may be a cause of bilirubin-type gallstones but is not a risk factor for gallbladder cancer; neither is biliary dyskinesia or autoimmune diseases.

2. **B.** A recent retrospective study of findings on MDCT associated with gallbladder cancer found two patterns most associated with finding malignancy at the time of surgery. A strongly enhancing thick inner layer and a weakly enhancing or nonenhancing outer layer of the gallbladder wall were shown to have a 52–55% incidence for gallbladder cancer. A single thick layer with heterogeneous enhancement on MDCT had an incidence of 35–38% for gallbladder cancer. PBM without bile duct dilatation has an incidence of biliary tract cancer of 37.9%, of which 93.2% of these were gallbladder cancer. Based on these data, prophylactic cholecystectomy is recommended for these patients. The incidence rates of malignancy in gallbladder polyps vary widely in published reports but range from 9.6–40% for polyps 10–20 mm. The wide variance is related to various imaging modalities used and populations studied. Polyps ≥10 mm, sessile polyps, and rapidly growing polyps are all recommendations for gallbladder removal.

The finding of gallbladder calcifications or a porcelain gallbladder was found to be associated with malignancy in 6% of cases in a recent systematic literature review. This is a far lower number than the historically quoted figure of approximately 25%. Attempts in the review were made to limit inherent biases in a review

of retrospective studies that favor overestimation, but this value likely still overestimates the true incidence. Given the incidence, the decision to perform a prophylactic cholecystectomy should not be absolute and should be weighed against the risks of surgery for the individual patient. The presence of gallstones is associated with an increased risk of gallbladder cancer. The size and volume of stone burden have been identified as potential risk factors for developing gallbladder cancer. However, there is no direct evidence of a causal relationship between gallstones and gallbladder cancer. The risk for gallbladder cancer development with a 3-cm or greater stone has been estimated to be a 2% risk over a 20-year period.

3. **D.** The patient has a T1b lesion or early gallbladder cancer. Surgical resection is the only curative therapy for gallbladder cancer. The consensus is for radical cholecystectomy for T1b or greater lesions. T1b tumors have been shown to have lymph node metastasis in 24% of cases. Lower recurrence rates and improved survival have been observed with radical resection including lymph nodes when compared to a simple cholecystectomy. A review of the SEER database showed that the evaluation of even a single lymph node improved overall survival and that radical resection without lymph node assessment was no better than cholecystectomy alone for early-stage gallbladder cancer. Neoadjuvant therapy has been evaluated in the setting of borderline and unresectable extra-hepatic biliary malignancies, with good results in survival and obtaining negative margins, but these studies did not address gallbladder cancer specifically and were confined to advanced disease. Adjuvant chemoradiation does have a role in select gallbladder cancer patients, especially with positive nodes or margins to improve local control.

4. **B.** Prognosis of gallbladder carcinoma is determined by the depth of tumor infiltration and the ability to obtain a tumor-free resection margin (R0). For T2 or greater, the definitive resection should include a minimal hepatic resection centered on the gallbladder bed and a regional lymphadenectomy. The majority of experts also extend this recommendation to T1b tumors, but some controversy persists. There is uniform agreement that cholecystectomy alone is sufficient for Tis and T1a tumors. There is also general agreement regarding several other technical points, such as resection of the common bile duct and the

need for port site excision. Regarding routine common bile duct excision with radical cholecystectomy, unless there is a direct invasion of the hepatoduodenal ligament and/or of the cystic duct, bile duct resection does not result in decreased recurrence or better overall survival and does not increase the number of nodes in the specimen. Peritoneal involvement with gallbladder cancer is common, and there is a theoretical adverse impact on this with pneumoperitoneum. However, the risk of port site recurrence is based on perforation of the gallbladder or extraction without a retrieval bag rather than the pneumoperitoneum. Port site excision does not improve overall or disease-free survival in large retrospective series. Port site excision does not need to be routinely performed during secondary procedures for gallbladder cancer discovered after laparoscopic cholecystectomy.

5. **D.** Although some studies have reported anatomical resection improves survival and R0 resection rate when compared to wedge resection, other reports have not demonstrated a benefit. The majority of these studies dealt with liver resection for liver metastases. There are a few studies looking at gallbladder cancer specifically. Pawlik et al. found that patients who underwent a major hepatic resection (e.g., formal segmentectomy of 4b + 5 or hemi-hepatectomy) had a similar risk of disease-specific death compared with patients who underwent hepatic wedge resection. Horiguchi et al. found the overall survival rate and disease-free survival rate at 5 years did not differ significantly between wedge resection and 4a + 5 resection group for T2 tumors. The available evidence in gallbladder cancer does not show a clear benefit to anatomic resection. As such, the surgeon's goal should be to resect all disease with negative histologic margins and choose the appropriate operation to achieve this with the fewest complications.

6. **C.** Adenomyomatosis is a somewhat uncommon (found in approximately 1% of cholecystectomies in one series) histologic change of the gallbladder lumen characterized by overgrowth of the mucosa and thickening of the muscularis layer. Additionally, intramural diverticula can form. These diverticula can herniate through the muscularis propria into the gallbladder wall forming Rokitansky-Aschoff sinuses, which are seen grossly as collections of bile within the gallbladder wall. In several series, gallbladder cancer has been identified at slightly increased rates in gallbladder specimens with adenomyomatosis. In one series, one quarter of patients with gallbladder cancer were found to have adenomyomatosis. In those patients, adenomyomatosis was associated with a significant increase in T stage, nodal positivity, and distant metastatic lesions. Kai et al. proposed that the imaging characteristics of adenomyomatosis may obscure the early detection of gallbladder cancer leading to a delay in diagnosis and more advanced lesions at the time of diagnosis. Based on the paucity of evidence for a causal link between adenomyomatosis and cancer, the decision to proceed to cholecystectomy should be based on the presence of symptoms.

7. **B.** Cholecystectomy should be offered to all symptomatic patients with polyps of any size, as these patients are likely to have symptom relief following removal. In patients with polyps <10 mm in size and without symptoms, a follow-up ultrasound in 6 months to assess for stability is reasonable. An increase in polyp size, regardless of the presence of symptoms, is an indication for surgery, even if the enlarged polyp is still <10 mm in size. Given that this patient is both symptomatic and has had an interval increase in polyp size, she should be strongly counseled to undergo cholecystectomy. Ursodeoxycholic acid is of little utility in decreasing the size of cholesterol polyps. Gallbladder cancers are frequently PET-avid, but a negative scan does not exclude malignancy in an otherwise concerning lesion.

BIBLIOGRAPHY

Araida T, Higuchi R, Hamano M, et al. Should the extrahepatic bile duct be resected or preserved in R0 radical surgery for advanced gallbladder carcinoma? Results of a Japanese Society of Biliary Surgery survey: A multicenter study. *Surg Today.* 2009;39:770–779.

Azuma T, Yoshikawa T, Araida T, Takasaki K. Differential diagnosis of polypoid lesions of the gallbladder by endoscopic ultrasonography. *Am J Surg.* 2001;181(1):65.

Cavallaro A, Piccolo G, Panebianco V, et al. Incidental gallbladder cancer during laparoscopic cholecystectomy: Managing an unexpected finding. *World J Gastroenterol.* 2012;18(30):4019–4027.

Corwin MT, Siewert B, Sheiman RG, Kane RA. Incidentally detected gallbladder polyps: is follow-up necessary?—long-term clinical and US analysis of 346 patients. *Radiology.* 2011;258(1):277–282.

Diehl AK. Gallstone size and the risk of gallbladder cancer. *JAMA.* 1983;250:2323–2326.

Fetzner UK, Holscher AH, Stippel DL. Regional lymphadenectomy strongly recommended in T1b gallbladder cancer. *World J Gastroent.* 2011;17(38):4347–4348.

Fuks D, Regimbeau JM, Pessaux P, et al. Is port-site resection necessary in the surgical management of gallbladder cancer? *J Visc Surg.* 2013;150:277–284.

Goetze TO, Paolucci V. Immediate re-resection of T1 incidental gallbladder carcinomas: a survival analysis of the German Registry. *Surg Endosc.* 2008;22:2462–2465.

Horiguchi A, Miyakawa S, Ishihara S, et al. Gallbladder bed resection or hepatectomy of segments 4 and 5 for pT2 gallbladder carcinoma: Analysis of Japanese registration cases by the study group for biliary surgery of the Japanese Society of Hepato-Biliary-Pancreatic Surgery. *J Hepatobiliary Pancreat Sci.* 2013;20(5):518–524.

Jensen EH, Abraham A, Habermann EB, et al. A critical analysis of the surgical management of early-stage gallbladder cancer in the United States. *J Gastrointest Surg.* 2009;13:722–727.

Jensen EH, Abraham A, Jarosek S, et al. Lymph node evaluation is associated with improved survival after surgery for early stage gallbladder cancer. *Surgery.* 2009;146:706–713.

Kai K, Ide T, Masuda M, et al. Clinicopathologic features of advanced gallbladder cancer associated with adenomyomatosis. *Virchows Archiv.* 2011;459(6):573–580.

Kim SJ, Lee JM, Lee JY, et al. Analysis of enhancement pattern of flat gallbladder wall thickening on MDCT to differentiate gallbladder cancer from cholecystitis. *AJR.* 2008;191:765–771.

Koga A, Watanabe K, Fukuyama T, Takiguchi S, Nakayama F. Diagnosis and operative indications for polypoid lesions of the gallbladder. *Arch Surg.* 1988;123(1):26–29.

Kwon W, Jang J-Y, Lee SE, et al. Clinicopathologic features of polypoid lesions of the gallbladder and risk factors of gallbladder cancer. *J Korean Med Sci.* 2009;24:481–487.

Lee J, Yun M, Kim KS, et al. Risk stratification of gallbladder polyps (1–2 cm) for surgical intervention with 18 F-FDG PET/CT. *J Nucl Med.* 2012;53:353–358.

Maker AV, Butte JM, Oxenberg J, et al. Is port site resection necessary in the surgical management of gallbladder cancer? *Ann Surg Oncol.* 2012;19:409–417.

Maringhini A, Moreau JA, Melton LJ, et al. Gallstones, gallbladder cancer, and other gastrointestinal malignancies. An epidemiologic study in Rochester, Minnesota. *Ann Intern Med.* 1987;107(1):30–35.

Marsh R DE W, Alonzo M, Bajaj S, et al. Comprehensive review of the diagnosis and treatment of biliary tract cancer 2012. Part II: multidisciplinary management. *J Surg Oncol.* 2012;106:339–345.

Miyazaki M, Takada T, Miyakawa S, et al. Risk factors for biliary tract and ampullary carcinomas and prophylactic surgery for these factors. *J Hepatobiliary Pancreat Surg.* 2008;15:15–24.

Nabatame N, Shirai Y, Nishimura A, Yokoyama N, Wakai T, Hatakeyama K. High risk of gallbladder carcinoma in elderly patients with segmental adenomyomatosis of the gallbladder. *J Exp Clin Cancer Res.* 2004;23(4):593–598.

Numata K, Oka H, Morimoto M, et al. Differential diagnosis of gallbladder diseases with contrast-enhanced harmonic gray scale ultrasonography. *J Ultrasound Med.* 2007;26:763–774.

Ootani T, Shirai Y, Tsukada K, Muto T. Relationship between gallbladder carcinoma and the segmental type of adenomyomatosis of the gallbladder. *Cancer.* 1992;69(11):2647–2652.

Pawlik TM, Gleisner AL, Vigano L, et al. Incidence of finding residual disease for incidental gallbladder carcinoma: implications for re-resection. *J Gastrointest Surg.* 2007;11:1478–1486.

Rodríguez-Fernández A, Gómez-Río M, Medina-Benítez A, et al. Application of modern imaging methods in diagnosis of gallbladder cancer. *J Surg. Oncol.* 2006;93(8):650–664.

Schnelldorfer T. Porcelain gallbladder: a benign process or concern for malignancy? *J Gastrointest Surg.* 2013;17:1161–1168.

Sugiyama M, Atomi Y, Yamato T. Endoscopic ultrasonography for differential diagnosis of polypoid gall-bladder lesions: analysis in surgical and follow-up series. *Gut.* 2000;46:250–254.

Vijayakumar A, Vijayakumar A, Patil V, et al. Early diagnosis of gallbladder carcinoma: an algorithm approach. *ISRN Radiol.* 2013; Article ID 239424:1–6.

Yamamoto, T. A study of cholesterol gallstone formation in cases of cholesterolosis of the gallbladder [author's translation]. *Nihon Shokakibyo Gakkai zasshi.* 1979;76(1):91.

27

Biliary Colic

Anne O'Shea and Timothy J. Vreeland

A 55-year-old obese female with no significant past medical history presents with a monthlong history of intermittent, sharp right upper quadrant (RUQ) abdominal pain, radiating to her mid-epigastrium. Her pain episodes last approximately 15 minutes, are associated with nausea without emesis, and seem to be exacerbated by food, especially greasy foods. She denies any associated fevers, chills, jaundice, acolic stools, or choluria. She has attempted to treat the episodic pain with Tums and Pepto-Bismol without relief and notes no change in, or pain with, bowel movements. Her past medical history is significant only for gastroesophageal reflux disease (GERD), she does not smoke or drink, and she denies any significant family history. Her vital signs are within normal limits and her abdominal exam is benign.

1. **Which of the patient's reported symptoms is part of the Rome Criteria IV for biliary pain?**

   A. Pain is sharp in nature.
   B. Pain is exacerbated by PO intake.
   C. Pain is not significantly relieved with bowel movements, acid suppression, or postural changes.
   D. Pain lasts 15 minutes.

2. **For laboratory workup, you order a complete blood count (CBC), basic metabolic panel (BMP), liver function tests (LFTs), and a lipase test. What results would you expect in this patient?**

   A. Elevated bilirubin with normal transaminases
   B. Elevated lipase
   C. Elevated white blood cell (WBC) count
   D. Normal hemoglobin and hematocrit (H&H) and normal WBC count

3. **Following lab work, what is the best initial study to determine the etiology of this patient's pain?**

   A. Computed tomography (CT) of the abdomen and pelvis
   B. RUQ ultrasound
   C. Esophagogastroduodenoscopy (EGD)
   D. Cholescintigraphy
   E. Abdominal x-ray

4. **The patient's imaging reveals multiple dependent subcentimeter gallstones, as well as a nondependent mass that does not move with positional changes, consistent with a gallbladder polyp measuring 0.9 cm. What is the most likely pathology of this mass?**

   A. Cholesterolosis
   B. Adenomyomatosis
   C. Gallbladder adenocarcinoma
   D. Adenoma
   E. Leiomyoma

5. **After discussing her options, the patient decides to undergo an elective laparoscopic cholecystectomy. You schedule her surgery for 3 weeks from now; however, a week before her surgery she presents to the ED with persistent RUQ pain, jaundice, and PO intolerance. Which of the following lab values, when elevated, is most predictive of choledocholithiasis?**

   A. Alkaline phosphatase (ALP)
   B. Total bilirubin
   C. Alanine aminotransferase (ALT)
   D. Aspartate aminotransferase (AST)

6. **The patient's labs are significant for a mildly elevated bilirubin, however. Her magnetic resonance cholangiopancreatography (MRCP) scan is negative for any gallstones in the common bile duct. She undergoes an uncomplicated cholecystectomy.**

   A. In patients with uncertain biliary anatomy or suspicion of bile duct injury during laparoscopic cholecystectomy, the procedure should immediately be converted to open to define anatomy.

   B. A critical view of safety should be obtained prior to the division of any structures.

   C. A laparoscopic total cholecystectomy via a fundus-first top-down approach should be performed when a critical view of safety cannot be obtained.

   D. In patients with significant cholecystitis and elevated white blood cell count, antibiotics should be started and cholecystectomy should be delayed by 4 weeks.

7. **The patient's pathology report reveals that the gallbladder polyp was, in fact, a papillary gallbladder adenocarcinoma invading into the lamina propria. The patient undergoes CT chest, abdomen, and pelvis scans for staging, which are negative. What is the next best step in management?**

   A. Extended right hepatectomy with regional lymphadenectomy

   B. Resection of hepatic segments IVB and V with regional lymphadenectomy

   C. No further surgical management

   D. Bile duct resection with hepaticojejunostomy

ANSWERS

1. **C.** The Rome criteria were developed to categorize and diagnose functional gastrointestinal disorders (FGIDs), disorders characterized by persistent, recurrent gastrointestinal (GI) symptoms without an identifiable anatomic or structural cause. The modified Rome IV classification was published in May 2016 and included certain criteria for biliary pain. The biliary pain criteria described does not apply to disorders with identifiable causes, like gallstones or other obstructive sources but rather is used to identify disorders of gut–brain interaction, such as functional gallbladder disorders like biliary dyskinesia and sphincter of Oddi dysfunction. Although they do not encompass all potential symptoms and presentations of any biliary-related pain, the Rome IV

criteria are still applicable to biliary disorders **with** identifiable anatomic or structural causes. However, it is important to recognize this limitation.

Biliary pain originates from the activation of visceral pain fibers usually stimulated by spasm of the gallbladder or luminal obstruction of the cystic duct. The pain can be located in the RUQ or epigastrium as the nerves that innervate the gallbladder originate in the celiac axis. Biliary pain will not be relieved by acid suppression or postural changes, and any pain relieved by acid suppression is likely secondary to GERD, gastritis, or peptic ulcer disease. Similarly, biliary pain will not be relieved by bowel movements; this is typical of pain secondary to irritable bowel syndrome. The specific nature of pain, that is, sharp, is not part of the Rome criteria, however, per the Rome criteria, biliary pain typically builds up to a steady level and is characterized as severe enough to interrupt daily activities or lead to an emergency department visit. In addition, benign biliary pain typically lasts at least 30 minutes before resolving, usually corresponding to the time in which a meal is digested and the secretion of cholecystokinin (CCK) subsides. Finally, while the exacerbation of pain with PO intake is characteristic of symptomatic cholelithiasis, as the secretion of CCK stimulates gallbladder contraction and stone impaction, the Rome criteria describe GI disorders without an identifiable anatomic cause; thus, exacerbation with PO intake is NOT part of these criteria.

2. **D.** This vignette is a classic presentation of uncomplicated biliary colic or symptomatic cholelithiasis. Biliary colic refers to pain secondary to temporary obstruction of the biliary tree usually caused by gallstones. In working up a patient with suspected pain of biliary origin, the most helpful laboratory tests include a CBC to evaluate for leukocytosis, LFTs to evaluate biliary physiology and look for evidence of hepatocellular injury, and a lipase test to rule out a pancreatic origin. Symptomatic cholelithiasis with only temporary occlusion of the cystic duct has no systemic manifestations and therefore would likely result in no lab abnormalities. Should this obstruction become prolonged, the resultant stasis, increased pressure and bacterial translocation will lead to the inflammation and infection termed acute cholecystitis. These patients typically report systemic symptoms and will exhibit a leukocytosis but normal LFTs. However, should a patient develop choledocholithiasis with a distal occlusion, the stasis of bile translates intrahepatically, resulting in a conjugated hyperbilirubinemia as well as elevated transaminases. Superimposed

infection from bacteria ascending from the GI tract produces acute cholangitis. Patients with cholangitis will typically report obstructive symptoms such as jaundice, acholic stools, and choluria, in addition to right upper quadrant pain and fever. This combination of symptoms is known as Charcot's triad (specifically jaundice, RUQ pain, and fever). The addition of hypotension and altered mental status comprises the Reynolds' pentad, which is indicative of **suppurative cholangitis**, essentially a worsening infection of the biliary system, and the development of sepsis from cholangitis. Finally, distal biliary obstruction at or near the sphincter of Oddi can result in stasis and back pressure in the pancreatic duct leading to inappropriate and excessive activation of intrapancreatic proteases and autodigestion of the pancreatic tissue, thus pancreatitis. Patients with gallstone pancreatitis appear systemically ill and have constant, visceral mid-epigastric pain that may radiate to the left and the back; often, this pain is improved with leaning forward and associated nausea and vomiting. Lab work will reveal leukocytosis and elevated lipase. Depending on the location of the distal biliary obstruction, these patients may also have elevated bilirubin and hepatic transaminases.

3. **B.** An RUQ ultrasound is the ideal initial imaging test to use in the setting of RUQ pain with suspected biliary pathology. It remains the most accurate test for distinguishing cholelithiasis and gallbladder sludge with a sensitivity of 97% and a specificity of 95%. Ultrasound can also be used to detect acute gallbladder inflammation, workup causes of biliary obstruction, and detect bile leaks following cholecystectomy. Furthermore, it is inexpensive, readily available, carries no radiation exposure, and noninvasive.

Based on the clinical presentation and lab results, you suspect the patient has symptomatic cholelithiasis. In order to rule in or out this diagnosis, imaging of the gallbladder is necessary to identify the presence or absence of gallstones and evaluate for any additional pathology. While abdominal plain films may be used to rapidly diagnose pathology, such as intraperitoneal free air or nephrolithiasis, less than 10% of gallstones are radio-opaque; therefore, x-ray is neither sensitive nor specific in the diagnosis of cholelithiasis. A CT scan is a useful modality to evaluate patients with abdominal pain and potential multisystem disease. However, it is not the most accurate test for diagnosing cholelithiasis with reported sensitivities ranging from 67–86%, and even lower for cholelithiasis without cholecystitis. Also, a CT scan is more expensive than ultrasound

and comes with unnecessary radiation. Nevertheless, abdominal CT scans can be useful in the diagnosis of acute cholecystitis using imaging findings such as pericholecystic fat stranding, mural stratification, pericholecystic enhancement, gallbladder distention, and wall thickening with sensitivities up to 92.5%.

Cholescintigraphy is a form of nuclear medicine hepatobiliary imaging that utilizes radiotracers, most commonly Tc-99m-IDA analogs, to assess the anatomy and function of the biliary tree. This hepatic iminodiacetic acid (IDA) imaging gives rise to the synonymous term hepatobiliary iminodiacetic acid (HIDA) scan. IDA radiotracers are injected intravenously, taken up by hepatocytes, and subsequently secreted into the biliary system. The absence of gallbladder visualization after an allotted amount of time is pathognomonic for cystic duct obstruction, which is indicative of acute cholecystitis. While this makes HIDA the most definitive test for diagnosing acute acalculous cholecystitis, it is not an ideal test for symptomatic cholelithiasis, which is defined by temporary cystic duct obstruction. An HIDA scan is typically ordered when clinical suspicion for acute cholecystitis is present, but US findings are equivocal. HIDA scans can also help with the diagnosis of biliary dyskinesia (low ejection fraction) or chronic cholecystitis (delayed filling of the gallbladder and/or slow biliary to bowel transit time). EGD can aid in ruling out other potential diagnoses, such as peptic ulcer disease, whose symptoms can mimic those of biliary colic, however, it is not the next-best test in the diagnosis of symptomatic cholelithiasis.

4. **A.** Unless impacted, gallstones should move with positional changes in the patient. On the other hand, gallbladder polyps are fixed, do not move with positional changes, and can be in a nondependent location within the gallbladder. Polypoid masses of the gallbladder can be nonneoplastic or neoplastic in nature. Of the nonneoplastic gallbladder polypoid masses, the most common is cholesterolosis resulting from cholesterol-laden macrophages in the lamina propria. These cholesterol masses can be multiple and depending on their location can lead to symptoms similar to those caused by gallstones. Cholesterolosis is also the most common polypoid lesion overall. Other benign etiologies of gallbladder polyps include adenomyomatosis, characterized by hyperplastic gallbladder mucosa occurring at Rokitansky-Aschoff sinuses and through the crypts

of Luschka in the gallbladder wall and extending into the lumen and the muscular layer of the gallbladder.

Of the neoplastic polypoid lesions of the gallbladder, adenomas are the most common, although less common than cholesterolosis. Gallbladder adenomas are benign epithelial tumors that can be classified as papillary or nonpapillary by histology and are considered premalignant in nature. The risk of adenocarcinoma increases as the size of the adenoma increases, with polyps ≥10 mm and those with rapid growth carrying reported risks of malignancy anywhere from 37–55%. A defining characteristic of neoplastic lesions on ultrasound is the presence of vascular flow within the lesion, which will not be seen in nonneoplastic lesions. Other benign neoplastic polypoid lesions of the gallbladder include leiomyomas, fibromas, and lipomas, all of which are exceeding rare. Finally, gallbladder adenocarcinoma is the most common malignant neoplastic lesion of the gallbladder, however, only 0.6% of polyps are malignant.

5. **A.** All of the listed lab values can be elevated in the setting of choledocholithiasis. Of the most common laboratory tests ordered to evaluate a patient with suspected choledocholithiasis, ALP has been identified as most predictive on multivariate logistic regression analysis. However, it is important to note that while not commonly ordered in the workup for choledocholithiasis, gamma-glutamyl transferase (GGT) has been implicated as the strongest biochemical predictor of choledocholithiasis (GGT OR 3.20 vs. ALP OR 2.03, p ≤ 0.001 and 0.001, respectively). Total bilirubin has a lower predictive value than either GGT or ALP as elevations in bilirubin can be caused by hemolytic disorders or any process impeding secretion of bile into the GI tract. Transaminitis, or elevations in AST and ALT, are not as sensitive as bilirubin for choledocholithiasis. AST and ALT can be elevated in a wide variety of conditions, including viral hepatitis, congestive heart failure, myocardial infarction, diabetes, acute hemolytic anemia, severe burns, and trauma.

It is important to note that while laboratory values can aid in the diagnosis of choledocholithiasis, they are relatively low in sensitivity and specificity and should therefore be coupled with imaging findings to make a clinical determination. Furthermore, because all liver tests can be elevated secondary to a wide variety of pathologies, their positive predictive value is comparatively low. Conversely, the negative predictive value of normal liver enzymes is relatively high. Therefore, normal liver function tests play a greater role in ruling out choledocholithiasis than elevated liver function tests play in diagnosing it.

6. **B.** As bile duct injuries are the most common serious complication of laparoscopic cholecystectomies, in 2014, the Society of American Gastrointestinal and Endoscopic Surgeons (SAGES) formed a safe cholecystectomy task force charged with creating a universal culture of safety in an attempt to decrease bile duct injuries. In 2020, SAGES went on to publish a multi-society practice guideline along with the Americas Hepato-Pancreato-Biliary Association (AHPBA), the International Hepato-Pancreato-Biliary Association (IHPBA), the Society for Surgery of the Alimentary Tract (SSAT), and the European Association for Endoscopic Surgery (EAES), based on a consensus conference devoted to the prevention of bile duct injuries during cholecystectomy. The multi-society practice guideline addressed a series of 18 key questions to provide evidence-based recommendations. The topics addressed included anatomic identification techniques, disease factors, surgical techniques, surgeon education, and intra-operative management of injury. The first question addressed by the consensus guideline was whether a critical view of safety technique should be used as opposed to other techniques (such as intraoperative cholangiogram, top-down, or infundibular approaches) to lower the risk of bile duct injury. From both large-sample single-institution studies and pooled bile duct injury incidence there exist lower than expected rates of common bile duct injuries with routine use of a critical view of safety. Given the above data and the fact that a critical view of safety is attainable in most dissections, SAGES recommends that surgeons at least attempt to obtain the critical view of safety in every case prior to dividing any structures (B). Although a critical view of safety is attainable in most laparoscopic cholecystectomies, there are instances where a critical view of safety cannot be achieved. In these instances, SAGES recommends a laparoscopic subtotal cholecystectomy over other techniques to include laparoscopic total cholecystectomy, converted open total vs. subtotal cholecystectomy, or a total cholecystectomy via a top-down approach based on percent of bile duct injuries, conversion to open rates, hospital LOS, wound infection, and re-operative rates (C).In cases of uncertain biliary anatomy or suspicion of bile duct injury, the consensus recommendation is to perform intraoperative biliary

imaging (such as intraoperative cholangiogram) to define anatomy, lower the risk of bile duct injury, and increase intra-operative recognition of bile duct injuries (A). In patients presenting with acute cholecystitis, the SAGES consensus guideline recommends early cholecystectomy, defined as within 72 hours of presentation. This recommendation is based largely off a single meta-analysis identifying that early cholecystectomy was associated with lower rates of wound infections, shorter hospital stays and lower complication rates (D).

7. **C.** Gallbladder cancer is an aggressive malignancy with a poor prognosis that usually manifests in the sixth or seventh decades of life and is two to three times more common in women. The predominant theory behind the development of gallbladder cancer is that chronic inflammation leads to increased cellular proliferation and subsequent malignant transformation. Therefore, gallstones, especially those greater than 3 cm, are considered a risk factor for gallbladder cancer. Gallbladder cancer is usually adenocarcinoma, with the papillary subtype having the most favorable prognosis. Because of the tendency for gallbladder cancer to form in the fundus, patients do not develop symptoms right away and therefore tend to have advanced disease at presentation. For gallbladder cancers identified at the time of cholecystectomy, management is based on staging according to the depth of penetration through the gallbladder wall and status of surgical margins.

Lesions that invade into the lamina propria but not the muscles are classified as T1a and do not require any further surgical management as long as an R0 resection has been achieved. According to the most recent National Comprehensive Cancer Network guidelines, cancers invading into the muscular layer of the gallbladder wall or farther ($\geq$T1b) should undergo hepatic resection with a regional lymphadenectomy. Although historically a formal segment IVB/V resection was performed, an increase in perioperative morbidity and the noninferiority of a nonanatomic resection has made IVB/V resection fall out of favor, with most surgeons resecting the tumor with a 2-cm margin of grossly normal liver based on imaging and intraoperative ultrasound. In reality, the answer of segment IVB/V would not be entirely incorrect if the tumor was T1b or greater as this is an area of active debate. Similarly, right hepatectomy is no longer performed for gall bladder cancer unless necessary to obtain adequate margins. Either way, formal resection would not be necessary for this patient given the stage of her cancer. Of note, although there is controversy around the type of liver resection necessary, it is clearly recommended that a lymphadenectomy be performed for all patients with $\geq$T1b gallbladder cancer. Finally, a bile duct resection with reconstruction should only be performed on patients with known malignancy in whom a negative cystic duct margin cannot be obtained on frozen section intraoperatively. Because our patient's cancer was found incidentally and margins were negative, this is not necessary in this case. Any bile duct resection in the setting of gallbladder cancer is of questionable benefit given the aggressive nature of the disease. Patients presenting with jaundice from gallbladder adenocarcinoma are generally considered unresectable.

BIBLIOGRAPHY

Bourgouin S, Truchet X, Lamblin G, De Roulhac J, Platel JP, Balandraud P. Dynamic analysis of commonly used biochemical parameters to predict common bile duct stones in patients undergoing laparoscopic cholecystectomy. *Surg Endosc.* 2017;31(11):4725–4734. doi:10.1007/s00464-017-5549-2.

Cameron JL. *Current Surgical Therapy.* 13th ed. Elsevier; 2019.

Farinon AM, Pacella A, Cetta F, Sianesi M. "Adenomatous polyps of the gallbladder" adenomas of the gallbladder. *HPB Surg.* 1991;3(4):251–258. doi:10.1155/1991/59324.

Hickman L, Contreras C. Gallbladder cancer: diagnosis, surgical management, and adjuvant therapies. *Surg Clin North Am.* 2019;99(2):337–355. doi:10.1016/j.suc.2018.12.008.

Kozuka S, Tsubone N, Yasui A, Hachisuka K. Relation of adenoma to carcinoma in the gallbladder. *Cancer.* 1982;50(10):2226–2234. doi:10.1002/1097-0142(19821115)50:10<2226::aid-cncr2820501043>3.0.co;2-3.

Lee SE, Jang JY, Lim CS, Kang MJ, Kim SW. Systematic review on the surgical treatment for T1 gallbladder cancer. *World J Gastroenterol.* 2011;17(2):174–180. doi:10.3748/wjg.v17.i2.174.

Michael Brunt L, Deziel DJ, Telem DA, et al. Safe cholecystectomy multi-society practice guideline and state-of-the-art consensus conference on prevention of bile duct injury during cholecystectomy. *Surg Endosc* 2020;34(7):2827-2855. DOI: 10.1007/s00464-020-07568-7.

National Comprehensive Cancer Network Clinical Practice Guidelines in Oncology: Hepatobiliary Cancer. August 4, 2020. https://www.nccn.org/professionals/physician_gls/pdf/hepatobiliary.pdf

Schmulson MJ, Drossman DA. What is new in Rome IV. *J Neurogastroenterol Motil.* 2017;23(2):151–163. doi:10.5056/jnm16214.

Shea JA, Berlin JA, Escarce JJ, et al. Revised estimates of diagnostic test sensitivity and specificity in suspected biliary tract disease. *Arch Intern Med.* 1994;154(22):2573–2581.

Thomas S, Jahangir K. Noninvasive imaging of the biliary system relevant to percutaneous interventions. *Semin Intervent Radiol.* 2016;33(4):277–282. doi:10.1055/s-0036-1592328.

Yang MH, Chen TH, Wang SE, et al. Biochemical predictors for absence of common bile duct stones in patients undergoing laparoscopic cholecystectomy. *Surg Endosc.* 2008;22(7):1620–1624. doi:10.1007/s00464-007-9665-2.

28

Biliary Tract—Cholangitis

Harry T. Aubin and Freeman Condon

A 70-year-old male presents to the emergency department with altered mental status. The family reports he was complaining of right upper quadrant abdominal pain prior to becoming altered mentally. On arrival, he is found to have a temperature of 102.5°F, a heart rate of 112, and systolic blood pressure of 80 despite 2 liters of crystalloid infusion. On exam, he is visibly jaundiced with tenderness in the right upper quadrant. He has three out of four systemic inflammatory response syndrome criteria. He is started on piperacillin/tazobactam and admitted to the intensive care unit for invasive monitoring and vasopressor support.

1. **Regarding this patient's constellation of symptoms, what is the most common cause?**

   A. Gallstones
   B. Biliary stricture
   C. Malignancy
   D. Alcohol abuse

2. **Regarding the pathophysiology of cholangitis, which of the following is correct?**

   A. A decrease in the production of IgG in the biliary mucosa leads to increased translocation.
   B. Intra-portal toxins and bacteria can enter through the biliary system due to stasis.
   C. Stones do not colonize with bacteria.
   D. Biliary stents do not contribute to cholangitis.

3. **Regarding the proper diagnostic workup, which noninvasive test has the highest sensitivity and specificity for detecting the most common cause?**

   A. Abdominal ultrasound
   B. Magnetic resonance cholangiopancreatography (MRCP)
   C. Computed tomography (CT) scan
   D. Hepatobiliary iminodiacetic acid (HIDA) scan

4. **Regarding the management of septic cholangitis caused by choledocholithiasis in this patient, which of the following is correct?**

   A. Urgent biliary tract decompression via endoscopic retrograde cholangiopancreatography (ERCP) should be successful 95% of the time.
   B. Percutaneous transhepatic cholangiography (PTC) is feasible for stone extraction, sphincterotomy, and stent placement.
   C. ERCP with a sphincterotomy is equivalent to cholecystectomy for reducing recurrence rates.
   D. Should ERCP and PTC fail or are not feasible, only laparoscopic choledochotomy and T-tube placement should be done because of the risk of open surgery.
   E. Broad-spectrum antibiotic therapy alone will generally provide adequate treatment.

5. **The described patient undergoes ERCP with successful clearance of the obstructing stone. A completion cholangiogram is performed demonstrating no further filling defects in the biliary tree. His septic physiology rapidly resolves, and he is downgraded to the medical/surgical ward. Which is true regarding his further management?**

   A. Provided a sphincterotomy was performed during the ERCP, there is no indication for cholecystectomy as recurrent choledocholithiasis is rare following sphincterotomy.

B. Cholecystectomy should be performed immediately following ERCP, preferably under the same anesthetic.

C. Cholecystectomy can be deferred for now but must be performed if he suffers another episode of choledocholithiasis or cholangitis.

D. Cholecystectomy should be performed during this admission once the patient has stabilized and recovered from his septic insult.

ANSWERS

1. A. Cholangitis is caused by obstruction of the biliary tree eventually leading to bile stasis and bacterial infection. The most common cause is gallstones, which account for about half of cases. Other causes include stenosis/biliary stricture (perhaps from chronic pancreatitis), malignancy, and biliary stents. Stents can cause obstruction from migration, occlusion, or colonization by bacteria, leading to bacterial overgrowth and translocation into the bloodstream.

2. B. Obstruction of the biliary tree via stricture/stenosis, stones, malignancy, or stent occlusion leads to increased biliary tract pressure. This pressure promotes stasis of bile and decreases the production of IgA in the bile tract mucosa. The lack of continuous bile flow, coupled with decrease mucosal protection, allows for bacterial translocation from the duodenum through the biliary tract. This static bile and gallstones provide a healthy growth medium for bacteria. The elevated intrabiliary pressure allows for translocation of these pathogens into the systemic circulation causing septicemia. Less commonly, bacteria and toxins can enter through the portal circulation into the bile due to an increase in biliary pressure.

The most common bacteria are gram-negative enteric pathogens: *E. coli*, *Klebsiella*, and *Enterobacter*. They carry a lipopolysaccharide that promotes cytokine release and leads to septic shock. *Enterococcus* is seen in a smaller set of cases.

3. B. MRCP is the best noninvasive test to confirm the presence of choledocholithiasis due to its high sensitivity (some studies quoting 100%) and nearly 100% specificity. If the test is positive, then this confirms the diagnosis. It also is helpful in evaluating for stricture and ampullary masses. An ultrasound is a good screening tool and can be used to evaluate for common bile duct dilatation to perhaps lend clinical suspicion to the presence of biliary obstruction. It is best used in identifying the presence of cholelithiasis/cholecystitis. However, it has a lower accuracy in identifying the presence of a choledocholith, roughly 80%.

A CT scan is less useful than ultrasound in detecting cholecystitis/common bile duct dilatation but is helpful at evaluating for ampullary masses as a cause of a dilated common bile duct.

HIDA scans are not useful in the setting of cholangitis as the biliary tract infection reduces the secretion of the radio-nucleotide-labeled marker into the biliary tree. It may show, however, obstruction with a lack of flow into the duodenum. It is also the definitive test for determining acute cholecystitis.

4. A. In cases of cholangitis without septic shock, a trial of antibiotic therapy is recommended as this can resolve symptoms and ensure stability in up to 80% of patients. Routine ERCP can be performed in this setting assuming the patient remains stable. This patient displays Reynold's pentad of fever, right upper quadrant pain, jaundice, altered mental status, and hypotension, the first three signs constituting Charcot's triad. This lends suspicion to suppurative cholangitis due to the patient's state of septic shock. Antibiotics, although required as initial therapy, are unlikely to completely resolve this patient's septic physiology. Emergent/urgent biliary tree decompression is warranted and must be performed to prevent excessive morbidity/mortality.

ERCP with sphincterotomy has shown upwards of a 95% success rate in stone extraction and decreasing the rate of recurrence of cholangitis. It is, however, not superior to cholecystectomy in decreasing rates of recurrence and thus cholecystectomy is recommended after the ERCP/sphincterotomy once the septic physiology has resolved.

Should ERCP fail, PTC is warranted as both of these procedures decrease the morbidity/mortality risk of a common bile duct exploration. PTC can be challenging if there is little intra-hepatic ductal dilatation, and it also does not allow sphincterotomy.

Common bile duct exploration is warranted should ERCP and PTC fail at decompressing the biliary tree. In the setting of a patient who is in septic shock, choledochotomy with stone extraction and T-tube placement is recommended as this allows for decompression of the biliary tree and allows for sepsis to resolve prior to performing cholecystectomy to limit the morbidity and mortality associated with both procedures. There are no data that the laparoscopic approach is superior in this setting. The exploration is performed through a choledochotomy on the common bile duct distal to the insertion of the cystic duct. Stay sutures are placed on either side of the choledochotomy, and using balloon catheters, fluoroscopy with basket retractors, and flushing, stone extraction is performed. In general, the choledochotomy should be roughly the size of the largest stone. It is best done in dilated ducts as the risk of stenosis is high in the setting of a common bile duct size of <6 mm.

A large-bore T-tube is placed and the choledochotomy repaired over the T-tube with 4-0 absorbable sutures. The tube is externalized, and bile is allowed to drain into an external bag. Due to a lack of reabsorption of bile, a patient with this procedure is prone to being deficient in fat-soluble vitamins (A, D, E, K). Vitamin K deficiency is the most worrisome as it can lead to a coagulopathy.

5. **D.** Recurrent choledocholithiasis following endoscopic sphincterotomy is common, with some series demonstrating rates of approximately 21% at 2 years. Cholecystectomy is therefore recommended for all patients medically fit to undergo an operation following an episode of calculus cholangitis. This operation is typically recommended to occur during the index hospitalization. Some authors have shown that cholecystectomy within 72 hours of successful ERCP is associated with a lower rate of postoperative complications than operations occurring greater than 72 hours after ERCP. Although early operation is recommended, it is important in cases of cholangitis associated with septic shock to ensure physiologic normalization to decrease the risks of surgery.

BIBLIOGRAPHY

Hui CK, Lai KC, Yuen MF, Ng M, Lai CL, Lam SK. Acute cholangitis–predictive factors for emergency ERCP. *Aliment Pharmacol Ther.* 2001 Oct;15(10):1633–1637.

Kim DI, Kim MH, Lee SK, et al. Risk factors for recurrence of primary bile duct stones after endoscopic biliary sphincterotomy. *Gastrointest Endosc.* 2001;54(1):42–48.

Kimura Y, Takada T, Kawarada Y, et al. Definitions, pathophysiology, and epidemiology of acute cholangitis and cholecystitis: Tokyo guidelines. *J Hepatobiliary Pancreat Surg.* 2007;14(1):15–26.

Lai EC, Mok FP, Tan ES, et al. Endoscopic biliary drainage for severe acute cholangitis. *N Engl J Med.* 1992;326(24): 1582–1586.

Lai EC, Tam PC, Paterson IA, et al. Emergency surgery for severe acute cholangitis. The high-risk patients. *Ann Surg.* 1990;211(1):55–59.

Leung JW, Sung JY, Costerton JW. Bacteriological and electron microscopy examination of brown pigment stones. *J Clin Microbiol.* 1989;27(5):915–921.

Salman B, Yılmaz U, Kerem M, et al. The timing of laparoscopic cholecystectomy after endoscopic retrograde cholangiopancreaticography in cholelithiasis coexisting with choledocholithiasis. *J Hepatobiliary Pancreat Surg.* 2009;16(6):832.

Schiphorst AH, Besselink MG, Boerma D, et al. Timing of cholecystectomy after endoscopic sphincterotomy for common bile duct stones. *Surg Endosc.* 2008 Sept;22(9):2046–2050.

Shimizu S, Yokohata K, Mizumoto K, Yamaguchi K, Chijiiwa K, Tanaka M. Laparoscopic choledochotomy for bile duct stones. *J Hepatobiliary Pancreat Surg.* 2002;9(2):201–205.

Singh A, Mann HS, Thukral CL, Singh NR. Diagnostic accuracy of MRCP as compared to ultrasound/CT in patients with obstructive jaundice. *J Clin Diagn Res.* 2014 Mar;8(3):103–107.

Snauwaert C, Laukens P, Dillemans B, et al. Laparoscopy-assisted transgastric endoscopic retrograde cholangiopancreatography in bariatric Roux-en-Y gastric bypass patients. *Endosc Int Open.* 2015;3(5):E458–E463.

Sung JY, Costerton JW, Shaffer EA. Defense system in the biliary tract against bacterial infection. *Dig Dis Sci.* 1992;37(5): 689–696.

Tsuchiya T, Sofuni A, Tsuji S, et al. Endoscopic management of acute cholangitis according to the TG 13. *Dig Endosc.* 2017;29:94–99.

29

Cholecystitis in Pregnancy

Alan P. Gehrich and Dylan Russell

A 32-year-old gravida 2 para 1 female at 24 weeks' gestation presents with acute onset of right upper quadrant (RUQ) and right upper flank pain with associated nausea and vomiting over the preceding 24 hours. She has no significant medical or surgical history. She has had one uncomplicated vaginal delivery. At the time of her evaluation, her temperature is 99.8°F, her heart rate is 110, and her respiratory rate is 24. Her exam documents a positive Murphy's sign and guarding in the RUQ. Laboratory studies show the following: white blood cell (WBC) count—20,000, hemaglobin and hematocrit—9/29, platelets—130,000, alanine aminotransferase (ALT)—60, and aspartate aminotransferase (AST)—90. Her bilirubin, lipase, and amylase levels are normal. Her urinalysis is within normal limits.

1. **Which of the following diagnoses is the most common disease in this pregnancy presenting with RUQ pain?**

   A. Acute fatty liver of pregnancy
   B. Cholecystitis
   C. Cholelithiasis
   D. Hemolysis, elevated liver enzymes, low platelets (HELLP) syndrome
   E. Appendicitis

2. **Which of the following statements is correct concerning acute fatty liver of pregnancy (AFLP)?**

   A. It most commonly presents during the second trimester of pregnancy.
   B. It commonly presents with serum aminotransferase levels similar to those found in gallbladder disease.

   C. It can present with hypoglycemia, which can help distinguish it from HELLP syndrome and gallbladder disease.
   D. In a preterm pregnancy, it is best to continue the pregnancy.

3. **Which of the following statements regarding radiographic imaging of biliary disease in pregnancy is correct?**

   A. Classic sonographic signs of biliary disease are altered in pregnancy.
   B. The risk of radiation exposure to the fetus with endoscopic retrograde cholangiopancreatography (ERCP) is high throughout pregnancy.
   C. The neuronal development of the fetus is most sensitive to radiation between 20–28 weeks' gestation.
   D. Exposure to less than 5 rad of ionizing radiation has not been associated with an increased risk of fetal anomalies or pregnancy loss.
   E. Magnetic resonance imaging (MRI) has a higher sensitivity and specificity in the diagnosis of cholecystitis than ultrasonography.

4. **In this patient, acute cholecystitis is diagnosed by ultrasound (US). Which of the following is correct regarding the treatment of this patient?**

   A. The risk of adverse effects of laparoscopy is high even with maximal intra-abdominal pressures limited to 9 mmHg.
   B. If left untreated, the most common complication of acute cholecystitis in pregnancy is gangrenous cholecystitis.

C. There are significant differences in preterm delivery rates with the laparoscopic technique.

D. Nonsteroidal anti-inflammatory drugs (NSAID) treatment for pain expected to last more than 48–72 hours is the pharmacologic option of choice after 30 weeks' gestation.

E. Beta-lactam antibiotics, such as ampicillin-sulbactam or piperacillin-tazobactam, are contraindicated in pregnant patients.

5. In this patient, which of the following statements regarding management of the pregnant patient is true?

A. Laparoscopic surgery should only be done during the second trimester.

B. Laparoscopic surgery should not be performed after 28 weeks of gestation.

C. She may undergo laparoscopic surgery safely during any trimester without an increased risk to the mother or fetus.

D. Her surgery should be postponed until after parturition as there is no increased risk to the mother or fetus.

6. You proceed to the operating room for laparoscopic cholecystectomy. How do you position the patient?

A. Supine

B. Right lateral decubitus or partial right lateral decubitus

C. Left lateral decubitus or partial left lateral decubitus

D. High lithotomy

7. This patient undergoes an uncomplicated laparoscopic cholecystectomy. On postoperative day 2, she develops increasing pain in her RUQ with fever and recurrent leukocytosis as well as elevated total bilirubin, transaminase, lipase, and amylase levels. An RUQ US documents dilated biliary ducts. Which of the following would be the most appropriate next step?

A. MRCP (magnetic resonance cholangiopancreaticography) scan

B. ERCP

C. Continued observation with antibiotic therapy

D. Repeat surgery with bile duct exploration

E. Delivery of the fetus

Answers

1. E. The most common surgical disease in pregnancy is appendicitis with an incidence of 1 in 1,000–2,000

pregnancies. Gallbladder disease is the second most common surgical disease in pregnancy with an incidence of 1 in 1,200 to 1 in 10,000. Theoretically, the incidence of gallbladder disease including cholelithiasis, cholecystitis, and cholangitis should be increased in pregnancy. The elevated level of serum estrogen seen in pregnancy increases cholesterol secretion, whereas the elevated level of progesterone reduces soluble bile acid secretion and slows the emptying of the gallbladder. Despite the predilection toward biliary sludge and stone formation, cholecystitis does not occur more frequently during pregnancy. Appendicitis occurs with equal frequency in each trimester, and the incidence is not increased in the gravid patient.

The differential diagnosis for RUQ abdominal pain is expanded in pregnancy. It includes gastrointestinal disorders, such as pancreatitis, peptic ulcer disease, hepatitis, and appendicitis, due to a superiorly displaced cecum, as well as pyelonephritis, nephrolithiasis, right lower lobe pneumonia, peptic ulcer disease, and myocardial infarction. Obstetric-specific diagnoses must also be included in the differential to include preeclampsia, HELLP syndrome, and AFLP. HELLP syndrome is a severe form of preeclampsia occurring in up to 8 of 1,000 pregnancies, presenting most commonly in the third trimester of pregnancy. This syndrome generally involves the characteristic hypertension and proteinuria seen with preeclampsia with evidence of liver dysfunction and a consumptive coagulopathy which can rapidly progress to fulminant disseminated intravascular coagulation (DIC). Patients with preeclampsia may present with right upper quadrant or epigastric pain due to liver involvement and in the most severe cases subcapsular hemorrhage or hepatic rupture. AFLP is a rare diagnosis, seen in 1 in 20,000 pregnancies.

This patient presents with findings consistent with an inflammatory intra-abdominal process. Cholecystitis, choledocholithiasis, and cholangitis lead the differential diagnosis. The physical exam findings are highly suggestive of gallbladder disease. WBC counts and alkaline phosphatase levels are routinely elevated during pregnancy and therefore may not be as specific for inflammation during the assessment of the gravid patient.

2. C. AFLP syndrome almost always presents in the third trimester with serum aminotransferase elevations up to 1,000 IU/L, which is generally higher than those found in gallbladder disease. AFLP can also present with hypoglycemia and renal failure, which is not characteristic of either HELLP or gallbladder disease. Findings of AFLP can still significantly overlap with those of HELLP, making it very difficult to distinguish these two syndromes. The treatment for both is the emergent delivery of the fetus.

3. **D.** Due to the acuity of presentation and the myriad of diagnoses in the differential, imaging is an essential component in the diagnostic evaluation. The risks of radiologic studies to the fetus must therefore be considered. Sonography is the appropriate first-line diagnostic modality in pregnancy for both biliary disease and appendicitis as this modality has a high diagnostic accuracy (90–100% for both diagnoses) and has no known risk to the fetus. Classic US findings include wall edema, pericholecystic fluid, calculi, and the sonographic Murphy's sign maintains its sensitivity and specificity in pregnancy. If US studies are nondiagnostic, MRI without contrast has become the confirmatory test for appendicitis. For biliary disease, an MRCP can be used in equivocal cases or in suspected cases of choledocholithiasis or cholangitis. It is not as sensitive as US for cholecystitis. Intraoperative cholangiogram in combination with cholecystectomy is an option for diagnostic evaluation after fetal organogenesis is complete in the second trimester and does not appear to increase the risk for preterm delivery or adverse fetal outcomes. If MRCP documents stone disease in the biliary tree, ERCP is considered a viable therapeutic option after the first trimester. The risks to the fetus with cholangiogram and ERCP can be reduced with shielding.

A CT scan of the abdomen, which is the preferred imaging modality for appendicitis in the nonpregnant patient, confers radiation levels of 5–10 rads, which approach the maximum permissible radiation dose for fetal exposure during pregnancy. Fetal exposure to ionizing radiation increases the risks of microcephaly, microphthalmia, mental retardation, growth restriction, and cataracts. The concern of ionizing radiation is greatest during organogenesis, which falls between 3–20 weeks of gestation. The described patient is at 24 weeks and therefore the risk of serious complications with ionizing radiation is limited. CT generally remains behind US and MRI on the imaging algorithm for both appendicitis and cholecystitis even in the patient with a fetus of advanced gestational age due to the disputed twofold increased risk of carcinogenesis (1:1000) in the fetus. CT imaging should, however, not be abandoned as a diagnostic modality, as the risk of delay in diagnosis far outweighs the risk of radiation. The consulting radiologist can design CT protocols to minimize the associated risks, and counseling can minimize the associated anxiety of the patient.

4. **B.** Initial nonsurgical management can be considered in hemodynamically normal pregnant patients experiencing cholelithiasis. This management plan generally involves bowel rest, intravenous hydration, and NSAID therapy. A short course (<48–72 hours) of indomethacin treatment can provide effective analgesia but is generally avoided in late pregnancy due to the potential adverse fetal effects. Use in the third trimester increases the risk of premature closure of the patent ductus arteriosis and oligohydramnios. Intravenous antibiotics to include ampicillin-sulbactam, piperacillin-tazobactam, and ticarcillin-clavulanate are not contraindicated in pregnant patients who need antibiotics for acute cholecystitis or choledocholithiasis.

Early surgery has been advocated for all types of biliary disease in pregnancy. If not treated, cholecystitis can lead to life-threatening complications, the most common of which is gangrenous cholecystitis followed by abscess formation, perforation, fistula, ileus, or emphysematous cholecystitis. For symptomatic cholelithiasis with no evidence of cholecystitis, surgery can be delayed. However, the literature reports that surgical management of symptomatic cholelithiasis in pregnancy is safe, decreases hospital days, reduces emergency department visits, and the rate of preterm deliveries.

Surgical management of biliary disease has been revolutionized with the advent of laparoscopy. The laparoscopic technique can be utilized safely in pregnancy across all trimesters depending on the comfort level of the surgeon. Although data are limited, laparoscopy does not confer an increased risk of adverse pregnancy outcomes to include preterm delivery as compared to laparotomy. An open-entry technique is recommended to prevent injury to the enlarged gravid uterus. Intra-abdominal pressure with pneumo-peritoneum should be limited to 10–12 mmHg to reduce the theoretical concern of fetal acidosis associated with the effect of CO_2. There is no indication for intraoperative fetal monitoring.

5. **C.** Surgeons previously recommended that non-emergent procedures during pregnancy should be avoided during the first and third trimesters to

minimize the risk of spontaneous abortion and preterm labor. This recommendation is not supported by good quality evidence. Multiple studies over nearly three decades have demonstrated that pregnant patients may undergo laparoscopic surgery safely during any trimester without an increased risk to the mother or fetus. The Society of American Gastrointestinal and Endoscopic Surgeons even publishes strong guideline statements that "laparoscopy can be safely performed during any trimester of pregnancy when operation is indicated" and "laparoscopic cholecystectomy is the treatment of choice in the pregnant patient with symptomatic gallbladder disease, regardless of trimester."

In this patient, with clear evidence of cholecystitis, surgical intervention is warranted to reduce the risk of serious complications. If complications such as cholangitis or gallstone pancreatitis develop in a pregnant patient, maternal mortality may approach 15% and fetal loss up to 60%.

6. **C.** When in the supine position, the gravid uterus compresses the inferior vena cava, resulting in decreased venous return from the lower extremities. This consequently reduces cardiac output due to decreased preload and results in maternal hypotension and placental hypoperfusion during surgery. These effects can be mitigated by placement in the left lateral decubitus position, which shifts the uterus off the inferior vena cava. A partial left lateral decubitus position can be utilized if a full left lateral decubitus position compromises abdominal access or performance of the procedure. Such positioning is generally only required after the first trimester as the small size of the uterus in early pregnancy does not compress the inferior vena cava.

7. **B.** Following cholecystectomy, this patient presents with findings consistent with choledocholithiasis, with associated gallstone pancreatitis and possible cholangitis. The best option in this case is ERCP with the option of sphincterotomy to decompress the biliary tract. This approach appears safe in pregnant patients with early-onset cholangitis with lower morbidity than conservative management. In this patient, repeat surgery with intraoperative cholangiography or bile duct exploration would be a backup option if the stones cannot be removed via ERCP. Percutaneous biliary tract decompression would be another option in a high-risk patient. MRCP is an

excellent and safe diagnostic test in pregnancy and is a viable option in patients when the diagnosis is uncertain; however, the US has proved the diagnosis.

In a case with a high suspicion of cholangitis, this step could delay therapy which could have severe consequences for both fetus and mother. More aggressive therapy for cholangitis is therefore indicated in pregnancy. Although conservative treatment with continued intravenous antibiotics and observation may be appropriate in the nongravid patient, the risks of this nonsurgical approach are higher in the gravid patient and predispose her to grave complications. Premature delivery of the fetus is not indicated for the treatment of biliary disease.

BIBLIOGRAPHY

Augustin G, Majerovic M. Non-obstetrical acute abdomen during pregnancy. *Eur J Obstet Gynecol Reprod Biol.* 2007;131(1):4–12.

Abbasi N, Patenaude V, Abenhaim H. Management and outcomes of acute appendicitis in pregnancy-population-based study of over 7000 cases. *BJOG.* 2014;121(12): 1509–1514.

Banks PA, Freeman ML, et al. Practice Guidelines in Acute Pancreatitis. *Am J Gastroenterol.* 2006;101(10): 2379–2400.

Chen MM, Coakley FV, Kaimal A, Laros RKJr. Guidelines for computed tomography and magnetic resonance imaging use during pregnancy and lactation. *Obstet Gynecol.* 2008; 112(2 Pt 1):333–340.

Dietrich CS, Hill CC, Hueman M. Surgical diseases presenting in pregnancy. *Surg Clin North Am.* 2008;88(2):403–419, vii–viii.

Gilat T, Konikoff F. Pregnancy and the biliary tract. *Can J Gastroenterol.* 2000;14(Suppl D):55D–59D.

Gilo NB, Amini D, Landy HJ. Appendicitis and cholecystitis in pregnancy. *Clin Obstet Gynecol.* 2009;52(4):586–596.

Gjelsteen AC, Ching BH, Meyermann MW, et al. CT, MRI, PET, PET/CT, and ultrasound in the evaluation of obstetric and gynecologic patients. *Surg Clin North Am.* 2008;88(2):361–390, vii.

Graham G, Baxi L, Tharakan T. Laparoscopic cholecystectomy during pregnancy: a case series and review of the literature. *Obstet Gynecol Surv.* 1998;53(9):566–574.

Khandelwal A, Fasih N, Kielar A. Imaging of acute abdomen in pregnancy. *Radiol Clin North Am.* 2013;51(6):1005–1022.

Kim YW, Zagorski SM, Chung MH. Laparoscopic common bile duct exploration in pregnancy with acute gallstone pancreatitis. *JSLS.* 2006;10(1):78–82.

Knight M, Nelson-Piercy C, Kurinczuk JJ, Spark P, Brocklehurst P. UK Obstetric Surveillance System. A prospective national study of acute fatty liver of pregnancy in the UK. *Gut.* 2008;57(7):951–956.

Koren G, Florescu A, Costei AM, Boskovic R, Moretti ME. Nonsteroidal antiinflammatory drugs during third trimester and the risk of premature closure of the ductus arteriosus: a meta-analysis. *Ann Pharmacother.* 2006;40(5):824–829.

Lu EJ, Curet MJ, El-Sayed YY, Kirkwood KS. Medical versus surgical management of biliary tract disease in pregnancy. *Am J Surg.* 2004;188(6):755–759.

Othman MO, Stone E, Hashimi M, Parasher G. Conservative management of cholelithiasis and its complications in pregnancy is associated with recurrent symptoms and more emergency department visits. *Gastrointest Endosc.* 2012;76(3):564–569.

Parangi S, Levine D, Henry A, Isakovich N, Pories S. Surgical gastrointestinal disorders during pregnancy. *Am J Surg.* 2007;193(2):223–232.

Pearl JP, Price RR, Tonkin AE, Richardson WS, Stefanidis D. SAGES guidelines for the use of laparoscopy during pregnancy. *Surg Endosc.* 2017;31(10): 3767–3782.

Reiss R, Nudelman I, Gutman C, Deutsch AA. Changing trends in surgery for acute cholecystitis. *World J Surg.* 1990;14(5):567–570, discussion 570–571.

Walcher T, Haenle MM, Kron M, et al. Pregnancy is not a risk factor for gallstone disease: Results of a randomly selected population sample. *World J Gastroenterol.* 2005;11(43): 6800–6806.

Wallace GW, Davis MA, Semelka RC, Fielding JR. Imaging the pregnant patient with abdominal pain. *Abdom Imaging.* 2012;37(5):849–860.

30

Liver Metastasis

Kevin M. Lin-Hurtubise, Robert L. Sheffler, and Travis Mason

A 60-year-old male presents with a 2-month history of rectal bleeding associated with anorexia and a 10-lb weight loss. He underwent a diagnostic colonoscopy revealing an ulcerated and circumferential right cecal mass; the biopsy returns as invasive adenocarcinoma. The staging computed tomography (CT) scan of the chest/abdomen/pelvis shows bilobar and peripheral liver masses ranging from 2–3 cm in diameter with a total of three masses, no regional or paraaortic adenopathy, and no other distant sites of disease. Percutaneous biopsy of a right lobar liver mass reveals metastatic adenocarcinoma, consistent with the colon as the primary site of malignancy. The patient has hypertension and hypercholesterolemia. He has no family history of colorectal cancer. His functional status is good.

1. **The best initial management in this patient is**
   A. neoadjuvant chemotherapy.
   B. concomitant right hemicolectomy and liver resection.
   C. right colectomy and then chemotherapy.
   D. radiofrequency ablation of liver tumors.
   E. hepatic intra-arterial chemotherapy.

2. **Regarding neoadjuvant chemotherapy used for metastatic colorectal cancer, which of the following statements is true?**
   A. XELOX (capecitabine and oxaliplatin) is less effective than 5-FU and leucovorin.
   B. FOLFOXIRI (leucovorin, 5-FU, oxaliplatin, irinotecan) is recommended over FOLFIRI (5-FU, leucovorin, and irinotecan).

   C. FOLFIRI increases overall survival compared to FOLFOX (5-FU, leucovorin, and oxaliplatin).
   D. Cetuximab plus multiagent chemo (FOLFOX or FOLFIRI) is best used for patients with the K-RAS mutant colorectal cancer.
   E. 5-FU and leucovorin are adequate.

3. **Contraindications to liver surgery for metastatic tumor resection include**
   A. a resection that would remove five hepatic segments.
   B. bilobar liver involvement.
   C. a resection that would require removal of 60% of the liver.
   D. a 4-cm liver lesion.
   E. a tumor involving the common hepatic artery.

4. **After successful resection of both the primary colon cancer and its liver metastases, the guidelines for surveillance include**
   A. occult fecal blood testing every 6 months.
   B. carcinoembryonic antigen (CEA) levels annually for the next 5 years.
   C. CT scans of thorax/abdomen/pelvis every 3 months for the next 5 years.
   D. surveillance colonoscopy 1 year after surgery, repeat in 3 years if no advanced adenomas found, then every 5 years.
   E. annual PET scan.

5. **For initially unresectable K-RAS mutant colorectal liver metastases, what percentage of patients will be resectable following neoadjuvant chemotherapy?**

A. About 5–10%
B. About 10–15%
C. About 30–35%
D. About 50–55%
E. About 70–75%

6. **In the described scenario, assume the patient received 6 cycles of FOLFOXIRI to assist with resectability of the liver metastases. On restaging CT scans the lesions in the right lobe of the liver have vanished. What is the next best step in management?**

A. Plan to proceed to the OR for a left-sided wedge resection and right lobectomy.
B. Obtain interval CT imaging of the liver in 3–6 months to see if the metastases reappear.
C. Obtain a preoperative MRI of the liver with Eovist contrast.
D. Proceed to the OR for liver resection, attempt to localize the vanished metastases with intraoperative liver ultrasound and, if this fails, proceed with blind hepatic sectionectomy.
E. Treat the patient with six additional cycles of chemotherapy and look for response in the left-sided lesion.

7. **In the described scenario, the left liver mass is 3 cm in segment 2, the two right liver masses are a 3-cm mass in segment 7, and 2-cm mass in segment 8 abutting the middle hepatic vein. There is a minimal response to six cycles of neoadjuvant chemotherapy. What is the best surgical plan for this patient?**

A. Proceed with a right hepatectomy and a left segmentectomy of 2, leaving the patient with a liver remnant of 24%.
B. Perform a two-stage operation with a segmentectomy of 2, followed by right portal venous embolization and interval right hepatic lobectomy.
C. Perform wedge resections of all three metastases, using a parenchyma-sparing strategy.

D. Perform a two-stage operation with a segmentectomy of 7 followed by left portal venous embolization and interval left trisectionectomy.
E. Perform a Y90 radioembolization of all three lesions to improve resectability prior to operation.

ANSWERS

1. **B.** Concomitant colon and liver resections would be preferable for this patient. If hepatic metastases are resectable on presentation, surgical resection should be considered rather than preoperative chemotherapy for medically fit patients with four or fewer metastases. The definition of resectable disease encompasses both the character of the metastatic lesions and the patient's overall health status. This patient has minimal comorbidities and a good functional status, rendering him a potentially good candidate for major abdominal surgery. The liver lesions in this scenario are considered resectable because of their overall number (4 or fewer), moderate size (only 2–3 cm), and its ideal peripheral liver location. Central or large metastatic liver lesions (>6 cm) that encroach on major liver vasculature, such as the hilum of the main portal vein would preclude liver resection. Unfortunately, no more than 20% of patients with isolated hepatic metastases are amenable to potential curative hepatic resection, but because of clear survival impact, surgical resection is the treatment of choice for resectable colorectal metastases to the liver.

There is an exception to this rule: if the metastatic tumor response to chemotherapy is expected to create a significantly less complex liver resection, then neoadjuvant therapy is recommended. The next recommended management option is an initial right hemicolectomy if the patient is already exhibiting gastrointestinal (GI) obstructive symptoms, followed by four to six cycles of chemotherapy (must be cognizant of potential hepatotoxicity if too much

Chemotherapeutic Regimen	5-FU	Leucovorin	Oxaliplatin	Irinotecan	Capecitabine
FOLFOX	+	+	+		
FOLFOXIRI	+	+	+	+	
FOLFIRI	+	+		+	
XELOX			+		+

chemotherapy is given), and then consideration of liver resection if still indicated. Radiofrequency ablation is not considered curative for larger liver metastases. Intra-arterial chemotherapy should be limited to centers with expertise in this modality.

2. **B.** The use of 5-FU (fluorouracil) and leucovorin have historically been the basis of adjuvant chemotherapy for Stage III colon cancer. Similarly for Stage II and III rectal cancer, 5-FU and leucovorin, along with radiation therapy, is recommended. Currently, for Stage III colon cancer, FOLFOX is considered the superior regimen over 5FU-Leucovorin, with improved survival but has an additional risk of peripheral neuropathy. For Stage IV disease, there seems to be increased response and better survival with the addition of biologic agents, such as cetuximab, panitumumab, and bevacizumab, or alkylating agents, such as oxaliplatin, and topoisomerase inhibitors, such as irinotecan to the 5FU-leucovorin regimen. The earlier table of chemotherapeutic regimens ± bevacizumab or cetuximab are acceptable for metastatic colorectal cancer treatment in the neoadjuvant setting. 5-FU and leucovorin alone are not adequate treatment for patients with metastatic colorectal disease.

According to the GONO and HORG trials, FOLFOXIRI was superior to FOLFIRI in increasing the chance of R0 resection (6% vs. 15% and 4% vs. 10%, respectively). The GONO trial also showed improved 5-year survival (23.4 months vs. 16.7 months).

The addition of biologic agents, cetuximab or panitumumab is recommended for patients with colorectal tumors exhibiting the K-RAS wild-type, which may increase the number of patients eligible for liver resection postchemotherapy (pt reevaluated for conversion to resectable disease every 2 months) to improve their outcomes. Cetuximab is not indicated in K-RAS mutant colorectal cancer.

For colorectal metastatic disease, FOLFOX or FOLFIRI are considered equally effective with different toxicity profiles. Capecitabine is an orally administered tumor-activated 5-FU prodrug.

3. **E.** Inadequate post-resection liver reserve is considered a contraindication for liver resection of colorectal metastases. That said, in healthy livers, up to 75% of the liver or up to six hepatic segments can be resected safely. The location of the tumor is also important as metastatic tumors invading the

common hepatic artery, common hepatic duct, main portal vein, or >3 hepatic veins would be considered contraindications. Extrahepatic involvement of the celiac, portal, or paraaortic nodes would also be considered a contraindication. Having bilobar disease or having more than four metastatic lesions that do not shrink with neoadjuvant chemotherapy was deemed inappropriate for liver resection based on OncoSurge statistical modeling.

4. **D.** Surveillance is an important aspect of cancer care to determine adequate initial management and to detect early recurrences. A patient would not be considered cured until they have survived at least 5 years after initial therapy. The clinical guidelines of surveillance for colon cancer patients have been put forth by the National Comprehensive Cancer Network, version 2.2020. Their recommendations include clinical assessments every 3–6 months for the first 2 years and then every 6 months for the next 3 years. This includes a serum CEA level at each clinic visit. A CT scan of the chest/abdomen/pelvis is recommended every 6–12 months for 5 years for patients at high risk of recurrence. Regarding colonoscopy, one is recommended 1 year after surgery. If no lesions or a simple adenoma is found (not advanced such as a villous polyp, polyp >1 cm, or high-grade dysplasia), a colonoscopy should be repeated in 3 years and then repeated every 5 years for the remainder of their lives. If an advanced or large adenoma is found (and subsequently removed completely via colonoscopy), then a repeat colonoscopy is recommended in 1 year. A positron emission tomography (PET) scan is reserved for instances in which the CEA is rising or lesions are seen on follow-up CT scans. Fecal occult blood testing is not required for surveillance.

5. **B.** For K-RAS mutant cancers, approximately 10–15% of patients will benefit from neoadjuvant chemotherapy in terms of ability to resect liver metastases. Two randomized studies, the GONO and HORG trials, showed modest improvement of liver resection rates from 6–15% and 4–10%, respectively.

Interestingly, in patients with K-RAS mutant cancer, neoadjuvant therapy with either FOLFOX or FOLFIRI with Cetuximab increases resectability of liver metastasis from 7.4–25.7%.

6. **C.** Vanishing liver metastases are an emerging problem in patients receiving neoadjuvant chemotherapy

for oligometastatic GI cancers. Liver MRI with Eovist contrast is the best preoperative modality for localizing vanishing metastases. What does Eovist do that allows for this better localization? This modality will decrease the need for non-therapeutic surgical explorations and blind liver sectionectomies. Right hepatic resection would remove too much parenchyma for potentially resolved right liver metastasis and would subject the patient to too much perioperative morbidity. There is no role for interval imaging as this would delay treatment of the patient's metastatic disease burden and possibly delay surgery for the primary cancer. Likewise, there is no role for continued chemotherapy in the setting of resectable liver disease as the additional chemotherapy may cause liver injury that may convert a resectable patient to nonresectable. Relying on exploration with intraoperative ultrasound would be the next best answer if the liver MRI shows no metastases. Many surgeons still advocate blind sectionectomy in the setting of disappearing metastases on all imaging modalities, although this is not a uniform standard of care. The rationale for this is that a complete pathologic response is only seen 60% of the time when vanishing liver metastases are resected.

7. **B.** A segmentectomy of 2 followed by right portal venous embolization and right hepatectomy the option that offers the best chance at cure with the least morbidity while leaving the patient with adequate liver reserve. Up-front resection of all three lesions that leaves a functional liver remnant less than 30% is not advised in patients who have received chemotherapy as it is thought that there is some underlying liver injury after chemotherapy. Although wedge resections and parenchyma sparing surgery are desirable for peripheral liver metastasis, the location of the segment 8 lesion by the middle hepatic vein would make wedge resection not feasible from a technical standpoint and would require a right lobectomy. Segmentectomy of 7 followed by left portal venous embolization and left trisectionectomy would be significantly more morbid than segmentectomy of 2 and interval right lobectomy. Y90 as a neoadjuvant therapy to improve resectability of hepatic metastases is still under investigation, and early series suggest that the complication rate after Y90 is much higher than without treatment. It is generally reserved for attempting to convert nonresectable liver metastases to resectable.

BIBLIOGRAPHY

Adam R, Aloia T, Levi F, et al. Hepatic resection after rescue cetuximab treatment for colorectal liver metastases, previously refractory to conventional systemic therapy. *J Clin Oncol.* 2007;25(29):4593–4602.

Andre T, Boni C, Navarro M, et al. Improved overall survival with oxaliplatin, fluorouracil, and leucovorin as adjuvant treatment in stage II or III colon cancer in the MOSAIC trial. *J Clin Oncol.* 2009;27(19):3109–3116.

Blazer D, Kishi Y, Maru DM, et al. Pathologic response to preoperative chemotherapy: a new outcome end point after resection of hepatic colorectal metastases. *J Clin Oncol.* 2008;26(33):5344–5351.

Bokemeyer C, Bondarenko I, Hartmann JT, et al. Efficacy according to biomarker status of ceftuximab plus FOLFOX-4 as first-line treatment for metastatic colorectal cancer: the OPUS study. *Ann Oncol.* 2011;22(7):1535–1546.

Bokemeyer C, Bondarenko I, Makhson A, et al. Fluorouracil, leucovorin, and oxaliplatin with and without ceftuximab in the first-line treatment of metastatic colorectal cancer. *J Clin Oncol.* 2009;27(5):663–671.

Carpizo D, Are C, Jarnagin W, et al. Liver resection for metastatic colorectal cancer in patients with concurrent extrahepatic disease: results in 127 patients treated at a single center. *Ann Surg Oncol.* 2009;16(8):2138–2146.

Colucci G, Gebbia V, Paoletti G, et al. Phase III randomized trial of FOLFIRI versus FOLFOX-4 in the treatment of advanced colorectal cancer: a multicenter study of the Gruppo Oncologico Dell'Ltalia Meridionale. *J Clin Oncol.* 2005;23(22):4866–4875.

Falcone A, Ricci S, Brunetti I, et al. Phase III trial of infusional fluorouracil, leucovorin, oxaliplatin, and irinotecan (FOLFOXIRI) compared with infusional flurouracil, leucovorin, and irinotecan (FOLFIRI) as first-line treatment for metastatic colorectal cancer: The Gruppo Oncologico Nord Ovest. *J Clin Oncol.* 2007;25(13):1670–1676.

Kadera B, D'Angelica M. Colorectal liver metastasis. *Deckerip Complex Gen Surg Oncol.* 2019 Jan;9:1–32.

Martin R, Augenstein V, Reuter NP, et al. Simultaneous versus staged resection for synchronous colorectal cancer liver metastases. *J Am Coll Surg.* 2009;208(5):842–850.

National Comprehensive Cancer Network. (n.d.). *NCCN Clinical Practice Guidelines in Oncology,* Version 1.2016. November 6, 2015. http://www.nccn.org/professionals/physician_gls/f_guidelines.asp

Poston G, Adam R, Alberts S, et al. OncoSurge: a strategy for improving resectability with curative intent in metastatic colorectal cancer. *J Clin Oncol.* 2005;23(28):7125–7134.

Reddy S, Pawlik TM, Zorzi D, et al. Simultaneous resections of colorectal and synchronous liver metastases: a multi-institutional analysis. *Ann Surg Oncol.* 2007;14(12):3481–3491.

Souglakos J, Androulakis N, Syrigos K, et al. FOLFOXIRI v. FOLFIRI as first-time treatment in metastatic colorectal cancer: a multicenter, randomized phase III trial from the

Hellenic Oncology Research Group (HORG). *Br J Cancer*. 2006;94(6):798–805.

Van Custem E, Kohne CH, Hitre E, et al. Ceftuximab and chemotherapy as initial treatment for metastatic colorectal cancer. *N Eng J Med*. 2009;360(14):1408–1417.

Wright, GP, Marsh, JW, Varma, MK, et al. Liver resection after selective internal radiation therapy with Yttrium-90 is safe and feasible: a bi-institutional analysis. *Ann Surg Oncol*. 2017;24(4):906–913.

31

Liver Cirrhosis

Travis Mason

A 55-year-old man with a known history of cirrhosis secondary to alcohol (ETOH) abuse presents with a several-month history of an increasing umbilical bulge. On exam he had a reducible umbilical hernia with a 3-cm fascial defect and shifting dullness and a fluid wave complete with moderate ascites. He denies any symptoms other than mild discomfort at the hernia. He denies any previous episodes of gastrointestinal (GI) bleed. History, physical exam, and serum laboratory evaluation of the patient shows a Child–Turcotte–Pugh (CTP) classification of 9 points or class B and a model for end-stage liver disease (MELD) score of 10. His platelets are 160,000, hemoglobin (HGB) is 12 g/dL, sodium level is 135 MeQ/L, and albumin is 3.0 ng/dL.

1. **Regarding evaluation and management of this patient's ascites, which of the following is true?**

    A. Variceal bleeding is the most common complication of cirrhosis.

    B. Paracentesis is the first step in the evaluation of this patient.

    C. Cessation of ETOH once ascites develop will have little impact on controlling ascites.

    D. Ascites is refractory in less than 5% of patients with ascites secondary to cirrhosis.

    E. Use of nonsteroidal anti-inflammatory drugs (NSAID), angiotensin-converting-enzyme (ACE) inhibitors, and angiotensin-receptor-blocking (ARB) drugs can prevent the progression to renal failure.

2. **Regarding umbilical hernia repair in patients with cirrhosis, which of the following is true?**

    A. Incidence of umbilical hernia is 20% in patients with cirrhosis and ascites.

    B. Large-volume paracentesis (LVP) decreases the risk of incarceration for umbilical hernias in the setting of refractory ascites.

    C. Nonoperative management of patients with umbilical hernia and ascites is the preferred management because of the morbidity and mortality associated with surgery.

    D. The use of synthetic mesh is contraindicated in repairing umbilical hernias in patients with cirrhosis and ascites.

    E. Complication rates are significantly higher in elective repair of umbilical hernia in cirrhotic patients when compared to noncirrhotic patients.

3. **Regarding morbidity and mortality in nonhepatic surgery in patients with liver cirrhosis, which statement is true?**

    A. Open surgery is preferred to laparoscopic surgery because of the concern for increased bleeding following laparoscopic procedures in cirrhotic patients.

    B. Elective pancreatic surgery in CTP class A and B has acceptable morbidity and mortality.

    C. Elective inguinal hernia repair is indicated for symptomatic inguinal hernias even in advanced liver disease with decompensated cirrhosis.

    D. Morbidity and mortality are higher for all surgical procedures in patients with liver cirrhosis when compared to patients without cirrhosis.

4. **The described patient presents to the emergency department several days after your evaluation with fever, abdominal pain, and ileus. His vitals are a temperature of 101°F, a heart rate of 90, and a systolic blood pressure of 100. On exam he is diffusely tender, without exam evidence of peritonitis, and has increased ascites. Plain films of the chest and abdomen show an ileus pattern, without obstruction and no free intraperitoneal air. Which of the following is true?**

   A. Administering broad-spectrum antibiotics as the first step is necessary to avoid circulatory collapse and hepatorenal syndrome.

   B. Multiple organisms would be found on paracentesis culture.

   C. Ascitic fluid analysis would expect to show neutrophils >100/mm^3.

   D. Administration of 1.5 g/kg of albumin on admission and 1 g/kg on day 3 has been shown to decrease mortality.

   E. A positive culture is necessary for diagnosis.

5. **The described patient undergoes elective umbilical hernia repair. On day 3 after the operation, he develops hematemesis and hypotension. Based on the most likely etiology of his upper GI hemorrhage, which of the following is true?**

   A. Propranolol plays an important role in the acute management of this problem by decreasing splanchnic blood flow.

   B. Transfusion to an HGB of 10 is the goal of resuscitation.

   C. The initiation of antibiotic therapy with Ceftriaxone or a fluoroquinolone is an important component of therapy.

   D. Transjugular intrahepatic shunt (TIPS) procedures have no role in the acute setting.

   E. Pharmacologic therapy should not be started until varices are confirmed by esophagogastroduodenoscopy (EGD).

6. **Which of the following answers is true regarding the preoperative optimization of a patient with liver cirrhosis?**

   A. Transfusing to a platelet count greater than 100,000 per microliter for any surgical procedure

   B. Use of preoperative spironolactone if the patient has altered platelet function on TEG

   C. Replenishment of vitamin K preoperatively

   D. Transfusion of von Willebrand's factor if preoperative fibrinogen is greater than 100

7. **Which of the following is true regarding perioperative morbidity and mortality from elective surgery in the cirrhotic patient population?**

   A. There is no difference in operative mortality between open and laparoscopic cholecystectomy in patients with liver cirrhosis.

   B. There is no difference in morbidity and mortality with laparoscopic appendectomy between cirrhotic and noncirrhotic patients.

   C. Complication rates are similar for umbilical hernia repair between cirrhotic and noncirrhotic patients.

   D. The mortality rate of colorectal surgery in cirrhotic patients is double the rate in noncirrhotic patients.

ANSWERS

1. **B.** The cessation of alcohol usually leads to improvement in liver function with alcohol-associated cirrhosis. One study found improvement of the Child–Pugh score was observed within 3 months in 66% of the abstinent patients. Ascites are the most common complication of cirrhosis, with 50% of compensated cirrhotics developing ascites over the course of 10 years. Paracentesis with appropriate ascitic fluid analysis is the first step in the evaluation of clinically apparent ascites. The serum-ascites albumin gradient with a value ≥1.1 g/dL is indicative of portal hypertension. Medical management with salt restriction and diuretics is highly effective in most patients with ascites. Refractory ascites occur in less than 20% of patients. The use of ACE inhibitors and ARB drugs can induce renal failure and hypotension increasing mortality in patients with ascites. NSAIDs impair the glomerular filtration rate due to a reduced renal perfusion secondary to the inhibition of renal prostaglandin synthesis leading to renal failure.

2. **A.** Umbilical hernia is present in 20% of patients with cirrhosis, and this is 10 times higher than the incidence in the overall population. The increased incidence is related to ascites, abdominal wall attenuation, and malnutrition. A sudden decrease in the number of ascites, as with TIPS or LVP, can lead to strangulation of an incarcerated umbilical hernia. Nonoperative management is associated with higher mortality when compared to elective repair. The higher mortality is related to the development of bowel incarceration or spontaneous rupture from necrosis of overlying skin (Flood syndrome) and

subsequent peritonitis developing during "watchful waiting." These complications force prompt repair in patients who are at very high risk for death with emergency surgery. A randomized study comparing umbilical hernia repair with or without prosthetic material in cirrhotic patients with symptomatic or complicated hernia found a decreased recurrence rate favoring prosthetic repair. The same study showed a nonsignificant increase in infections in the prosthetic group, but no mesh had to be removed in any of the cases. Morbidity in elective repair of umbilical hernia is similar between cirrhotics and noncirrhotics.

3. **C.** Patients with advanced decompensated cirrhosis frequently have severe symptoms because of ascites entering the hernia sac both in the standing position and when recumbent, making it difficult to relieve symptoms. Patients with decompensated cirrhosis have been shown to benefit the most in terms of improved quality of life and the procedures can be done with minimal morbidity. Laparoscopic cholecystectomy has been shown to be safe in patients with Childs–Turcotte class A and B cirrhosis and is associated with less blood loss and shorter hospital stay when compared to open cholecystectomy. Similar benefits are seen favoring laparoscopic appendectomy over open appendectomy. The data are limited for patients with Child's C classification. Pancreatic surgery is associated with an increased risk of postoperative complications in patients with liver cirrhosis. The mortality in Child's A patients is similar to noncirrhotics but the mortality for Child's B patients is prohibitive. Although morbidity is higher for cirrhotics when compared to noncirrhotics for most procedures, some procedures such as inguinal hernia repair have similar morbidity even for advanced liver disease. Mortality in Child's A patients is often fairly similar to noncirrhotics for a variety of procedures ranging from pancreatic surgery to cardiac surgery.

4. **D.** This patient most likely has spontaneous bacterial peritonitis (SBP). The use of IV albumin in cirrhotics with SBP in addition to antibiotics has been shown to decrease in-hospital mortality from 29% to 10% compared to antibiotics alone. The effect is more pronounced for patients with a creatinine greater than 1 mg/dL or a bilirubin greater than 4 mg/dL. Ascitic fluid testing should be done prior to the initiation of antibiotics because 86% of cultures will be negative even after a single dose of antibiotics. The finding of

multiple organisms from a diagnostic paracentesis should prompt consideration of a secondary peritonitis not SBP. The findings of neutrophils >100/mm^3 with lactate dehydrogenase greater than the upper limit of normal for serum, glucose less than 50 mg/dL, and ascitic protein >1 g/dL are associated with secondary peritonitis. A cirrhotic patient with signs and symptoms of SBP should be treated empirically regardless of culture results. The cultures are important for narrowing of antibiotic coverage given the increasing emergence of resistant organisms.

5. **C.** Variceal bleeding accounts for 70% of all upper GI bleeding in patients with cirrhosis. Antibiotic prophylaxis in cirrhotic patients with GI bleeding has been shown to decrease the risk of bacterial infections, rebleeding, and overall mortality. Nonselective beta-blockers (propranolol) do reduce portal blood flow by decreasing cardiac output (B-1 effect) and, more important, by producing splanchnic vasoconstriction (B-2 effect) and play a role in preventing variceal bleeding. However, they should not be used in the acute setting as they will decrease blood pressure and will blunt a physiologic response to bleeding. The goal for transfusion is for hemoglobin to be approximately 7–8 g/dL. This is based on studies showing aggressive restoration of blood volume leads to increases in portal pressure and subsequent rebleeding and mortality. TIPS procedures are very effective in controlling bleeding in the 10–20% of patients who fail pharmacologic and endoscopic therapy. Early placement of TIPS within 24–48 hours after admission has been shown to improve survival in patients at the highest risk of rebleeding (Child's C and patients with a hepatic venous pressure gradient over 20 mmHg). Vasoconstrictor therapy (vasopressin ± nitroglycerin, terlipressin, somatostatin, or octreotide) is considered first-line therapy and should be started at the time of admission in any patient with suspected variceal hemorrhage even prior to EGD.

6. **A.** Transfusion of platelets over 100,000 is only required for higher-risk surgical procedures in cirrhotic patients. Please list 2-3 higher-risk procedures. A platelet count over 50,000 is acceptable for lower-risk surgical procedures. The use of desmopressin in uremic patients, the replenishment of vitamin K preoperatively, the use of cryoprecipitate to replete clotting factors, and the routine use of antibiotics preoperatively are all within current guidelines for

the preoperative preparation of a cirrhotic patient for surgery.

Von Willebrand's factor binds with factor VIII and helps promote platelet plug formation that helps with clotting in those missing this clotting protein. Fibrinogen is produced by the liver and is converted by thrombin to fibrin to help form clots. Patients with fibrinogen less than 200 mg/dL are at risk of bleeding. Cryoprecipitate is used to replenish low fibrinogen.

7. B. Laparoscopic appendectomy is one of the few surgeries with a similar complication profile between cirrhotic and noncirrhotic patients. Open cholecystectomy has a 1–7-fold increase in mortality in cirrhotic patients whereas laparoscopic cholecystectomy is similar between the two groups. Although low in both groups, morbidity and mortality are higher for both open and laparoscopic umbilical hernia repairs in cirrhotic patients. The mortality of colorectal surgery in cirrhotic patients reported in the literature is 3–6 times higher than the mortality rate of noncirrhotic patients.

BIBLIOGRAPHY

Akriviadis EA, Runyon BA. Utility of an algorithm in differentiating spontaneous from secondary bacterial peritonitis. *Gastroenterology.* 1990;98(1):127–133.

Ammar SA. Management of complicated umbilical hernias in cirrhotic patients using permanent mesh: randomized clinical trial. *Hernia.* 2010;14(1):35–38.

Bernard B, Grange JD, Khac EN, Amiot X, Opolon P, Poynard T. Antibiotic prophylaxis for the prevention of bacterial infections in cirrhotic patients with gastrointestinal bleeding: a meta-analysis. *Hepatology.* 1999;29(6):1655–1661.

Belghiti J, Durand F. Abdominal wall hernias in the setting of cirrhosis. *Semin Liver Dis.* 1997;17(3):219–226.

de Goede B, Klitsie PJ, Lange JF, Metselaar HJ, Kazemier G. Morbidity and mortality related to non-hepatic surgery in patients with liver cirrhosis: a systematic review. *Best Pract Res Clin Gastroenterol.* 2012;26(1):47–59.

Dokmak S, Aussilhou B, Belghiti J. Umbilical hernias and cirrhose. *J Visc Surg.* 2012;149(5 Suppl):e32–e39.

Eker HH, van Ramshorst GH, de Goede B, et al. A prospective study on elective umbilical hernia repair in patients with liver cirrhosis and ascites. *Surgery.* 2011;150(3):542–546.

El-Awadi S, El-Nakeeb A, Youssef T, et al. Laparoscopic versus open cholecystectomy in cirrhotic patients: a prospective randomized study. *Int J Surg.* 2009;7(1):66–69.

European Association for the Study of the Liver. EASL Clinical Practice Guidelines on the management of patients with decompensated cirrhosis. *J Hepatol.* 2018;69:406–460.

Garcia-Pagan JC, Caca K, Bureau C, et al. Early use of TIPS in patients with cirrhosis and variceal bleeding. *N Engl J Med.* 2010;362(25):2370–2379.

Garcia-Tsao G, Sanyal AJ, Grace ND, Carey W, Practice Guidelines Committee of the American Association for the Study of Liver Diseases, Practice Parameters Committee of the American College of Gastroenterology. Prevention and management of gastroesophageal varices and variceal hemorrhage in cirrhosis. *Hepatology.* 2007;46(3):922–938.

Gines P, Quintero E, Arroyo V, et al. Compensated cirrhosis: natural history and prognostic factors. *Hepatology.* 1987;7(1):122–128.

Gray SH, Vick CC, Graham LA, Finan KR, Neumayer LA, Hawn MT. Umbilical herniorrhaphy in cirrhosis: improved outcomes with elective repair. *J Gastrointest Surg.* 2008;12(4):675–681.

Liou IW. Management of end-stage liver disease. *Med Clin North Am.* 2014;98(1):119–152.

Lopez-Delgado, J, Ballus, J, Esteve, F, et al. Outcomes in abdominal surgery in patients with liver cirrhosis. *World J Gastroenterol.* 2016 Mar 7;22(9):2657–2667.

Marsman HA, Heisterkamp J, Halm JA, Tilanus HW, Metselaar HJ, Kazemier G. Management in patients with liver cirrhosis and an umbilical hernia. *Surgery.* 2007;142(3):372–375.

Neeraj, N, Tsoi, K, Marshall, J. Should albumin be used in all patients with spontaneous bacterial peritonitis? *Can J of Gastroenterol.* 2011;25(7):373–376.

Northup, PG, Friedman, LS, Kamath, PS. AGA Clinical Practice Update on surgical risk assessment and perioperative management in cirrhosis: expert review. *Clin Gastroenterol Hepatol.* 2019;17:595–606.

Patti R, Almasio PL, Buscemi S, Fama F, Craxi A, Di Vita G. Inguinal hernioplasty improves the quality of life in patients with cirrhosis. *Am J Surg.* 2008;196(3):373–378.

Perez-Ayuso RM, Arroyo V, Planas R, et al. Randomized comparative study of efficacy of furosemide versus spironolactone in nonazotemic cirrhosis with ascites. Relationship between the diuretic response and the activity of the renin-aldosterone system. *Gastroenterology.* 1983;84(5 Pt 1):961–968.

Puggioni A, Wong LL. A metaanalysis of laparoscopic cholecystectomy in patients with cirrhosis. *J Am Coll Surg.* 2003;197(6):921–926.

Runyon BA, AASLD. Introduction to the revised american association for the study of liver diseases practice guideline management of adult patients with ascites due to cirrhosis 2012. *Hepatology.* 2013;57(4):1651–1653.

Runyon BA, Montano AA, Akriviadis EA, Antillon MR, Irving MA, McHutchison JG. The serum-ascites albumin gradient is superior to the exudate-transudate concept in the differential diagnosis of ascites. *Ann Intern Med.* 1992;117(3):215–220.

Sort P, Navasa M, Arroyo V, et al. Effect of intravenous albumin on renal impairment and mortality in patients with cirrhosis and spontaneous bacterial peritonitis. *N Engl J Med.* 1999;341(6):403–409.

Stanley MM, Ochi S, Lee KK, et al. Peritoneovenous shunting as compared with medical treatment in patients with alcoholic cirrhosis and massive ascites. Veterans Administration cooperative study on treatment of alcoholic cirrhosis with ascites. *N Engl J Med.* 1989;321(24):1632–1638.

Telem DA, Schiano T, Divino CM. Complicated hernia presentation in patients with advanced cirrhosis and refractory ascites: management and outcome. *Surgery.* 2010;148(3):538–543.

Trotter JF, Suhocki PV. Incarceration of umbilical hernia following transjugular intrahepatic portosystemic shunt for the treatment of ascites. *Liver Transpl Surg.* 1999;5(3):209–210.

Warnick P, Mai I, Klein F, et al. Safety of pancreatic surgery in patients with simultaneous liver cirrhosis: a single center experience. *Pancreatology.* 2011;11(1):24–29.

Veldt BJ, Laine F, Guillygomarc'h A, et al. Indication of liver transplantation in severe alcoholic liver cirrhosis: quantitative evaluation and optimal timing. *J Hepatol.* 2002;36(1):93–98.

32

Pancreatitis and Pancreatic Cysts

Kiran Lagisetty and Joy Sarkar

SCENARIO 1

A 56-year-old male presents to the emergency department, complaining of acute onset of intense boring epigastric pain radiating to his back. He is unable to find a comfortable position in which to lie in bed. The patient is afebrile and hemodynamically normal, and his laboratory analysis is significant for a serum lipase of 1,300, serum glucose of 260 mg/dL, lactate dehydrogenase (LDH) of 375 IU/L, aspartate aminotransferase (AST) of 350 IU/L, total bilirubin of 0.9 mg/dL, and a white blood cell (WBC) count of 18,000.

1. **In order to diagnose acute pancreatitis, two out of three of which of the following criteria are required?**

    A. Epigastric pain, radiologic evidence of pancreatitis, serum lipase at least two times normal.

    B. Epigastric pain, radiologic evidence of pancreatitis, serum amylase at least three times normal.

    C. Cholelithiasis, radiologic evidence of pancreatitis, serum lipase at least three times normal.

    D. Epigastric pain, cholelithiasis, serum lipase at least two times normal.

2. **Which of the following conditions is most likely the etiology of this patient's condition?**

    A. Hypertriglyceridemia
    B. Cholelithiasis
    C. HIV infection
    D. Pancreatic head mass
    E. Antibiotic usage

3. **A right upper quadrant ultrasound is performed, demonstrating a gallbladder wall thickness of**

2 mm, multiple small gallstones, and sludge. Which of the following is the most appropriate management of this finding?

    A. Endoscopic retrograde cholangiopancreatography (ERCP) with sphincterotomy, followed by cholecystectomy

    B. Nothing-by-mouth (NPO) status until resolution of pancreatitis, then cholecystectomy in 6 weeks

    C. Cholecystectomy within 24 hours of admission

    D. Antibiotics until resolution of leukocytosis, then cholecystectomy prior to discharge

    E. Supportive care until resolution of symptoms, then cholecystectomy prior to discharge

4. **Which of the following conditions associated with acute pancreatitis increases the mortality rate from 1% to 10–20%?**

    A. Necrosis of greater than one-fourth of the pancreas

    B. Inflammation of the entire pancreas on a computed tomography (CT) scan

    C. Development of a pseudocyst

    D. Fluid in the lesser sac

5. **A 7-cm acute peripancreatic fluid collection was identified on a CT scan prior to discharge. It was managed expectantly, and a repeat CT scan was obtained 6 weeks after admission. Which of the following would be criteria for drainage of a pseudocyst?**

    A. No evidence of malignancy on the CT scan and only a simple 5-cm pseudocyst persists

    B. Decrease in size from 7 cm to only 4 cm

    C. Persistence of abdominal pain

D. Cholelithiasis

E. No communication between the pseudocyst and a pancreatic duct such that the pseudocyst cannot drain

SCENARIO 2

A 67-year-old female undergoing a contrasted CT scan of the abdomen and pelvis for right lower quadrant abdominal pain is incidentally found to have a cyst in the head of her pancreas. The cyst measures 4 cm, and the main pancreatic duct measures 8 mm. Laboratory analysis demonstrates a WBC count of 85,000, lipase of 25 U/L, total bilirubin of 0.7 mg/dL, alkaline phosphatase of 74 U/L, and carbohydrate antigen (CA) 19-9 of 5 U/mL.

6. **What is the next best step in the management of the pancreatic cyst?**

A. Endoscopic ultrasound with fine-needle aspiration (FNA)

B. Repeat CT scan in 3 months

C. ERCP with brushing

D. Percutaneous biopsy/aspiration

E. Magnetic resonance cholangiopancreatography (MRCP) followed by surgical resection

7. **Which of the following correctly matches the type of pancreatic cyst to its imaging or pathology findings?**

A. Serous cystadenoma; unilocular cyst, containing fluid high in bicarbonate

B. Retention cyst; wall formed by granulation tissue, containing fluid rich in amylase

C. Intraductal papillary mucinous neoplasm; mucin-secreting columnar epithelium and "ovarian-type" stroma within the cyst capsule

D. Pancreatic pseudocyst; septated cyst with honeycomb appearance containing clear fluid

E. Mucinous cystic neoplasm; calcified cyst wall, containing fluid high in CEA

ANSWERS

1. **B.** At least two of the following criteria are required to diagnose acute pancreatitis: characteristic abdominal pain, radiologic evidence of pancreatitis, and/or serum amylase or lipase level at least three times normal.

2. **B.** Each of the mentioned conditions is known to cause pancreatitis. The most common etiologies are

gallstone- and alcohol-related. Hypertriglyceridemia >1,000 mg/dL is the third-most common. Other known causes of acute pancreatitis include HIV infection, certain medications like antibiotics, carcinoma, parasites, and trauma.

3. **E.** Gallstone pancreatitis is managed with cholecystectomy, but the optimal timing depends on disease severity. In patients with mild pancreatitis and no evidence of biliary obstruction, cholecystectomy should be performed during the index admission after the pancreatitis has clinically resolved. In patients with severe disease, a 6-week interval should be granted prior to cholecystectomy. There is no evidence to support the claim that enteral feeding exacerbates pancreatic inflammation, and in patients with mild pancreatitis, immediate enteral feeding should be initiated. For biliary obstruction without cholangitis, it is reasonable to delay ERCP up to 48 hours, as spontaneous stone passage may occur, obviating the need for intervention. If cholangitis is suspected, urgent ERCP should be performed as soon as possible. In this patient with no evidence of cholangitis, cholecystitis, or infected pancreatic necrosis, there is no indication for antibiotics.

4. **D.** Mild acute pancreatitis is associated with a mortality rate of about 1%. Acute pancreatitis in conjunction with any of the listed complications is considered severe acute pancreatitis and increases the mortality rate to 10–20%; necrosis of greater than one third of the pancreas, organ failure to include a systolic blood pressure ≤90 mmHg, serum creatinine >2.9 mg/dL, gastrointestinal blood loss >500 mL within a 24-hr period, or PaO_2 ≤60 mmHg. The development of a necrosis, an abscess, or a pseudocyst also represents severe acute pancreatitis and, thus, also increases the mortality rate.

5. **C.** Approximately 50% of pancreatic pseudocysts will resolve spontaneously after about 4–6 weeks and should therefore be managed expectantly. Repeat CT scan after 6 weeks should be obtained to ensure the pseudocyst is resolving. Indications for intervention are clinical symptoms, cyst enlargement or persistence over 6 cm, ductal communication, and suspected malignancy. An interval of 6 weeks is generally recommended to give time for the pseudocyst wall to "mature" into a thick, fibrous rind. The presence of cholelithiasis is not an indication for operative intervention of a pancreatic pseudocyst.

6. **A.** Pancreatic cysts can be broadly classified into simple (true) cysts, pseudocysts, and cystic neoplasms. The latter may be benign or have malignant potential. Multiple guidelines exist for the diagnosis, evaluation, and surveillance of cystic neoplasms to include the American Gastroenterological Association, the International Association of Pancreatology, and the American College of Gastroenterology, among others. While the guidelines vary in the exact definitions of high-risk stigmata, most societies agree that a cyst size ≥ 3 cm, dilated main pancreatic duct (MPD), and solid component (mural nodule) are features concerning for malignancy that warrant additional evaluation with endoscopic ultrasound and FNA. Most guidelines additionally agree that obstructive jaundice and/or atypical cytology are then indications for surgery. Because this patient has at least two high-risk factors (cyst size >3 cm and MPD >5 mm), observation with interval CT scans is not appropriate. ERCP may provide further characterization of pancreatic ductal dilation and allow for sampling or clearance of mucus in the duct but would provide a limited characterization of the cyst itself if there is no communication between the cyst and the pancreatic ducts.

7. **E.** The various types of pancreatic cysts can be differentiated by their appearances on axial imaging, endoscopic ultrasound, and pathological evaluation. Retention cysts, also called true or simple cysts, have a cyst wall made of normal pancreatic cells (ductal and centroacinar). Pancreatic pseudocysts lack a true wall; rather, the "wall" is formed of fibrous and granulation tissue. Their fluid is usually dark and high in amylase and other pancreatic enzymes, as well as bicarbonate. Serous cystadenomas have a septated "honeycomb" appearance on imaging, and occasionally a central calcified scar. The fluid is clear, serous, and low in CEA and mucin content, and the pathognomonic finding is cuboidal, glycogen-rich cells in the epithelium that stain PAS-positive. Mucinous cystic neoplasms (MCNs) are also septated, but the fluid is thick and difficult to aspirate due to the high mucin content and has a high CEA level. They are also characterized by columnar or cuboidal mucinous epithelial cells and an "ovarian-type" stroma, and the cyst wall may be calcified in some areas. Unlike MCNs, intraductal papillary mucinous neoplasms (IPMNs) occupy the pancreatic ducts themselves and lack the "ovarian-type" stroma. Due to mucus plugging of the ducts, the characteristic imaging finding with IPMNs is diffuse or segmental dilation of the main pancreatic duct or side branches.

BIBLIOGRAPHY

Beger H, Matsuno S, Cameron J. *Diseases of the Pancreas: Current Surgical Therapy*. Springer; 2008.

Hasan A, Visrodia K, Farrell JJ, Gonda TA. Overview and comparison of guidelines for management of pancreatic cystic neoplasms. *World J Gastroenterol*. 2019;25(31):4405–4413.

Karoumpalis I, Christodoulou DK. Cystic lesions of the pancreas. *Ann Gastroenterol*. 2016;29(2):155–161.

33

Head of Pancreas Mass

Phillip M. Kemp Bohan and Timothy J. Vreeland

A 60-year-old male with no significant medical history except for smoking presents with 1 week of painless jaundice. He denies any symptoms of obstruction, weight loss, or fatigue. Initial labs show a mild elevation in transaminases to less than 1.5 times normal values and a bilirubin of 8 mg/dL. A right upper quadrant (RUQ) ultrasound was obtained that shows dilated intra- and extra-hepatic bile ducts and a dilated gallbladder without stones. The pancreas is not well visualized secondary to overlying bowel gas.

1. **What would be the next best step in the evaluation of this patient?**
   A. Magnetic resonance cholangiopancreatography (MRCP)
   B. Multidetector thin-cut computed tomography (CT) scan with pancreatic and portal venous phases
   C. Whole-body positron emission tomography (PET) scan
   D. Endoscopic retrograde cholangiopancreatography (ERCP)

2. **The described patient is found to have a 2-cm mass in the head of the pancreas that is hypodense on contrast-enhanced series. There is no evidence of vascular contact or adenopathy. He has no evidence of metastatic disease on a CT scan. His carbohydrate antigen (CA) 19-9 level is elevated to 1.5 times the normal level. He is in good physical condition with no significant comorbidities that would limit his surgical options. The initial endoscopic ultrasound (EUS) biopsy is nondiagnostic. An**

IgG4 level is checked and within normal limits. What is the next most appropriate step?
   A. PET scan to evaluate for occult metastatic disease
   B. ERCP and stenting of the bile duct, decompression, and resection in 4 weeks
   C. Repeat EUS and fine-needle aspiration (FNA) biopsy of the mass to confirm the diagnosis prior to resection
   D. Proceed to pancreaticoduodenectomy

3. **The described patient is instead noted to have a 3-cm mass in the head of the pancreas that abuts greater than 180 degrees of the superior mesenteric vein (SMV) with occlusion of a short segment. There is no evidence of metastatic disease. An EUS-guided FNA biopsy was obtained showing adenocarcinoma. What is the most appropriate management for this patient?**
   A. Neoadjuvant chemoradiation
   B. Immediate pancreaticoduodenectomy with resection and reconstruction of the involved SMV followed by adjuvant chemoradiation
   C. Palliative chemotherapy
   D. Prophylactic surgical biliary and gastric bypasses prior to initiating palliative chemotherapy

4. **Which of the following is true for patients undergoing neoadjuvant therapy for resectable or borderline resectable adenocarcinoma of the pancreas?**

   Which of the following is true regarding neoadjuvant therapy for an adenocarcinoma of the pancreas?
   A. Significantly decreased local recurrence rate
   B. Lower rate of lymph node positivity

C. Significantly increased overall survival
D. Same rate of R0 resections

ANSWERS

1. **B.** Given the lack of stones, painless presentation, and age of the patient, the most likely diagnosis is a periampullary neoplasm. The next step in workup is obtaining axial imaging to assess for malignancy and determining the radiographic stage of the cancer (resectable, borderline resectable, locally advanced). The thin-cut CT scan is the best test for both establishing the cause of biliary obstruction and determining the radiographic stage. Consensus guidelines recommend multidetector CT angiography of the abdomen with a dedicated pancreatic protocol that captures the pancreatic and portal venous phases of contrast enhancement with thin (submillimeter) sections (B). Another appropriate answer (not listed) would be a contrast-enhanced, multiphasic, pancreas-protocoled magnetic resonance imaging (MRI) of the abdomen. MRI and multidetector CT have similar rates of sensitivity and specificity for determining the local extent of disease and vascular involvement, and the choice of axial imaging is often institution-dependent. MRCP (A) would not be the correct choice as this would give details of the ductal anatomy but not the relationship between the tumor and the vasculature, which is required for radiographic staging. MRCP should be used only in conjunction with a pancreas-protocoled MRI. FDG-PET/CT (C) can improve rates of detection of metastatic disease but should not be used as a tool for determining local staging or resectability. Again, PET/CT does not give details about the relationship between the tumor and surrounding vasculature. ERCP/EUS (D) is likely to be a part of most patients' staging but should not be done before axial imaging. Once axial imaging is complete, EUS with biopsy is usually used to establish tissue diagnosis. EUS also offers the opportunity for lymph node sampling but is unable to evaluate for distant metastatic spread. ERCP can also be a therapeutic intervention for patients requiring decompression of the biliary tree (particularly those who will require neoadjuvant therapy) but, again, should not be done prior to axial imaging.

2. **D.** This patient has a mass consistent with resectable pancreatic cancer and is an appropriate surgical candidate. It is somewhat controversial whether this patient needs any tissue diagnosis at all, but most

would at least make one attempt at EUS and endoscopic biopsy. In this setting, it would be important to rule out autoimmune pancreatitis (IgG4). With a nondiagnostic biopsy, the next best would be to proceed to surgery (D). A PET/CT scan to look for metastatic disease (A) is recommended only for high-risk patients (borderline resectable, significantly elevated CA 19-9 A PET/CT scan to look for metastatic disease (A) is recommended only for high-risk patients (borderline resectable, significantly elevated CA 19-9 level, or large primary tumor/nodes) or large primary tumor/nodes). Although FNA (C) is highly sensitive and specific for diagnosis and often used, given the history, imaging characteristics, and a negative IgG4 (which would identify patients with autoimmune pancreatitis), repeat sampling would not be recommended. Preoperative biliary stent placement (B) is only mandated in patients with severe jaundice/pruritus (bilirubin >12–15), cholangitis, or those who are going to receive neoadjuvant chemotherapy. Prophylactic stent placement for patients with mild/moderate symptoms who are receiving upfront surgery should be avoided as stent placement may increase rates of postoperative complications. Neoadjuvant therapy (E) for resectable pancreatic cancer remains controversial at this time. If neoadjuvant chemotherapy is pursued, the patient should be referred to a large academic center for consideration for clinical trial enrollment; in that case, EUS with FNA and ERCP with stent placement would be mandatory.

3. **A.** This patient has borderline resectable pancreatic cancer (>180 degrees of SMV involvement) and would benefit from neoadjuvant chemotherapy. Relative to up-front surgery (B), administration of neoadjuvant therapy in patients with borderline resectable cancer is associated with more R0 resections and disease-free survival in a randomized trial, as well as improved overall survival in retrospective series (no randomized trials to date). Resectability is determined by the relationship of the tumor to the major nearby arterial and venous structures, with resection status denoted as either resectable, borderline resectable, or locally advanced. Recent American Society of Clinical Oncology (ASCO) guidelines recommend neoadjuvant therapy for all patients with borderline resectable and locally advanced cancers. Treatment for patients with resectable disease remains controversial, with most

patients still receiving up-front surgery followed by adjuvant chemotherapy. The ASCO guideline does recommend neoadjuvant chemotherapy be "considered" for those patients with resectable disease. This patient should not receive palliation (C) given that many patients with borderline resectable cancer will make it to surgical resection after neoadjuvant therapy. The use of endoscopic biliary drainage has largely replaced surgical bypass procedures for biliary obstruction (D). Self-expandable metal stents have relatively low rates of reintervention (although higher than surgical bypass) and are significantly cheaper, associated with shorter lengths of hospital stay, and obviously less invasive. Metal stents are preferred to plastic stents (improved long-term patency, lower complication rates, fewer reinterventions) for patients who will require biliary decompression for longer than a month. This patient does not have gastric outlet obstruction or duodenal obstruction, so gastrojejunostomy (D) is not needed. In the case of significant gastric outlet or duodenal obstruction secondary to a pancreatic head mass, endoscopic placement of a duodenal stent and surgical creation of a gastrojejunostomy carry similar success rates. Endoscopic stent placement is less invasive and preferred in the palliative setting but is not preferred for patients with potentially resectable disease because stents frequently migrate and can cause a local inflammatory response in the future surgical field.

4. B. The recent PREOPANC trial randomized patients with either resectable or borderline resectable pancreas cancer to receive either preoperative chemoradiation or upfront surgery. Preoperative chemoradiation therapy was associated with improved disease-free survival, longer time to local recurrence (A), and a lower incidence of patients with pathologic nodal disease (B). The resection rate was slightly lower in the neoadjuvant group, although this did not reach significance (61% vs. 72%, p = 0.06). The R0 resection rate (D) was higher in the neoadjuvant chemoradiation group (71% vs. 40%, p < 0.001). However, there was no significant benefit in overall survival (C). Of note, when comparing patients who made it to resection after neoadjuvant to those who made it through up-front resection and received postoperative chemotherapy, there was improved survival amongst the patients who received neoadjuvant therapy. A recent meta-analysis that compared neoadjuvant therapy to up-front

surgery also found that neoadjuvant therapy resulted in lower overall resection rates but improved overall survival (18.8 months vs. 14.8 months). An improvement in overall survival was also shown in a National Cancer Database–derived study that evaluated neoadjuvant versus adjuvant therapy for patients with borderline resectable disease (25.7 months vs 19.6 months, p < 0.001). The concept behind providing neoadjuvant therapy instead of up-front resection is to distinguish between patients with intrinsically aggressive disease who would not benefit from a morbid operation and those patients with less aggressive disease for whom surgical resection can provide a survival benefit. Improved R0 resection rates and decreased nodal positivity contribute to the improved local recurrence rates seen in patients who receive neoadjuvant chemotherapy prior to resection.

BIBLIOGRAPHY

Al-Hawary MM, Francis IR, Chari ST, et al. Pancreatic ductal adenocarcinoma radiology reporting template: consensus statement of the society of abdominal radiology and the american pancreatic association. *Gastroenterology.* 2014;146(1):291–304.e291.

Almadi MA, Barkun A, Martel M. Plastic vs. self-expandable metal stents for palliation in malignant biliary obstruction: a series of meta-analyses. *Am J Gastroenterol.* 2017;112(2): 260–273.

Banafea O, Mghanga FP, Zhao J, Zhao R, Zhu L. Endoscopic ultrasonography with fine-needle aspiration for histological diagnosis of solid pancreatic masses: a meta-analysis of diagnostic accuracy studies. *BMC Gastroenterol.* 2016;16:108.

Bolm L, Petrova E, Woehrmann L, et al. The impact of preoperative biliary stenting in pancreatic cancer: a casematched study from the German nationwide pancreatic surgery registry (DGAV StuDoQ|Pancreas). *Pancreatology.* 2019;19(7):985–993.

Chawla A, Molina G, Pak LM, et al. Neoadjuvant therapy is associated with improved survival in borderline-resectable pancreatic cancer. *Ann Surg Oncol.* 2020;27(4):1191–1200.

Farma JM, Santillan AA, Melis M, et al. PET/CT fusion scan enhances CT staging in patients with pancreatic neoplasms. *Ann Surg Oncol.* 2008;15(9):2465–2471.

Khorana AA, Mangu PB, Berlin J, et al. Potentially curable pancreatic cancer: American Society of Clinical Oncology Clinical Practice Guideline. *J Clin Oncol.* 2016;34(21): 2541–2556.

Lee ES, Lee JM. Imaging diagnosis of pancreatic cancer: a state-of-the-art review. *World J Gastroenterol.* 2014;20(24): 7864–7877.

Ma KW, Chan ACY, She WH, et al. Efficacy of endoscopic self-expandable metal stent placement versus surgical bypass for inoperable pancreatic cancer-related malignant biliary obstruction: a propensity score-matched analysis. *Surg Endosc.* 2018;32(2):971–976.

Macedo FI, Ryon E, Maithel SK, et al. Survival outcomes associated with clinical and pathological response following neoadjuvant FOLFIRINOX or gemcitabine/nab-paclitaxel chemotherapy in resected pancreatic cancer. *Ann Surg.* 2019;270(3):400–413.

Miyasaka Y, Ohtsuka T, Kimura R, et al. Neoadjuvant chemotherapy with gemcitabine plus nab-paclitaxel for borderline resectable pancreatic cancer potentially improves survival and facilitates surgery. *Ann Surg Oncol.* 2019;26(5):1528–1534.

Pancreatic Adenocarcinoma. NCCN Clinical Practice Guidelines in Oncology. 2020. Accessed March 18, 2020. https://www.nccn.org/professionals/physician_gls/pdf/pancreatic.pdf.

Qayyum A, Tamm EP, Kamel IR, et al. ACR Appropriateness criteria® staging of pancreatic ductal adenocarcinoma. *J Am Coll Radiol.* 2017;14(11s):S560–S569.

Santhosh S, Mittal BR, Bhasin DK, et al. Fluorodeoxyglucose-positron emission tomography/computed tomography performs better than contrast-enhanced computed tomography for metastasis evaluation in the initial staging of pancreatic adenocarcinoma. *Ann Nucl Med.* 2017;31(8):575–581.

Shridhar R, Takahashi C, Huston J, Meredith KL. Neoadjuvant therapy and pancreatic cancer: a national cancer database analysis. *J Gastrointest Oncol.* 2019;10(4):663–673.

Timmermann L, Rosumeck N., Klein F, et al. Neoadjuvant chemotheraphy enhances local postoperative histopathological tumour stage in borderline resectable pancreatic cancer—a matched-pair analysis. *Anticancer Res.* 2019;39(10):5781–5787.

Treadwell JR, Zafar HM, Mitchell MD, Tipton K, Teitelbaum U, Jue J. Imaging tests for the diagnosis and staging of pancreatic adenocarcinoma: a meta-analysis. *Pancreas.* 2016;45(6):789–795.

Truty et al: Truty MJ, Kendrick ML, Nagorney DM, Smoot RL, Cleary SP, Graham RP, Goenka AH, Hallemeier CL, Haddock MG, Harmsen WS, Mahipal A, McWilliams RR, Halfdanarson TR, Grothey AF. Factors Predicting Response, Perioperative Outcomes, and Survival Following Total Neoadjuvant Therapy for Borderline/Locally Advanced Pancreatic Cancer. *Ann Surg.* 2021 Feb 1;273(2):341-349. doi: 10.1097/SLA.0000000000003284. PMID: 30946090.

Uemura et al: Uemura S, Iwashita T, Iwata K, Mukai T, Osada S, Sekino T, Adachi T, Kawai M, Yasuda I, Shimizu M. Endoscopic duodenal stent versus surgical gastrojejunostomy for gastric outlet obstruction in patients with advanced pancreatic cancer. *Pancreatology.* 2018 Jul;18(5):601-607. doi: 10.1016/j.pan.2018.04.015. Epub 2018 May 3. PMID: 29753623.

Versteijne E, Suker M, Groothuis K, et al. Preoperative chemoradiotherapy versus immediate surgery for resectable and borderline resectable pancreatic cancer: results of the Dutch randomized phase III PREOPANC trial. *J Clin Oncol.* 2020:Jco1902274.

Versteijne E, Vogel JA, Besselink MG, et al. Meta-analysis comparing upfront surgery with neoadjuvant treatment in patients with resectable or borderline resectable pancreatic cancer. *Br J Surg.* 2018;105(8):946–958.

Ye et al: Ye M, Zhang Q, Chen Y, Fu Q, Li X, Bai X, Liang T. Neoadjuvant chemotherapy for primary resectable pancreatic cancer: a systematic review and meta-analysis. HPB (Oxford). 2020 Jun;22(6):821-832. doi: 10.1016/j.hpb.2020.01.001. Epub 2020 Jan 27. PMID: 32001139 .

Yoshida Y, Fukutomi A, Tanaka M, et al. Gastrojejunostomy versus duodenal stent placement for gastric outlet obstruction in patients with unresectable pancreatic cancer. *Pancreatology.* 2017;17(6):983–989.

34

Spleen/Idiopathic Thrombocytopenic Purpura

C.T. Grayson

A 53-year-old female with a 3-week history of melena presents to her primary care provider and is found to have scattered ecchymoses, heme-positive stool, and a platelet count of 45,000. Colonoscopy screening was performed 1 year ago and was negative. She does not take any medications. Other than mild anemia, laboratory workup is otherwise unremarkable. Peripheral smear and bone marrow biopsy are negative, which do not demonstrate an underlying malignancy. She is diagnosed with idiopathic thrombocytopenic purpura (ITP).

After 8 weeks of prednisone therapy and the addition of intravenous immunoglobulin (IVIG), the patient's platelet count ranges from 20,000–40,000 and she has ongoing mucosal bleeding. She has been sent for a surgical consultation to discuss the possibility of splenectomy.

1. **Which of the following statements characterizes ITP?**

   A. Endothelial damage triggers the deposition of platelets and fibrin in small arterioles and capillaries, leading to microvascular thrombotic events.

   B. IgG autoantibodies directed against platelet fibrinogen receptors cause increased platelet destruction via removal by macrophages.

   C. Abnormal myeloid precursor cells are hyperplastic, resulting in splenic sequestration of platelets and associated thrombocytopenia.

   D. Peripheral blood smears show schistocytes, nucleated red blood cells, and basophilic stippling.

   E. Renal failure and neurologic complications are both seen in late stages.

2. **Which of the following statements about steroid-refractory ITP is correct?**

   A. Rituximab therapy can be used as an alternative to splenectomy and has an equivalent response rate.

   B. Approximately 98% of patients who undergo splenectomy are found to have a permanent response with no need for further therapy.

   C. Significant splenomegaly is seen in ITP patients who do not respond to medical therapy.

   D. Plasmapheresis is a first-line therapy for steroid-refractory ITP and should be initiated before considering splenectomy.

   E. Although the initial response rate to splenectomy is in the range of 85–90%, the relapse rate over the next 5 years can be as high as 25%.

3. **Regarding the preoperative and intraoperative management of patients undergoing splenectomy for ITP, which of the following statements is correct?**

   A. Platelet transfusion should be initiated once anesthesia is induced and continued into postoperative day (POD) 1 until the platelet count rises above 50,000.

   B. Patients should be vaccinated in the holding area just prior to surgery.

   C. The splenic hilar vessels are often divided simultaneously with suture ligatures or a vascular load on a linear stapler device.

   D. Accessory spleens can be present in 10–30% of patients.

   E. Laparoscopic splenectomy is less effective in identifying and removing accessory spleens.

4. **Which of the following statements is true regarding postoperative complications after splenectomy for ITP?**

    A. Overwhelming postsplenectomy infection (OPSI) is seen in approximately 5% of children and 15% of adults, regardless of vaccination status.

    B. Splenectomy is associated with an increased risk of abdominal venous thromboembolism within the first 90 days after surgery.

    C. Patients treated with medical therapy alone are at an equivalent risk for venous thromboembolism as are those who undergo splenectomy.

    D. It is standard of care for patients to take daily prophylactic antibiotics for at least a 5-year period following splenectomy.

    E. Rates of bleeding and infectious complications are similar in ITP cases that show a response to splenectomy and in those that do not.

5. **Which of the following statements best characterizes the current role of thrombopoietin (TPO) receptor agonists in the treatment of ITP?**

    A. These agents are third-line therapies in cases of symptomatic thrombocytopenia and commonly induce remission of ITP.

    B. TPO receptor agonists are effective at increasing platelet counts and can be used preoperatively to boost platelet counts in preparation for splenectomy.

    C. TPO receptor agonists are commonly used in conjunction with steroids as first-line therapy for ITP.

    D. TPO receptor agonists are given in the postoperative period to increase the chances of a therapeutic response to splenectomy.

    E. TPO receptor agonists require weekly intravenous infusions.

6. **Which of the following is true regarding minimally invasive procedures for splenectomy in the setting of ITP?**

    A. Robot-assisted laparoscopic splenectomy has demonstrated improved remission of ITP compared to a standard laparoscopic splenectomy.

    B. When compared to open splenectomy, laparoscopic splenectomy for ITP is associated with a reduction in overall morbidity.

    C. Splenomegaly is a limiting factor in the use of minimally invasive surgery for ITP.

    D. Open splenectomy remains the standard of care for ITP because it leads to higher remission rates.

7. **Which of the following is true regarding quality-of-life (QOL) measures in patients with ITP?**

    A. Decreased QOL is explained entirely by symptomatic bleeding events in ITP patients.

    B. QOL measures are lowest on initial diagnosis and tend to improve over time.

    C. Decreased QOL measures in ITP occur independently of platelet counts.

    D. Evidence suggests that TPO agonist therapy can improve QOL measures.

ANSWERS

1. **B.** ITP is an acquired, immune-mediated disorder that involves the splenic production of IgG autoantibodies. These autoantibodies target fibrinogen receptors on platelets and result in subsequent clearance of the platelets by phagocytic cells. More recently, the term *primary immune thrombocytopenia* has also been used to describe this condition, reflecting the immune-mediated nature of the disease and the large proportion of cases that do not involve overt signs of bleeding. In addition, research has shown that impaired platelet production and T-cell-mediated effects may also play a role in the pathophysiology of ITP. Peripheral blood smears in cases of ITP tend to be within normal limits.

    Thrombotic thrombocytopenic purpura (TTP) is a condition in which endothelial damage triggers the deposition of platelets and fibrin in small arterioles and capillaries, leading to microvascular thrombotic events. A patient with TTP will manifest microangiopathic hemolytic anemia, fever, and severe thrombocytopenia and will commonly suffer from neurologic complications and renal failure. A peripheral blood smear will demonstrate schistocytes, nucleated red blood cells, and basophilic stippling.

    Primary myelofibrosis (PMF) is a malignant disorder in which patients suffer from significant splenomegaly and cytopenias. The underlying cause of the condition is related to hyperplasia of an abnormal myeloid precursor cell, resulting in marrow fibrosis and subsequent extramedullary hematopoiesis.

2. **E.** According to a recent consensus report on the investigation and management of primary immune thrombocytopenia, 80% of patients respond to splenectomy, and this response persists in 66% of patients through at least 5 years following surgery.

Unfortunately, 20–30% of initial responders can experience relapses requiring additional medical or surgical therapy in the short or long term, and up to 20% of patients do not respond at all. These numbers are relatively consistent in laparoscopic and open approaches and across multiple studies.

Rituximab is used as a second-line therapy in older patients with more comorbidities and who are not ideal surgical candidates. It has also been used for patients who prefer nonoperative management. Rituximab is a monoclonal antibody directed against the B-cell surface protein CD20. A 40–50% response rate is seen initially, but relapses are common and the response rate at 5 years is 20%.

Plasmapheresis is a first-line therapy for TTP but is not indicated in ITP. Splenomegaly should prompt workup for other diagnoses, as the spleen is usually normal in size in cases of ITP.

3. **D.** Accessory spleens can be present in 10–30% of patients and are most commonly found at the splenic hilum, the tail of the pancreas, within the splenocolic and gastrosplenic ligaments, in the omentum, or in the paraduodenal area. Both laparoscopic and open approaches can be effective in identifying accessory spleens.

Platelet transfusion should be initiated after the splenic artery is ligated in order to prevent platelet consumption. The splenic vessels should ideally be ligated separately to prevent arteriovenous fistula formation. Vaccination against encapsulated organisms (*Haemophilus influenzae*, *Neisseria meningitides*, *Klebsiella pneumonia*) should be performed in the 2- to 4-week period prior to surgery, 14 days after surgery, or at the time of discharge from the hospital. If patients were previously on rituximab therapy, vaccinations may need to be delayed for up to 3 months to allow for B-cell recovery.

4. **B.** In a retrospective review of 9,976 patients with ITP, 1,762 who underwent splenectomy, the incidence of thrombotic events was evaluated. An increased risk of portal vein or mesenteric vein thrombosis was seen in the first 90 days after splenectomy but not after 90 days when compared to patients who underwent medical therapy alone. There was an increased risk of venous thromboembolism in both the early and late periods in the splenectomy group.

No consensus has been reached in terms of the benefit or duration of antibiotic prophylaxis.

Studies have shown that asplenic patients carry a lifelong risk of OPSI, and this risk is highest in the first 2 years after surgery. Children are at a higher risk than adults (5% vs. 0.9%), and OPSI is reported to have a 50% mortality rate. A retrospective analysis of 233 patients with ITP who underwent splenectomy showed that, in a 10-year follow-up period, a stable response to splenectomy was associated with a lower rate of infectious and bleeding complications.

5. **B.** TPO receptor agonists are used for persistent thrombocytopenia despite first- and second-line medical and surgical therapy, and they do not induce remission. They stimulate the production of megakaryocytes and subsequently platelets in the bone marrow by activating the TPO receptor. Upon cessation of the medication, platelet counts begin to fall again. These medications are considered maintenance therapy and require ongoing use in refractory cases of ITP. Romiplostim is administered as a once-weekly subcutaneous injection and eltrombopag is given as a once-daily pill.

TPO agonists can be used in the preoperative setting in order to boost platelet counts in preparation for splenectomy. They have also been used in patients who are not good candidates for rituximab therapy secondary to infectious risks. Patients who do not want to have surgery or are not good candidates can also use TPO agonists as chronic maintenance therapy. Using these agents in the postoperative period is not standard unless a relapse occurs, and they do not increase the chances of responding to a splenectomy.

Although previous TPO-based therapeutics, such as recombinant human TPO and PEG-rHuMGDF, were associated with cross-reactivity, no such reaction exists with the newer agents that do not share any sequence homology with human TPO. Romiplostin is only available as a subcutaneous injection, but eltrombopag is administered as a daily oral medication. Long-term maintenance therapy of eltrombopag was demonstrated in the recently published EXTEND trial. Adverse events were uncommon, although they included thromboembolic events and hepatobiliary events. Eltrombopag can be used in patients who are taking steroids or other medications for TPO, but many patients in the trial were able to discontinue steroid use while on eltrombopag, with use dropping from 29% to 18%.

6. B. The role of laparoscopic splenectomy in ITP has increased dramatically since its introduction in 1991. A systematic review demonstrated improvements in blood loss, postoperative complications, and hospital length of stay in all patients, and these conclusions were also demonstrated in the ITP subgroup. Additionally, the remission rate in ITP patients was comparable between open and laparoscopic surgery. Splenomegaly is not typically present in the setting of ITP. In addition, these same trends have been demonstrated in patients with splenomegaly for other indications, so splenomegaly is neither an absolute nor relative contraindication to laparoscopic splenectomy. There are no head-to-head trials comparing robotic to laparoscopic splenectomy. Early observational reports demonstrate a possible advantage of robotic over laparoscopic splenectomy in the setting of splenomegaly, in that robotic surgery leads to fewer cases being converted to open. However, the role of robotic surgery in the setting of ITP is not yet clearly defined.

7. D. ITP impacts patient QOL measures in measurable ways, and this impact is not just due to symptoms of bleeding and bruising. QOL measures in ITP tend to get worse in the first 6 months to 1 year after diagnosis, although some improvement is noted in chronic refractory cases 5 years out from diagnosis. Even in the absence of active bleeding or bruising events, the patient's knowledge of low platelet counts can lead to fear of bleeding occurrences and can negatively impact QOL, in part because it leads to avoidance of physical and social activities. Fatigue plays a significant role in the physical and emotional toll of ITP and may impact up to 45% of patients. Other less obvious ramifications include suspicions of domestic abuse due to frequent bruising, sexual dysfunction related to bleeding risk, and cancellation of elective surgery due to decreased platelet counts. Treatment side effects are a significant mediator of decreased QOL, particularly among patients on steroid therapy. There is some limited evidence suggesting that treatment with both romiplostim and eltrombopag QOL scores were significantly improved compared to placebo treatment. However, TPO agonist therapy did not appear to impact fatigue in these studies.

BIBLIOGRAPHY

Beauchamp RD, Holzman MD, Fabian TC, et al. The spleen. In: Townsend CM, Beauchamp RD, Evers M, et al., eds. *Sabiston Textbook of Surgery: The Biological Basis of Modern Surgical Practice.* 18th ed. WB Saunders; 2008.

Boyle S, White RH, Brunson A, Wun T. Splenectomy and the incidence of venous thromboembolism and sepsis in patients with immune thrombocytopenia. *Blood.* 2013;121(23):4782–4790.

Cheng Ji, Tao K, Peiwu, Y. Laparoscopic splenectomy is a better surgical approach for spleen-relevant disorders: a comprehensive meta-analysis based on 15-year literature. *Surg Endosc.* 2016;30:4575–4588.

Cavaliere D, Solaini L, di Pietrantonio D, et al. Robotic vs laparoscopic splenectomy for splenmegaly: a retrospective comparative cohort study. *Int J Surg.* 2018 July;55:1–4.

Khan M, Mikhael J. A review of immune thrombocytopenic purpura: focus on the novel thrombopoietin agonists. *J Blood Med.* 2010;1:21–31.

Mikhael J, Northridge K, Lindquist K, Kessler C, Deuson R, Danese M. Short-term and long-term failure of laparoscopic splenectomy in adult immune thrombocytopenic purpura patients: a systematic review. *Am J Hematol.* 2009;84(11):743–748.

Moulis G, Sailler L, Sommet A, Lapeyre-Mestre M, Derumeaux H, Adoue D. Rituximab versus splenectomy in persistent or chronic adult primary immune thrombocytopenia: an adjusted comparison of mortality and morbidity. *Am J Hematol.* 2013;89(1):41–46.

Patel NY, Chilsen AM, Mathiason MA, Kallies KJ, Bottner WA. Outcomes and complications after splenectomy for hematologic disorders. *Am J Surg.* 2012;204:1014–1020.

Provan D, Stasi R, Newland AC, et al. International consensus report on the investigation and management of primary immune thrombocytopenia. *Blood.* 2010;115(2):168–186.

Taghizadeh M, Muscarella P. Splenectomy for hematologic disorders. In: Cameron JL, Cameron AM, eds. *Current Surgical Therapy.* 10th ed. Elsevier Saunders; 2011:473–479.

Trotter P, Hill QA. Immune thrombocytopenia: improving quality of life and patient outcomes. *Patient Relat Outcome Meas.* 2018;27(9):369–384.

Vecchio R, Marchese S, Intagliata E, Swehli E, Ferla F, Cacciola E. Long-term results after splenectomy in adult idiopathic thrombocytopenic purpura: comparison between open and laparoscopic procedures. *J Laparoendosc Adv Surg Tech A.* 2013;23(3):192–198.

Vianelli N, Palandri F, Polverelli N, et al. Splenectomy as a curative treatment for immune thrombocytopenia: a retrospective analysis of 233 patients with a minimum follow up of 10 years. *Haematologica.* 2013;98(6):875–880.

Wong RSM, Sale MN, Khelif A, Salama A, Portella MSO, Burgess P, Bussel JB. Safety and efficacy of long-term treatment of chronic/persistent ITP with eltrombopag: final results of the EXTEND study. *Blood.* 2017;130(23):2527–2536.

Zeng Y, Duan X, Xu J, Ni X. TPO receptor agonist for chronic idiopathic thrombocytopenic purpura. *Cochrane Database Syst Rev.* 2011 Jul;6(7):CD008235.

35

Small Bowel Obstruction

Patrick Golden and Emily Ofstun

You are called to the emergency department (ED) to see a 54-year-old female with a chief complaint of abdominal pain with nausea and vomiting. Reviewing her ED record reveals she has a heart rate of 112, a blood pressure of 154/96, and a normal temperature of 98.6°F. On exam the patient appears to be in mild distress with a distended abdomen. The patient states that the pain started 48 hours before, is intermittent and crampy, and is now getting worse. She states that she has been vomiting now for about the last 24 hours and is unable to keep any fluids down. She does not remember the last time she passed flatus or had a bowel movement. The patient has been in the ED for about half an hour, her labs are still pending, and no imaging studies have been done. Her past medical history is significant for hypertension, hyperlipidemia, chronic kidney disease, and diet-controlled type 2 diabetes. Her past surgical history is significant for two previous C-sections 20 years ago, a laparoscopic cholecystectomy, and an open sigmoidectomy for complicated diverticulitis. The patient denies ever having symptoms like this before.

1. **Following fluid resuscitation with two liters of crystalloid, the heart rate downtrends to 90 and the blood pressure remains normal. Which of the following is the next best step in the management of this patient?**

   A. To the operating room immediately for a diagnostic laparoscopy with possible exploratory laparotomy

   B. Admission to the surgical floor and then continue IV fluids and perform abdominal exams every 4 hours

   C. Placement of a nasogastric tube and obtaining an acute abdominal series

   D. Immediate computed tomography (CT) scan of the abdomen and pelvis with PO and IV contrast.

   E. Discharge to home from the ED with close clinic follow-up within 48 hours

2. **You obtain radiologic studies that show several dilated loops of small bowel. Which of the following is the most common cause of these imaging findings in this patient?**

   A. Small bowel ileus

   B. Mechanical small bowel obstruction

   C. Mechanical colonic obstruction

   D. Acute colonic pseudo-obstruction

   E. Gastric outlet obstruction

3. **Which of the following is the most common cause of mechanical small bowel obstruction (SBO)?**

   A. Adhesions

   B. Strictures

   C. Hernias

   D. Gallstones

   E. Tumors

4. **Twenty-four hours have now passed since the described patient was admitted and had a nasogastric (NG) tube and Foley catheter placed. Since that time, her NG tube output has been 1.6 liters of bilious fluid, and her urinary output has been around 1.1 cc/kg/hr. Her creatinine has remained at her baseline of 1.5. You have also obtained an abdominal CT scan that demonstrates**

a clear transition point suspected to be a single adhesive band. The patient's pain and physical exam only worsen intermittently. Her heart rate is in the 90s, and her blood pressure is holding steady. Which of the following is true?

A. The presence of small bowel "fecalization" on the CT scan of the abdomen and pelvis with IV/oral contrast predicts the need for an operation.

B. If this patient had her sigmoidectomy 4 weeks ago, she would still be a candidate for nonoperative management.

C. A laparotomy is indicated.

D. If a laparoscopic approach is chosen within the first 48 hours of admission, it is more likely to be completed without conversion.

E. One can continue observation in this patient for up to 3 days without increasing morbidity.

5. **A decision is made to proceed to surgery 24 hours later because the patient developed a fever and leukocytosis. Which of the following is true regarding surgical management?**

A. The laparoscopic approach is associated with longer operating times.

B. The laparoscopic approach may be associated with decreased mortality.

C. The rate of major complications is similar for both the laparoscopic and open approaches.

D. The optical view approach is recommended for this patient.

E. The laparoscopic approach has no effect on postoperative length of stay.

6. **Exploratory laparoscopy is attempted. The transition point is identified as a section of bowel with densely matted adhesions. You are having difficulty obtaining adequate visualization while taking down the adhesions. Which of the following is true regarding the conversion of laparoscopic lysis of adhesions to an open exploratory laparotomy?**

A. Conversion to the open approach is only recommended after an intraoperative complication has occurred

B. More than 70% of laparoscopic SBO cases are converted to open.

C. Early conversion is associated with significantly less morbidity than conversion in reaction to an intra-operative complication.

D. Laparoscopically treated patients have similar hospital lengths of stay as patients who require conversion.

E. Laparoscopically experienced surgeons have a far smaller conversion rate than less experienced surgeons.

7. **You are able to obtain better visualization and complete this patient's case laparoscopically. Prior to discharging home, she asks you what the chances are of this happening again. The rate of recurrence for the laparoscopic approach is roughly**

A. 10% or less.

B. 20%.

C. 30%.

D. 45%.

E. 75% or more.

ANSWERS

1. **C.** This patient is presenting with symptoms most consistent with some type of bowel obstruction. This patient has received 2 liters of crystalloid with an appropriate response in her heart rate, but she still requires an NG tube. Given her lack of peritonitis, imaging studies are appropriate, and an acute abdominal series is adequate, especially given this patient's history of chronic kidney disease and an as-yet-unknown creatinine level.

Answer A is not appropriate given that she does not have peritonitis and her workup is not yet complete. Given that she is responding to resuscitation, this patient should be given the chance to see if her symptoms resolve with nonoperative management. Answer B is not appropriate in that this patient still has a workup to be done with labs and imaging as the diagnosis is still unclear at this time.

Answer D is not appropriate in that while CT has a high specificity and sensitivity for bowel obstructions and can locate points of blockage, her creatinine is unknown, and with her history of kidney disease and likely kidney injury from dehydration, a contrast load would not be advisable. An acute abdominal series is fast, and with careful interpretation, the diagnosis of a small bowel obstruction can still be made. A noncontrast CT scan, however, would be a reasonable option as it would not risk an insult to the kidneys, and it may determine an internal hernia, which would be an indication for surgical intervention. Answer E is not appropriate as this patient still requires workup.

2. **A.** Small bowel ileus is, by far, the most common form of intestinal dilation as it is seen after many surgical procedures whether they are performed in the abdomen or not. The exact etiology of the ileus is unclear but is probably multifactorial, taking into account anesthesia and narcotic usage. Viral ileus can also be seen in cases of gastroenteritis. Ileus is most times self-limited and resolves with or without NG tube decompression and keeping the patient in NPO status.

Answer B, mechanical SBO, is the second-most common cause of these findings and, 90% of the time, is due to adhesions, hernias, or cancer, although gallstones, bezoars, and parasitic worms have also been reported. Mechanical colonic obstruction, while usually more severe in its presentation, only accounts for about 10% of all mechanical obstructions. The usual causes of this are cancer, volvulus, or diverticulitis resulting in a stricture.

Answer D, acute colonic pseudo-obstruction, is much less common and is usually seen in older, debilitated, or institutionalized patients who are on numerous medications, and Answer E, gastric outlet obstruction, is a less common form of obstruction and is usually seen with gastric/duodenal/pancreatic malignancies or gastric ulcers. These would not, however, result in intestinal dilatation.

3. **A.** Until the early to mid-1900s, the leading cause of mechanical SBO was due to hernias, but over the past century, that has now switched to postoperative adhesions accounting for more than 75% of all mechanical SBOs.

Hernias are the second-most common cause of mechanical SBOs, and in the absence of a surgical history, the presence of an incarcerated inguinal, umbilical, or incisional hernia needs to be ruled out. The remaining answer choices have all been shown to cause mechanical bowel obstructions, although their incidence is low.

4. **E.** This patient's physical exam and clinical status are largely unchanged. As such, she is a candidate for nonoperative management for up to 72 hours. Patients who have had abdominal surgery within 6 weeks before the episode of SBO, patients with signs of strangulation (fever, tachycardia, leukocytosis,

metabolic acidosis, continuous pain), and patients with irreducible hernias are NOT candidates for nonoperative management. On CT scan, the lack of small bowel fecalization, free intraperitoneal fluid, and mesenteric edema predict the need for urgent laparotomy. As she is not exhibiting signs of peritonitis, ischemia, or strangulation she is most appropriately a candidate for continued observation. If, after 72 hours, if there is no improvement in her status, an operation is indicated. Until then, there is no increase in morbidity or mortality with observation. There are no data suggesting that earlier intervention with a laparoscopic approach will reduce morbidity, mortality, or conversion rates.

5. **B.** In a study published in 2014 on more than 9,600 patients using the National Surgical Quality Improvement Database, laparoscopic intervention for small bowel obstructions was shown to have decreased operative time (77.2 vs. 94.2 min) and decreased length of stay (4.7 vs. 9.9 days). Additionally, the laparoscopic approach was less likely to develop major complications, with an odds ratio of 0.7. Additionally, the laparoscopic approach showed a lower 30-day mortality rate (1.3% vs. 4.7%). As such, if the surgeon feels comfortable, the laparoscopic approach may be a safer alternative for the surgical management of SBOs caused by adhesive disease. When accessing the abdomen in a patient with previous abdominal incisions, the recommended technique for gaining the pneumoperitoneum and placing the initial trocar is via the Hasson or open technique.

6. **C.** In a study of 537 patients comparing morbidity/mortality after conversion of laparoscopic to open surgery for lysis of adhesions for various reasons, it was found that reactive conversion (i.e., conversion in reaction to an intraoperative complication such as an unintentional enterotomy) was associated with significantly higher postoperative morbidity rates than early conversion (conversion due to inadequate visualization, working space, etc.). Postoperative morbidity was 39.2% for reactive conversions versus 11.9% for early conversions. Thus, early conversion should be strongly considered if difficulties arise during the case.

Answer A, there is a low threshold for conversion to the open approach given higher morbidity rate if conversion after an intraoperative complication occurs.

Answer B, Conversion rates vary from 15–52% between sources. This study estimated the conversion rate at 32%. A study of 2,009 patients estimated the conversion rate at 29%. This study also reported a success rate for laparoscopic surgery of 73.4% when a single adhesive band was reported as the cause of the obstruction.

Answer D, Laparoscopically treated patients have shorter lengths of stay than those who underwent conversion, by an average of 6 days in this study. If conversion was due to an intraoperative complication, length of stay was 9 days greater than laparoscopically treated patients.

Answer E, In this same study, laparoscopically experienced surgeons (100 or more laparoscopic cases) had similar rates of conversion as less experienced surgeons.

7. **A.** A study of 62 patients comparing the laparoscopic approach to conservative management found a recurrence rate in the laparoscopic group of 6.2%. The recurrence rate in the conservative management group was significantly higher at 32.6%. Another study of 110 patients found a similar SBO recurrence rate of 8.2% after laparoscopic lysis of adhesions. B–E likely overestimate the recurrence rate, although C, 30%, may be a reasonable estimate for the recurrence rate of SBO with conservative management.

BIBLIOGRAPHY

Arnaoutakis GJ, Eckhauser FE. Small Bowel Obstruction. In: Cameron L, Cameron AM. *Cameron Current Surgical Therapy*. 10th ed. Elsevier Saunders; 2011:93–97.

Cirocchi R, Abraha I, Farinella E, Montedori A, Sciannameo F. Laparoscopic versus open surgery in small bowel obstruction. *Cochrane Database Syst Rev*. 2010;2:CD007511.

Dindo D, Schafer M, Muller MK, Clavien PA, Hahnloser, D. Laparoscopy for small bowel obstruction: the reason for conversion matters. *Surg Endosc*. 2010;24:792–797.

Di Saverio S, Coccolini F, Galati M, et al. Bologna guidelines for diagnosis and management of adhesive small bowel obstruction (ASBO): 2013 update of the evidence-based guidelines from the world society of emergency surgery ASBO working group. *World J Emerg Surg*. 2013;8(1):42.

Helton WS, Fisichella, PM. Intestinal Obstruction. In: Souba WW, Fink MP Jurkovich GJ, Kaiser LP, Pearce WH, Pemberton JH, et al. eds. *ACS Surgery Principles and Practice*. 6th ed. WebMD Professional Publishing; 2007:514–534.

Kelly KN, Iannuzzi JC, Rickles AS, Garimella V, Monson JR, Fleming FJ. Laparotomy for small-bowel obstruction: first choice or last resort for adhesiolysis? A laparoscopic approach for small-bowel obstruction reduces 30-day complications. *Surg Endosc*. 2014;28(1):65–73.

O'Connor DB, Winter DC. The role of laparoscopy in the management of acute small-bowel obstruction: a review of over 2,000 cases. *Surg Endosc*. 2012;26:12–17.

Pearl JP, Marks JM, Hardacre MJ, Ponsky JL, Delaney CP, Rosen MJ. Laparoscopic treatment of complex small bowel obstruction: is it safe? *Surg Innov*. 2008;15(2):110–113.

Soper NJ. Access to Abdomen. In: Soper NJ, Scott-Conner, Carol EH, eds. *SAGES Manual: Volume 1 Basic Laparoscopy and Endoscopy*. Springer; 2012.

Soybel DI, Landman WB. Ileus and bowel obstruction. In: Mulholland MW, Lillemoe KD, Doherty GM, et al. eds. *Greenfield's Surgery Scientific Principles and Practice*. 5th ed. Lippincott Williams & Wilkins; 2011:748–772.

Suh SW, Choi YS. Laparoscopy for small bowel obstruction caused by single adhesive band. *JSLS*. 2016;20(30): e2016.00048.

Yao S, Tanaka E, Ikeda A, Murrakami T, Okumoto T, Harada T. Outcomes of laparoscopic management of acute small bowel obstruction: a 7-year experience of 110 consecutive cases with various etiologies. *Surg Today*. 2017;47(4):432–439.

36

Illicit Drug-Induced Abdominal Pain

Bonnie B. Hunt and Stuart Reynolds

SCENARIO 1

A 26-year-old male with no significant past medical history presents to the emergency department in distress, complaining of chest discomfort and severe epigastric pain of sudden onset 3 hours prior to presentation. He denies aenny prior surgical intervention and has no prior medical history. On social history, he endorses recent cocaine use that evening. The patient has a heart rate of 130 and a respiratory rate of 24. On physical exam, the patient has a diffusely tender abdomen with rigidity.

1. **Which of the following is true regarding complications of stimulant drug abuse?**

    A. Perforated gastroduodenal ulcer is unlikely to occur without a known history of ulcer disease.

    B. Acute abdominal processes are the most common complications of stimulant drug abuse.

    C. An ileus is the most well-documented acute abdominal complication of cocaine abuse.

    D. Systemic vasoconstriction may cause multiple gastrointestinal complications.

2. **Which radiographic study would most readily provide the diagnostic finding for the diagnosis in the patient presentation provided?**

    A. Computed tomography (CT) scan

    B. Abdominal ultrasound

    C. Upright chest radiograph

    D. Angiography

3. **After making the preceding diagnosis, which of the following would be the most appropriate intervention?**

    A. Fluid resuscitation, gastric decompression via nasogastric tube, and antibiotic therapy for *Helicobacter pylori* infection

    B. Abdominal washout, debridement of ulcerated tissue, and omental patch closure

    C. Truncal vagotomy with pyloroplasty

    D. Truncal vagotomy with antrectomy and Billroth I or II reconstruction

4. **In addition to the surgical management of the perforated ulcer, what, if any, adjunctive management should be included in the patient's care?**

    A. Nothing, pathophysiology is directly related to the stimulant drug and management directed at repair of the acute perforation.

    B. Empiric triple or quadruple therapy for *H. pylori*

    C. Ulcer biopsy for *H. pylori* infection and triple or quadruple therapy only with the presence of bacteria

    D. Pharmacologic vasodilation to reverse effects of stimulant physiology

5. **If a patient presents with mesenteric ischemia secondary to stimulant drug abuse, along with peritonitis or acidosis, after resuscitation, which of the following represents appropriate management?**

    A. Exploratory laparotomy with resection of necrotic bowel and vasodilation

    B. Endovascular thrombolysis and arterial stenting

    C. Operative superior-mesenteric-artery (SMA) embolectomy

    D. Aortomesenteric arterial bypass

SCENARIO 2

A 32-year-old male with no significant past medical history presents to the emergency department with a 3-hour history of abdominal pain and chest pain associated with intractable nausea and vomiting. He states he has had this nausea and emesis before, but they were always self-limited and not this severe. He has a significant surgical history for a laparoscopic cholecystectomy and a social history of chronic marijuana use. His last usage was earlier today. He endorses regular bowel movements and normal flatus. His last bowel movement was dark. On exam, he is mildly tender in the epigastric region without rebound or guarding and breath sounds are equal bilaterally throughout. A chest x-ray is obtained and does not demonstrate any abnormalities. His emesis is bilious with some blood recently, which prompted his evaluation. His vitals demonstrate a blood pressure of 125/64, a heart rate of 104, and a respiratory rate of 16.

6. **What is the next best diagnostic step?**

    A. Upper endoscopy
    B. Gastrografin swallow study
    C. CT scan with IV contrast
    D. Emergent exploratory laparotomy

7. **What is the most likely diagnosis?**

    A. Boerhaave syndrome
    B. Mallory Weiss tear
    C. Pneumothorax
    D. Small bowel obstruction

8. **Thus far, the work has included a gastrografin swallow, a CT scan of the chest and abdomen, and an urgent endoscopy, but no pathology was found except for a small tear at the gastroesophageal junction. What is the most likely underlying etiology?**

    A. Psuedoachalasia
    B. Cameron's ulcer
    C. Hyperemesis cannabinoid syndrome
    D. Alcohol abuse

ANSWERS

1. **D.** Illicit drugs, such as cocaine and methamphetamine, are highly addictive central nervous system stimulants that produce a rapid euphoria secondary to elevated levels of the monoamine transmitters dopamine, serotonin, and norepinephrine.

Immediate effects of stimulant use include wakefulness, increased physical activity, decreased appetite, tachypnea, tachycardia, hypertension, and hyperthermia. The most common and well-known serious side effects of stimulant drug abuse include cardiac and neurologic complications, such as myocardial infarction, arrhythmias, and cerebral vascular accidents. Additionally, pulmonary and psychiatric complications are common. Although less common, acute abdominal complications related to both cocaine and methamphetamine are well documented in the medical and surgical literature. The two most commonly documented gastrointestinal complications are perforated peptic ulcer and mesenteric ischemia, both thought to be secondary to splanchnic vasoconstriction via activated alpha-1 receptors following rapid elevation in norepinephrine. Gastroduodenal perforation after stimulant drug abuse may be the initial presentation of ulcer disease, and the clinician should have a high index of suspicion for such when a patient presents with acute abdomen and a history of stimulant abuse, despite the lack of ulcer disease in the patient's history. Less commonly, methamphetamines can cause paralytic ileus.

2. **C.** The diagnosis of a perforated gastroduodenal ulcer, in conjunction with an appropriate history, is confirmed by the finding of pneumoperitoneum, most quickly visualized on the upright chest x-ray under the hemidiaphragm(s) or on the left lateral decubitus abdominal x-ray. In some cases of perforated ulcer of the anterior duodenal wall, free air and the fish-eye sign may be demonstrated via ultrasound. In approximately 25% of perforated peptic ulcer presentations, free air will not be visualized. A CT scan will demonstrate inflammatory changes surrounding the perforated ulcer and is highly sensitive for evidence of micro-perforation (free air or fluid). However, in diagnosing a perforated peptic ulcer for which plain film did not already reveal pneumoperitoneum, a CT scan did not demonstrate additional diagnostic utility within the first 6 hours. Had the patient's acute abdomen also presented with hematochezia in the setting of stimulant drug abuse, mesenteric ischemia would be higher on the differential, diagnosed by a CT abdominal angiogram. In the setting of stimulant drug abuse and an acute abdomen, it is important for the provider to obtain imaging to evaluate for the presence of pneumoperitoneum, indicating possible perforated peptic ulcer.

3. **B.** In the absence of free air or shock, a trial of nonoperative management may lead to spontaneous closure of approximately 50% of perforations. Nonoperative management of a perforated peptic ulcer presenting with free air and a surgical abdomen would not be appropriate; surgical intervention is indicated. With the success of medical therapy directed toward *H. pylori* and gastric acid suppression, surgical goals for perforated ulcers have been increasingly moved away from the traditional options for acid-reducing operations to management of the acute complication with omental patch closure of the perforation, with or without primary closure. Gastroduodenal ulcerations presenting in conjunction with stimulant drug abuse in particular often occur at a younger age and without a known history of ulcer disease. Although the prevalence of *H. pylori* is still high in stimulant-associated perforated ulcers, the path to perforation is promoted by vasoconstriction and focal ischemia. Given this pathophysiology, the indication for acid-reducing surgery remains limited to perforations in patients who have failed medical therapy prior to perforation.

4. **C.** The traditional approach to perforated gastroduodenal ulcer, outside of stimulant drug use, presumes that the vast majority of perforated ulcers involve *H. pylori* infection. As such, standard treatment includes surgical management of the acute complication as well as empiric treatment for *H. pylori* with triple or quadruple therapy. Standard triple therapy for *H. pylori* infection includes a proton pump inhibitor and dual antibiotic coverage with clarithromycin plus amoxicillin or metronidazole; quadruple therapy includes a proton pump inhibitor, dual antibiotic coverage with tetracycline plus metronidazole, and bismuth subsalicylate. Perforated gastroduodenal ulcers following stimulant drug abuse may occur with or without previous symptoms of peptic ulcer disease. Despite a lack of previous symptoms, there is evidence to show that up to 80% of these ulcers are positive for *H. pylori* per intraoperative biopsy. However, despite the potential presence of *H. pylori*, a key component in the acute perforation is vasoconstriction leading to focal ischemia, ultimately causing ulcer perforation in patterns different from standard ulcer behavior, notably at younger ages. Given the potential multifactorial ulcer etiology in the setting of perforation following stimulant drug use, the result of *H. pylori* testing on intraoperative ulcer biopsy can direct the inclusion of triple or quadruple therapy following surgical intervention. Despite the vasoconstrictive physiology in stimulant drug–related perforations, treatment recommendations are directed at repair of the perforation rather than vasodilation.

5. **A.** Acute mesenteric ischemia (AMI) may result from arterial occlusion via embolus or thrombus (65%), venous occlusion (10%), or nonocclusive etiologies (25%). Prompt diagnosis of AMI is strongly correlated to outcomes, as a delay in intervention results in morbidity up to 50%. Selective mesenteric catheter angiography is the traditional diagnostic gold standard; however, abdominal CT angiography with intravenous contrast can provide a faster diagnosis with decreased procedural risk to the patient. Endovascular thrombolysis and arterial stenting can be effective at restoring splanchnic perfusion in acute arterial thrombosis; however, acute embolic arterial occlusions typically do not respond to thrombolytic therapy (which may also result in secondary distal embolization from fragmented portions of the embolus) and require laparotomy with SMA embolectomy. Splanchnic vasoconstriction secondary to catecholamine release in stimulant drug use is a rare cause of acute nonocclusive mesenteric ischemia (ANOMI), and impacts the major arterial sources of bowel perfusion, the SMA, and the IMA, as well as smaller collaterals. Thrombolysis, embolectomy, and bypass have no role in the management of these cases. Intra-arterial vasodilator therapy can be effective at restoring bowel perfusion. Regardless of the AMI etiology, with evidence or suspicion of peritonitis or bowel ischemia or infarction, urgent exploratory laparotomy and resection of necrotic bowel are imperative, typically conducted according to damage control principles with subsequent exploration for the reassessment of tenuous bowel. Additionally, major abdominal vessels and mesenteric perfusion can be assessed by direct vessel palpation.

6. **B.** Given the patient's history of intractable nausea and vomiting associated with chest pain and abdominal pain, the next-best diagnostic test would be a thin barium swallow study for evaluation of esophageal perforation. The patient is hemodynamically stable with hematemesis. Gastrografin followed by thin barium swallow study is the gold standard for evaluation of possible. Gastrografin will identify 80%

of intrathoracic perforations. The thin barium will identify 90% (Foley, Gollub). An upper endoscopy is needed for evaluation of the esophageal tear, but a perforation should be ruled out before. A CT will demonstrate intra-abdominal and intrathoracic free air if present but will not be able to identify the location of perforation.

7. **B.** A Mallory-Weiss tear is the most expected diagnosis given hematemesis and chest pain in the setting of intractable vomiting. Given his stable vitals and a normal chest x-ray, there is low suspicion for frank perforation. A swallow study should not show any contrast extravasation and an upper endoscopy should be performed to identify the location and likelihood of rebleeding. While usually single in nature, multiple mucosal tears have been identified in up to 27%. Their most common location is at the gastroesophageal junction. Boerhaave syndrome would typically have a left pleural effusion and a more clinically ill patient. An esophagram would demonstrate an esophageal leak. An occult pneumothorax suspicion is low with a normal respiratory rate, a normal chest x-ray, and no signs of respiratory distress. A small bowel obstruction is considered given his previous surgical history but is not the best answer given his normal bowel function.

8. **C.** Hyperemesis cannabinoid syndrome is intractable nausea/vomiting without an obvious organic cause in the setting of marijuana use. There is frequent associated incidence of hot bathing that previously relieved symptoms. Most management involves fluid resuscitation and anti-emetic medications to control symptoms. Hiatal hernias have not shown a significant difference in the prevalence of Mallory-Weiss syndrome and are not considered a predisposing factor for a tear. An esophagogastroduodenoscopy (EGD) would have diagnosed a Cameron's ulcer, which is an ulcer associated with an incarcerated paraesophageal hernia. Excessive alcohol use can certainly be associated with vomiting and a Mallory-Weiss tear, but this patient's history does not indicate chronic alcohol abuse, although it should be on this patient's differential. Pseudoachalasia can cause vomiting, but it is associated with a mass or a foreign body (an adjustable gastric band) that causes dysmotility and obstructive symptoms of the esophagus. The treatment would be removal of the mass or foreign body. Neither of these are seen on a CT scan or EGD.

BIBLIOGRAPHY

Albertson TE, Derlet RW, Van Hoozen BE. Methamphetamine and the expanding complications of amphetamines. *West J Med.* 1999;170:214–219.

Baker RJ. In: Fischer JE, Jones DB, Pomposeli FB, et al. eds. *Mastery of Surgery.* 6th ed. Wolters Kluwer Health; 2011:892.

Brannan TA, Soundararajan S, Houghton BL. Methamphetamine-associated shock with intestinal infarction. *Med Gen Med.* Dec 29;6(4):6.

Carlson T, Plackett, T, Gagliano RA, et al. Crystal methamphetamine-induced paralytic ileus. *Hawai'i J Med Pub Health.* 2012 Feb;71(2):44–45.

Chander B, Aslanian HR. Gastric perforations associated with the use of crack cocaine. *Gastroenterol Hepatol (NY).* 2010;6(11):733–735.

Chey WD, Wong BCY. American college of gastroenterology guideline on the management of helicobacter pylori infection. *Am J Gastroenterol.* 2007;102(8):1808–1825.

Corral JE, Keihanian T, Kröner PT, Dauer R, Lukens FJ, Sussman DA. Mallory Weiss syndrome is not associated with hiatal hernia: a matched case-control study. *Scand J Gastroenterol.* 2017;52(4):462–464. doi:10.1080/00365521.2016.1267793

Dunser MW, Hasibeder WR. Sympathetic overstimulation during critical illness: adverse effects of adrenergic stress. *J Intensive Care Med.* 2009;24:293–316.

Feliciano DV, Ojukwu JC, Rozycki GS, et al. The epidemic of cocaine-related juxtapyloric perforations: with a comment on the importance of testing for *Helicobacter pylori. Ann Surg.* 1999;229:801–804.

Foley MJ, Ghahremani GG, Rogers LF. Reappraisal of contrast media used to detect upper gastrointestinal perforations: comparison of ionic water-soluble media with barium sulfate. *Radiology.* 1982;144(2):231–237.

Gollub MJ, Bains MS. Barium sulfate: a new (old) contrast agent for diagnosis of postoperative esophageal leaks. *Radiology.* 1997;202(2):360–362.

Grassi R, Romano S, Pinto A, et al. Gastroduodenal perforations: conventional plain film, US and CT findings in 166 consecutive patients. *Eur J Radiol.* 2004;50(1):30–36.

Herr RD, Caravati EM. Acute transient ischemic colitis after oral methamphetamine ingestion. *Am J Emerg Med.* 1991;9:406–409.

Herskowitz MM, Gilego V, Ward M, et al. Cocaine-induced mesenteric ischemia: treatment with intra-arterial papaverine. *Emerg Radiol.* 2002;9(3):172–174.

Huang SP, Wang HP, Lee YC, et al. Endoscopic hemoclip placement and epinephrine injection for Mallory-Weiss syndrome with active bleeding. *Gastrointest Endosc.* 2002;55(7):842–846. doi:10.1067/mge.2002.124560

Kish SJ. Pharmacologic mechanism of crystal meth. *CMAJ.* 2008;178:1679–1682.

Knauer CM. Mallory-Weiss syndrome. Characterization of 75 Mallory-Weiss lacerations in 528 patients with upper gastrointestinal hemorrhage. *Gastroenterology.* 1976;71(1):5–8.

Mulholland MW. In: Mulhollond MW, Lillemoe KD, Goherty GM, et al. eds. *Greenfield's Surgery: Scientific Principles and Practice*. 5th ed. Lippincott Williams & Wilkins; 2010:699–703.

Ng EK, Lam YH, Sung JJ, et al. Eradication of *Helicobacter pylori* prevents recurrence of ulcer after simple closure of duodenal ulcer perforation: Randomized controlled trial. *Ann Surg*. 2000;231(2):153–158.

Nirula R. Acute mesenteric ischemia. *Surg Clin North Am*. 2014;94(1):165–181.

Nirula R. Gastroduodenal perforation. *Surg Clin North Am*. 2014;94(1):31–34.

Osorio J, Farreras N, Ortiz DeZárate L, et al. Cocaine-induced mesenteric ischaemia. *Dig Surg*. 2000;17(6):648–651.

Pecha RE, Prindiville T, Pecha BS, et al. Association of cocaine and methamphetamine use with giant gastroduodenal ulcers. *Am J Gastroenterol*. 1996;91:2523–2527.

Reginelli A, Iacobellis F, Berritto D, et al. Mesenteric ischemia: the importance of differential diagnosis for the surgeon. *BMC Surg*. 2013;13(Suppl 2):S51.

Shanti CM, Lucas CE. Cocaine and the critical care challenge. *Crit Care Med*. 2003;31(6):1851–1859.

Sugawa C, Benishek D, Walt AJ. Mallory-Weiss syndrome. A study of 224 patients. *Am J Surg*. 1983;145(1):30–33. doi:10.1016/0002-9610(83)90162-9

Sun S, Zimmermann AE. Cannabinoid hyperemesis syndrome. *Hosp Pharm*. 2013;48(8):650–655. doi:10.1310/hpj4808-650

Trompeter M, Brazda T, Remy CT, et al. Non-occlusive mesenteric ischemia: etiology, diagnosis, and interventional therapy. *Eur Radiol*. 2002;12(5):1179–1187.

Yamaguchi Y, Yamato T, Katsumi N, et al. Endoscopic hemoclipping for upper GI bleeding due to Mallory-Weiss syndrome. *Gastrointest Endosc*. 2001;53(4):427–430. doi:10.1067/mge.2001.111774

Yuan Y, Wang C, Hunt RH. Endoscopic clipping for acute nonvariceal upper-GI bleeding: a meta-analysis and critical appraisal of randomized controlled trials. *Gastrointest Endosc*. 2008;68(2):339–351. doi:10.1016/j.gie.2008.03.1122

37

Carcinoid Tumors

Christopher G. Yheulon

A 50-year-old otherwise healthy male presents to the emergency room with nausea, vomiting, and abdominal pain. He has had a 1-month history of chronic intermittent abdominal pain. He has no prior history of abdominal surgeries and had a normal colonoscopy earlier this year. His vital signs are within normal limits. On exam, his abdomen is soft and nondistended, with mild diffuse abdominal tenderness. There are no hernias present. His laboratory exam is unremarkable. He undergoes an abdominal computed tomography (CT) scan that demonstrates an area of intussusception in the distal small bowel with thickening and calcification of the adjacent mesentery (shown).

1. **What is the best next step in diagnosis?**

   A. Small bowel follow-through
   B. Abdominal magnetic resonance imaging (MRI)
   C. Capsule endoscopy
   D. Barium enema
   E. Diagnostic laparoscopy

2. **What is the most likely malignant pathologic diagnosis?**

   A. Adenocarcinoma
   B. Carcinoid tumor
   C. Lymphoma

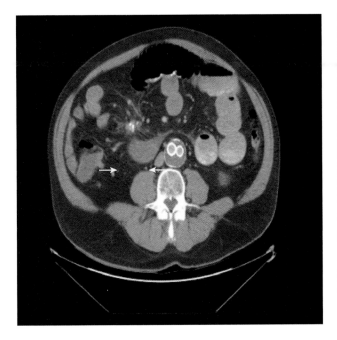
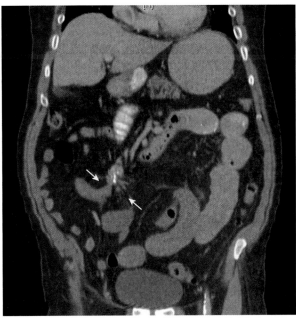

D. Small bowel sarcoma

E. Small bowel gastrointestinal stromal tumor (GIST)

3. **After you complete your diagnostic workup, you take the patient to the operating room for a diagnostic laparoscopy. You identify a 4-cm solid mass in the mid-ileum. The adjacent mesentery appears thickened and foreshortened. There is no evidence of metastatic disease. You perform a resection with primary anastomosis. In the recovery room, the patient has profound flushing, altered mental status, and hypotension refractory to fluid resuscitation. What is the next best step in management?**

A. Initiation of vasopressors

B. Broad spectrum antibiotics

C. IV octreotide

D. Stress dose corticosteroids

E. Transfusion of packed red blood cells (PRBCs)

4. **The patient ultimately recovers well and is discharged. What labs should be ordered for surveillance of recurrence and metastatic disease?**

A. Chromogranin A and urine 5-HIAA

B. Carcinoembryonic antigen (CEA) and carbohydrate antigen (CA) 19-9

C. Plasma VMA and metanephrines

D. Follicle stimulating hormone (FSH) and luteinizing hormone (LH) testing

E. AFP and HCG

5. **Three years later, on a surveillance CT scan, the patient is noted to have multiple new liver masses. Imaging is consistent with metastatic disease. What is the best treatment option?**

A. Systemic chemotherapy

B. Metastasectomy

C. Hepatic artery embolization

D. External beam radiation

E. Observation

6. **Prior to treatment of the metastases, the patient is recommended to undergo cardiac evaluation. Which is the most likely finding on an echocardiogram?**

A. Aortic stenosis

B. Mitral regurgitation

C. Tricuspid regurgitation

D. Tricuspid stenosis

E. Pulmonary regurgitation

7. **Despite continued maximal somatostatin therapy, appropriate treatment of the liver metastases, and stable radiographic findings, the patient still has elevated 5-HIAA levels and refractory diarrhea. Which medication type may benefit the patient the most?**

A. Bile acid sequestrant (cholestyramine)

B. Tryptophan hydroxylases inhibitor (Telotristat)

C. 5-HT3 antagonist (Odansetron)

D. Antidiarrheal (Loperamid)

E. Opiates (tincture of opium)

ANSWERS

1. **E.** Intussusception in an adult is typically due to a pathologic lead point. Only 8–20% of intussusceptions are idiopathic. Malignancy accounts for up to 30% of cases of adult intussusception. Benign causes for intussusception include Meckel's diverticulum, postoperative adhesions, lipomas, adenomatous polyps, and intestinal tubes (i.e., jejunostomy). Although advanced imaging techniques may provide additional information, surgery remains the definitive modality for diagnosis and treatment of adult intussusceptions.

   This differs from intussusception in a child, which is typically idiopathic or associated with a viral infection. Nonoperative enema reduction is the treatment of choice of uncomplicated intussusception in children and has a success rate of 90%. Surgery is reserved for children with evidence of shock, peritonitis, or failed enema reduction.

2. **B.** The most common small bowel malignancy is carcinoid tumor (37.4%), followed by adenocarcinoma (36.9%), lymphoma (17.3%), and stromal tumor (8.4%). The most frequent location of carcinoid tumors is the ileum, followed by the duodenum, and, least frequently, in the jejunum.

3. **C.** This patient has developed carcinoid crisis. A carcinoid crisis is a phenomenon that occurs after manipulation of tumor masses, during induction of anesthesia, and after administration of chemotherapy but can also occur in up to 11% of patients with metastatic disease. Significant amounts of serotonin, histamine, and other mediators cause the characteristics of profound flushing, extreme changes in blood pressure, bronchoconstriction, arrhythmias, and mental status changes. If the condition is associated

with hypotension, it is usually refractory to fluid resuscitation but can be treated with the infusion of plasma and the use of octreotide.

If the diagnosis of carcinoid is made preoperatively, steps can be taken to reduce the risk of carcinoid crisis, including administering antihistamines and octreotide. Octreotide is a long-acting somatostatin analogue. In addition to reducing the release of gastrointestinal (GI) hormones, it reduces the amount of serotonin released from tumor cells. Regardless, intraoperative carcinoid events are difficult to predict, and there is no standard octreotide administration regimen available.

4. **A.** Chromogranin A is a protein associated with neuroendocrine cells and tumors. It is useful for monitoring disease response and progression in patients with carcinoid tumors. Plasma chromogranin A levels are an independent predictor of survival. 5-HIAA is the primary urinary metabolite of serotonin. Measuring these levels are useful for the diagnosis, monitoring, and prognosis of patients with carcinoid tumors. There is also reduced survival among patients with elevated Urine 5-HIAA levels, and the degree of elevation is correlated with the degree of carcinoid symptoms.

CEA is a marker for colon and pancreatic cancer. CA 19-9 is a marker for pancreatic cancer. Plasma VMA and metanephrines are useful in the diagnosis of pheochromocytoma. FSH and LH are hormones released by the pituitary gland that are not particularly useful in tumor surveillance. AFP and bHCG can be used to identify testicular cancer.

5. **B.** Many different chemotherapy regimens for carcinoid tumors have been investigated, with response rates ranging only from 0–33%. Chemotherapy has not been shown to improve survival but is typically used for control of symptoms caused by metastases.

Surgery for metastatic carcinoid disease has been shown to relieve symptoms related to intestinal obstruction and ischemia. Multiple studies have shown that surgery provides an improved control of carcinoid syndrome symptoms. In addition, cytoreductive surgery including liver metastases has shown to improve survival when compared to observation, systemic chemotherapy, and hepatic artery embolization.

In 2006, Osborne et al. demonstrated that patients who underwent cytoreductive resection for metastatic carcinoid tumor had better complete symptom relief (69% vs. 59%) and a significantly longer mean survival (43 vs. 24 months) when compared to patients undergoing embolization.

6. **C.** Approximately half of patients with long-standing elevation in serum serotonin levels will have evidence of cardiac valvular disease on echocardiogram. Because of this, patients with a known history of carcinoid tumor should undergo echocardiogram prior to planned invasive procedures.

Right-sided valvular disease predominates, with tricuspid regurgitation being by far the most common abnormality. Left-sided disease is uncommon (<10%), although is still possible via a patent foramen ovale with a right-to-left shunt.

7. **B.** Patients with refractory diarrhea in the setting of persistently elevated 5-HIAA levels and otherwise stable disease should be maximized on somatostatin therapy. If somatostatin therapy is maximized, tryptophan hydroxylase inhibitors (Telotristat) have been shown to significantly reduce bowel movements when compared to the placebo.

Bile acid sequestrants may benefit patients with a history of carcinoid who have had a terminal ileal resection. Opiates, antidiarrheals, and ondansetron may improve refractory diarrhea symptoms. However, limited data exist regarding these treatments in refractory carcinoid patients.

BIBLIOGRAPHY

Bilimoria KY, Bentrem DJ, Wayne JD, Ko CY, Bennett CL, Talamonti MS. Small bowel cancer in the United States: changes in epidemiology, treatment, and survival over the last 20 years. *Ann Surg.* 2009;249(1):63–71.

Chambers AJ, Pasieka JL, Dixon E, Rorstad O. The palliative benefit of aggressive surgical intervention for both hepatic and mesenteric metastases from neuroendocrine tumors. *Surgery.* 2008;144(4):645–651; discussion 651–653.

Davar J, Connolly HM, Caplin ME, et al. Diagnosing and managing carcinoid heart disease in patients with neuroendocrine tumors: an expert statement. *J Am Coll Cardiol.* 2017;69(10):1288–1304.

Kulke MH. Clinical presentation and management of carcinoid tumors. *Hematol Oncol Clin North Am.* 2007;21(3): 433–455; vii–viii.

Mancuso K, Kaye AD, Boudreaux JP, et al. Carcinoid syndrome and perioperative anesthetic considerations. *J Clin Anesth.* 2011;23(4):329–341.

Marinis A, Yiallourou A, Samanides L, et al. Intussusception of the bowel in adults: a review. *World J Gastroenterol.* 2009;15(4):407–411.

Modlin IM, Kidd M, Latich I, Zikusoka MN, Shapiro MD. Current status of gastrointestinal carcinoids. *Gastroenterology*. 2005;128(6):1717–1751.

Musunuru S, Chen H, Rajpal S, et al. Metastatic neuroendocrine hepatic tumors: resection improves survival. *Arch Surg (Chicago, Ill: 1960)*. 2006;141(10):1000–1004; discussion 1005.

Naraev BG, Halland M, Halperin DM, Purvis AJ, O'Dorisio TM, Halfdanarson TR. Management of diarrhea in patients with carcinoid syndrome. *Pancreas*. 2019;48(8): 961–972.

Osborne DA, Zervos EE, Strosberg J, et al. Improved outcome with cytoreduction versus embolization for symptomatic hepatic metastases of carcinoid and neuroendocrine tumors. *Ann Surg Oncol*. 2006;13(4):572–581.

Rorstad O. Prognostic indicators for carcinoid neuroendocrine tumors of the gastrointestinal tract. *J Surg Oncol*. 2005;89(3):151–160.

38

Mesenteric Ischemia

Danielle E. Smith

An 81-year-old female with a history of hypertension, diabetes mellitus, atrial fibrillation, and obesity presents to the emergency department with acute onset abdominal pain, nausea, vomiting, and hematochezia. Previous operations include a laparoscopic appendectomy. The patient's medication list includes Coumadin; however, she admits to missing doses over the last week. On physical exam, the patient appears to be in significant distress due to pain. She is writhing in pain, but her abdomen is soft, mildly tender, and nondistended. Laboratory analysis is remarkable for a white blood cell count of 21×10^9/mL and a lactate of 3.5 mmol/L. Abdominal radiography is unremarkable. A computed tomography angiography (CTA) is significant for absence of flow distal to the origin of the superior mesenteric artery (SMA).

1. **What is the likely etiology for this SMA occlusion?**

   A. Splanchnic vasoconstriction
   B. Embolic occlusion of the mesenteric circulation
   C. Acute thrombosis of the mesenteric circulation
   D. Hypercoagulable state
   E. Mesenteric venous thrombosis (MVT)

2. **Associated risk factors with acute mesenteric ischemia include which of the following?**

   A. Hyperlipidemia
   B. Obesity
   C. Advanced age
   D. Cardiac implantable electronic device (CIED) placement
   E. Hemodialysis

3. **What is the optimal management approach for this patient?**

   A. Therapeutic anticoagulation
   B. Intra-arterial thrombolytics
   C. Supportive care with avoidance of vasopressors and optimization of fluid status
   D. Mesenteric bypass
   E. Surgical embolectomy

4. **During surgical exploration, the bowel is assessed for viability, and 50 cm of small bowel is resected. What is the most reliable means of determining bowel viability after revascularization?**

   A. Second-look laparotomy
   B. Acid-base status
   C. Intraoperative Doppler ultrasound
   D. Transcutaneous oxygen measurement
   E. Resection of all necrotic and marginal appearing bowel during the initial exploration

5. **A significant proportion of morbidity and mortality in mesenteric ischemia is due to the subsequent development of**

   A. multi-organ dysfunction syndrome (MODS) due to intestinal reperfusion injury.
   B. mesenteric restenosis.
   C. malignancy.
   D. malnutrition.
   E. recurrent thrombosis.

6. **The collateral network between the celiac artery and superior mesenteric artery is primarily through the**

   A. marginal artery of Drummond.
   B. superior and inferior pancreaticoduodenal arteries.
   C. the arc of Riolan.

  D. meandering mesenteric arteries.

  E. hypogastric arteries.

7. A rare condition that can cause mesenteric ischemia is

  A. aortic dissection.

  B. radiation arteritis.

  C. median arcuate ligament syndrome.

  D. autoimmune arteritis.

ANSWERS

1. B. There are four distinct pathophysiologies for mesenteric ischemia: arterial thromboembolism, hypoperfusion syndrome, acute arterial thrombosis on chronic ischemia, and venous thrombosis. Arterial types are classified as acute or chronic. Acute mesenteric ischemia (AMI) is due to either thromboembolism or hypoperfusion syndromes, also known as nonocclusive mesenteric ischemia (NOMI). Acute-on-chronic mesenteric ischemia is due to thrombotic occlusion in the setting of atherosclerotic disease. Finally, there is one classification for venous mesenteric ischemia, which is due to MVT.

The most common type is arterial embolism, composing approximately 50% of cases. The classic presentation is acute onset periumbilical abdominal pain out of proportion to physical exam findings. A retrospective study of patients with AMI who underwent surgery found the most frequent presenting symptom was abdominal pain (95%), with nausea (44%), vomiting (35%), and diarrhea (35%) to follow. Patients with thrombotic occlusion, acute-on-chronic mesenteric ischemia, typically have a history of chronic postprandial abdominal pain and weight loss due to "food fear." It is common in the elderly population with diffuse atherosclerosis leading to relative ischemia after meals.

Patients with mesenteric hypoperfusion, or NOMI, are usually critically ill patients who present with a slower onset of diffuse abdominal pain related to splanchnic vasoconstriction in a low-flow state. Those with MVT may have various, nonspecific abdominal complaints insidious in onset that progressively worsen over time. Further diagnosis of mesenteric ischemia relies on associated risk factors, which will be discussed below, as well as laboratory analysis and imaging. One study found the mean white blood cell count to be elevated in 98% of patients, and greater than 20×10^9/mL in over half of the patients. Lactate was also elevated in greater than 90% of patients and greater than 3 mmol/L in more than 60% of patients. Imaging may include abdominal X-rays, duplex ultrasonography, CTA, magnetic resonance angiography (MRA), and contrast angiography. Contrast angiography is considered the gold standard providing both diagnostic and therapeutic options; however, CTA and MRA are commonly used as well.

Abdominal X-rays may show fluid-filled loops of bowel with bowel wall edema. Endoscopy may be useful for acute or chronic ischemia in which the duodenum and right colon may have evidence of ischemia. Classic angiographic patterns exist that assist in the diagnosis of mesenteric ischemia. First, the SMA is the most common site of embolism due to its high basal flow rate and anatomic angle of takeoff from the aorta. Second, the emboli typically lodge distal to the middle colic branch and the jejunal branches. It appears as an oval-shaped clot surrounded by contrast in a noncalcified segment. On the other hand, the thrombus in acute-on-chronic mesenteric ischemia typically forms at the atherosclerotic plaque, most commonly at the origin of the mesenteric vessel, causing a complete absence of flow. It will appear as a clot superimposed on a heavily calcified occlusive lesion at the ostium. NOMI is caused by hypoperfusion or a low-flow state; thus, angiographic findings include the absence of large vessel occlusion with evidence of sequential focal vasospasm. Finally, MVT findings include bowel wall thickening, delayed passage of contrast into the portal system, and a lack of opacification of the portal vein. It is better diagnosed with CTA with portal phase enhancement.

2. E. Associated risk factors for AMI are essential to the diagnosis. General risk factors for AMI include hypertension, tobacco use, peripheral vascular disease, and coronary artery disease. Arterial embolic occlusion is most commonly associated with a cardiac source such as atrial fibrillation leading to atrial appendage thrombus. Other causes include valvular disease and left ventricular mural thrombus due to previous myocardial infarction (MI) and subsequent hypokinesis. Arterial thrombosis involves a slow progression of atherosclerosis until a critical stenosis and subsequent thrombosis develops; thus, patients will have other manifestations of atherosclerotic disease. Low flow states can result in acute or acute-on-chronic ischemia and have been associated with MI, recent cardiac surgery, and acute viral illness. NOMI is also related to low flow states but without focal occlusion. Patients in cardiogenic or septic shock, those with vasopressor infusions, or patients with toxic pharmacologic ingestion have all been implicated as inciting events for NOMI. Dialysis patients with excessive fluid removal are also at risk. In contrast, MVT is often due to systemic disease related to hypercoagulable states such as malignancy, trauma, medications, and hypercoagulable syndromes. Hyperlipidemia may contribute to vascular disease but has very little role in acute occlusion. Obesity has an increased risk for a venous thrombotic event but is not an independent risk factor for AMI. Advanced age alone does not portend to AMI. Cardiac implantable electronic devices have been reported to have pulmonary embolisms and strokes but not AMI.

3. **E.** Treatment goals in AMI include restoration of normal pulsatile flow and resection of nonviable bowel. Open surgery and endovascular intervention can both restore flow; however, open laparotomy versus laparoscopy may be required to assess bowel viability and is mandatory with peritonitis unless palliative management is planned. The progression of endovascular technology and skill over the last decade has made an endovascular or hybrid approach more common and more accepted. One retrospective study of more than 4,000 patients compared outcomes for endovascular versus open surgery in the treatment of AMI. Endovascular intervention had a decreased mortality and shorter length of hospital stay when compared to open surgery. Other studies report decreased morbidity and mortality for endovascular intervention in acute thrombotic occlusions while others still report no difference in mortality between the groups. Retrograde open mesenteric stenting is an alternative to open surgical bypass with similar outcomes but shorter operative times. Some vascular surgeons argue retrograde open mesenteric stenting should be first-line therapy in acute cases and appropriate operator expertise. Endovascular or a hybrid approach requires a vascular center with appropriate facilities and support in place to be successful.

Surgical embolectomy is the standard treatment for arterial embolic occlusion. The occlusion is not likely amenable to thrombolytic therapy as it is a relatively organized cardiac thrombus. Furthermore, thrombolytics risks distal embolization and bowel infarction. The standard surgical approach is a transverse arteriotomy with thromboembolectomy using a 3- or 4-Fr Fogarty catheter. In patients without peritonitis, endovascular aspiration embolectomy is a treatment option. Furthermore, catheter-directed thrombolysis is an alternative option in cases of incomplete aspiration embolectomy or distal embolization. Thrombotic arterial occlusion can be managed endovascularly with stenting and/or thrombolytic therapy as this is a fresh thrombus. However, the patient may require exploratory laparotomy if bowel ischemia is a concern. Revascularization usually precedes bowel resection and treatment of the underlying stenosis or occlusive lesion is typically done during the same procedure.

Open surgical management involves surgical bypass of the occlusion and may be necessary in unsuccessful embolectomy as well. Retrograde bypass from the infrarenal aorta or iliac artery is preferred due to easier exposure and less hemodynamic changes as it avoids supraceliac cross-clamp. However, retrograde bypass may produce inferior results. Antegrade bypass from the suprarenal aorta is less susceptible to kinking; however, it may be more difficult due to postsurgical adhesive disease and calcific atherosclerotic disease. A hybrid approach with SMA thrombectomy followed by retrograde stenting of the lesion is also an option.

NOMI is preferably managed nonoperatively with the optimization of fluid status and cardiac output and the limitation of vasoconstrictors. Interestingly, one study found that 40% of patients with NOMI had a potentially treatable SMA stenotic lesion; thus, angiography should be performed if possible. Other potential causes of NOMI that should be addressed include aortic dissection or abdominal compartment syndrome which is commonly seen after ruptured abdominal aortic aneurysm repair. The mainstay of MVT treatment is therapeutic systemic anticoagulation and further workup to identify the underlying cause. For the few patients that fail medical management, endovascular options do exist, but there are no studies with comparative data. In all cases, clinical deterioration with peritonitis or any concern for bowel ischemia requires surgical exploration to assess bowel viability.

4. **A.** Regardless of surgical approach or methods to assess bowel perfusion at initial exploration,

a second-look laparotomy is essential in the management of AMI. Published criteria for a second-look laparotomy include low flow state, bowel resection, and mesenteric thromboembolectomy. The key is to plan the return to the operating room 24–48 hours after initial exploration no matter what the patient's condition. After resuscitation and correction of acid-base imbalances, patients' conditions may improve drastically; however, there is still the risk for necrotic bowel requiring resection. Clearly necrotic bowel must be resected at the initial operation; however, a marginally perfused bowel needs further evaluation to limit the risk of excessive bowel resection and potentially short gut syndrome. Pulse exam, intraoperative Doppler ultrasound, fluorescein, and transcutaneous oxygen measurements are all intraoperative diagnostic options to assess bowel viability after revascularization, but second-look laparotomy is the most reliable means of determining the viability of marginally perfused bowel after revascularization.

5. **A.** Mesenteric ischemia has a poor prognosis with mortality rates reported at approximately 30% for embolic and thrombotic ischemia and 80% for NOMI. Diagnostic delays may be the most important prognostic factor, but comorbidities may place patients at further cardiac risk and postoperative complications. A significant proportion of morbidity and mortality is due to the subsequent development of MODS in relation to mesenteric ischemia and reperfusion. Intestinal reperfusion injury leads to the synthesis and release of inflammatory mediators, the formation of reactive oxygen species, and cell membrane instability, which ultimately causes remote organ injury. Overall MVT does have a better prognosis than other forms of mesenteric ischemia; however, long-term prognosis for MVT is based on the underlying pathology. Thus, malignancy is associated with shorter survival.

6. **B.** There is abundant collateral flow between the mesenteric arteries, such that a progressive reduction of flow in one or two mesenteric arteries is typically well tolerated. However, if there is poor collateralization or acute occlusion the result may be profound mesenteric ischemia. The primary collateral network between the celiac artery and SMA is through the superior and inferior pancreaticoduodenal arteries. The marginal artery of Drummond, the arc of Riolan, and other collateral vessels, such as the meandering mesenteric arteries, may provide collateral flow between the inferior mesenteric artery (IMA) and SMA. The hypogastric arteries and hemorrhoidal network provide collateral flow to the IMA and hindgut.

7. **C.** Median arcuate ligament syndrome (MALS), or celiac artery compression syndrome, is a compressive syndrome of the celiac artery and plexus by the diaphragm on expiration. Most patients are young females 20–40 years of age. Abdominal symptoms are nonspecific but is typically localized to the upper abdomen, precipitated by meals, and is often associated with recent weight loss. In athletes, the pain may be exercise-induced rather than postprandial. MALS is a diagnosis of exclusion and often includes arterial duplex or angiography for diagnosis. Surgical therapy was traditionally done via midline laparotomy to ensure a thorough exploration of the abdomen to exclude other causes of pain. After exploration, the surgery proceeds with skeletonization of the aorta at the level of the celiac axis by division of the tendinous diaphragmatic bands, celiac plexus fibers, and enlarged lymphatics. Finally, the artery is assessed for adequate flow after release. The first report of a laparoscopic release in 2000 has since changed the standard surgical approach to a laparoscopic release with additional arterial interventions as needed per vascular surgery. Robotic-assisted median arcuate ligament release has been increasingly performed by several institutions with similar outcomes to laparoscopic release.

BIBLIOGRAPHY

Acosta S, Bjorck M. Modern treatment of acute mesenteric ischaemia. *Br J Surg.* 2014;101(1):e100–e108.

Acosta S, Alhadad A, Ekberg O. Findings in multi-detector row CT with portal phase enhancement in patients with mesenteric venous thrombosis. *Emerg Radiol.* 2009;16(6): 477–482.

Acosta S, Ogren M, Sternby NH, Bergqvist D, Bjorck M. Fatal nonocclusive mesenteric ischaemia: population-based incidence and risk factors. *J Intern Med.* 2006;259(3):305–313.

Andraska E, Haga L, Li X, Avgerinos E, Singh M, Chaer R, Madigan M, Eslami MH. Retrograde open mesenteric stenting should be considered as the initial approach to acute mesenteric ischemia. Published April 4, 2020. *J Vasc Surg.*

Arthurs ZM, Titus J, Bannazadeh M, et al. A comparison of endovascular revascularization with traditional therapy for the treatment of acute mesenteric ischemia. *J Vasc Surg.* 2011;53(3):698–704; discussion 704–705.

Atkins MD, Kwolek CJ, LaMuraglia GM, Brewster DC, Chung TK, Cambria RP. Surgical revascularization versus endovascular therapy for chronic mesenteric ischemia: a comparative experience. *J Vasc Surg.* 2007;45(6):1162–1171.

Beaulieu RJ, Arnaoutakis KD, Abularrage CJ, Efron DT, Schneider E, Black JH 3rd. Comparison of open and endovascular treatment of acute mesenteric ischemia. *J Vasc Surg.* 2014;59(1):159–164.

Belkin M, Owens C, Whittemore A, Donaldson M, Conte M, Gravereaux E. Mesenteric ischemia. In: Townsend C, Beauchamp R, Evers B, Mattox K, eds. *Sabiston textbook of surgery.* 18th ed. Saunders Elsevier; 2008.

Bobadilla JL. Mesenteric ischemia. *Surg Clin North Am.* 2013;93(4):925–940, ix.

Coelho J, Hosni A, Claus CM, Aguilera Y, Abot GP, Freitas A, Costa M. Treatment of median arcuate ligament syndrome: outcome of laparoscopic approach. Published May 18, 2020. *Arq Bras Cir Dig.*

Harnik IG, Brandt LJ. Mesenteric venous thrombosis. *Vasc Med.* 2010;15(5):407–418.

Kasirajan K, O'Hara PJ, Gray BH, et al. Chronic mesenteric ischemia: Open surgery versus percutaneous angioplasty and stenting. *J Vasc Surg.* 2001;33(1):63–71.

Khrucharoen U, Juo YY, Chen Y, Jimenez JC, Dutson EP. Short- and intermediate-term clinical outcome comparison between laparoscopic and robotic-assisted median arcuate ligament release. *J Robot Surg.* 2020;14(1);123–129.

Kibbe M, Hassoun H. Acute mesenteric ischemia. Souba WW, Mitchell P, Fink MD, et al. eds. *ACS Surgery: Principles and Practice.* 6th ed. 2014;1016–1026.

Lee H, Ko EH, Lai M, et al. Delineating the relationships among the formation of reactive oxygen species, cell membrane instability and innate autoimmunity in intestinal reperfusion injury. *Mol Immunol.* 2014;58(2):151–159.

Lin PH, Ruth BL, Lumsden AB. Treatment of acute visceral artery occlusive cisease. In: Greald TS, Zelenock B. eds. *Mastery of Vascular & Endovascular Surgery.* Lippincott Williams & Wilkins; 2006:293–299.

Moore EE, Moore FA, Franciose RJ, Kim FJ, Biffl WL, Banerjee A. The postischemic gut serves as a priming bed for circulating neutrophils that provoke multiple organ failure. *J Trauma.* 1994;37(6):881–887.

Paladino NC, Inviati A, Di Paola V, et al. Predictive factors of mortality in patients with acute mesenteric ischemia. A retrospective study. *Ann Ital Chir.* 2014 May–Jun;85(3):265–270.

Park WM, Gloviczki P, Cherry KJ Jr, et al. Contemporary management of acute mesenteric ischemia: factors associated with survival. *J Vasc Surg.* 2002;35(3):445–452.

Roayaie S, Jossart G, Gitlitz D, Lamparello P, Hollier L, Gagner M. Laparoscopic release of celiac artery compression syndrome facilitated by laparoscopic ultrasound scanning to confirm restoration of flow. *J Vasc Surg.* 2000;32(4):814–817.

Rose SC, Quigley TM, Raker EJ. Revascularization for chronic mesenteric ischemia: comparison of operative arterial bypass grafting and percutaneous transluminal angioplasty. *J Vasc Interv Radiol.* 1995;6(3):339–349.

Ryer EJ, Kalra M, Oderich GS, et al. Revascularization for acute mesenteric ischemia. *J Vasc Surg.* 2012;55(6):1682–1689.

Sise MJ. Acute mesenteric ischemia. *Surg Clin North Am.* 2014;94(1):165–181.

Tallarita T, Oderich GS, Macedo TA, et al. Reinterventions for stent restenosis in patients treated for atherosclerotic mesenteric artery disease. *J Vasc Surg.* 2011;54(5):1422–1429.e1.

Yanar H, Taviloglu K, Retaken C, et al. Planned second-look laparoscopy in the management of acute mesenteric ischemia. *World J Gastroenterol.* 2007;13(24):3350–3353.

39

Appendicitis

Erik Criman

You are called to the emergency department to evaluate a 25-year-old woman complaining of abdominal pain starting 12 hours prior to presentation. She initially characterized the pain as a periumbilical discomfort, but now it is sharp and localizes to her right lower quadrant. A review of systems is positive for a temperature elevation (measured at 38°C at home), anorexia, and nausea without emesis. The patient denies diarrhea, melena, and hematochezia. Her past medical history, past surgical history, social history, and family history are all unremarkable. The patient's last menstrual period was 3 weeks ago. She does not take any medications and has no allergies. Measurement of her vital signs demonstrates a temperature of 37.8°C, a heart rate of 88 beats per minute, a blood pressure of 118/74 mmHg, respiratory rate of 18 breaths per minute, and oxygen saturation of 98% on room air. Physical examination is normal except for focal tenderness to palpation most prominent at McBurney's point.

1. **What is the most important laboratory test to order for this patient?**

   A. Complete blood count
   B. Type and screen
   C. Prothrombin time (PT) and partial thromboplastin time (PTT)
   D. Human chorionic gonadotropin
   E. Complete metabolic panel

2. **Regarding the clinical manifestations of this diagnosis, which of the following is correct?**

   A. The location of the appendiceal tip has little to do with determining the presenting symptoms.

   B. Only 25% of adult patients with acute appendicitis will present with a "classic" history.
   C. A clinical diagnosis of acute appendicitis is more accurate in men than in women.
   D. The appendiceal obstruction is not the hypothesized pathogenesis of acute appendicitis.
   E. A delay in diagnosis and/or surgical intervention is the most common cause of complicated (gangrenous or perforated) appendicitis rather than a patient's delay in seeking medical attention.

3. **Regarding the use of imaging in acute appendicitis, which of the following is correct?**

   A. Ultrasound is the most specific imaging study available.
   B. Selective imaging has been used to lower the accepted negative appendectomy rate to less than 20%.
   C. Confirmatory imaging is not required to make the diagnosis of acute appendicitis in all cases prior to definitive management.
   D. The most accurate ultrasound finding in acute appendicitis is the presence of mesenteric lymphadenopathy.
   E. For pregnant women, magnetic resonance imaging (MRI) is not recommended.

4. **Regarding nonoperative management of acute appendicitis, which of the following is correct?**

   A. Nonoperative management has been definitively shown to be cost-effective.
   B. Surgical management is a standard of care for acute appendicitis in the United States.

C. No trials have demonstrated a potential benefit to medical management.

D. Nonoperative management has consistently been shown to reduce the length of stay.

E. The presence of a fecalith on imaging does not predispose a patient to fail nonoperative management.

5. **A decision is made to take the patient to the operating room for a laparoscopic appendectomy. Regarding possibilities that may occur during the operation, which of the following is correct?**

A. If the appendix appears normal, it should NOT be removed.

B. If a subcentimeter mass is identified at the appendiceal tip, one should perform an ileocecectomy.

C. If an enterotomy occurs during trocar placement, one should perform a bowel resection.

D. If a free rupture of the appendix with fecal contamination of the peritoneal cavity has occurred, one should do a washout only at this operation.

E. If one encounters a perforated appendix, leaving a drain has not been shown to reduce the rate of abscess formation.

6. **Intraoperatively, the patient's appendix is found to be perforated with a small, contained phlegmon. Which of the following is most correct regarding the duration of her postoperative antibiotic course?**

A. Plan to trend the patient's CBC postoperatively and discontinue antibiotics when this value returns to the normal range.

B. Keep the patient hospitalized for 7 days of antibiotics.

C. Following appendectomy, plan for a fixed 4-day course of antibiotics.

D. Discontinue antibiotics immediately after surgery.

E. Discharge the patient on 14 days of antibiotics.

7. **Your patient returns to the emergency department 6 days after surgery with recurrent right lower quadrant abdominal pain, oral intolerance, fever, and leukocytosis. Which of the following is a risk factor for the development of intra-abdominal abscess following laparoscopic appendectomy?**

A. Complicated appendicitis

B. Surgical resident performing the procedure

C. American Society of Anesthesiologists (ASA) class

D. Gender

E. Case duration longer than 60 minutes

ANSWERS

Acute inflammation of the vermiform appendix, first described by Fitz in 1886, is one of the most common causes of the acute abdomen encountered by the general surgeon. Anatomically, this structure is a true diverticulum of the cecum as it contains all layers of the colonic wall. It receives its arterial supply from the appendiceal artery (a terminal branch of the ileocolic artery). It is invariably found at the base of the cecum at the convergence of the taenia coli. This structure is histologically distinct from the cecum in that it contains lymphoid tissue in the mucosa and submucosa. Epidemiologically, acute appendicitis presents most commonly in the second generation of life, is 1.4 times more common in men, is 1.5 times more common in whites, and is 11.3% more common in the summer months. The estimated lifetime risk of acute appendicitis is 8.6% for males and 6.7% for females. The hypothesized pathogenesis of acute appendicitis is that of appendiceal obstruction. This may be caused by a fecalith, true calculi, lymphoid hyperplasia, masses (both benign and malignant), or infectious processes. When the appendix becomes obstructed, increased intraluminal pressure causes localized ischemia, leading eventually to perforation and localized abscess formation or generalized peritonitis.

1. **D.** All women of childbearing age must have a pregnancy test for two reasons. First, it narrows the differential diagnosis. The differential diagnosis for acute right lower quadrant pain is extensive, especially in a female of childbearing age. It includes such entities as inflammatory bowel disease (Crohn's disease, ulcerative colitis), ileitis, epiploic appendagitis, cecal diverticulitis, Meckel's diverticulitis, and renal colic. Specific to women, obstetrical diagnoses (pregnancy, ectopic pregnancy) and gynecologic diagnoses (ruptured ovarian cyst, endometriosis, pelvic inflammatory disease, tubo-ovarial abscess, Mittelschmerz, ovarian torsion) are in play. A rectal examination along with pelvic examination in women or genitourinary examination in men should be considered. Second, the result of this test will most directly impact the diagnostic workup and management of the patient. If the patient is found to be pregnant and is still suspected to have acute appendicitis, the diagnostic study of choice will change (ultrasound vs. MRI

over computerized tomography [CT]), teratogenic medications should be avoided, and fetal heart tones will be documented both before and after anesthesia.

2. **C.** Clinical diagnosis of acute appendicitis is more accurate in men than it is in women. Although the overall accuracy of a clinical diagnosis of acute appendicitis is given as approximately 80%, this value is significantly higher in men than in women because acute obstetric and gynecologic pathology may confound the diagnosis. The anatomic location of the appendix, along with the time of the presentation, determines the clinical manifestations of acute appendicitis. Furthermore, the "classic" presentation of appendicitis (vague periumbilical discomfort followed by nausea and anorexia followed by migration of the pain to the right lower quadrant) only occurs in 50–60% of presentations. Interestingly, patient delay in seeking medical attention is cited as the most common cause for the intraoperative findings of gangrenous or perforated appendicitis. The other factor that heavily influences delay in diagnosis is the patient's age. Appendicitis often presents atypically in children (particularly those younger than 3 years of age) and the elderly (defined as those patients older than 60 years). Adult patients who are obese, diabetic, or immunologically compromised may also present in an atypical manner. A high index of suspicion is required to make the diagnosis in these patient populations.

3. **C.** Confirmatory imaging is not required to diagnose acute appendicitis, and there is evidence to suggest that waiting for imaging only serves to delay definitive management in cases where there is little doubt of the history, physical exam, and laboratory evaluation. While historically the negative appendectomy rate was accepted as 10% for men and 20% for women, this value has been reduced to less than 10%, with the selective use of preoperative imaging (primarily CT) in cases where the diagnosis is not clinically apparent. CT is the most specific imaging modality available, with an estimated specificity of >95%. Regarding ultrasound, an appendiceal diameter of 6 mm or greater has been set as the threshold for making the diagnosis of acute appendicitis in an individual with coexistent right lower quadrant pain. MRI is recommended for pregnant women when the transabdominal ultrasound is nondiagnostic for acute appendicitis.

4. **B.** Surgical management remains the standard of care for acute appendicitis in the United States. Appendectomy, increasingly done using a laparoscopic approach, has become an extremely safe procedure with a reported intraoperative complication rate of 0.7% and a general postoperative complication rate of 1.5%. In the adult literature, there has recently been some promising research including several randomized, prospective trials that collectively have documented nonoperative management has an aggregate treatment failure rate and recurrence rate (adjudged as crossing over to operative management) ranging from 14–32% at 2 years. For those who are successfully managed nonoperatively, reviews have demonstrated decreased morbidity, decreased pain, and a reduced amount of sick leave and disability. Unfortunately, there has also been evidence that those who fail conservative management more often present with abscess or perforation (about 30%). Nonoperative management has not proved to be cost-effective because of an associated longer length of stay along, with the cost of readmission and crossover to the operative arm. The presence of a fecalith is considered a contraindication to nonoperative management because this finding has an association with treatment failure, recurrence, and complicated appendicitis.

5. **E.** There is no evidence that drains reduce complications (e.g., abscess formation, wound infection) following appendectomy for any stage of appendicitis. If a normal-appearing appendix is encountered intraoperatively, care should be taken to perform a thorough evaluation of the peritoneal cavity. Most authors recommend incidental appendectomy to remove appendicitis from the differential going forward. It should be noted that even if the appendix appears normal, final pathology will not infrequently demonstrate inflammation consistent with a diagnosis of acute appendicitis. Appendiceal tumors are rare and only found in 1% of appendectomy specimens. Of these, carcinoid tumors are the most common (>50%), and 90% are located at the appendiceal tip. If the tumor is less than 2 cm, an appendectomy is adequate. If the tumor is greater than 2 cm in size or there is a question of incomplete resection (positive margins, grossly positive lymph nodes), the National Comprehensive Cancer Network recommendation is initial appendectomy followed by reexploration and right partial

colectomy if the staging evaluation is negative for metastatic disease.

An enterotomy may be repaired primarily if it is identified at the time of the original operation. Although operative management of appendiceal phlegmon or abscess at the time of presentation is controversial, thorough washout and appendectomy (either laparoscopically or via laparotomy) without drain placement is indicated for cases of fecal peritonitis caused by free rupture of the appendix.

6. **C.** Although high-quality evidence exists to guide the choice of antimicrobial agent in the setting of complicated intra-abdominal infection, there has historically been little consensus regarding the optimum duration of treatment. The STOP-IT Trial was a multicenter randomized controlled trial published in 2015 and did much to guide surgeons on this latter point. After obtaining source control, the study's investigators randomized patients to receive either a fixed 4 ± 1-calendar-day course of antibiotics (experimental group) or a variable course that added 2 ± 1 calendar days to the patient's course after resolution of fever, leukocytosis, and oral intolerance (control group). The experimental group received a median of 4 days of antibiotics while the control group received a median 8-day course. There was no difference between the groups in terms of surgical site infection, recurrent intra-abdominal infection, or death within 30 days following the source control procedure.

7. **A.** Development of an intra-abdominal abscess following laparoscopic appendectomy remains a well-known complication despite advances in surgical technique and antibiotic therapy. The overall incidence is quoted as less than 1% for uncomplicated appendicitis and as high as 20% for complicated appendicitis. Following multivariate analysis on a cohort of European patients, the only significant factor associated with the development of an intra-abdominal abscess after laparoscopic appendectomy was the presence of complicated appendicitis. All other factors studied (resident surgeon, ASA class, gender, age older than 35, diabetes, symptoms more than 48 hours, operative duration, Alvarado score greater than 7, C-reactive protein >100 mg/L) were not significantly different between groups.

BIBLIOGRAPHY

Addiss DG, Shaffer N, Fowler BS, Tauxe RV. The epidemiology of appendicitis and appendectomy in the United States. *Am J Epidemiol.* 1990;132(5):910.

Binenbaum SJ, Goldfarb MA. Inadvertent enterotomy in minimally invasive abdominal surgery. *JSLS.* 2006;10(3): 336–340.

Birnbaum BA, Wilson SR. Appendicitis at the millennium. *Radiology.* 2000;215(2):337–348.

Brügger L, Rosella L, Candinas D, Güller U. Improving outcomes after laparoscopic appendectomy: a population-based, 12-year trend analysis of 7446 patients. *Ann Surg.* 2011;253(2):309.

Chiarugi M, Buccianti P, Decanini L, et al. What you see is not what you get. A plea to remove a "normal" appendix during diagnostic laparoscopy. *Acta Chir Belg.* 2001;101(5):243.

Connor SJ, Hanna GB, Frizelle FA. Appendiceal tumors: Retrospective clinicopathologic analysis of appendiceal tumors from 7970 appendectomies. *Dis Colon Rectum.* 1998;41(1):75.

Daehlin L. Acute appendicitis during the first three years of life. *Acta Chir Scand.* 1982;148(3):291.

Di Saverio S, Sibilio A, Giorgini E, Biscardi A, Villani S, Coccolini F, et al. The NOTA Study (Non-Operative Treatment for Acute Appendicitis): prospective study on the efficacy and safety of antibiotics (amoxicillin and clavulanic acid) for treating patients with right lower quadrant abdominal pain and long-term follow-up of conservatively treated suspected appendicitis. *Ann Surg.* 2014 Jul;260(1):109–17.

Fitz, RH. Perforating inflammation of the vermiform appendix with special reference to its early diagnosis and treatment. *Am J Med Sci.* 1886;92:321.

Horattas MC, Guyton DP, Wu D. A reappraisal of appendicitis in the elderly. *Am J Surg.* 1990;160(3):291.

Jeffrey RB Jr, Laing FC, Townsend RR. Acute appendicitis: sonographic criteria based on 250 cases. *Radiology.* 1988;167(2):327.

Lasek A, Pedziwiatr M, Wysoki M, et al. Risk factors for intraabdominal abscess formation after laparoscopic appendectomy – results from the Pol-LA (Polish Laparoscopic Appendectomy) multicenter large cohort study. *Wideochir Inne Tech Maloinwazyjne.* 2019;14(1):70–78.

Lee SL, Walsh AJ, Ho HS. Computed tomography and ultrasonography do not improve and may delay the diagnosis and treatment of acute appendicitis. *Arch Surg.* 2001;136(5): 556.

McCutcheon BA, Chang DC, Marcus LP, et al. Long-term outcomes of patients with non-surgically managed uncomplicated appendicitis. *JACS.* 2014;218:905.

National Comprehensive Cancer Network. Neuroendocrine Tumors (Version 2.2014). Accessed April 30, 2014. http://www.nccn.org/professionals/physician_gls/pdf/neuroendocrine.pdf

Park JS, Jeong JH, Lee JI, Lee JH, Park JK, Moon HJ. Accuracies of diagnostic methods for acute appendicitis. *Am Surg.* January 2013;79(1):101–106.

Parks NA, Schroeppel TJ. Update on imaging for acute appendicitis. *Surg Clin North Am.* 2011;91(1):141–154.

Petrowsky H, Demartines N, Rousson V, Clavien PA. Evidence-based value of prophylactic drainage in gastrointestinal surgery: A systematic review and meta-analyses. *Ann Surg.* 2004;240(6):1074.

Pittman-Waller VA, Myers JG, Stewart RM, Dent DL, Page CP, Gray GA, et al. Appendicitis: why so complicated? Analysis of 5755 consecutive appendectomies. *Am Surg.* 2000; 66(6):548.

Sawyer RG, Claridge JA, Nathens AB, et al. Trial of short-course antimicrobial therapy for intraabdominal infection. *N Engl J Med.* 2015;372:1996–2005.

Shindoh J, et al. Predictive factors for negative outcomes in initial non-operative management of suspected appendicitis. *J Gastrointest Surg.* 2010;14(2):309–314.

Varadhan KK, Neal KR, Lobo DN, et al. Safety and efficacy of antibiotics compared with appendectomy for treatment of uncomplicated, acute appendicitis: meta-analysis of randomized controlled trials. *BMJ.* 2012;344:e2156

Wagner PL, Eachempati SR, Soe K, Pieracci FM, Shou J, Barie PS. Defining the current negative appendectomy rate: for whom is preoperative computed tomography making an impact? *Surgery.* 2008;144(2):276.

Wilms I, de Hoog D, de Visser D, Janzing H. Appendectomy versus antibiotic treatment for acute appendicitis. *Cochrane Review of Syst Rev.* 2011. doi:10.1002/14651858.CD008359. pub2

40

Colon Cancer

Suzanne Gillern

A 51-year-old female presents to your office for pain-less hematochezia. She is otherwise feeling well and has no other past medical or surgical history. She has never had a colonoscopy. She is adopted and unaware of her family history.

1. **The patient is in the process of finding her biological family and is inquiring about risk factors for colon cancer. Which of the following is true?**

   A. All newly diagnosed colorectal cancers under age 70 should be evaluated for the mismatch repair deficiency of Lynch syndrome.
   B. In families with suspected familial adenomatous polyposis (FAP) syndrome, screening should start in the third decade of life and be done every 5 years.
   C. In patients at risk for attenuated FAP (AFAP), the average age of onset of colon cancer is the same as with FAP.
   D. In patients with Peutz-Jeghers syndrome, COX-2 inhibitors have been shown to slow the progression to cancer.
   E. In serrated polyposis syndrome, the polyps are typically hyperplastic in nature and thus, this syndrome is not associated with an increased risk of malignancy development.

2. **On physical exam, the patient has a body mass index (BMI) of 32 kg/m². Digital rectal exam reveals no masses, and on anoscopy, she has an external and internal hemorrhoid. The rest of her exam is normal. What is your next step in management?**

   A. Hemorrhoidectomy
   B. Colonoscopy
   C. Follow-up in 6 months after dietary modifications (daily fiber intake 25–35g/day and water intake of 64 oz per day).
   D. Computed tomography (CT) abdomen/pelvis
   E. Hemorrhoid banding

3. **On your chosen exam, you are able to evaluate the entire colon. A 4-cm sessile polyp is found at 20 cm from the anus with a flexible scope. You biopsy the lesion and place a tattoo to mark the location. Pathology reveals poorly differentiated adenocarcinoma. Further testing reveals the tumor is MSI-instable (microsatellite instability–instable) and, on immunohistochemistry testing, demonstrates a mismatch repair gene deficiency of *MSH2*. What other cancer is this patient at highest risk of getting?**

   A. Endometrial cancer
   B. Brain cancer
   C. Adrenal cancer
   D. Pancreatic cancer
   E. Ovarian cancer

4. **When the patient returns to your clinic to discuss biopsy results, you perform a rigid proctoscopy and are unable to see the tattoo when you insert the scope in 15 cm. What is your next step in management?**

   A. Magnetic resonance imaging (MRI) scan of the pelvis
   B. Refer to an oncologist for neoadjuvant chemoradiation

C. Positron emission tomography (PET)/CT scan

D. Chest x-ray

E. CT scan of the chest/abdomen/pelvis

5. On imaging, there is no evidence of metastasis or pathologic lymph nodes. Which operation is the standard of care for this patient, and what you should recommend?

A. Endoscopic mucosal resection of the tumor

B. Low anterior resection with diverting loop ileostomy

C. Sigmoidectomy

D. Total colectomy with ileorectal anastomosis and hysterectomy w/ bilateral salpingo-oophorectomy

E. Total colectomy with ileorectal anastomosis

6. Prior to performing the selected operation, what is the appropriate bowel preparation to give your patient?

A. Mechanical bowel preparation alone

B. Preoperative oral antibiotics alone

C. Enemas alone

D. Mechanical and oral antibiotics bowel preparation

E. No bowel preparation

7. The patient is prepared for surgery. You plan to perform a laparoscopic resection. Which of the following is true regarding laparoscopic approaches?

A. The robotic-assisted laparoscopic approach has the least amount of blood loss.

B. A single-incision laparoscopic approach has less pain compared to other laparoscopic approaches.

C. The laparoscopic approach has higher rates of port site/wound recurrences versus an open approach.

D. The laparoscopic approach has fewer deep surgical site infections than does an open approach.

E. A single-incision laparoscopic approach has a shorter length of hospital stay.

ANSWERS

1. A. Hereditary syndromes of the gastrointestinal (GI) tract account for 5–10% of GI malignancies including colon cancer. There are several known such syndromes: Lynch syndrome (LS; formerly hereditary nonpolyposis colorectal cancer, or HNPCC), adenomatous polyposis syndromes (APSs), including FAP,

AFAP, and MUTYH-associated polyposis (MAP); Peutz-Jegher syndrome (PJS), juvenile polyposis syndrome (JPS), Cowden syndrome (CS), serrated/hyperplastic polyposis syndrome (SPS), and the conditions of hereditary pancreatic cancer and gastric cancer. All these syndromes increase the risk of colorectal cancer development and in the case of the FAPs, all these patients will progress to malignancy.

LS: This is the most common hereditary syndrome and these patients have a mismatch repair gene mutation. The average age of colorectal cancer diagnosis is 44–61 years (sporadic cancer is 69 years). LS is also hallmarked by right-sided colon predominance and a rapid progression from adenomatous polyp to cancer (35 months). All newly diagnosed colorectal cancer patients should be genetically screened for LS mutations. For those family members at risk, screening with colonoscopy should begin at 20–25 years and continue at least every 2 years.

APSs: There are three variants: FAP, attenuated-FAP AFAP, and molecular adenomatous polyposis (MAP). One hundred percent of FAP patients will go on to develop colon cancer with an average onset of 39–41 years of age. This condition is hallmarked by >100 synchronous polyps. Colon cancer screening should begin at age 10–12 via colonoscopy and should continue annually, and fortunately, screening with subsequent surgery can eliminate the mortality from this disease. In AFAP, the number of colonic polyps is reduced to about 50%, and correspondingly, the average age of malignant onset is higher at 58 years and occurs in about 69% of patients with AFAP. Screening is recommended to begin in the third decade of life and continued every 1–2 years. In MAP patients, cancer develops in 41% to 100% of patients with an average age of onset of 58 years. There are typically 20–99 synchronous polyps. Here, *MUTYH* is a base excision repair gene, and its mutation causes the oncogenesis. In addition to other malignancies, APSs are associated with desmoid tumors.

Prophylactic colectomy, meaning total colectomy with ileo-rectal anastomosis or total proctocolectomy with ileal pouch-anal anastomosis, should be considered in the late teens and early 20s and if there is evidence of high-grade dysplasia, polyps >10 mm in diameter, marked increases in polyp number from one exam to the next, and if symptoms are present.

PJS: PJS is hallmarked by hamartomatous polyps of the GI tract and mucocutaneous pigmentation. Colon cancer develops in 39% of patients with an age of onset of 42–44. More commonly patients will present with abdominal pain due to one of the hamartomatous polyps causing an intussusception. This typically occurs in younger patients. Those with a suspected diagnosis or at risk should have a screening colonoscopy and esophagogastroduodenoscopy (EGD, for duodenal and gastric cancer risk) at age 8. If polyps are found and can be controlled endoscopically, then surveillance is recommended for every 3 years. If no polyps are found and the patient is asymptomatic, the next screening by endoscopy can be delayed until 18 years of age and then every 3 years. While COX-2 inhibitors are theoretically believed to eliminate polyps, there is no conclusive evidence that they are helpful in doing so.

JPS: JPS is defined by the presence of five or more juvenile polyps in the GI tract, which can present in the first decade of life. The average age of diagnosis for JPS is 18 years of age, with the mean age of colon cancer onset being 34 years of age. By this age, 17–22% of carriers will have developed colon cancer. Endoscopic screening with both EGD and colonoscopy should begin at age 12, with surveillance done every 1–3 years.

CS: Of CS patients, 95% have colonic polyps, typically hamartomatous in nature, and they can be numerous, even over 100. CS is also associated with ganglioneuromas, and it carries a 9–16% increased risk for colon cancer. Screening should begin at age 15 and continued every 1–2 years.

SPS: SPS was previously known as hyperplastic polyposis syndrome when it was felt the only types of polyps present were serrated hyperplastic ones, but in fact, the polyps can be adenomatous also. All the polyps are serrated, however. The diagnosis can be confirmed clinically in patients who have >5 serrated polyps proximal to the sigmoid colon with at least 2 of them being >10 mm, any number of serrated polyps proximal to the sigmoid colon and a first degree relative with the diagnosis, or >20 serrated polyps distributed throughout the colon. While SPS is felt to increase the risk of colorectal cancer, the exact risk is unknown. The screening age is unknown but once it is diagnosed, a colonoscopy is recommended every 1–3 years.

2. **B.** The initial workup for this 51-year-old patient who presents with painless hematochezia should be a colonoscopy. Complete endoscopic evaluation of the colon is indicated in the following patients

with hemorrhoids and rectal bleeding: age ≥50 if no complete examination within 10 years, age ≥40 or 10 years younger than the age at diagnosis with history positive for a first-degree relative with colorectal cancer or advanced adenoma diagnosed at age >60 years, age ≥40 or 10 years younger than the age at diagnosis with the history positive for two first-degree relatives with advanced adenomas or colorectal cancer, positive fecal immunochemical testing (FIT) or FIT fecal DNA testing.

FIT and stool DNA testing are other screening tests used to detect the presence of cancer or advanced adenomas. Both are considered specific and sensitive in the detection and absence of colorectal cancer, but their exact role has yet to be defined. It is likely they would be used as screening tools in average-risk patients. Positive FIT or stool DNA tests would prompt the performance of a colonoscopy.

Hemorrhoidectomy and/or hemorrhoid banding should be deferred until a full workup of the hematachezia has been performed as well as an attempt of conservative management with dietary modifications. Dietary modifications are the first-line therapy for patients with symptomatic hemorrhoid disease. Increasing fiber and water (25–35 g/day of fiber and >64 oz of water per day), as well as maintaining proper stool habits (avoidance of straining and limiting time on the toilet), provide symptomatic relief of haemorrhoids in nearly 80% of patients. Recommending these modifications to this patient is appropriate; however, it would be inappropriate to defer reevaluation of this patient, who is in need of a colonoscopy now. Hemorrhoid banding may be offered to patients with grade I and II and select patients with grade III internal hemorrhoidal disease who fail medical treatment. A hemorrhoidectomy is recommended for patients with symptoms resulting from external hemorrhoids or combined internal and external haemorrhoids with prolapse after a trial of dietary modifications is made.

There is no role for a CT scan of the abdomen/pelvis at this time as this is not an effective screening tool for colon and rectal lesions. CT virtual colonoscopy would not be the first diagnostic method in this patient as it is generally used as a screening tool only for either asymptomatic patients or patients who cannot tolerate sedation. Additionally, CT colonography has not proven to be as accurate as conventional colonoscopy for lesions <10 mm in diameter.

3. **A.** LS is associated with many other malignancies besides colon cancer. The lifetime risk of getting colon cancer with LS is reported as up to 69% in men and 52% in women by the age of 70 years.

Endometrial cancer is the next most common cancer that this patient is at risk for. The average risk of getting endometrial cancer with LS ranges from 18–60% with a mean age of diagnosis at 50 years. Although less prevalent than endometrial cancer in LS, there is a risk of ovarian cancer of up to 12% in female patients.

LS is also associated with pancreas and different brain cancers. Although the risk of pancreatic and brain cancer with LS is greater than the general population, it occurs in approximately 4% or fewer of the patients with LS. LS is also associated with cancers of the stomach, small bowel, urinary tract, breast, and prostate cancers. There is no association between adrenal cancer and LS.

4. **E.** Disease workup is recommended prior to proceeding to surgery in cases of colon cancer. The NCCN guidelines recommend a CT scan of the chest, abdomen, and pelvis. A chest x-ray is no longer adequate to rule out possible metastasis to the lungs. Routine preoperative imaging has been shown to change the treatment plan or operative plan in up to 14% of patients. In addition to identifying metastatic disease, preoperative imaging can be helpful with T stage, nodal status, and location of the lesion. All patients should also obtain a preoperative carcinoembryonic antigen level to assist with surveillance after treatment is complete.

The rigid proctoscopy was performed to ensure that this was not a rectal cancer. When measuring the distance from the anus with a flexible scope, it can be unreliable. Any patient who has a lesion suspected to be on the left side or sigmoid colon should undergo a rigid proctoscopy to ensure the lesion is not in the rectum, which would significantly alter the workup as well as treatment of this cancer. In the case of rectal cancer, rigid proctoscopy is noted to be better to determine the actual distance of the lesion from the anal verge to help with operative planning.

If this lesion was in the rectum, it would be appropriate to perform an MRI scan of the pelvis to determine T and N stage. Any clinical T3 or T4 lesions and any abnormal nodes seen on the MRI scan are an indication for neoadjuvant chemoradiation therapy. This lesion is in the sigmoid colon (not visible on rigid proctoscopy), and therefore, MRI or referral for neoadjuvant chemoradiation is not appropriate.

A PET scan is more routinely used after resection of colon cancers to determine recurrence, but this is not mandatory. A PET scan/CT colonography is recommended if the proximal colon cannot be examined due to an obstructing lesion or if metastatectomy is anticipated.

5. **D.** For this individual with LS and colon cancer, a total colectomy is recommended for cancer risk reduction. There is a high risk of metachronous colon cancer with LS, and multiple studies have demonstrated a significantly reduced degree of metachronous cancer risk reduction with a segmental colectomy when compared to a total colectomy with ileorectal anastomosis. However, despite the inferior cancer risk reduction, a segmental colectomy may be considered in patients who are concerned about the differences in bowel function after surgery. If a patient elects for segmental bowel resection of the colon cancer, they should undergo an annual colonoscopy for surveillance.

In addition, a hysterectomy and bilateral salpingo-oophorectomy should be offered to woman with LS undergoing a colectomy, especially if they have finished childbearing. The 2014 LS guidelines by the US Multi-Society Task Force on Colorectal Cancer recommend hysterectomy and bilateral salingo-oopherectomy in all women aged older than 40 or have finished childbearing. This is a personal decision that should be made by the patient, after weighing the risks and benefits of undergoing this additional procedure, but the role of the surgeon is to initiate these discussions to allow the patient to make an informed decision.

A low anterior resection would be utilized if this was a rectal cancer. Because a rigid proctoscopy was appropriately performed prior to surgery and demonstrated the mass was not in the rectum; therefore, a low anterior resection is not required.

An endoscopic mucosal resection would be inappropriate in this setting for many reasons. It would fail to evaluate the lymph nodes and potentially lead to incomplete treatment of colon cancer. In addition, due the risk of metachronous lesions, a local resection is not recommended.

6. **D.** Elective colon and rectal surgery has a historically high rate of surgical site infection (SSI), ranging

from 5.4–23.2%. Mechanical bowel preparation combined with preoperative oral antibiotics is recommended for elective colorectal resections. In combination, this preparation strategy reduces the rate of SSI, anastomotic leak, readmission, and length of stay when compared to all other methods of bowel preparation to include no bowel preparation.

Preoperative mechanical bowel preparation alone provides no difference in postoperative complications when compared to no bowel preparation and therefore provides no benefit when utilized without preoperative oral antibiotics. There are no conclusive data available to suggest the use of preoperative oral antibiotics alone, without a mechanical preparation, provides any benefit or is equivalent to the use of both the oral antibiotics and mechanical preparation. There are limited data looking into the use of enemas alone, but there is nothing in the literature to suggest it is equivalent or superior to the combination of oral antibiotic and mechanical bowel preparation.

7. **E.** Laparoscopic colonic resection continues to be more popular, and it has proved advantages of decreased hospital length of stay, less postoperative pain, decreased superficial surgical site infection, and decreased nonsurgical complications. While robot-assisted laparoscopic surgery is touted to decrease blood loss because of superior vision and articulation of instruments, there is no proof that any surgical outcomes, including operative time, associated injury, postoperative pain, need for reoperation, and leak, are superior with the use of a robot. Additionally, using the robot is theoretically felt to decrease discomfort and injury to the surgeon, but this has yet to be proven. Indeed, there is no proven advantage with use of a robot in laparoscopic surgery.

Single incision laparoscopic surgery, also known as single port access surgery or laparoscopic single site surgery, was touted to reduce postoperative pain, decrease recovery time, and improve cosmetic outcomes, as all the laparoscopic instruments would be placed through a single <4-cm incision. SILS is technically more demanding than traditional laparoscopic techniques. When compared to standard multiport laparoscopy, the SILS approach is associated with a shorter length of stay.

Initially, the use of laparoscopic surgery for colon cancer resection was felt to increase the rate of port-site metastases, but this has not proved to be true. There is no increase in metastatic disease with the use of laparoscopy. Furthermore, the laparoscopic approach is equivalent to the open one in terms of oncologic outcomes.

BIBLIOGRAPHY

Bailey CE, Hu C-H, You YN, Kaur H, Ernst RD, Chang GJ. Variation in positron emission tomography use after colon cancer resection. *J Oncol Pract*. 2015;11(3): 363–372.

Davis BR, Lee-Kong SA, Migaly J, Feingold DL, Steele SR. The American Society of Colon and Rectal Surgeons Clinical Practice Guidelines for the management of hemorrhoids. *Dis Colon Rectum*. 2018;61:284–292.

Giardiello FM, Allen JI, Axilbund JE, et al. Guidelines on genetic evaluation and management of Lynch syndrome: a consensus statement by the US Multi-Society Task Force on Colorectal Cancer. *Dis Colon Rectum*. 2014;57: 1025–1048.

Herzig DO, Buie WD, Weiser MR, et al. Clinical practice guidelines for the surgical treatment of patients with Lynch Syndrome. *Dis Colon Rectum*. 2017;60:137–143.

Järvinen HJ, Renkonen-Sinisalo L, Aktán-Collán, K, et al. Ten years after mutation testing for Lynch syndrome: cancer incidence and outcome in mutation-positive and mutation-negative family members. *J Clin Oncol*. 2009;27: 4793–4797.

Kijima S, Saski T, Nagata K, Utano K, Lefore AT, Sugimoto H. Preoperative evaluation of colorectal cancer using CT colonography, MRI and PET/CT. *World J Gastroenterol*. 2014;20(45):16964–16975.

Kuhry E, Schwenk WF, Gaupset R, Romild U, Bonjer HJ. Long-term results of laparoscopic colorectal cancer resection. *Cochrane Database Syst Rev*. 2008;16(2): 498–504.

Maggiori L, Gaujoux S, Tribillon E, Bretangnol F, Panis Y. Single-incision laparoscopy for colorectal resection: a systematic review and meta-analysis of more than a thousand procedures. *Colorectal Dis*. 2012;4(10):643–654.

Martín-López JE, Beltrán-Calvo C, Rodríguez-López R, Molina-López T. Comparison of the accuracy of CT colonography and colonoscopy in the diagnosis of colorectal cancer. *Colorectal Dis*. 2014;16(3):82–89.

Mauchley DC, Lynge DC, Langdale LA, Stelzner, MG, Mock CN, Billingsley KG. Clinical utility and cost-effectiveness of routine preoperative computed tomography scanning in patients with colon cancer. *Am J Surg*. 2005;189(5):512–517.

Migaly J, Bafford AC, Francone TD, et al. The American Society of Colon and Rectal Surgeons Clinical Practice Guidelines for the use of bowel preparation in elective colon and rectal surgery. *Dis Colon Rectum*. 2019;62:3–8.

Rex DK, Boland CR, Dominitz JA, et al. Colorectal cancer screening: recommendations for physicians and patients from the US Multi-Society Task Force on Colorectal Cancer. *Am J Gastroenterol*. 2017;112:1016–1030.

Sali L, Falchini M, Taddei A, Mascalchi M. Role of preoperative CT colonography in patients with colorectal cancer. *World J Gastroenterol.* 2014;20(14):3795–3803.

Stracci F, Zorzi M, Grazzini G. Colorectal cancer screening: Tests, strategies, and perspectives. *Front Public Health.* 2014;2:210.

Syngal S, Brand RE, Church JM, et al. ACG Clinical Guideline: genetic testing and management of hereditary gastrointestinal cancer syndromes. *Am J Gastroenterol.* 2015;110:223–262.

Trinh BB, Jackson NR, Hauch AT, Hu T, Kandil E. Robotic versus laparoscopic colorectal surgery. *JSLS.* 2014;18(4):e00187.

Vasen HF, Möslein G, Alonso A, et al. Guidelines for the clinical management of familial adenomatous polyposis. *Gut.* 2008;57:704–713.

Young H, Knepper B, Moore EE, Johnson JL, Mehler P, Price CS. Surgical site infection after colon surgery: National Healthcare Safety Network risk factors and modeled rats compared with published risk factors and rates. *J Am Coll Surg.* 2012;214:852–859.

41

Crohn's Disease

Jace J.P. Franko and Andrew T. Schlussel

A 28-year-old woman with a history of Crohn's disease and remote ileocecectomy presents to the emergency department with worsening diarrhea, >20 bowel movements a day, and a 10% loss in body weight over the past 6 weeks. She has previously been managed on 5-aminosalicylic acid and infliximab. Her vital signs on evaluation are significant for a heart rate of 105 beats per minute and a temperature of 100.6°F. Her abdomen is soft with mild left low quadrant tenderness, and her rectal exam is normal. Her white blood cell count is $15 \times 10^3/\mu L$. She undergoes a computed tomographic (CT) enterography that shows an ileosigmoid fistula with a surrounding 3-centimeter rim-enhancing fluid collection that abuts the abdominal wall, and a more proximal ileoileal fistula. There is no free air or free fluid.

1. **A surgical intervention should be offered for which of the following presentations of Crohn's disease?**
   A. Enteroenteric fistulas with mild symptoms
   B. Medically managed disease but on two medications
   C. New inflammatory changes of the terminal ileum on radiographic findings
   D. Ileosigmoid fistula and associated diarrhea and malnutrition
   E. Intra-abdominal abscess

2. **In the absence of symptoms, malnutrition, and diarrhea, which of the following is the best option for this patient?**
   A. Ileocecectomy
   B. Enterectomy with primary hand-sewn anastomosis
   C. Enterectomy with stapled anastomosis
   D. Nonoperative management
   E. Proximal diversion

3. **Surgical management of the ileosigmoid fistula in this patient is best approached with which of the following techniques?**
   A. En bloc resection of all inflamed tissue with proximal diversion
   B. Debridement and primary closure of fistula site on sigmoid colon if there are no secondary signs of inflammation
   C. Enterectomy, debridement of fistula tract, and segmental colectomy
   D. Small bowel resection with primary anastomosis alone
   E. No surgical indications

4. **Which of the following is true regarding the medical management of enteroenteric fistulas?**
   A. Infliximab has demonstrated some benefit in the closure of intra-abdominal fistulas.
   B. Infliximab has a higher rate of closure for intra-abdominal fistulas compared to perianal fistulas.
   C. There is no role for anti-tumor necrosis factor (TNF) agents in the setting of Crohn's disease.
   D. There is no risk in postoperative anastomotic complications with preoperative use of an anti-TNF agent.

5. **Which of the following is true regarding the development of cancer in Crohn's disease?**

A. There is a higher rate of Crohn's-associated malignancy in a fistula tract compared to a stricture.

B. The risk of colon cancer in Crohn's disease is no greater than the general population.

C. Surveillance colonoscopy is not indicated in a patient with an ileosigmoid fistula.

D. Colon cancer in the setting of Crohn's disease should be managed similar to the general population.

E. Subtotal colectomy with ileorectal anastomosis has better outcomes in Crohn's disease than a segmental colectomy.

6. **Following an initial trial of antibiotics and nonoperative management, the patient clinically decompensates. An acute abdominal series is obtained and reveals free air under the diaphragm. The patient is taken to the operating room, where a large perforation is identified in the sigmoid colon. There is purulent peritonitis, edematous-appearing small intestine, and inflammatory changes surrounding only the sigmoid colon consistent with segmental Crohn's colitis. Which is the best surgical option for this patient?**

A. Suture closure of the perforated segment, intraabdominal drain placement, and intensive care unit resuscitation

B. Sigmoidectomy with end colostomy and primary repair of the small intestine involved in the fistula

C. Total abdominal colectomy with ileorectal anastomosis and resection of small intestine involved in the fistula

D. Total abdominal colectomy with J-pouch and resection of the small intestine involved in the fistula

E. Resection of the small intestine involved in the fistula with intraabdominal lavage and drain placement

7. **The patient is currently without symptoms of malnutrition and diarrhea related to the known enterocolonic fistulas but now presents with a small bowel obstruction 3 years following her laparoscopic ileocecectomy. Screening colonoscopy with intubation of the ileum was performed 8 months prior, with circumferential narrowing at the anastomosis that is negative for malignancy. She is hemodynamically stable, with a CT scan revealing a short stricture at the ileocolic**

anastomosis. What are the most likely etiology and best treatment option for this patient?

A. Anastomotic stricture secondary to narrowed afferent limb—endoscopic dilation

B. Anastomotic stricture secondary to ischemia—resection and primary anastomosis

C. Anastomotic stricture secondary to Crohn's inflammation—endoscopic dilation

D. Anastomotic stricture secondary to Crohn's inflammation—increase medical management of underlying Crohn's disease

E. Anastomotic stricture secondary to malignancy—staging and oncologic resection

ANSWERS

1. **D.** Crohn's disease was first described in 1932. It involves inflammation of the entire gastrointestinal tract from mouth to anus, and 50% of patients present with ileocolic disease. The Vienna system, published in 2000, is most commonly used for the classification of Crohn's disease. It includes (1) penetrating or fistulizing; (2) stricturing; and (3) non-penetrating, nonstricturing Crohn's disease. Surgical management of this disease is reserved for patients who fail medical treatment or who present with complications that include hemorrhage, perforation, abscess, fistula, strictures, malignancy, and slowed growth in children. Fistulas that result in dehydration and malnutrition due to poor absorption in the small bowel should also be considered for surgery. Percutaneous drainage of an intraabdominal abscess in an otherwise stable patient should be considered prior to an operative intervention.

2. **D.** Patients with Crohn's disease often undergo multiple abdominal operations, with 40–55% requiring an operation 10 years following their diagnosis and 75% requiring surgery in their lifetime. Surgery is not recommended for asymptomatic enteroenteric fistulas. However, exacerbation of diarrhea with associated malnutrition is an indication for resection.

3. **B.** A systematic approach to the surgical management of Crohn's disease is critical to the preservation of bowel length. Nutrition should be optimized as tolerated, and preoperative studies to include esophagogastroduodenoscopy, colonoscopy, and CT enterography should be considered. It is critical to determine the site of inflammation, as oftentimes, the

colon only needs to be debrided with primary closure of the fistula site. Only the diseased portion of the colon or small bowel should be removed. However, healthy bowel should be excised if the fistula is compromising the mesentery. Resection should only be performed back to grossly normal appearing bowel.

4. **A.** Infliximab is a human chimeric antibody directed against the pro-inflammatory cytokine TNF. This therapy was one of the original monoclonal antibodies to show an improvement in symptoms, complete endoscopic remission, and a decreased need for surgery in Crohn's disease. Infliximab has been used in the treatment of fistulizing Crohn's disease. In a review of 26 patients with fistulizing Crohn's disease, infliximab alone was able to result in a complete closure; however, only one was intra-abdominal.

The ACCENT II study published in 2004 evaluated the maintenance dosing of infliximab in patients with fistulizing Crohn's who responded to induction therapy. The majority of patients had perianal fistulas. This study showed complete fistula closure in 36% of patients at 54 weeks. When evaluated by location, approximately 97% of perianal fistulas had complete closure, demonstrating superior outcomes compared to intra-abdominal fistulas.

Anti-TNF agents will impede the immune response following surgery. El-Hussuna and colleagues performed a systemic review of postoperative complications following the use of anti-TNF alpha agents within 3 months prior to an operation. Fourteen studies were reviewed, and overall, there was no difference in anastomotic complications (7.6% vs. 8.2% in the control groups). In a subgroup analysis, studies determined to have a lower chance of bias identified a greater risk of adverse events with the administration of anti-TNF agents.

5. **D.** The risk of colorectal cancer in Crohn's disease is a controversial topic, with some reports of up to a 20-fold increase in risk compared to the general population. Lovasz and colleagues in 2013 demonstrated the rate of colorectal cancer to be 5.5% after 5 years and 7.5% after 10 years of disease duration, with a greater prevalence in stricturing disease. Furthermore, it was recommended to employ closer endoscopic surveillance compared to the general population following diagnosis.

Surveillance colonoscopy for Crohn's disease is recommended at similar time intervals as ulcerative colitis: beginning 8–10 years after disease onset for pancolitis, 15 years for left-sided disease, and then annually after 30 years following diagnosis. Surgical management of a Crohn's associated malignancy should be treated like the general population with segmental resection and associated lymphadenectomy. There have been reports that recommend subtotal colectomy in the setting of a Crohn's associated colorectal cancer due to the risk of synchronous and metachronous lesions.

6. **B.** In patients with segmental Crohn's colitis and perforation requiring surgery, the procedure of choice is segmental colectomy with end colostomy and Hartmann pouch. If the patient is hemodynamically normal, performing a primary anastomosis with proximal fecal diversion may be considered. If there was evidence of fulminant Crohn's colitis the treatment of choice is a total abdominal colectomy with end ileostomy. Extrafascial placement of the rectosigmoid stump or a buried mucous fistula should be considered based on the degree of inflammation as this may result in a lower rate of pelvic septic complications. Abdominal drains, as well as transanal drainage of the rectal stump, may further reduce the risk of pelvic sepsis. Answer E is referencing laparoscopic lavage as it has been previously studied in the setting of Hinchey III diverticulitis. Based on 1-year results from the SCANDIV trial, this intervention did not demonstrate improved outcomes, and long-term follow-up analysis by Sneiders et al. reports diverticulitis-related events occurring up to 6 years after the index procedure. Nonetheless, laparoscopic lavage should only be considered in patients with diverticulitis, not Crohn's disease.

7. **C.** Timing is an important factor when considering the etiology of anastomotic strictures, especially in the setting of Crohn's disease. It is unlikely for a technical error to present 3 years postoperatively, and instead supports progressive/persistent inflammation secondary to the underlying Crohn's disease. Although there is an increased incidence of malignancy at the anastomosis site, this is unlikely with a negative colonoscopy 8 months prior.

To evaluate the management of fibrostenotic Crohn's disease, Hassan and colleagues performed a systematic review of 13 retrospective studies, including 347 patients, with 74% having a postsurgical stricture. The authors report a mean time from disease diagnosis to stricture formation of 13 years, with an average stricture length of 2.7 cm. Endoscopic dilation was technically successful in 86% of cases, with long-term efficacy reaching 58% over 33 months. In a review of over 2,000 dilations across 25 studies, Morar et al. reported a complication rate of 4%, including hemorrhage and perforation. Dilation is a relatively safe procedure when performed by an experienced endoscopist. This should be considered as the initial procedure of choice to provide therapeutic improvement of a mechanical small bowel obstruction while also simultaneously allowing for improved medical management of the underlying Crohn's disease for preserving bowel length. If resection and primary anastomosis is ultimately required, the anastomosis can be constructed per provider preference. A meta-analysis performed by Guo and colleagues determined that end-to-end, side-to-side, and end-to-side anastomoses are equivalent and can be constructed with staples or sutures without increasing the risk of anastomotic leak or endoscopic, clinical, and operative recurrence.

BIBLIOGRAPHY

Carter FM, McLeod RS, Cohen Z. Subtotal colectomy for ulcerative colitis: complications related to the rectal remnant. *Dis Colon Rectum.* 1991;34:1005–1009.

Castellano TJ, Frank MS, Brandt LJ, Mahadevia P. Metachronous carcinoma complicating Crohn's disease. *Arch Intern Med.* 1981;141(8):1074–1075.

Cooper DJ, Weinstein MA, Korelitz BI. Complications of Crohn's disease predisposing to dysplasia and cancer of the intestinal tract: considerations of a surveillance program. *J Clin Gastroenterol.* 1984;6(3):217–224.

Crohn BB, Ginzburg L, Oppenheimer GD. Regional ileitis: a pathologic and clinical entity. 1932. *Mt Sinai J Med.* 2000;67(3):263–268.

El-Hussuna A, Krag A, Olaison G, Bendtsen F, Gluud LL. The effect of anti-tumor necrosis factor alpha agents on postoperative anastomotic complications in Crohn's disease: a systematic review. *Dis Colon Rectum.* 2013;56(12):1423–1433.

Gasche C, Scholmerich J, Brynskov J, et al. A simple classification of Crohn's disease: report of the working party for the world congresses of gastroenterology, Vienna 1998. *Inflamm Bowel Dis.* 2000;6(1):8–15.

Guo Z, Li Y, Zhu W, Gong J, Li N, Li J. Comparing outcomes between side-to-side anastomosis and other anastomotic configurations after intestinal resection of patients with Crohn's disease: a meta-analysis. *World J Surg.* 2013;37:893–901.

Hassan C, Zullo A, De Francesco V, et al. Systematic review: endoscopic dilation in Crohn's disease. *Aliment Pharmacol Ther.* 2007;26:1457–1464.

Jess T, Winther KV, Munkholm P, Langholz E, Binder V. Intestinal and extra-intestinal cancer in Crohn's disease: follow-up of a population-based cohort in Copenhagen County, Denmark. *Aliment Pharmacol There.* 2004;19(3):287–293.

Lovasz BD, Lakatos L, Golovics PA, et al. Risk of colorectal cancer in Crohn's disease patients with colonic involvement and stenosing disease in a population-based cohort from Hungary. *J Gastrointestin Liver Dis.* 2013;22(3):265–268.

Lu KC, Hunt SR. Surgical management of Crohn's disease. *Surg Clin North Am.* 2013;93(1):167–185.

McKee RF, Keenan RA, Munro A. Colectomy for acute colitis: is it safe to close the rectal stump? *Int J Colorectal Dis.* 1995;10:222–224.

Morar PS, Faiz O, Warusavitarne J, et al. Systematic review with meta-analysis: endoscopic balloon dilation for Crohn's disease strictures. *Aliment Pharmacol Ther.* 2015;42:1137–1148.

Ng RL, Davies AH, Grace RH, Mortensen NJ. Subcutaneous rectal stump closure after emergency subtotal colectomy. *Br J Surg.* 1992;79:701–703.

Peters CP, Eshuis EJ, Toxopeus FM, et al. Adalimumab for Crohn's disease: long-term sustained benefit in a population-based cohort of 438 patients. *J Crohns Colitis.* 2014;8(8):866–875.

Peyrin-Biroulet L, Loftus EV Jr, Colombel JF, Sandborn WJ. The natural history of adult Crohn's disease in population-based cohorts. *Am J Gastroenterol.* 2010;105(2):289–297.

Poritz LS, Rowe WA, Koltun WA. Remicade does not abolish the need for surgery in fistulizing Crohn's disease. *Dis Colon Rectum.* 2002;45(6):771–775.

Sands BE. New therapies for the treatment of inflammatory bowel disease. *Surg Clin North Am.* 2006;86(4):1045–1064.

Sands BE, Anderson FH, Bernstein CN, et al. Infliximab maintenance therapy for fistulizing Crohn's disease. *N Engl J Med.* 2004;350(9):876–885.

Schultz JK, Wallon C, Blecic L, et al. One-year results of the SCANDIV randomized clinical trial of laparoscopic lavage versus primary resection for acute perforated diverticulitis. *Br J Surg* 2017;104:1382–1392.

Sneiders D, Lambrichts DPV, Swank HA, et al. Long-term follow-up of a multicentre cohort study on laparoscopic peritoneal lavage for perforated diverticulitis. *Colorectal Dis.* 2019;21:705–714.

Steele SR. Operative management of Crohn's disease of the colon including anorectal disease. *Surg Clin North Am.* 2007;87(3):611–631.

Strong SA, Koltun WA, Hyman NH, Buie WD. Standards Practice Task Force of the American Society of Colon and Rectal Surgeons. Practice parameters for the surgical management of Crohn's disease. *Dis Colon Rectum.* 2007;50(11):1735–1746.

Teeuwen PH, Stommel MW, Bremers AJ, van der Wilt GJ, de Jong DJ, Bleichrodt RP. Colectomy in patients with acute colitis: a systematic review. *J Gastrointest Surg.* 2009;13:676–686.

Trickett JP, Tilney HS, Gudgeon AM, Mellor SG, Edwards DP. Management of the rectal stump after emergency sub-total colectomy: which surgical option is associated with the lowest morbidity? *Colorectal Dis.* 2005;7:519–522.

Warren S, Sommers S. Cicatrizing enteritis as a pathologic entity; analysis of 120 cases. *Am J Pathol.* 1948;24(3):475–501.

42

Diverticulitis

Kelli Tavares and Erik Roedel

A 47-year-old obese man presents to the emergency department with a 2-day history of sharp, constant left lower quadrant pain that is worse with straining and is associated with subjective fevers. This is the patient's first episode of pain. His vital signs are normal, and he is in no distress. You are able to elicit moderate tenderness in the left lower quadrant on exam, and a complete blood count shows a mild leukocytosis of 13,000/μL.

1. **Regarding the patient described, what is the single best study to obtain to confirm your suspected diagnosis?**
   A. Plain abdominal X-rays
   B. Magnetic resonance imaging (MRI) of the abdomen
   C. Computed tomographic (CT) scan of the abdomen and pelvis with IV and oral contrast
   D. CT scan of the abdomen and pelvis with rectal contrast
   E. Abdominal ultrasound

2. **Regarding the treatment of acute, uncomplicated, sigmoid diverticulitis in a reliable patient, what is the most appropriate treatment plan?**
   A. Discharge with pain medication
   B. Discharge with oral (PO) antibiotics and close follow-up
   C. Admission, IV antibiotics, and bowel rest
   D. Urgent exploratory laparotomy and resection of the involved colon
   E. Discharge with PO antibiotics and planned laparoscopic resection in 6–8 weeks

3. **Regarding the indications for elective colon resection after an episode of uncomplicated diverticulitis, which of the following is the strongest indication?**
   A. A patient with continued chronic symptoms that fail to resolve with antibiotics
   B. If the first episode occurs in a patient younger than the age 50
   C. After the second episode of uncomplicated diverticulitis
   D. After the first episode in order to prevent future perforation and abdominal sepsis
   E. After three documented cases of uncomplicated diverticulitis

4. **Regarding a similar patient who presents without signs of sepsis but on imaging has evidence of complicated diverticulitis with a 6-cm pelvic abscess, what is the best treatment plan?**
   A. Discharge with PO antibiotics and close follow-up
   B. Percutaneous drainage
   C. Laparoscopic washout with drain placement
   D. Laparoscopic washout with drain placement and planned laparoscopic resection in 6–8 weeks
   E. Resection of the diseased segment with end colostomy

5. **Regarding a patient who presents with similar symptoms and early signs of sepsis and an abdominal exam consistent with diffuse peritonitis, what is the best course of action?**

A. Percutaneous drainage
B. Laparoscopic washout with drain placement
C. Laparoscopic washout with drain placement and planned laparoscopic resection in 6–8 weeks
D. Proximal diversion *without* resection
E. Resection of the diseased segment

6. **Which of the following statements is true regarding the surgical approach to a patient undergoing surgery for diverticulitis?**

    A. The laparoscopic approach has been demonstrated to be superior with improved outcomes when compared to the open approach in the *acute* setting.
    B. Every patient undergoing emergent surgery should undergo a Hartmann's procedure.
    C. Patients who undergo a Hartmann's procedure are significantly less likely to undergo stoma reversal compared to patients that initially undergo primary anastomosis with diverting ileostomy.
    D. Ureteral stents are routinely indicated in the elective setting to reduce the risk of ureteral injury.

7. **One year later, you see the described patient in clinic. He has had no further episodes of diverticulitis; however, he complains of dysuria and that he feels like he is passing air when he urinates. What is the most likely diagnosis?**

    A. Coloenteric fistula
    B. Colonic stricture
    C. Colovesical fistula
    D. Recurrent acute diverticulitis

ANSWERS

1. **C.** Multi-slice CT has become the standard imaging modality to confirm the diagnosis of sigmoid diverticulitis. It has been shown to have a sensitivity and specificity as high as 98% and 99%, respectively, with intravenous and intraluminal contrast. A CT scan is useful to confirm the diagnosis of diverticulitis, determine disease severity, and guide treatment. Despite the accuracy of cross-sectional imaging in the detection of diverticulitis, it may provide a diagnostic dilemma, as radiographically a colonic neoplasm can appear similar. Therefore, colonoscopy is recommended after the acute process has subsided.

    Plain radiographs of the abdomen are inexpensive, easily available, and expose the patient to minimal radiation. However, they offer limited diagnostic information in the evaluation of diverticulitis. MRI and ultrasound may be a useful alternative in a patient where a CT scan or intravenous contrast is contraindicated. Ultrasound in some studies has diagnostic accuracy up to 97%; however, it is limited by operator variability, patient discomfort, and inability to accurately make an alternative diagnosis. MRI is not limited by the same issues as ultrasound and has a sensitivity and specificity as high as 92–94% in some studies.

2. **B.** Recent publications have questioned the pathophysiology of uncomplicated diverticulitis and have disputed the need for antibiotics in these cases. However, current guidelines recommend that the standard treatment of acute uncomplicated diverticulitis in the United States is outpatient antibiotic therapy. This is supported by the American Society of Colon and Rectal Surgeons (ASCRS) and will continue until there is significant evidence supporting the safety of outpatient management without antibiotics. To be a candidate for outpatient therapy the patient must be stable, non-toxic, reliable, able to maintain an adequate enteral diet, and have uncomplicated disease. Finally, the patient should have close interval follow-up to ensure their symptoms are improving.

3. **A.** The current indications for elective resection in diverticulitis include chronic symptoms, complicated disease, inability to rule out a malignancy, and patient specific factors. The surgical management of uncomplicated diverticulitis has changed. Previous retrospective studies, performed prior to the use of CT scan, reported recurrence in one third of patients after an uncomplicated episode. Recent data has shown not only a lower recurrence rate, 13–23%, but, more important, a low risk of complicated disease and a need for emergent surgery. Due to these findings, the ASCRS recommends against routine sigmoid resection for the indications of two or more uncomplicated episodes, age <50, or to prevent complicated disease in the future. The guidelines recommend that each patient be evaluated individually regarding their overall health, age, access to care, number, severity, and frequency of episodes, as well as the impact of each episode on the patient's quality of life. These multiple factors should be weighed against the risks associated with elective resection. Thoughtful counseling can be performed

with the patient, and an informed decision can be made.

As a subgroup, immunocompromised patients have been found to be at a higher risk of mortality with nonoperative treatment; therefore, surgeons should have a lower threshold for resection in this patient population.

4. **B.** The treatment of complicated diverticulitis with an associated abscess has drastically changed with the advent of image-guided percutaneous drainage. A treatment plan of antibiotics with selective drainage has been shown to allow up to 75% of patients with a diverticular abscess to avoid urgent surgery. Percutaneous drainage is beneficial as a bridge for stable patients without signs of peritonitis that would have previously needed an urgent operation. Drainage provides patients the opportunity of an elective single-stage resection, the avoidance of surgery in the acute inflammatory stage, a lower risk of ostomy placement, and an overall decrease in morbidity and mortality.

Currently, there are no data to support the outpatient management of acute complicated diverticulitis. Regarding the decision for elective resection after an episode of complicated diverticulitis, the ASCRS recommends that resection should be considered in all patients who are appropriate candidates for surgery. However, CT scan findings of a phlegmon or extraluminal gas alone does not indicate complicated disease. Finally, there are insufficient data to show that laparoscopic lavage is a safe alternative to resection in patients with purulent or feculent peritonitis. The ASCRS does not currently support operative therapy without resection for the treatment of diverticulitis.

5. **E.** The treatment for patients with complicated diverticulitis with evidence of purulent or feculent peritonitis is an operative approach with resection of the diseased bowel. There is ongoing research in Europe to determine if there is a role for laparoscopic lavage in patients with severe complicated diverticulitis. However, as stated earlier, the ASCRS does not currently support non-resectional therapy except in the rare circumstance that the abdomen is too hostile for extirpation of the colon. Previous literature has evaluated diversion without resection, but this technique was shown to have an increased rate of postoperative peritonitis as compared to resection.

In general, the extent of resection should include the entire sigmoid colon with a proximal margin of soft and pliable descending colon. Although not all the diverticula need to be removed, it is important to ensure that none are included in the anastomosis if one is performed. The distal aspect of the specimen should include a margin of normal rectum in order to reduce the risk of recurrence.

The decision to perform a primary anastomosis with or without protective ileostomy versus end colostomy in the setting of emergent surgery for diverticulitis is currently being debated. There is nonrandomized and retrospective data that supports primary anastomosis. It was found to be safe and not associated with worse outcomes in the setting of complicated diverticulitis. The inherent selection bias in these studies has prevented the surgical community from making broad recommendations regarding primary anastomosis in the setting of emergent colectomy for diverticulitis.

6. **C.** Multiple studies have demonstrated that patients who undergo a Hartmann's procedure for acute diverticulitis are less likely to undergo stoma reversal when compared to patients that undergo primary anastomosis with diverting ileostomy. Although it appears morbidity and mortality are similar when comparing the two operative approaches, only about 50–60% (even as low as 28.3% in one study), of these patients will undergo stoma reversal within the first year following index operation. Answer A is incorrect; there is no *clear* evidence that a laparoscopic approach is superior to an open approach in the acute setting. A *Cochrane Systematic Review* published in 2017 included an analysis of three randomized control trials examining the use of laparoscopic versus open resection in patients with acute diverticulitis. The authors ultimately concluded that there was insufficient evidence to support or refute a laparoscopic approach over an open approach. The ASCRS guidelines state that a laparoscopic approach is preferred in the setting of *elective* colectomy given improved short-term outcomes, increased quality-of-life scores, and decreased rates of subsequent ventral hernias when compared to open surgery. Answer B is incorrect. The decision to perform primary anastomosis with diversion versus Hartmann's procedure should be individualized based on patient characteristics and surgeon experience. Answer D is incorrect. The incidence of ureteral injury is less than 1% in the

elective setting; therefore, the ASCRS does not recommend the routine use of ureteral stents in these cases.

7. C. The patient is complaining of pneumaturia and dysuria, which are concerning for a colovesical fistula. Diverticular fistulas are the most common cause of colovesical fistulas, but the overall occurrence is rare. Most commonly patients will present with dysuria or recurrent urinary tract infections, pneumaturia, or fecaluria. There is no gold standard for diagnostic imaging; however, a CT scan with oral or rectal contrast seems to be the preferred method of diagnosis. Other methods include cystoscopy and colonoscopy to attempt to visualize the fistula tract and rule out malignant fistula. Treating all diverticular fistulas involves surgical resection of the fistula tract and involved segment of colon. Managing the other involved organ is dependent on the organ itself, the location of the fistula, and the degree of inflammation.

BIBLIOGRAPHY

Abbas S. Resection and primary anastomosis in acute complicated diverticulitis, a systematic review of the literature. *Int J Colorectal Dis.* 2007;22(4):351–357.

Abraha I, Binda GA, Montedori A, Arezzo A, Cirocchi R. Laparoscopic versus open resection for sigmoid diverticulitis. *Cochrane Database Syst Rev.* 2017;11:CD009277.

Acuna SA, Wood T, Chesney TR, Dossa F, Wexner SD, Quereshy FA, Chadi SA, Baxter NN. Operative strategies for perforated diverticulitis: a systematic review and meta-analysis. *Dis Colon Rectum.* 2018;61(12):1442–1453.

Alonso S, Pera M, Pares D, et al. Outpatient treatment of patients with uncomplicated acute diverticulitis. *Colorectal Dis.* 2010;12(10):e278–e282.

Ambrosetti P, Chautems R, Soravia C, Peiris-Waser N, Terrier F. Long-term outcome of mesocolic and pelvic diverticular abscesses of the left colon: a prospective study of 73 cases. *Dis Colon Rectum.* 2005;48(4):787–791.

Ambrosetti P, Jenny A, Becker C, Terrier TF, Morel P. Acute left colonic diverticulitis-compared performance of computed tomography and water-soluble contrast enema: Prospective evaluation of 420 patients. *Dis Colon Rectum.* 2000;43(10):1363–1367.

Anaya DA, Flum DR. Risk of emergency colectomy and colostomy in patients with diverticular disease. *Arch Surg.* 2005;140(7):681–685.

Baker ME. Imaging and interventional techniques in acute left-sided diverticulitis. *J Gastrointest Surg.* 2008;12(8):1314–1317.

Broderick-Villa G, Burchette RJ, Collins JC, Abbas MA, Haigh PI. Hospitalization for acute diverticulitis does not mandate routine elective colectomy. *Arch Surg.* 2005;140(6):576–581; discussion 581–583.

Chabok A, Pahlman L, Hjern F, Haapaniemi S, Smedh K, AVOD Study Group. Randomized clinical trial of antibiotics in acute uncomplicated diverticulitis. *Br J Surg.* 2012;99(4):532–539.

Constantinides VA, Tekkis PP, Athanasiou T, et al. Primary resection with anastomosis versus Hartmann's procedure in nonelective surgery for acute colonic diverticulitis: a systematic review. *Dis Colon Rectum.* 2006;49(7):966–981.

Constantinides VA, Tekkis PP, Senapati A, Association of Coloproctology of Great Britain Ireland. Prospective multicentre evaluation of adverse outcomes following treatment for complicated diverticular disease. *Br J Surg.* 2006;93(12):1503–1513.

de Korte N, Ulna C, Boermeester MA, et al. Use of antibiotics in uncomplicated diverticulitis. *Br J Surg.* 2011;98(6):761–767.

Destigter KK, Keating DP. Imaging update: Acute colonic diverticulitis. *Clin Colon Rectal Surg.* 2009;22(3):147–155.

Dozois EJ. Operative treatment of recurrent or complicated diverticulitis. *J Gastrointest Surg.* 2008;12(8):1321–1323.

Eglinton T, Nguyen T, Raniga S, et al. Patterns of recurrence in patients with acute diverticulitis. *Br J Surg.* 2010;97(6):952–957.

Etzioni DA, Chiu VY, Cannom RR, et al. Outpatient treatment of acute diverticulitis: rates and predictors of failure. *Dis Colon Rectum.* 2010;53(6):861–865.

Feingold D, Steele SR, Lee S, et al. Practice parameters for the treatment of sigmoid diverticulitis. *Dis Colon Rectum.* 2014;57(3):284–294.

Forgione A, Leroy J, Cahill RA, et al. Prospective evaluation of functional outcome after laparoscopic sigmoid colectomy. *Ann Surg.* 2009;249(2):218–224.

Hall JF, Roberts PL, Ricciardi R, et al. Long-term follow-up after an initial episode of diverticulitis: what are the predictors of recurrence? *Dis Colon Rectum.* 2011;54(3):283–288.

Holmer C, Lehmann KS, Engelmann S, et al. Long-term outcome after conservative and surgical treatment of acute sigmoid diverticulitis. *Langenbecks Arch Surg.* 2011;396(6):825–832.

Hwang SS, Cannom RR, Abbas MA, Etzioni D. Diverticulitis in transplant patients and patients on chronic corticosteroid therapy: a systematic review. *Dis Colon Rectum.* 2010;53(12):1699–1707.

Janes S, Meagher A, Frizelle FA. Elective surgery after acute diverticulitis. *Br J Surg.* 2005;92(2):133–142.

Lameris W, van Randen A, Bipat S, et al. Graded compression ultrasonography and computed tomography in acute colonic diverticulitis: meta-analysis of test accuracy. *Eur Radiol.* 2008;18(11):2498–2511.

Melchoir S, Cudovic D, Jones J, Thomas C, Gilitzer R, Thuroff J. Diagnosis and surgical management of colovesical fistulas due to sigmoid diverticulitis. *J Urol.* 2009;182(3):978–982.

Salem L, Flum DR. Primary anastomosis or Hartmann's procedure for patients with diverticular peritonitis? *A systematic review. Dis Colon Rectum.* 2004;47(11):1953–1964.

Sarma D, Longo WE, NDSG. Diagnostic imaging for diverticulitis. *J Clin Gastroenterol.* 2008;42(10):1139–1141.

Shabanzadeh DM, Wille-Jorgensen P. Antibiotics for uncomplicated diverticulitis. *Cochrane Database Syst Rev.* 2012;11:CD009092.

Stollman N, Raskin JB. Diverticular disease of the colon. *Lancet*. 2004;363(9409):631–639.

Thaler K, Baig MK, Berho M, et al. Determinants of recurrence after sigmoid resection for uncomplicated diverticulitis. *Dis Colon Rectum*. 2003;46(3):385–388.

Zeitoun G, Laurent A, Rouffet F, et al. Multicentre, randomized clinical trial of primary versus secondary sigmoid resection in generalized peritonitis complicating sigmoid diverticulitis. *Br J Surg*. 2000;87(10): 1366–1374.

43

Colon, Rectum, and Anus—Rectal Cancer

Tiffany P. Wheeler

A 48-year-old white man presents to your office with a history of seven months of intermittent painless blood per rectum with bowel movements, which was diagnosed as internal hemorrhoids by his primary care provider. He has no other medical problems and has an unknown family history because he was adopted as an infant. On your digital and anoscopic evaluations, you find scant bloody mucous, no pathologic hemorrhoids, no other anal diseases, and the visualized area of rectal mucosa is normal.

1. What is the next best step in his evaluation?

A. Immunohistochemical fecal occult blood test
B. Guaiac fecal occult blood test
C. Colonoscopy
D. Computed tomographic (CT) colonography
E. Flexible sigmoidoscopy

2. A flexible endoscopic examination demonstrates an endoscopically unresectable mass lesion concerning for cancer located approximately 14 cm from the anal verge and a biopsy is performed. Which is the next best step for evaluating the lesion?

A. CT scan of the pelvis
B. Rigid proctoscopy
C. Serum carcinoembryonic antigen (CEA) level
D. Hepatic function tests
E. Fusion positron emission tomography (PET)/ CT scan of the chest, abdomen, and pelvis

3. A colonoscopy shows no other lesions. High-resolution CT scans of the chest, abdomen, and

pelvis do not demonstrate distant disease, and recommended blood tests demonstrate only a mild anemia. Pathologic evaluation returns a diagnosis of moderately differentiated adenocarcinoma, about 9 cm from the anal verge. What, if any, tests remain to complete the pretreatment staging?

A. Transabdominal liver ultrasound
B. KRAS mutation genotype
C. Fusion PET/CT scan of the chest, abdomen, and pelvis
D. No further evaluation is necessary.
E. Magnetic resonance imaging (MRI) of the pelvis

4. Preoperative staging reveals a 4 cm moderately differentiated adenocarcinoma T2N1M0 located at 9 cm from the anal verge. What is the preferred treatment strategy?

A. Preoperative chemotherapy followed by chemoradiation therapy followed by full-thickness transanal excision of the primary lesion
B. Low anterior resection of the rectum followed by chemotherapy or chemoradiation therapy based on a pathologic evaluation of the resection specimen
C. Preoperative chemotherapy followed by chemoradiation therapy followed by low anterior resection of the rectum
D. Chemoradiation followed by low anterior resection of the rectum
E. Preoperative chemotherapy followed by chemoradiation therapy followed full-thickness transanal excision of the primary lesion.

5. **Regarding additional testing to evaluate the patient, which is recommended for all rectal cancer patients younger than age 50?**

   A. Somatic APC gene sequencing
   B. Tumor gene sequencing
   C. Circulating tumor cells
   D. Hypermethylation analysis of tumor DNA
   E. Mismatch repair protein analysis and/or microsatellite instability analysis

6. **The patient in the scenario successfully undergoes chemoradiation and low anterior resection of the rectum for his T2N1MO (Stage IIIA) rectal cancer. At his follow-up appointment, what will you tell him regarding surveillance guidelines?**

   A. Proctoscopy (with endoscopic ultrasound [EUS] or MRI with contrast) every 3–6 months for the first 2 years and then every 6 months for a total of 5 years *and* a colonoscopy at 1 year after surgery
   B. Colonoscopy at 1 year after surgery
   C. History and physical every 3–6 months, CEA every 3–6 months, CT scan of the chest/abdomen/pelvis every 6–12 months, *and* colonoscopy in 1 year after surgery.
   D. History and physical every 3–6 months, CEA every 3–6 months, CT scan of the chest/abdomen/pelvis every 6–12 months, colonoscopy in 1 year after surgery, *and* PET/CT scan in 1 year
   E. Colonoscopy at 1 year after surgery and CEA every 3–6 months

7. **At his 1-year follow-up, his CT chest/abdomen/pelvis scan is reviewed, and he is found to have distal metastasis. Which of the following locations is the most likely site for distal metastasis in rectal cancer?**

   A. Liver
   B. Lung
   C. Brain
   D. Bone
   E. Small intestine

8. **Which of the following has been shown to prolong survival in patients with colorectal liver metastasis?**

   A. Chemotherapy alone
   B. Hepatic resection
   C. Portal vein embolization
   D. Radiofrequency ablation
   E. High-intensity focused ultrasound

ANSWERS

1. **C.** The diagnostic concern in this patient is primarily cancer as the most likely other causes of painless rectal bleeding have been ruled out based on in-office evaluation. Other likely diagnoses to consider would be some form of colitis or bleeding diverticulosis, but these are less likely due to the lack of abdominal symptoms, bleeding only with bowel movements. From the choices listed, the immunohistochemical fecal occult blood test (iFOBT) and Guaiac fecal occult blood test (gFOBT) are designed to detect blood in the gastrointestinal (GI) tract; therefore, they do not advance the patient's workup as he has visible gross blood in his bowel movements. Both flexible sigmoidoscopy and colonoscopy can be used to diagnose and biopsy cancers, but only colonoscopy can evaluate the entire colon and possibly treat the source of the bleeding. In a comparison of four diagnostic strategies for adult rectal bleeding, colonoscopy was the best overall strategy. CT colonography is controversial in its utility in colorectal cancer screening, but it is not recommended in the evaluation of the symptomatic patient with sensitivity not equivalent to fiberoptic endoscopy.

2. **B.** The location of the lesion is critical for the next phases of the evaluation and management of this tumor as there are significant differences in the evaluation and management of certain stages of colon versus rectal cancers, as well as very proximal versus middle and distal rectal cancers. Flexible endoscopy is notoriously unreliable regarding the accurate measurement of a distal lesion and generally overestimates the distance from the verge. Rigid proctoscopy is mandatory for any lesion in the rectum or recto-sigmoid junction, as it is reliable in its results. It ideally should be performed by the operating surgeon. Tumors with the distal-most aspect located above 12 cm from the anal verge are diagnosed as colon cancer and below 12 cm are diagnosed as rectal cancer. However, tumors diagnosed in the rectum from 10.1–11.9 cm from the anal verge can be treated as colon cancers as there seems to be no benefit for local control from neoadjuvant or adjuvant chemoradiation therapy. CT is part of the staging of colorectal cancer, but CT of the pelvis alone is incomplete for staging. Serum CEA is indicated until a colon or rectal cancer is diagnosed by biopsy, but it is not the next best step. Furthermore, it does not advance the patient's evaluation at this time. Hepatic function

tests are unhelpful and not indicated unless there is coexistent liver disease. PET/CT scan does not replace a high-resolution CT of the chest, abdomen, and pelvis with oral and IV contrast and is generally not indicated in the initial evaluation of colon and rectal cancer.

3. **E.** The lesion is now clearly a rectal adenocarcinoma with no evidence of distant metastasis, giving us a stage of TxNxM0. What we need next are the tests that determine the T and N status in order to generate our treatment plan, thereby making the choice of no further evaluation wrong. The best test listed is the MRI of the pelvis. This test gives the most accurate assessment of tumor depth and presence of nodal metastasis without the user variability of endorectal ultrasound. It is also the best test to assess the possibility of a threatened circumferential radial margin by the invasion of or near to the mesorectal fascia.

Given the normal CT of the abdomen, there is no indication for the liver ultrasound, and again, there is generally no indication for the PET/CT in the initial staging of colorectal cancer, especially if a normal high-resolution CT scan is normal. KRAS mutation from wild type is useful for predicting whether biologic therapy will be useful but only in patients with metastatic disease, which this patient does not have.

4. **D.** The patient now can be staged as Stage IIIA and the lower edge of the tumor is below 10 cm from the anal verge. Based on current guidelines, this patient should have neoadjuvant chemoradiation therapy followed by low anterior resection using a total mesorectal approach, with a distal margin 4 cm from the tumor. The transanal excision choices are incorrect based on nodal status and tumor size of 4 cm and location of the lower edge above 8 cm from the anal verge. The choice for low anterior resection (LAR) first then chemoradiation is wrong because in patients who can tolerate the neoadjuvant therapy, there is an absolute decrease in local recurrence of about 7% (6–13%) in these patients who get chemoradiation prior to operation compared to after the operation and is backed by category 1 data. The choice with chemotherapy, then chemoradiation, and then LAR is an option for care but not preferred in this situation.

5. **E.** The patient has no knowledge of his family history, nor any timely way to get it, thereby making a preoperative determination of his risk for a hereditary colorectal cancer syndrome by Bethesda or Amsterdam criteria impossible. Approximately 2–4% of rectal cancers are known to be due to hereditary nonpolyposis colorectal cancer (HNPCC) syndrome or Lynch syndrome. This syndrome is caused by germline mutation in any one of a number of genes involved with the process of DNA mismatch repair (MMR). Impairment of the MMR results in an accumulation of length alterations in simple repeated DNA fragments called microsatellites. This accumulation leads to a state of genetic instability termed microsatellite instability (MSI). The syndrome is further characterized by an increased incidence of cancers in the female genital system and the urinary system, as well as data supporting an increase in brain, pancreatic and gastric cancers in certain families. The Evaluation of Genomic Applications in Practice and Prevention (EGAPP) working group of the Centers for Disease Control and Prevention found it to be cost-effective for MMR and/or MSI testing for all colorectal cancers in patients younger than 50 years of age, and many cancer centers in the United States test all patients under 70 and all patients regardless of age if the Bethesda or Amsterdam criteria are met. Somatic APC gene sequencing is used to diagnose an index mutation in the familial adenomatous polyposis (FAP) syndrome. Tumor gene sequencing may be useful in some settings but not before performing the more rapid and cheaper testing for Lynch syndrome. The presence of circulating tumor cells is being studied as a diagnostic tool for cancer and cancer recurrence but currently is not routinely used. Hypermethylation analysis of tumor DNA is not routinely done and is suggested as the cause of cancer for patients with MMR protein abnormality detected in hMSH1 and a BRAF mutation rather than a somatic mutation. This is the same for colon cancers.

6. **C.** Per National Comprehensive Cancer Network guidelines, the recommended surveillance screening for patients who were successfully treated for Stage III rectal cancer include a complete history and physical every 3–6 months for 2 years and then every 6 months for a total of 5 years, CEA levels every 3–6 months for 2 years, then every 6 months for a total of 5 years, CT chest/abdomen/pelvis every 6–12 months for a total of 5 years and a colonoscopy 1 year after surgery. PET/CT scan is not recommended for surveillance of any stage rectal cancer.

Surveillance for a lesion that required local transanal excision only is proctoscopy (with EUS or MRI with contrast) every 3–6 months for the first 2 years and then every 6 months for a total of 5 years AND colonoscopy at 1 year after surgery. For stage I disease that is not amenable to transanal resection, the appropriate surveillance is to repeat colonoscopy at 1 year after surgery.

7. **A.** Of the choices listed, the liver is the most likely site of metastasis for rectal cancer. Peritoneal metastasis is also a common site. At the time of initial diagnosis, 5% of patients will have peritoneal carcinomatosis, and 11% will have liver metastasis. One study reports that up to 70% of metastatic lesions will be in the liver. Due to the route of spread, metastasis can also be seen in the lung. Venous drainage from the distal rectum bypasses the portal system and therefore is likely to spread to the lungs first, whereas the venous drainage from the proximal rectum and colon enters into the portal system and acts as the transport for liver metastasis. Overall, the liver is the most common site for rectal cancer metastasis.

8. **B.** Hepatic resection is the only treatment that can provide the possibility of prolonged survival or even cure for colorectal liver metastasis. There are multiple adjunct treatments (including chemotherapy, radiofrequency ablation, cryotherapy, and high-intensity focused ultrasound) that may allow for downsizing of tumors or help increase the future liver remnant but have not been shown to prolong survival without hepatic resection. The 5-year survival rates after liver resection for colorectal metastasis vary but have been reported to be as high as 71%.

BIBLIOGRAPHY

Adam R, Kitano Y. Multidisciplinary approach of liver metastases from colorectal cancer. *Ann Gastroenterol Surg.* 2019;3(1):50–56. doi:10.1002/ags3.12227

Adams RB, Aloia TA, Loyer E, Pawlik TM, Taouli B, Vauthey JN. Selection for hepatic resection of colorectal liver metastases: expert consensus statement. *HPB (Oxford).* 2013;15(2):91–103. doi:10.1111/j.1477-2574.2012.00557.x

Allen E, Nicolaidis C, Helfand M. The evaluation of rectal bleeding in adults. A cost-effectiveness analysis comparing four diagnostic strategies. *J Gen Intern Med.* 2005 Jan;20(1):81–90. PMID:15693933.

Bipat S, Glas AS, Slors FJ, et al. Rectal cancer: Local staging and assessment of lymph node involvement with endoluminal US, CT, and MR imaging—a meta-analysis. *Radiology.* September 2004;232(3):773–783.

Evaluation of Genomic Applications in Practice and Prevention (EGAPP) Working Group. Recommendations from the EGAPP Working Group: genetic testing strategies in newly diagnosed individuals with colorectal cancer aimed at reducing morbidity and mortality from Lynch syndrome in relatives. *Genet Med.* January 2009;11(1):35–41.

Garden OJ, Rees M, Poston GJ, et al. Guidelines for resection of colorectal cancer liver metastases. Gut. 2006;55(Suppl 3):iii1–8. doi:10.1136/gut.2006.098053

Misiakos EP, Karidis NP, Kouraklis G. Current treatment for colorectal liver metastases. *World J Gastroenterol.* 2011;17(36):4067–4075. doi:10.3748/wjg.v17.i36.4067

National Comprehensive Cancer Network. NCCN Clinical Practice Guidelines in Oncology Rectal Cancer v3. 2014. https://www.nccn.org/professionals/physicians_gls/pdf/rectum.pdf.

National Comprehensive Cancer Network. NCCN Clinical Practice Guidelines in Oncology Colorectal Cancer Screening v2. 2013. https://www.nccn.org/professionals/physicians_gls/pdf/colon.pdf.

National Comprehensive Cancer Network. NCCN Clinical Practice Guidelines in Oncology—Rectal Cancer. 2020. https://www.nccn.org/professionals/physician_gls/pdf/rectal.pdf

Pretzsch E, Bösch F, Neumann J, et al. Mechanisms of Metastasis in Colorectal Cancer and Metastatic Organotropism: Hematogenous versus Peritoneal Spread. *J Oncol.* 2019 Sept 19;7407190. doi:10.1155/2019/7407190

Riihimäki M, Hemminki A, Sundquist J, Hemminki K. Patterns of metastasis in colon and rectal cancer. *Sci Rep.* 2016;6:29765. doi:10.1038/srep29765

Sauer R, Becker H, Hohenberger W, et al. Preoperative versus postoperative chemoradiotherapy for rectal cancer. *N Engl J Med.* 2004 Oct 21;351(17):1731–1740.

Thomassen I, van Gestel YR, Lemmens VE, de Hingh, IH. Incidence, prognosis, and treatment options for patients with synchronous peritoneal carcinomatosis and liver metastases from colorectal origin. *Dis Colon Rectum.* 2013;56(12):1373–1380. doi:10.1097/DCR.0b013e3182a62d9d

44

Peri-Rectal Abscess

Ryan Bram

A 40-year-old woman presents with a 5-day history of worsening gluteal and rectal pain. Her pain is dull and constant, and she describes a sensation of rectal fullness. She has fevers and chills. She has had no changes in bowel habits and denies constipation. She denies purulence, hematochezia, melena, or incontinence. She has some discomfort with defecation but no pain. She denies a history of inflammatory bowel disease, hemorrhoids, or rectal prolapse. She denies trauma to the area. She is not sexually active. Her significant past medical and surgical history includes an appendectomy. In the emergency department, she is febrile to 102.3°F, her heart rate is 103, and her blood pressure is 120/83. She has some induration and erythema 4–5 cm laterally and anterior to the anal verge on the right with tenderness, no fluctuance, normal sphincter tone, no masses, and no induration. No fistula openings are visible. Laboratory workup is significant only for a white blood cell count of 19.2.

1. **What would be the expected course of a fistula-in-ano (if present)?**
   A. Radial to the posterior midline
   B. Curvilinear to the anterior midline
   C. Radial to the anterior midline
   D. Curvilinear to the posterior midline

2. **What is the preferred operative management of horseshoe abscesses?**
   A. Intravenous antibiotics
   B. Presacral drainage
   C. Incision and drainage with counter-incision
   D. Single incision and drainage
   E. Transabdominal drainage

3. **Regarding the outcomes of treatment for anal fistula, which of the following is correct?**
   A. There is no difference in fistula closure rate with fibrin glue versus standard fistulotomy, but those who underwent fibrin glue placement have shorter recovery times.
   B. Fistulas occur in 66% of patients who have perirectal abscesses.
   C. Noncutting setons have an increased risk of incontinence.
   D. All anterior fistulas in females should be managed with a cutting seton.

4. **Regarding perirectal abscesses, which of the following is correct?**
   A. Horseshoe abscesses can occur in two planes and usually require imaging for diagnosis.
   B. Immunocompromised patients can be managed with bedside incision and drainage and intravenous antibiotics.
   C. Crohn's disease is responsible for the majority of perirectal abscesses.
   D. Necrotizing soft tissue infection of the perianal and perineal areas has a mortality rate approaching 50%.

5. **Regarding perirectal abscesses, which of the following is correct?**
   A. Supralevator abscesses can be a complication of diverticulitis.
   B. Perianal abscesses always require a counter incision.

C. Fistulas encountered at the time of incision and drainage of a perirectal abscess should be surgically repaired.

D. External manifestations of intersphincteric abscesses generally include a fistula track.

6. **When evaluating a neutropenic patient with a perirectal abscess which of the following findings is the strongest indication for surgical drainage?**

A. Platelets <50,000

B. Skin necrosis overlying a well-defined fluctuant mass

C. Absolute neutrophil count under 500 cell/μL

D. Fever improving with IV antibiotics

7. **When considering surgical management of a perirectal abscess with fistula, which of the following fistula characteristics would suggest a complex fistula and therefore indicate seton placement for staged management?**

A. Fistula with multiple tracts

B. Subcutaneous fistula

C. Involvement of <10% of the external sphincter

D. Any anteriorly located fistula

ANSWERS

1. **D.** According to Goodsall's rule, the transverse anal line generally dictates the course of a fistula track. External orifices of a fistula track posterior to the transverse anal line course in a curvilinear fashion to the posterior midline. External orifices anterior to the transverse anal line generally course in a radial fashion to the anterior midline. However, if a fistula is present greater than 2–3 cm from the anal verge, their course does not follow the traditional radial course to the anterior midline. They typically produce curvilinear tracks that may end at the posterior midline or just lateral to the posterior midline. This patient's area of induration and erythema foci is approximately 4–5 cm from the anal verge and thus could be considered a long anterior fistula track; therefore, D is correct.

2. **C.** Horseshoe abscesses encompass almost the entire circumference of the rectum and can occur in the supralevator plane, the ischiorectal plane, and the intersphincteric plane. Each area of concern dictates the clinical management. Intravenous antibiotics are not adequate treatment for suppurative perirectal disease and may predispose the patient to worsening perirectal sepsis.

Presacral drainage is not the recommended treatment for horseshoe abscesses and is reserved for rectal injuries in the settings of trauma. Single incision and drainage may be effective in certain abscesses but is generally not recommended in horseshoe abscesses. Drainage may be inadequate or ineffective and counter-incisions are preferred, which also includes unroofing of the external sphincter complex. This same modality is also preferred in the setting of a horseshoe fistula.

Transabdominal drainage may be warranted in certain clinical scenarios involving supralevator abscesses when the origin of the abscess is intraabdominal in nature. Transabdominal drainage for a cryptoglandular abscess runs the risk of inadequate drainage and transsphinctertic fistula formation, along with the risk of systemic sepsis due to inadequate drainage.

3. **A.** Fistula-in-ano represents a common chronic problem after perirectal abscess. Fibrin glue and conventional fistulotomy have similar outcomes for rates of recurrence and closure of fistula tracks, but fibrin glue insertion may have shorter return-to-work times. Fistulas occur in up to 25–50% of patients who have perirectal abscesses. Setons are placed to promote drainage of fistulas and to facilitate fibrosis of the fistula track. Cutting setons are gradually tightened by the surgeon in the outpatient setting, which eliminates the fistula while gradually dividing the sphincter complexes, putting the patient at risk for incontinence.

Noncutting setons have a significantly reduced risk of incontinence when compared to cutting setons, with some studies suggestive of preservation of continent function, and generally are accepted for treating high intersphincteric fistula tracks.

4. **D.** As stated earlier, horseshoe abscesses can occur in the supralevator plane, the ischiorectal plane, and the intersphincteric plane. Imaging is not necessary for the diagnosis but does provide a helpful adjunct to clinical correlation.

Immunocompromised patients should generally not be managed in the outpatient setting after incision and drainage of a perirectal abscess. They may or may not manifest systemic or local signs of inflammation and can present with delayed diagnoses of sepsis or necrotizing soft tissue infection. These patients are generally managed with inpatient admission, incision and drainage, and intravenous antibiotic therapy. If the abscess is a superficial perianal one, then incision, drainage, and packing may be performed with close follow-up.

Crohn's disease manifests in several different ways and can certainly be the inciting factor for perirectal abscesses and complex fistula disease. However, the most common cause of perirectal suppuration is cryptoglandular formation of infection. Other causes include malignancy, trauma, and hidradenitis suppuritiva.

Necrotizing soft tissue infection of the perirectal and perineal region is a life-threatening process, as is the disease in any soft tissue location. Intersphincteric abscesses can often go unnoticed or misdiagnosed and can result in a delayed diagnosis. In areas without access to health care, perirectal disease can progress rapidly as well. Infection can worsen and spread through soft tissue planes, progressing to a necrotizing soft tissue infection or Fournier's gangrene, requiring wide local debridement. In some cases, the debridement is large enough that a diverting colostomy is required for wound healing. Mortality rates with necrotizing soft tissue infection are approximately 40–50%.

5. **A.** Supralevator abscess can occur as a result of intra-abdominal pathology such as diverticular abscesses, malignancy, or trauma. Perianal abscesses usually are superficial, simple abscesses without fistula tracks and are treated with a single cruciate incision with packing.

Fistulas encountered at the time of a perirectal abscess are common. However, fistulotomy is generally not performed in the acute setting as no improved clinical outcome has been documented with acute management. Intersphincteric abscesses generally have a more insidious clinical course and plague the patient, with complaints of vague discomfort without external manifestations. Induration and tenderness can be elicited on a digital rectal examination, but other findings are often inconsistent. This type of abscess requires

an exam under anesthesia for adequate treatment modalities.

6. **B.** Management of a perianal abscess in a neutropenic patient is difficult, and recent data suggest a multidisciplinary approach. There is debate as to the need for surgical intervention, but according to Badgwell et al., who analyzed the largest series of neutropenic patients with perirectal abscess the physical exam findings most often associated with operative intervention were abscess formation and erythema with odds ratios of 10.5 and 3.1, respectively. There are also data to suggest medical management alone for these patients, but it is limited to small retrospective case series. Regardless of this, there seems to be consensus that surgical management should be perused in the case of obvious fluctuance, erythema, tissue necrosis, and worsening clinical picture despite IV antibiotics.

7. **A.** Managing complex fistulas depends on fistula anatomy, medical comorbidities like inflammatory bowel disease, and surgeon preference. It is common practice for a draining seton to be placed during the initial period of inflammation and then to schedule further surgical intervention once the acute phase of inflammation has resolved. This practice partly comes from a small prospective trial by Van der Hagen et al. in which patients with trans-, supra-, and extrasphincteric fistulas underwent a two-stage surgical treatment of anal fistula to include seton placement followed by mucosal advancement flap. There was only one failure and a fistula recurrence rate of 22%. It was thought that through the seton placement the local inflammatory reaction was allowed time to heal so that the tissue used during definitive repair was healthier, thus leading to a better outcome. Recently a systematic review of 26 studies found a similar recurrence rate of 21% for mucosal advancement flap, thus proving its effectiveness for complex fistula treatment. Other characteristics of a complex fistula track include any fistula involving more than 30% of the external sphincter, suprasphincteric fistula, extrasphincteric or high fistulas, proximal to the dentate or pectinate line; recurrent fistulas; fistulas related to inflammatory bowel disease, tuberculosis, or HIV; and fistulas secondary to local radiation treatments.

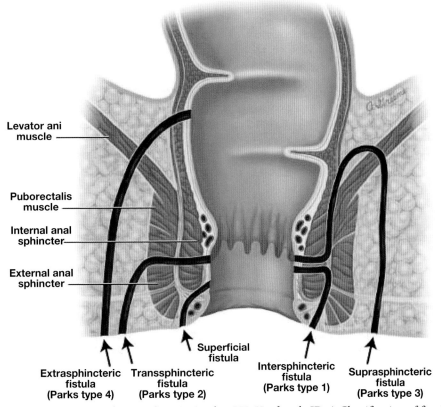

Source: Reproduced, with permission, from Parks AG, Gordon PH, Hardcastle JD. A Classification of fistula-in-ano. Br J Surg. 1976;63(1):1–12.

Parks described four types of anorectal fistulas that originate from cryptoglandular infections. Fistulas can have a complicated anatomy with one or more extensions and accessory tracts. The original Parks's classification did not include a superficial fistula tract. Type 1 is an intersphincteric fistula that travels along the intersphincteric plane. Type 2 is a transsphincteric fistula that encompasses a portion of the internal and external sphincter. Type 3 is a suprasphincteric fistula that encompasses the entire sphincter apparatus. Type 4 is an extrasphincteric fistula that extends from a primary opening in the rectum, encompasses the entire sphincter apparatus, and opens onto the skin overlying the buttock.

BIBLIOGRAPHY

Badgwell BD, Chang GJ, Rodriguez-Bigas MA, et al. Management and outcomes of anorectal infection in the cancer patient. *Ann Surg Oncol.* 2009;16:2752–2758.

Balciscueta Z, Uribe N, Balciscueta I, Andreu-Ballester JC, García-Granero E. Rectal advancement flap for the treatment of complex cryptoglandular anal fistulas: a systematic review and meta-analysis. *Int J. Colorectal Dis.* 2017;32(5):599–609.

Rizzo JA, Naig AL, Johnson EK. Anorectal abscess and fistula-in-ano: evidence-based management. *Surg Clin North Am.* 2010;90(1):45–68.

Sullivan PS, Moreno C. A multidisciplinary approach to perianal and intra-abdominal infections in the neutropenic cancer patient. *Oncology.* 2015;29:581–590.

Van Der Hagen SJ, Baeten CG, et al. Staged mucosal advancement flap for the treatment of complex anal fistulas: pretreatment with noncutting Setons and in case of recurrent multiple abscesses a diverting stoma. *Colorectal Dis.* 2005;7(5):513–518.

Vogel JD, Johnson EK, Morris AM, et al. Clinical practice guideline for the management of anorectal abscess, Fistula-in-ano, and rectovaginal fistula. *Dis Colon Rectum.* 2016;59(12):1117–1133.

Cirocco WC, Reilly JC. Challenging the predictive accuracy of Goodsall's rule for anal fistulas. *Dis Colon Rectum.* 1992 June;35(6):537–542.

Chung W, Kazemi P, Ko D, et al. Anal fistula plug and fibrin glue versus conventional treatment in repair of complex anal fistulas. *Am J Surg.* 2009 May;197(5):604–608. doi:10.1016/j.amjsurg.2008.12.013

Dunn KM, Rothenberger DA. Colon, rectum, and anus. In: Brunicardi, CF, et al. eds. *Schwartz's Principles of Surgery.* 9th ed. McGraw Hill Co.; 2010:1060–1064.

Henrichsen S, Christiansen J. Incidence of fistula-in-ano complicating anorectal sepsis: a prospective study. *Br J Surg.* 1986;73:371–372.

Huber P Jr, Kissack AS, Simonton CT. Necrotising soft-tissue infection from rectal abscess. *Dis Colon Rectum.* 1983; 26(8):507–511.

Nelson, H. Anus. In: Townsend CM et al. eds. *Sabiston Textbook of Surgery.* 19th ed. Elsevier; 2012:1392–1396.

North JH Jr, Weber TK, Rodriguez-Bigas MA, Meropol NJ, Petrelli NJ. The management of infectious and noninfectious anorectal complications in patients with leukemia. *J Am Coll Surg.* 1996 Oct;183(4):322–328.

Pezim ME. Successful treatment of horseshoe fistula requires deroofing of deep postanal space. *Am J Surg.* 1994 May;167(5):513–515.

Sentovich SM. Fibrin glue for anal fistulas: long-term results. *Dis Colon Rectum.* 2003 Apr;46(4):498–502.

Vial M, Parés D, Pera M, Grande L. Faecal incontinence after seton treatment for anal fistulae with and without surgical division of internal anal sphincter: a systematic review. *Colorectal Dis.* 2010 Mar;12(3):172–178. doi:10.1111/j.1463-1318.2009.01810.x.

45

Breast Mass

Anita Mamtani and Zakiya Shakir

SCENARIO 1

A 57-year-old otherwise healthy female presents to your clinic to discuss the results of her recent screening mammogram. She has had unremarkable screening mammograms since the age of 40. She has two aunts with breast cancer and recently heard that her 35-year-old niece was diagnosed with invasive ductal adenocarcinoma. She reports no palpable masses noticed on breast self-exams, no nipple drainage, no breast skin changes, and no other concerning constitutional symptoms.

1. **The patient requests counseling on various genetic syndromes, given the young age of her recently diagnosed niece. Which of the following is correctly matched?**
   A. *BRCA1*—chromosome 13q—increased female and male breast cancer risk
   B. *BRCA1*—chromosome 17q—increased female breast and ovarian cancer risk
   C. *BRCA2*—chromosome 17q—increased female and male breast cancer risk
   D. Li-Fraumeni syndrome—PTEN mutation—increased breast, nervous system, and gastrointestinal (GI) tract cancers
   E. Peutz-Jehgers syndrome—KRAS mutation—increased breast and colon cancer, mucocutaneous lesions

2. **The patient's screening mammogram reveals a 1.1-cm density in the subareolar region of her left breast. She promptly undergoes a diagnostic mammogram with ultrasound for further**

evaluation of the lesion, which the radiologist classifies as BIRADS 4B. She has no palpable lesion on physical exam. The most appropriate next step is
   A. repeat mammography in 6 months.
   B. magnetic resonance imaging (MRI) of the breast.
   C. genetic screening for inherited mutations.
   D. stereotactic core needle biopsy.

3. **Pathology reveals lobular carcinoma in situ (LCIS). The patient now seeks advice on her overall risk of cancer. Which of the following is true?**
   A. LCIS has a 40% lifetime risk of development into lobular carcinoma.
   B. LCIS has an increased risk of malignancy in either breast.
   C. LCIS is a precursor to malignancy.
   D. LCIS becomes lobular carcinoma.

4. **The patient opts to proceed with prophylactic bilateral mastectomies. In a discussion of operative details, she mentions that her niece, who had Stage I invasive ductal carcinoma with positive estrogen receptor status, underwent a lumpectomy with radiation. Which of the following is true?**
   A. All patients benefit from chemotherapy, regardless of nodal status.
   B. Adjuvant therapy with tamoxifen results in significant prolongation of disease-free and overall survival in patients with *HER2/neu* gene overexpression.
   C. The purpose of radiation is to decrease the risk of distant metastasis.

D. Patients with early-stage breast cancer who undergo lumpectomy with sentinel lymph node biopsy followed by radiation have similar survival rates as those who undergo formal axillary lymph node dissection.

E. Aromatase inhibitors may be helpful for adjuvant therapy in premenopausal women.

5. **At her follow-up visit after her operation, the patient reports feeling a sensation of numbness in her upper inner arm. She has full motor strength of the extremity, and the remainder of her arm has normal sensation. Her incisions appear to be healing well. What is the most likely etiology of this?**

A. Injury to cutaneous branches of the brachial plexus

B. Injury to the thoracodorsal nerve

C. Injury to the intercostobrachial nerve

D. Disruption of the lymphatic network

E. Occult postoperative seroma in the axilla

SCENARIO 2

A 40-year-old female with no medical or surgical history presents to your office to discuss a palpable left breast mass. She first noticed it 2 months ago; it is nontender, and it has increased in size. Her screening mammogram was normal 1 year ago, and she has no family history of breast cancer. On exam, the mass is 4 cm, well defined, and mobile. She has no other masses in either breast and no adenopathy, nipple discharge, or skin changes.

6. **Based on the provided information, what findings would you expect on a diagnostic mammogram?**

A. Branching linear calcifications

B. Spiculated mass with distortion of architecture

C. Oval mass with well-circumscribed margins

D. A cluster of pleomorphic calcifications

7. **You discuss the potential treatment options with the patient. What is the next step in confirming the diagnosis?**

A. Bilateral breast mammogram

B. Ultrasound with core needle biopsy

C. Left breast MRI with stereotactic biopsy

D. No further workup needed; follow with serial breast exam and ultrasound

8. **The biopsy results show "stromal atypia with mild cellularity." Which of the following is true?**

A. This is a radial scar and can be observed with serial ultrasound and exam.

B. This is a Phyllodes tumor and requires surgical excision.

C. This is a fibroadenoma and can be observed with serial ultrasound and exam.

D. This is an invasive lobular cancer and requires surgical excision.

9. **Given the biopsy results, what recommendations would you now provide?**

A. Modified radical mastectomy

B. Observation with clinical breast exam and ultrasound in 6 months

C. Lumpectomy with negative margins and sentinel lymph node biopsy

D. Wide excision with 1-cm margins

ANSWERS

1. **B.** The *BRCA1* gene is located on chromosome 17q and confers an increased risk of female breast and ovarian cancer.

Breast cancer is the most common cancer in women and is second to lung cancer as a cause of death in women, with a lifetime risk of 1 in 8. Risk factors for developing breast malignancy include a family history of breast cancer, early menarche, late menopause, personal history of breast or uterine cancer, and nulliparity. The Gail model is a tool designed to calculate breast cancer risk by assessing risk factors including personal medical history, reproductive history, and history of breast cancer among first-degree relatives, and translating these into a score to estimate the risk of developing invasive breast cancer over set periods.

Approximately 10% of breast cancers are hereditary in nature. Genes and syndromes implicated in hereditary *BRCA* include, among others, the BRCA1 (chromosome 17q, increased female breast and ovarian cancer risk) and BRCA2 mutations (chromosome 13q, increased ovarian cancer, and female and male breast cancer risk), Li-Fraumeni syndrome (p53 mutation, increased breast cancer, sarcoma, leukemia, brain tumors), Cowden's syndrome (PTEN mutation, increased breast, nervous system, and GI tract cancers), and hereditary nonpolyposis colon cancer (mismatch repair defect, increased colon, endometrial, ovarian, and breast cancers).

2. **D.** For BIRADS 4 or 5 lesions detected on screening studies, stereotactic core biopsy is considered the preferred first step in pathologic diagnosis.

Clinical features concerning for breast cancer include fixed/firm palpable masses, nipple retraction, skin changes, and unilateral nipple discharge. Annual mammography is valuable as a screening tool in women ≤40 years in age, although is limited in women younger than 35 due to increased breast density. Concerning mammographic findings include an architectural distortion, developing asymmetry, mass (with partially or ill-defined margins), or a cluster of microcalcifications with amorphous, linear, branching patterns. Screening mammography in women 50 years and older has decreased breast cancer mortality by 33%. Ultrasound may be used to distinguish solid and cystic masses. MRI is available as an adjunctive tool but cannot replace mammography or ultrasound. Fine needle aspiration yields simple cytological results but cannot distinguish carcinoma in situ from invasive cancer because it does not include information about architecture. Core biopsy is considered the preferred first step in pathologic diagnosis, particularly for palpable lesions and for lesions detected on screening studies. In general, a two-step approach of initial biopsy followed by definitive operation, if indicated, is the preferred pathway of management.

3. **B.** LCIS is not considered a precancerous lesion but is associated with an increased risk of malignancy in either breast. LCIS is not considered a precursor to invasive adenocarcinoma but is associated with a 20–30% risk of ductal adenocarcinoma in either breast. Tamoxifen can decrease this risk, and depending on tumor biology and individual patient risk, management that may be advised includes close observation with serial monitoring, chemoprevention with tamoxifen, or prophylactic bilateral mastectomies.

Ductal carcinoma in situ (DCIS) is considered a precursor to ductal adenocarcinoma, the most common histologic type of breast cancer, and is associated with a significant increase in the risk of ipsilateral cancer. Ten to twenty percent of patients with newly discovered DCIS already have associated invasive carcinoma, and when untreated, 40–60% of these patients will develop ipsilateral invasive ductal carcinoma. Lobular carcinoma comprises a smaller 10% of all invasive breast cancers. Inflammatory breast cancer is yet rarer and with the worst prognosis of all breast cancer types, comprising 5% of cases, with a characteristic rapid onset of pain, visible breast edema, skin changes ("peau d'orange"), and a median survival of 36 months. Skin biopsy alone often reveals unique tumor invasion of lymphatic channels.

4. **D.** Multiple large randomized studies with long-term follow-up including the National Surgical Adjuvant Breast and Bowel Project (NSABP) trials and Milan series showed that disease-free and overall survival rates are similar in Stage I and II patients treated with lumpectomy with axillary dissection followed by radiation, and those treated by modified radical mastectomy. This led to breast-conserving surgery with radiation to be a safe and less morbid course of treatment for patients with amenable, early-stage breast cancer. This has been the historical approach to early breast cancer. The Z11 trial showed that patients treated with breast conservation therapy (lumpectomy + SLN biopsy + radiation therapy) and who had a positive sentinel lymph node had the same survival as those who underwent completion axillary lymph node dissection for the positive node. This further decreased the morbidity of breast cancer surgery. This makes D the correct answer.

Upon discovering a new diagnosis of breast cancer, the stage must clearly be determined before initiating treatment. Surgery is indicated for Stage I–III disease, while Stage IV (metastatic) disease is generally managed with medical and/or radiation therapies. The purpose of surgery is to obtain local control by either lumpectomy or mastectomy and evaluate nodal burden. Lumpectomy may be done with or without preoperative mammographic needle localization. Types of mastectomy include simple (removal of all breast tissue), radical (removal of all breast tissue, pectoralis major, pectoralis minor, and an axillary node dissection), and modified radical (removal of all breast tissue, pectoralis fascia only, and an axillary node dissection). If nodes are clinically negative, the preferred method for staging axillary lymph nodes is sentinel node biopsy, which is performed with methylene blue or 99mTc sulfur colloid, a radiopharmaceutical taken up by lymphatic capillaries, transported to the sentinel node, and then phagocytosed by macrophages. A formal axillary dissection is generally indicated in the case of clinically positive nodes or completion axillary dissection in the case of clinically negative nodes with failed sentinel mapping. The currently evolving realm of neoadjuvant chemotherapy, with the potential for downstaging both the breast mass and the nodal metastases, continues to change the landscape of breast cancer surgery.

Radiation is used to decrease the risk of local recurrence, particularly when used as adjuvant to breast-conserving surgery. Chemotherapy typically consists of anthracycline and taxane agents and may be helpful for patients with positive nodal status and a high risk of relapse but may generally be excluded in patients with small tumors and negative lymph nodes. Hormonal therapy has been known to decrease risk of recurrence and mortality in patients with estrogen receptor-positive (ER+) tumors. Tamoxifen, a selective ER modulator, reduces recurrence and contralateral disease (side effects include increased risk of endometrial cancer, thromboembolism, and stroke). Adjuvant therapy with tamoxifen has been shown to lead to a significant prolongation of disease-free and overall survival in ER+ disease, regardless of nodal status. Anastrazole is an aromatase inhibitor that may be used in patients with contraindications to tamoxifen and only in postmenopausal women as they do not produce sufficient estrogen opposition in premenopausal women. Trastuzumab is a monoclonal HER2 antibody that may be used as adjuvant therapy in both pre- and postmenopausal women who have overexpression of the *HER2/neu* gene.

Stage is the best indicator of prognosis. When limited to the breast only, there is a 99% cure rate; however, 5-year survival decreases to 66–87% based on surveillance, epidemiology, and end results (SEER) data with axillary spread. The tumor, node, metastasis (TNM) model is the most widely accepted staging method. T0 implies no evidence of a primary tumor, and it includes in situ lesions, T1 is a mass ≤2 cm, T2 is a mass from 2–5 cm, T3 is a mass >5 cm, and T4 is a mass with chest wall invasion, skin edema or ulceration, or inflammatory breast cancer.

N0 implies negative lymph nodes, N1 means positive mobile ipsilateral axillary lymph nodes, N2 is fixed or matted ipsilateral axillary nodes, and N3 is ipsilateral infraclavicular, supraclavicular, or internal mammary nodes. There is also pathologic N-staging based on the number of histologically positive lymph nodes.

M0 disease implies no metastatic disease, and M1 means metastatic disease is present. The most common locations for breast cancer metastasis are bone, lung, and brain.

5. **C.** Injury to the intercostobrachial nerve, the lateral cutaneous branch of the second intercostal nerve, results in numbness of the medial upper arm. The anatomic borders of the breast are the second rib superiorly, sixth to seventh rib inferiorly, sternal border medially, and midaxillary line laterally. The parenchyma of the breast is comprised of glandular lobes in a radial pattern, each with a ductal system ending at the nipple, and a surrounding connective tissue framework made by the suspensory ligaments of Cooper. The most common distribution of cancer is the upper outer quadrant (45%), followed by subareolar (25%), upper inner (15%), lower outer (10%), and lower inner (5%).

The blood supply of the breast includes perforator branches from the internal mammary artery, branches from the posterior intercostal arteries, and axillary artery branches including the lateral thoracic and pectoral branches of the thoracoacromial artery. Venous drainage parallels the arterial supply. The axillary lymph nodes drain 75–85% of lymph from the breast, with the remainder draining to parasternal/internal mammary lymph nodes. There are three levels of lymph nodes: level I (lateral to pectoralis minor), level II (deep to pectoralis minor), and level III (medial to pectoralis minor). Nerves present in the axillary fat pad, and to be mindful of during dissection, include the long thoracic nerve (innervating the serratus anterior, with injury resulting in a "winged scapula"), the thoracodorsal nerve (innervating the latissimus dorsi, with injury resulting in weak adduction and internal rotation), the intercostobrachial nerve (providing sensation to the upper inner arm, with injury resulting in paresthesia or numbness), and the medial and lateral anterior thoracic nerves (innervating the pectoralis muscles, with injury resulting in weakness).

6. **C.** This lesion likely represents a fibroadenoma, the most common benign tumor of the breast. Fibroadenoma is characterized by the proliferation of fibroblasts that can compress ductal elements. It is typically described as a mobile mass with well-defined margins on clinical breast exam and on imaging. The interpretation of mammographic findings helps determine the underlying pathology, as well as treatment options. Branching linear

calcifications and pleomorphic calcifications usually represent DCIS. A spiculated mass with architectural distortion is concerning for a ductal carcinoma but could also represent a benign entity, such as a radial scar.

7. **B.** Ultrasound evaluation is recommended in addition to a diagnostic mammogram for the workup of any palpable mass in a patient older than 30 years. Given the relatively large size of this mass and its rate of growth, a core needle biopsy is indicated. A bilateral mammogram would be helpful in screening the contralateral breast for abnormalities but would not confirm the diagnosis of the mass. A stereotactic biopsy is not necessary if the mass is palpable and able to be visualized under ultrasound. If the mass were smaller in size and stable in its growth pattern, observation with annual clinical breast exam and annual mammogram would be acceptable.

8. **B.** While fibroadenomas represent the proliferation of stroma of the breast, Phyllodes tumors (previously known as cystosarcoma phyllodes) represent a fibroepithelial lesion with a sarcomatous appearance. Pathology review will demonstrate increased cellularity of the stroma and epithelium. They are a rare entity, with an incidence of 0.3–1% of all breast tumors. Patients with Li-Fraumeni syndrome are at an increased risk of developing these tumors. Phyllodes tumors are difficult to differentiate from fibroadenomas on either mammogram or ultrasound; core needle biopsy is also unreliable, and these lesions often require excisional biopsy for diagnostic confirmation. They are characterized as benign, borderline, or malignant based on the histology and degree of cellularity. Rapid growth of a painless breast mass, a size >3 cm, and imaging evidence of a fibroadenoma should prompt concern for Phyllodes tumor.

9. **D.** The main factor in preventing recurrence of Phyllodes tumor is the surgical margin of resection. The National Comprehensive Cancer Network guidelines recommend a >1-cm margin of tumor-free resection and follow-up with an annual clinical breast exam and imaging for 3 years. There is no utility to performing lymph node sampling, as

a Phyllodes tumor does not spread via lymphatic channels. Rather, it tends to recur locally, with a local failure rate of up to 22%, and can involve the chest wall, at which point reexcision is indicated. Metastatic disease (most commonly to the lungs) is treated as metastatic soft tissue sarcoma, including radiation and chemotherapy.

BIBLIOGRAPHY

American College of Radiology. Practice guideline for the breast conservation therapy in the management of invasive breast carcinoma. *J Am Coll Surg.* 2007;205(2):362–376.

American Society of Breast Surgeons. Official Statement: Management of Fibroadenomas. 2008.

Bao T, Prowell T, Stearns V. Chemoprevention of breast cancer: tamoxifen, raloxifene, and beyond. *Am J Ther.* 2006;13(4):337–348.

Bartella L, Smith CS, Dershaw DD, et al. Imaging breast cancer. *Radiol Clin North Am.* 2007;45(1):45–67.

Chan K, Morris GJ. Chemoprevention of breast cancer for women at high risk. *Semin Oncol.* 2006;33(6):642–646.

Chang J, Denham L, Dong EK, Malek K, Lum SS. Trends in the diagnosis of phyllodes tumors and fibroadenomas before and after release of WHO Classification Standards. *Ann Surg Oncol.* 2018;25(10):3088–3095. doi:10.1245/s10434-018-6622-3

Giuliano AE, Hunt KK, Ballman KV, et al. Axillary dissection vs no axillary dissection in women with invasive breast cancer and sentinel node metastasis: a randomized clinical trial. *JAMA.* 2011;305(6):569–575.

King TA, Morrow M. Breast disease. In: Mulholland MW, Lillemoe KD, Doherty GM, et al. eds. *Greenfield's Surgery: Scientific Principles and Practice.* 5th ed. Lippincott, Williams & Wilkins; 2011:2635–2701.

Li J, Tsang JY, Chen C, et al. Predicting outcome in mammary phyllodes tumors: relevance of clinicopathological features. *Ann Surg Oncol.* 2019;26(9):2747–2758. doi:10.1245/s10434-019-07445-1

National Comprehensive Cancer Network. Breast Cancer (version 5.2020). 2020. https://www.nccn.org/professionals/physician_gls/pdf/breast_blocks.pdf

National Comprehensive Cancer Network. Breast Cancer Screening and Diagnosis (version 1.2019). 2019. https://www.nccn.org/professionals/physician_gls/pdf/breast-screening.pdf

Patel RR, Sharma CG, Jordan VC. Optimizing the antihormonal treatment and prevention of breast cancer. *Breast Cancer.* 2007;14(2):113–122.

Strode M, Khoury T, Mangieri C, Takabe K. Update on the diagnosis and management of malignant Phyllodes tumors of the breast. *Breast.* 2017;33:91–96. doi:10.1016/j.breast.2017.03.001

46

Ductal Carcinoma in Situ

Ashley Chinn

A 42-year-old woman presents with extensive new calcifications on screening mammography. She undergoes stereotactic core biopsy that reveals ductal carcinoma in situ (DCIS), intermediate grade, with comedonecrosis. Estrogen receptor status is positive (ER+). She has no significant past medical history, and there is no family history of cancer.

1. **Which of the following is a risk factor for this patient having occult invasion?**
   A. +ER receptor status
   B. Palpable mass on clinical exam
   C. DCIS that spans a diameter larger than 3 cm
   D. Intermediate grade histology
   E. Contralateral disease

2. **Which of the following statements is correct?**
   A. For patients undergoing breast conservation therapy (BCT) for DCIS, the optimal margin width is 10 mm.
   B. Adjuvant radiation does not decrease the risk of recurrence after lumpectomy for DCIS.
   C. Adjuvant radiation increases survival in patients undergoing BCT for DCIS.
   D. Risk of death after any treatment for DCIS is less than 2% after 10 years and is usually secondary to recurrence as invasive disease.
   E. Approximately 10% of ipsilateral breast recurrences after lumpectomy alone or in conjunction with radiation are invasive disease.

3. **Regarding the role of sentinel lymph node biopsy (SLNB) in DCIS, which of the following statements is correct?**

A. An SLNB does not need to be performed if this patient undergoes a mastectomy for her DCIS.
B. By definition, DCIS is noninvasive disease; therefore, an SLNB should never be performed.
C. An SLNB has an almost negligible risk of lymphedema.
D. An SLNB should be considered at the time of lumpectomy for DCIS located in the axillary tail of the breast.
E. An SLNB should only be considered if a patient has DCIS in the setting of a mass.

4. **Regarding imaging in DCIS, which of the following is correct?**
   A. Approximately 50% of all mammography-detected breast cancers are DCIS.
   B. Magnetic resonance imaging (MRI) estimates of the size and extent of DCIS often correlate with pathologic evaluation.
   C. DCIS often extends beyond the area of calcification seen on a mammography.
   D. MRI is better than mammography for distinguishing DCIS from benign, atypical proliferative lesions or microinvasion.
   E. MRI is not helpful in identifying multicentric disease and synchronous disease in the contralateral breast.

5. **Regarding adjuvant tamoxifen for DCIS, which of the following statements is correct?**
   A. Tamoxifen (TMX) improves both local recurrence and survival rates in DCIS.
   B. TMX has no significant effect on survival in invasive breast cancer.

C. Side effects of TMX include an increased risk of ovarian cancer.

D. Tamoxifen is equally effective in ER+ lesions as in ER− lesions.

E. In women undergoing breast conservation therapy for DCIS, TMX decreases invasive and noninvasive breast cancer events for both the ipsilateral and contralateral breast.

6. **When considering adjuvant anastrozole for DCIS, which of the following statements is correct?**

A. Anastrozole should be used in postmenopausal PR-positive DCIS.

B. The side effects of anastrozole include an increased risk of ovarian cancer.

C. When compared with TMX, anastrozole improved estimated cancer-free survival at 10 years.

D. Anastrozole is superior to TMX in terms of overall survival.

7. **Regarding prognosis in DCIS, which of the following is correct?**

A. The risk of recurrence of DCIS decreases with age.

B. ER receptor positivity predicted a higher risk of death.

C. The risk of development of metastases and/or death in a patient with pure DCIS is 5%.

D. A papillary growth pattern of DCIS is a strong predictor for the risk of ipsilateral breast recurrence after treatment.

ANSWERS

1. B. Because of sampling error, after surgical excision of a lesion diagnosed on core biopsy, DCIS is upgraded to invasive cancer in approximately 10–20%. Risk factors for occult invasive disease include the presence of a mass, the extent of DCIS greater than 5 cm, comedonecrosis, or a high-grade histology.

DCIS represents a heterogeneous spectrum of disease involving the abnormal proliferation of epithelial cells confined to the breast ducts. Unlike invasive cancer, DCIS is bounded by the basement membranes and does not invade beyond its ductal origin or into the neighboring tissues. Although studies of the natural progression of DCIS are lacking, the consensus is that in-situ disease represents an intermediary between normal breast tissue and invasive disease. However, its behavior is highly variable, ranging from indolent low-grade lesions that may never progress to invasion to high-grade lesions that may harbor foci of invasive cancer. This nonobligate progression and variation in biologic behavior have raised dilemmas in clinical management with some patients being overtreated for the disease.

2. D. The mortality for patients with DCIS after excision is low (less than 2% in 10 years based on population studies) but is generally secondary to recurrence as invasive disease. Almost half of recurrences after treatment for DCIS occur in the form of invasive disease. Therefore, the fundamental goals of management are to prevent recurrence and to minimize treatment-related morbidity. DCIS can be treated by either mastectomy or BCT. Mastectomy should be considered in patients with extensive or multicentric disease, in whom the breast volume to tumor volume ratio is low and lumpectomy with reasonable cosmesis cannot be achieved, or in whom lumpectomy fails to achieve negative margins. Most patients, however, can and should be considered for BCT.

Optimal margins for lumpectomy remain controversial. Studies suggest a decrease in recurrence rates after lumpectomy alone with increased margin width up to 10 mm, with no additional benefit to margins wider than 10 mm. However, this benefit is eradicated when radiation is added to lumpectomy, and the consensus is that margin width greater than or equal to 2 mm is adequate, with some advocating the absence of cancer at the inked margin as the definition of a negative margin.

Given the variable behavior of DCIS, there have been extensive efforts to identify a subgroup of patients with indolent disease for whom radiation can be safely eliminated after lumpectomy. Such efforts have thus far resulted in conflicting data. Therefore, radiotherapy remains the standard of care for patients with DCIS who undergo BCT. The prospective National Surgical Adjuvant Breast and Bowel Project (NSABP) B-06 trial demonstrated significant decreases in recurrence rate with adjuvant radiation in BCT for invasive disease. There were some women in this study who were initially thought to have invasive disease. However, on review of their biopsy specimens, they were determined to have DCIS instead.

These women were found to have a significant reduction in recurrence rates, including recurrence as invasive disease. The NSABP B-17 study was subsequently designed to evaluate radiotherapy specifically in patients with DCIS. This study found a significant reduction in recurrence rates with adjuvant radiation for noninvasive disease. In neither invasive nor in-situ disease was there a demonstrated survival benefit to adjuvant radiotherapy. The European Organisation for Research and Treatment of Cancer (EORTC) 10753 trial was a large European study that corroborated similar findings.

3. **D.** Although, by definition, DCIS is a noninvasive disease, given the significant chance of upgrading to invasive disease after surgical excision, an SLNB to evaluate for possible nodal metastases has been advocated in certain scenarios. Although it is reasonable to consider an SLNB in patients who have risk factors for occult invasive disease to avoid a second operation should they be upgraded to invasive disease after excision, many patients would undergo unnecessary axillary sampling. SLNB is not entirely benign, and there is about a 6% risk of lymphedema. Because an SLNB can be performed subsequent to a lumpectomy, an SLNB is not advocated at the time of initial excision for most patients. The consensus, however, is to perform an SLNB if a patient is to undergo mastectomy for DCIS. In this situation, removal of the breast precludes a subsequent SLNB should the final pathology reveal invasive disease. These patients would then require axillary lymph node dissection. For the same reason, patients whose DCIS is located in the axillary tail of the breast should be considered for an SLNB at the time of initial excision as lymphatic drainage to the axilla may be disrupted during excision and may decrease the likelihood of successful localization of an SLN subsequently. Most patients, however, can and should undergo an SLNB subsequent to a final pathological determination of invasive disease.

4. **C.** Most cases of DCIS are discovered on a screening mammography and DCIS now accounts for approximately 20% of all screening-detected breast cancers. DCIS most often presents mammographically as microcalcifications, sometimes with branching corresponding to intraductal disease.

Mammography is limited in that DCIS often extends beyond the area of microcalcifications seen on imaging. Thus, up to 15–20% of women undergoing lumpectomy for DCIS may be subjected to reexcision to obtain negative margins. In addition, up to 40% of DCIS lesions grow discontinuously, which can make complete excision difficult. This is a postulated reason as to why adjuvant breast irradiation is effective in decreasing recurrence rates after excision.

Given the limitations of mammography, MRI has been studied as an alternate imaging modality. MRI tends to have high sensitivity but low specificity in breast cancer imaging. Given its high sensitivity, it may be helpful in identifying multicentric or synchronous disease in the contralateral breast. However, it appears to be no better than mammography for distinguishing DCIS from benign proliferative lesions, and MRI estimates of lesion size and extent correlate only moderately well with pathological findings, both over- and underestimating the size of the DCIS.

5. **E.** Given the role of estrogen in the pathogenesis of breast cancer, strategies targeting the estrogen pathway have been investigated as possible adjuncts to breast cancer therapy. Tamoxifen is a selective estrogen receptor modulator. Although it is an estrogen receptor agonist at some sites such as the bone and endometrium, it has potent antagonist effects in breast tissue. Studies had demonstrated the benefit of tamoxifen as adjuvant therapy in invasive disease, including decreased local recurrence and breast cancer mortality rates. The NSABP B-24 study was designed to investigate tamoxifen in the setting of DCIS. In this study, patients undergoing lumpectomy and radiation for DCIS were subsequently randomized to receive tamoxifen or a placebo. Tamoxifen was administered in the treatment group at 10 mg twice a day for 5 years. The median follow-up was 74 months, and patients in the tamoxifen arm had 37% fewer breast cancer events overall and there was both an ipsilateral and contralateral breast benefit. There was no benefit in terms of overall survival. Adverse effects of tamoxifen include an increased incidence of thromboembolic events and endometrial cancer. A subsequent subset analysis demonstrated that the benefit of tamoxifen was limited to those with ER-positive disease.

DCIS represents a very heterogeneous group of lesions that have a variable clinical course lending challenges to the management of this disease. Almost all patients with DCIS will be cured of the disease, and adjuvant radiation and endocrine therapy have

DCIS	LCIS
Nonobligate precursor to invasive cancer.	Risk factor for invasive cancer, both lobular and ductal. Risk is elevated for both the ipsilateral and contralateral breast. Consider hormone modulators to decrease risk.
Often diagnosed with mammography as microcalcifications.	Often mammographically occult and found incidentally on biopsy for other reasons. Consider MRI.
Usually unilateral but multifocality is common.	Often bilateral and multifocal
Surgical treatment is with lumpectomy or mastectomy.	Surgical excision is indicated if found on core needle biopsy secondary to the risk of sampling error (DCIS or invasive cancer nearby is frequently found). If found on surgical excision, no further excision is necessary since it is not treated as a precursor lesion.
Adjuvant radiotherapy is indicated if treated with lumpectomy.	No adjuvant radiotherapy

further improved recurrence rates. With further understanding of the biology of the subtypes of DCIS, we will be able to better tailor therapy to individual patients.

6. **C.** Anastrozole is a potent and nonselective aromatase inhibitor and a reasonable alternative to tamoxifen for postmenopausal women with ER-positive DCIS to reduce the risk of breast cancer. It is also used off-label for the treatment of recurrent ovarian and endometrial cancer. Notable adverse reactions associated with aromatase inhibitors include a loss of bone mineral density, fractures, and increased ischemic cardiovascular events. The choice between anastrozole and TMX should be individualized based on patient preference, side-effect profile, and menopausal status. However, the double-blind randomized, phase 3, NSABP B-35 trial showed that compared with TMX, anastrozole provided a significant improvement in breast cancer–free interval, mainly in women younger than 60 years of age. The study enrolled more than 3,000 postmenopausal women with ER-positive DCIS who underwent BCT; at a median follow-up of 9 years, when compared to TMX, anastrozole resulted in
   - a lower incidence of subsequent breast cancer events (i.e., recurrent DCIS or subsequent invasive breast cancer; 90 vs. 122 events, respectively; HR 0.73), including a lower rate of invasive breast cancer (43 vs. 69 cases; HR 0.62).
   - improved estimated breast cancer–free survival at 10 years (93.1 vs. 89.1%).

   - no significant difference in either disease-free survival (235 vs. 260 events; HR 0.89, 95% CI 0.75–1.07) or overall survival (OS; 98 vs. 88 deaths; HR 1.11, 95% CI 0.83–1.48). The estimated 10-year overall survival was approximately 92% for both groups.

7. **A.** The risk of development of metastases and/or death in a patient with pure DCIS is rare (<1%), and in an analysis of more than 100,000 patients with DCIS enrolled in the surveillance, epidemiology, and end results database, the 20-year breast cancer mortality among women with DCIS was 3.3%. In this study, the predictors of higher risk of death included young age, high grade, and black ethnicity. Estrogen receptor positivity predicted a lower risk of death (HR 0.53, 95% CI 0.41–0.69). Pathology is another useful tool in predicting recurrence and invasion. The traditional method for classifying DCIS lesions is primarily based on the growth pattern (architectural features) of the tumor and recognizes five major types: comedo, cribriform, micropapillary, papillary, and solid type. The comedo type is more often associated with invasion and the degree of comedo necrosis in patients with DCIS appears to be a strong predictor for the risk of ipsilateral breast recurrence after treatment. Papillary was not a strong predictor of recurrence. In a separate, prospective observational study, which included almost 3,000 patients, the risk of recurrence of DCIS was shown to decrease with age. These types of findings and considerations should be incorporated into the risk/benefit discussions of treatment options with patients.

BIBLIOGRAPHY

Alfred C. Ductal carcinoma in situ. In: Harris JR, Lippman ME, Morrow M, Osborne CK. eds. *Diseases of the Breast.* 4th ed. Lippincott-Raven; 2009:321.

Allred DC, Anderson SJ, Paik S, et al. Adjuvant tamoxifen reduces subsequent breast cancer in women with estrogen receptor-positive ductal carcinoma in situ: a study based in NSABP Protocol B-24. *J Clin Oncol.* 2012;30:1268–1273.

Bijker N, Meijnen P, Peterse JL, et al. Breast-conserving treatment with or without radiotherapy in ductal carcinoma in situ: ten-year results of European Organisation for Research and Treatment of Cancer randomized phase III trial 10853 – a study by the EORTC Breast Cancer Cooperative Group and EORTC Radiotherapy Group. *J Clin Oncol.* 2006;24:3381–3387.

Burak WE Jr, Owens KE, Tighe MB, et al. Vacuum-assisted stereotactic breast biopsy: histologic underestimation of malignant lesions. *Arch Surg.* 2000;135:700–7073.

Cronin PA, Olcese C, Patil S, et al. Impact of age on risk of recurrence of ductal carcinoma in situ: outcomes of 2996 women treated with breast-conserving surgery over 30 years. *Ann Surg Oncol.* 2016 Sep;23(9):2816–2824.

Dunne C, Burke JP, Morrow M, et al. Effect of margin status on local recurrence after breast conservation and radiation for ductal carcinoma in situ. *J Clin Oncol.* 2009;27: 1615–1620.

Eastell R, Adams JE, Coleman RE, et al. Effect of anastrozole on bone mineral density: 5-year results from the anastrozole, tamoxifen, alone or in combination trial 18233230. *J Clin Oncol.* 2008;26(7):1051–1057.

Ernster VL, Barclay J, Kerlikowske K, et al. Mortality among women with ductal carcinoma in situ of the breast in the population-based Surveillance, Epidemiology and End Results program. *Arch Intern Med.* 2000;160:953–958.

Fisher B, Constantino JP, Remond C, et al. A randomized clinical trial evaluating tamoxifen in the treatment of patients with node-negative breast cancer who have estrogen-receptor-positive tumors. *N Engl J Med.* 1989;320:479–484.

Fisher B, Costantino JP, Wickerham DL, et al. Tamoxifen for the prevention of breast cancer: current status of the National Surgical Adjuvant Breast and Bowel Project P-1 Study. *J Natl Cancer Inst.* 2005;97:1652–1662.

Fisher B, Dignam J, Wolmark N, et al. Lumpectomy and radiation therapy for the treatment of intraductal breast cancer: findings from National Surgical Adjuvant Breast and Bowel Project B-17. *J Clin Oncol.* 1998;16:441–452.

Fisher B, Dignam J, Wolmark N, et al. Tamoxifen in treatment of intraductal breast cancer: National Surgical Adjuvant Breast and Bowel Project B-24 randomized controlled trial. *Lancet.* 1999;353:1993–2000.

Fisher B, Redmond C, Poisson R, et al. Eight-year results of a randomized clinical trial comparing total mastectomy and lumpectomy with or without irradiation in the treatment of breast cancer. *N Engl J Med.* 1989;320:822–828.

Fisher ER, Dignam J, Tan-Chiu E, et al. Pathologic findings from the National Surgical Adjuvant Breast Project (NSABP) eight-year update of Protocol B-17: intraductal carcinoma. *Cancer.* 1999;86(3):429.

Huo L, Sneige N, Hunt KK, et al. Predictors of invasion in patients with core-needle biopsy-diagnosed ductal carcinoma in situ and recommendations for a selective approach to sentinel lymph node biopsy in ductal carcinoma in situ. *Cancer.* 2006;107:1760–1768.

Hwang ES, Kinkel K, Esserman LJ, et al. Magnetic resonance imaging in patients diagnosed with ductal carcinoma in situ: value in the diagnosis of residual disease, occult invasion, and multicentricity. *Ann Surg Oncol.* 2003;10:381–388.

Kaufmann M, Morrow M, von Minckwitz G, et al. Loco-regional treatment of primary breast cancer: consensus recommendations from an international expert panel. *Cancer.* 2010;116:1184–1191.

Kerlikowske K, Molinaro A, Cha I, et al. Characteristics associated with recurrence among women with ductal carcinoma in situ treated by lumpectomy. *J Natl Cancer Inst.* 2003;95:1692–1702.

King TA, Farr GH Jr, Cederbom GJ, et al. A mass on breast imaging predicts coexisting invasive carcinoma in patients with a core biopsy diagnosis of ductal carcinoma in situ. *Am Surg.* 2001;67:907–912.

MacDonald HR, Silverstein MJ, Mabry H, et al. Local control inductal carcinoma in situ treated by excision alone: incremental benefit of larger margins. *Am J Surg.* 2005;190:521–525.

Margolese RG, Cecchini RS, Julian TB, et al. Anastrozole versus tamoxifen in postmenopausal women with ductal carcinoma in situ undergoing lumpectomy plus radiotherapy (NSABP B-35): a randomised, double-blind, phase 3 clinical trial. *Lancet.* 2016;387(10021):849.

McLaughlin SA, Wright MJ, Morris KT, et al. Prevalence of lymphedema in women with breast cancer 5 years after sentinel lymph node biopsy or axillary dissection: objective measurements. *J Clin Oncol.* 2008;26:5213–5219.

Narod SA, Iqbal J, Giannakeas V, et al. Breast cancer mortality after a diagnosis of ductal carcinoma in situ. *JAMA Oncol.* 2015;1(7):888.

Roses RE, Arun BK, Lari SA, et al. Ductal carcinoma-in-situ of the breast with subsequent distant metastasis and death. *Ann Surg Oncol.* 2011 Oct;18(10):2873–2878.

Silverstein MJ, Lagios M, Groshen S, et al. The influence of margin width on local control of ductal carcinoma in situ of the breast. *N Engl J Med.* 1999;340:1455–1461.

Vanderwalde LH, Dang CM, Bresee C, et al. Discordance between pathologic and radiologic tumor size on breast MRI may contribute to increased re-excision rates. *Am Surg.* 2011;77:1361–1363.

47

Inflammatory Breast Cancer

Ranjna Sharma and Leah Brazer

A 42-year-old female presents to your office with an erythematous and edematous left breast that she reports as occurring acutely over the last 2 weeks. She is not breast-feeding. She denies any recent trauma or source of infection. She presented to her primary care physician last week who administered a trial of antibiotics for presumed cellulitis, without any improvement in symptoms. Upon physical exam, you note an erythematous, edematous, left breast with clinical findings of peau d'orange and a mass underlying the area of clinical change. The left breast appears larger than the right breast. You are able to appreciate fullness in the left axilla. You order dedicated breast imaging. Her diagnostic mammogram shows skin thickening and trabecular distortion in the left breast, with increased tissue density in the retroareolar region. An ultrasound of the left breast shows a 6-cm vague irregular mass in the retroareolar region, with two enlarged left axillary lymph nodes. A skin punch biopsy is performed in your office and it demonstrates cancer cells infiltrating the dermal lymphatics. A core needle biopsy of the mass reveals invasive ductal carcinoma. A fine-needle aspiration of an enlarged left axillary lymph node shows ductal breast carcinoma. A staging work-up is negative for any distant sites of disease. You discuss the treatment modalities of surgery, chemotherapy, and radiation therapy as part of her treatment plan.

1. **What surgical procedure will this patient have?**
   A. Mastectomy
   B. Mastectomy with sentinel lymph node biopsy
   C. Modified radical mastectomy
   D. Radical mastectomy

2. **What impact does the addition of neoadjuvant chemotherapy have on the outcome of patients with inflammatory breast cancer?**
   A. It decreases the risk of developing a contralateral breast cancer in the future.
   B. It decreases the risk of developing a concurrent ovarian cancer.
   C. It increases effectiveness of endocrine therapy.
   D. It improves survival.

3. **What is the role of radiation therapy in this clinical scenario?**
   A. It results in decreased incidence of local recurrence.
   B. It improves response to endocrine therapy.
   C. It improves response to chemotherapy.
   D. It prevents distant metastases.

4. **What is the usual order of treatments delivered?**
   A. Surgery, radiation therapy, chemotherapy
   B. Radiation therapy, surgery, chemotherapy
   C. Chemotherapy, surgery, radiation therapy
   D. Radiation therapy, chemotherapy, surgery

5. **What is the underlying pathophysiology in inflammatory breast cancer contributing to the skin changes that are noted on a clinical exam?**
   A. Infection (mastitis/abscess)
   B. Tumor emboli obstructing the dermal lymphatic vessels
   C. Localized dermatitis
   D. Congestive heart failure causing skin edema
   E. Concurrent non-Hodgkin lmphoma

6. **Which of the following information obtained from the core needle biopsy would help to direct the treatment of this patient?**

   A. Hormone receptor status of the tumor
   B. Oncotype DX
   C. The presence or absence of microcalcifications
   D. The presence or absence of comedo necrosis

7. **The patient is now status postoncologic resection of her inflammatory breast cancer. She presents to your office for follow-up postoperatively. Her incisions are healing well and she has returned to many of her normal daily activities. What is the next best step in management?**

   A. Monthly self-breast examinations with screening mammograms every 2 years
   B. History and physical examination every 3 to 6 months with alternating breast magnetic resonance imaging (MRI) and diagnostic mammograms every 6 months for the first 3 years
   C. History and physical examination every 3 to 6 months with yearly diagnostic mammograms for the first 3 years after primary therapy
   D. Annual mammograms

ANSWERS

1. **C.** This patient will have a modified radical mastectomy (MRM), which comprises a simple mastectomy and axillary lymph node dissection. The borders of the mastectomy portion of the procedure are superiorly to the clavicle and deltopectoral groove, laterally to the latissimus muscle, inferiorly to the upper edge of the rectus sheath, and medially to the sternal border. The posterior border is the fascia overlying the pectoralis major muscle. The mastectomy should resect any residual gross disease and obtain negative surgical margins. The surgical plan must remove all skin changes. The mastectomy skin flaps must be closed without tension. The borders of an axillary lymph node dissection are the axillary vein superiorly, the pectoralis major muscle anteriorly, the subscapularis muscle posteriorly, the serratus anterior muscle medially, and the latissimus dorsi muscle laterally. Within these anatomic boundaries, dissection will occur, which will excise the Level 1 and Level 2 axillary lymph nodes.

   Inferiorly, the dissection should be carried out to the fourth or fifth rib. The Level 1 nodes are located lateral to the pectoralis minor muscle and the Level 2 nodes are located posterior to this muscle. A modified radical mastectomy for a patient with IBC with metastases to the axillary lymph nodes will remove the affected skin, generalized disease process in the breast, and involved lymph nodes. This will contribute to improved local control of the disease process. A sentinel lymph node biopsy is not indicated since there is already known disease in the axillary nodes. Consequently, to control regional disease, a complete axillary lymph node dissection must be done.

2. **D.** The introduction of neoadjuvant chemotherapy has significantly improved clinical outcomes in patients with IBC. It is used to downstage the tumor to allow surgical resection to be more successful by decreasing the likelihood of leaving residual disease behind. Anthracycline-based regimens show a survival benefit. A regimen containing cyclophosphamide, 5-fluorouracil, and either doxorubicin or epirubicin is generally used. Taxanes are also administered. The combination of anthracycline and taxane regimens increases the rate of clinical response to chemotherapy and shows improvement in survival and prognosis. If HER2/neu is overexpressed, then trastuzumab is given for 1 year, which contributes to increased pathologic complete response (pCR). The skin changes of erythema and edema in IBC will generally improve when a patient is responding to neoadjuvant chemotherapy. If a pCR can be achieved, survival is increased. The improvement in survival is seen in both disease-free survival and overall survival.

3. **A.** Radiation therapy is administered after MRM; thus, it is post-mastectomy radiation therapy (PMRT). PMRT is given to improve local control of the disease process and decrease the risk of local recurrence seen in patients with IBC due to high local disease burden at the time of diagnosis. Administration of PMRT is known to decrease the risk of recurrence on the chest wall, mastectomy scar, and regional lymph node basins. It is delivered to the chest wall and regional lymph node basins in the axilla, infraclavicular, supraclavicular, and internal mammary regions in standard fractionation, with a boost to the chest wall scar. Any area with pretreatment skin involvement should receive radiation to decrease the risk of local recurrence.

4. **C.** IBC is treated with a multidisciplinary/multimodality approach, combining local and systemic

treatments. Local treatment modalities are surgery and radiation therapy, whereas chemotherapy and endocrine therapy are utilized as systemic therapies. However, in regard to endocrine therapy, most IBCs are ER/PR negative, so there would be no role for endocrine therapy in those patients. This combination and order of neoadjuvant chemotherapy, MRM, and PMRT will improve local disease control, thus decreasing risk of local recurrence. MRM is most effective if a patient has a good clinical response (decrease in skin erythema and edema) to neoadjuvant chemotherapy, and particularly so in patients who have a pCR to neoadjuvant chemotherapy. This multimodality treatment plan has improved survival, particularly disease-free survival.

5. **B.** In IBC, tumor emboli invade the dermal lymphatic vessels, causing an obstruction, which leads to the edema, induration, and peau d'orange appearance. The emboli invade vessels in the papillary and reticular dermis.

6. **A.** Once tissue is obtained from a core needle biopsy, the tumor will be evaluated for hormone receptors. Human epidermal growth factor receptor 2 (HER2) is overexpressed in up to 60% of cases of inflammatory breast cancer. Patients with tumors that have overexpression of HER2 should receive directed therapy with Trastuzumab in addition to systemic chemotherapy. Prospective studies have shown that the addition of Trastuzumab to an anthracycline-based chemotherapy regimen in women with locally invasive breast cancer, including those with inflammatory breast cancer, significantly improves pCR.

The Oncotype DX genomic assay is a prognostic assay used to identify patients who are most and least likely to benefit from adjuvant chemotherapy. It does not apply in inflammatory breast cancer. It is only indicated in patients without nodal involvement, who are estrogen receptor (ER) positive, and are HER2 negative. All patients with inflammatory breast cancer will receive adjuvant chemotherapy, so performing an Oncotype DX assay plays no role in directing patient treatment.

Microcalcifications can be seen in atypical breast lesions, ductal carcinoma in situ (DCIS), and invasive ductal carcinoma. However, the presence or absence of microcalcifications will not affect the treatment of inflammatory breast cancer. Comedo necrosis can be seen with DCIS, not inflammatory breast cancer.

7. **C.** The approach to the surveillance of inflammatory breast cancer after primary treatment is the same as that for noninflammatory breast cancer. Surveillance includes a history and physical examination every 3 to 6 months for the first 3 years, every 6 to 12 months for years 4 and 5, and then annually thereafter. A mammogram of the contralateral breast should be obtained yearly.

There is some controversy around the recommendation for women to perform monthly self-breast exams. *The performance of monthly self-breast exams is neither universally encouraged nor discouraged.* Screening mammograms every year to every 2 years are recommended by expert groups for the screening of breast cancer and would not be appropriate for surveillance in a patient who has undergone treatment for inflammatory breast cancer.

Breast MRIs alternating with mammograms every 6 months is the breast cancer *screening recommendation for women who are at high risk for breast cancer.* High-risk patients include those known to have a BRCA mutation, those with a first-degree relative who has a known BRCA mutation but the patient has not been tested themselves, lifetime risk of developing breast cancer of >20% to 25%, patients with a history of radiation to the chest between age 10 and 30, and patients with Li-Fraumeni syndrome or Cowden and Bannayan-Riley-Ruvalcaba syndromes. Breast MRIs alternating with diagnostic mammography every 6 months is not appropriate for surveillance of inflammatory breast cancer.

Close follow-up for patients after primary treatment of inflammatory breast cancer is required and no further follow-up or simply just an annual examination would not be standard of care.

BIBLIOGRAPHY

ASCO 2006 update of the breast cancer follow-up and management guideline in the adjuvant setting. *J Oncol Pract.* 2006;2(6):317–318.

Dawood S, Merajver S, Viens P, et al. International expert panel on inflammatory breast cancer: consensus statement for standardized diagnosis and treatment. *Ann Oncol.* 2011;22(3):515–523.

Duskin H, Cristofanilli M. Inflammatory breast cancer. *J Natl Compr Canc Netw.* 2011;9:233–241.

Hunt, KK, Mittendorf, EA. Diseases of the breast. In: Townsend CM Jr, Beauchamp, RD, Evers BM, et al. eds. *Sabiston Textbook of Surgery: The Biological Bases of Modern Surgical Practice.* 2nd ed. Elsevier; 2017: 820–864.

Khan AJ, Haffty BG. Postmastectomy radiation therapy. In: Kuerer HM, ed. *Kuerer's Breast Surgical Oncology.* McGraw-Hill; 2010: 995–1008.

Li BD, Sicard MA, Ampil F, et al. Trimodal therapy for inflammatory breast cancer: a surgeon's perspective. *Oncology.* 2010;79:3–12.

Makower D, Sparano JA. How do I treat inflammatory breast cancer? *Curr Treat Options Oncol.* 2013;14:66–74.

McVeigh TP, Kerin, MJ. Clinical use of the Oncotype DX genomic test to guide treatment decisions for patients with invasive breast cancer. *Breast Cancer: Targets and Therapy.* 2017;9:393–400.

National Comprehensive Cancer Network Guidelines Version 2.2011. Inflammatory breast cancer, IBC-1. NCCN breast cancer clinical practice guidelines in oncology. Available at http://www.nccn.org/professionals/physician_gls/PDF/breast.pdf. Accessed June 1, 2014.

National Comprehensive Cancer Network Guidelines Version 3.2020. NCCN clinical practice guidelines in oncology: breast cancer. Available at https://www.nccn.org/professionals/physician_gls/pdf/breast.pdf.

Negron Gonzalez V, Oh JL, Cristofanilli M. Inflammatory breast cancer. In: Kuerer HM, ed. *Kuerer's Breast Surgical Oncology.* McGraw-Hill; 2010: 927–936.

Neuman HB, Van Zee KJ. Axillary lymph node dissection. In: Kuerer HM, ed. *Kuerer's Breast Surgical Oncology.* McGraw-Hill; 2010: 679–691.

Rao R, Leitch AM. Modified radical mastectomy and techniques for avoiding skin necrosis. In: Kuerer HM, ed. *Kuerer's Breast Surgical Oncology.* McGraw-Hill; 2010: 693–697.

Recht A, Edge SB, Solin LJ, et al. Postmastectomy radiotherapy: guidelines of the American Society of Clinical Oncology. *J Clin Oncol.* 2001;19(5):1539–1569.

Rehman S, Reddy CA, Tendulkar RD. Modern outcomes of inflammatory breast cancer. *Int J Radiation Oncol Biol Phys.* 2012;84(3):619–624.

Robertson FM, Bony M, Yang, W, et al. Inflammatory breast cancer: the disease, the biology, the treatment. *CA Cancer J Clin.* 2010;60:351–375.

Saigal K, Hurley J, Takita C, et al. Risk factors for locoregional failure in patients with inflammatory breast cancer treated with trimodality therapy. *Clin Breast Cancer.* 2013;13(5):335–343.

Saslow D, Boetes C, Burke W, et al. American Cancer Society Guidelines for breast screening with MRI as an adjunct to mammography. *CA: A Cancer J Clin.* 2007;57(2):75–89.

Yamauchi H, Woodward, WA, Ueno, NT. Inflammatory breast cancer: what we know and what we need to learn. *The Oncologist.* 2012:17(7):891–899.

Zellars R. Post-mastectomy radiotherapy. *Clin Adv Hematol Oncol.* 2009;7(8):533–543.

48

Breast Reconstruction

Ally Ha

A 42-year-old female with a history of left thoracotomy, open cholecystectomy, and diastasis recti recently underwent core-needle biopsy of a palpable 4-cm left breast mass in the upper outer quadrant that revealed invasive ductal carcinoma on pathology. On physical exam, she has no other palpable lesions and no clinical lymphadenopathy. Metastatic workup is negative. She would like to discuss mastectomy and reconstruction options.

1. **Regarding reconstruction, which of the following is correct?**

   A. Autologous tissue reconstruction is preferred over implant reconstruction.

   B. Breastfeeding is not recommended after implant reconstruction due to possible silicone leakage into breast milk.

   C. Cancer surveillance is adequate even with reconstruction.

   D. Smoking is an absolute contraindication for autologous tissue reconstruction.

   E. Immediate autologous and implant reconstruction significantly delays subsequent adjuvant therapy.

2. **The patient inquires about a nipple-sparing mastectomy. Which of the following is a contraindication to this procedure?**

   A. 3-cm tumor

   B. Paget's disease

   C. A large tumor-to-areola distance

   D. Positive axillary lymph nodes

   E. Multifocal disease

3. **Which of the following is an advantage of autologous tissue reconstruction over implant reconstruction?**

   A. Better symmetry with the contralateral breast

   B. Shorter operating time

   C. Shorter inpatient hospitalization

   D. Lower potential for the need of blood transfusion

   E. Less chance for flap loss

4. **The patient is interested in a left mastectomy with autologous reconstruction. What is the best option in this patient?**

   A. Pedicled Transverse Rectus Abdominus Myocutaneous (TRAM) flap

   B. Free TRAM flap

   C. Latissimus dorsi flap

   D. Deep Inferior Epigastric Perforator (DIEP) flap

5. **The patient undergoes a left skin-sparing mastectomy and sentinel lymph node biopsy with tissue expander placement at the time of surgery. Which of the following factors would increase the patient's risk of complications associated with implant reconstruction?**

   A. 5-cm tumor

   B. Four positive lymph nodes

   C. Sentinel lymph node biopsy containing micrometastases

   D. 1-mm negative margins

ANSWERS

1. **C.** Autologous or implant breast reconstruction has not been shown to decrease the ability to detect local

or locoregional breast cancer recurrence. Multiple studies have shown that reconstruction after mastectomy with a variety of methods does not adversely affect the incidence or time to detection of recurrent breast cancer. Furthermore, reconstruction does not change recommended surveillance methods. It is debatable whether immediate breast reconstruction delays adjuvant therapy due to a higher likelihood of postoperative wound complications, but this has not been shown to impact cancer-specific survival.

The choice between autologous or implant reconstruction and its timing is influenced by a number of factors, including patient preference, comorbidities, previous surgeries, body habitus (availability of autologous tissue), and radiation therapy. While heavy smoking is not an absolute contraindication for autologous tissue reconstruction, it does influence the type of available autologous options. Therefore, the preoperative discussion about the various reconstruction options and informed consent process is critical to a patient's reconstructive expectations, success, and satisfaction.

The possibility of implants affecting breast milk has been addressed in studies comparing silicone levels in breast milk from women with or without silicone gel breast implants. There is no evidence of elevated silicone in breast milk or any other substance that would be deleterious to infants. Therefore, all mothers with implants should attempt breastfeeding.

2. B. The literature suggests that the nipple-sparing mastectomy is oncologically safe with a clearly defined set of pathologic parameters. Absolute contraindications to nipple-sparing mastectomy include inflammatory breast cancer, tumors involving the nipple-areolar complex, and tumors that present with pathologic nipple discharge.

3. A. Autologous reconstruction involves the transfer of vascularized muscle, subcutaneous tissue, and skin to the mastectomy defect. Tissue can be transferred on a vascular pedicle or as a free flap requiring a microsurgical anastomosis. Autologous reconstruction typically allows for a more natural-appearing breast contour than implant reconstruction and frequently eliminates the need for contralateral symmetry procedures. Consequently, it is associated with fewer revision surgeries. Furthermore, for patients who have undergone radiation therapy, delayed autologous tissue reconstruction is preferred because tissue-expander/implant reconstruction in previously irradiated tissues has a higher risk of capsular contraction, malposition, poor cosmesis, and implant exposure. Disadvantages of autologous reconstruction include longer operative times, longer inpatient hospitalizations, potentially higher need for blood transfusion, morbidity associated with the donor site, and the potential for total flap loss.

4. D. A pedicled TRAM flap utilizes the superior deep epigastric vessels and involves the tunneling of the entire rectus abdominus muscle and fascia, resulting in significant abdominal wall weakness. The superior epigastric vessels are not as robust as the inferior epigastric vessels, so in patients with higher risks (i.e., diabetics and smokers), the deep inferior epigastric vessels can be ligated 2 weeks prior to the planned reconstruction to allow the vascular choke vessels to dilate. Surgeries that disrupt the vascular supply (i.e., subcostal or paramedian incisions) are a contraindication to this flap option.

Transverse Rectus Abdominis Myocutaneous (TRAM) Flap Surgery

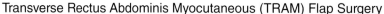
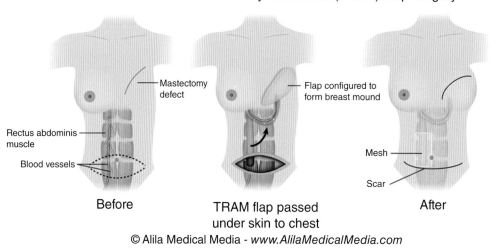

Mastectomy defect

Rectus abdominis muscle

Blood vessels

Before

TRAM flap passed under skin to chest

Flap configured to form breast mound

Mesh

Scar

After

© Alila Medical Media - www.AlilaMedicalMedia.com

A free TRAM flap utilizes the deep inferior epigastric vessels that are anastomosed to the thoracodorsal vessels in the axilla or the internal mammary vessels in the chest wall. A minimal amount of rectus abdominus muscle and fascia is required in this option, which minimizes the donor site morbidity and abdominal wall weakness. This option would be inferior to a DIEP flap, which completely spares the rectus muscle.

The latissimus dorsi muscle can be used as a myocutaneous or a muscle-only flap. While it can be used without an implant in patients with smaller breasts, this muscle flap usually provides inadequate autologous tissue for complete reconstruction, so it is typically used in combination with a permanent implant following a period of tissue expansion. Patients who have undergone prior thoracotomy are not candidates for this option and those who have undergone axillary node dissection should be considered for preoperative computed tomography (CT) angiography to ensure patency of the thoracodorsal vessels. Sacrifice of the latissimus dorsi muscle generally results in minimal functional deficits, except for certain competitive athletes.

In a DIEP flap, the perforating vessels are dissected completely from the rectus muscle and transferred to the chest wall as a free flap. These flaps have longer pedicle lengths and completely spare the rectus muscle, resulting in less abdominal wall morbidity when

Free TRAM Flap Surgery

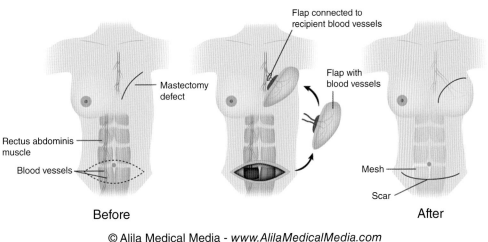

Flap connected to recipient blood vessels

Mastectomy defect

Flap with blood vessels

Rectus abdominis muscle

Blood vessels

Mesh

Scar

Before

After

© Alila Medical Media - *www.AlilaMedicalMedia.com*

Latissimus Dorsi Flap

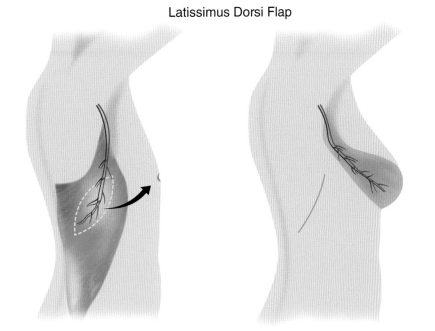

© Alila Medical Media - *www.AlilaMedicalMedia.com*

Deep Inferior Epigastric Perforator Flap

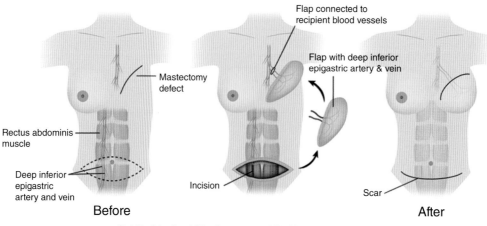

© Alila Medical Media - www.AlilaMedicalMedia.com

compared with TRAM flaps. Previous extensive abdominal wall surgeries (i.e., ventral hernia repairs) and abdominoplasties are contraindications due to disruption of the vascular supply.

5. B. Because of the local tissue effects of radiation therapy, autologous tissue options are preferred over implant-based techniques in previously irradiated patients. It is, however, recommended to wait 6 to 12 months following radiation to perform a microvascular anastomosis.

According to the 2020 NCCN guidelines on invasive breast cancer, for patients with T1-3, N0-1, M0 disease who undergo mastectomy with surgical axillary staging, those with positive margins for which re-excision is not feasible, tumors >5 cm (pT3), or one to three positive axillary lymph nodes (pN1) should consider radiation therapy while those with four or more positive lymph nodes (pN2) should receive radiation therapy to the chest wall, infraclavicular region, supraclavicular area, internal mammary nodes, and any part of the axillary bed at risk. Micrometastasis and 1-mm negative margins are not absolute indications for adjuvant radiation therapy.

BIBLIOGRAPHY

Adesiyun TA, Lee BT, Yueh JH, et al. Impact of sequencing of postmastectomy radiotherapy and breast reconstruction on timing and rate of complications and patient satisfaction. *Int J Radiat Oncol Biol Phys.* 2011;80:392.

Bezuhly M, Temple C, Sigurdson LJ, et al. Immediate post mastectomy reconstruction is associated with improved breast cancer-specific survival: evidence and new challenges from the Surveillance, Epidemiology, and End Results database. *Cancer.* 2009;115(20):4648–4654.

Black CK, Graziano FD, Fan KL, et al. Combining abdominal flaps and implants in the breast reconstruction patient: a systematic and retrospective review of complications and outcomes. *Plast Reconstr Surg.* 2019;143:495e.

Chang EI, Liu TS, Festekjian JH, et al. Effects of radiation therapy for breast cancer based on type of free flap reconstruction. *Plast Reconstr Surg.* 2013;131:1e–8e.

Fitoussi AD, Berry MG, Famà F, et al. Oncoplastic breast surgery for cancer: analysis of 540 consecutive cases. *Plast Reconstr Surg.* 2010;125:454.

Fosnot J, Fischer JP, Smartt JM Jr, et al. Does previous chest wall irradiation increase vascular complications in free autologous breast reconstruction? *Plast Reconstr Surg.* 2011;127:496.

Gucwa A, Harper JG, Lind DS. Chapter 5: Breast procedures. In: Ashley SW, ed. *ACS Surgery [Online]*. Decker Intellectual Properties; 2009.

Kwon DS, Kelly CM, Ching CD. Invasive breast cancer. In: Feig BW, Ching CD, eds. *MD Anderson Surgical Oncology Handbook*. 5th ed. [Kindle edition]. Lippincott Williams & Wilkins; 2012.

Losken A, Dugal CS, Styblo TM, Carlson GW. A meta-analysis comparing breast conservation therapy alone to the oncoplastic technique. *Ann Plast Surg.* 2014;72:145.

Mirzabeigi MN, Smartt JM, Nelson JA, et al. An assessment of the risks and benefits of immediate autologous breast reconstruction in patients undergoing postmastectomy radiation therapy. *Ann Plast Surg.* 2013;71:149.

Nahabedian MY. Breast reconstruction after mastectomy: indications, technique, and results. In: Cameron JL, Cameron AM, eds. *Current Surgical Therapy: Expert Consult.* 10th ed. Online. Elsevier Health Sciences; 2011.

Nahabedian MY, Momen B. The impact of breast reconstruction on the oncologic efficacy of radiation therapy: a retrospective analysis. *Ann Plast Surg.* 2008;60:244.

National Comprehensive Cancer Network. Breast cancer (version 3.2020). https://www.nccn.org/professionals/physician_gls/pdf/breast.pdf.

Namnoum JD. Breast reconstruction: TRAM flap techniques. In: Thome CH, ed. *Grabb and Smith's Plastic Surgery*. 6th ed. Lippincott Williams & Wilkins; 2007: 641–647.

Reddy S, Colakoglu S, Curtis MS, et al. Breast cancer recurrence following post mastectomy reconstruction compared to mastectomy with no reconstruction. *Ann Plast Surg*. 2011;66(5):466–471.

Rietjens M, Urban CA, Rey PC, et al. Long-term oncological results of breast conservative treatment with oncoplastic surgery. *Breast*. 2007;16:387–395.

Semple JL. Breast-feeding and silicone implants. *Plast Reconstr Surg*. 2007;120:123S.

Spear SL, Onyewu C. Staged breast reconstruction with saline-filled implants in the irradiated breast: recent trends and therapeutic implications. *Plast Reconstr Surg*. 2000;105:930.

49

Adrenal Gland Tumors

Yong Choi

A 35-year-old female presents with a 3-cm mass in the left adrenal gland that was incidentally found on a computed tomography (CT) scan done for diffuse abdominal pain. The patient reports intermittent increases in blood pressure but she does not take any anti-hypertensive medications. She has no other complaints. She has no significant past medical history and her only past surgery is a laparoscopic appendectomy 15 years ago. She does have a sister who had a total thyroidectomy for medullary carcinoma of the thyroid gland. She is referred to the general surgery clinic by her primary care physician for evaluation of this left adrenal gland.

1. **Regarding the workup of this adrenal mass, which of the following is correct?**

   A. Diagnosis of Cushing's syndrome is suggested by suppression of plasma cortisol levels after an overnight low-dose dexamethasone test.

   B. Patients with primary cortisol producing adenomas have elevated cortisol levels and low plasma adrenocorticotropic hormone (ACTH).

   C. The risk of adrenal carcinoma is increased due to the size of this adrenal mass.

   D. Percutaneous biopsy of this mass is critical in making the diagnosis.

2. **Due to the history of intermittent hypertension, the patient is evaluated for a pheochromocytoma. Which of the following is correct?**

   A. Plasma-free metanephrine levels but not normetanephrine levels are sensitive markers for pheochromocytoma.

   B. Monoamine oxidase inhibitors (MAOIs) can falsely elevate plasma-free metanephrine and normetanephrine levels.

   C. Pheochromocytoma on a CT scan is represented by venous phase enhancement exclusively.

   D. Pheochromocytomas represent the majority of incidentalomas found on a CT scan.

3. **In relation to perioperative considerations in patients with adrenal tumors, which of the following is true?**

   A. In patients with pheochromocytoma, beta blockade should be initiated prior to alpha-adrenergic blockade.

   B. Tumor manipulation may stimulate sudden catecholamine release during the surgery.

   C. Patients with an aldosterone secreting adrenal tumor will most likely have hyperkalemia.

   D. Patients with cortisol producing tumor should not receive heparin due to their coagulopathy.

4. **Which of the following is correct regarding the natural history/treatment of the adrenal mass in this patient?**

   A. Due to the size of the mass (3 cm), the patient should be taken for an adrenalectomy even if the mass is nonfunctional.

   B. Since the patient has a family history of medullary carcinoma of the thyroid, she should be taken for an adrenalectomy.

   C. Metastatic cancer presenting as a true adrenal incidentaloma is common.

   D. This patient can be followed with serial CT scans.

5. **Which of the following statements on operative treatment/technique is correct?**

   A. The right adrenal vein is identified as it enters directly into the vena cava.

   B. Laparoscopic adrenalectomy should not be performed if the patient has adrenal carcinoma.

   C. For benign disease, laparoscopic adrenalectomy is clearly superior over the open adrenalectomy.

   D. Posterior retroperitoneal approach has a higher risk of injury to the liver and spleen compared to the transabdominal approach.

6. **The patient tells you that she has been researching robotic use in surgical procedures. Which of the following is a true statement regarding robotic adrenalectomies?**

   A. There is a low conversion rate of robotic adrenalectomies to an open procedure.

   B. The robotic approach has an equivalent overall cost compared to the laparoscopic approach.

   C. Robotic adrenalectomy has a lower learning curve than traditional laparoscopic surgery.

   D. Robotic adrenalectomy has a shorter hospital stay.

ANSWERS

1. **B.** The diagnosis of Cushing's syndrome can be accomplished by a dexamethasone suppression test. Patients with Cushing's syndrome fail to suppress plasma cortisol levels after an overnight low-dose dexamethasone suppression test. In addition, these patients have an elevated 24-hour urine-free cortisol level. Once diagnosis of Cushing's syndrome is confirmed, further tests can be performed to identify the cause.

   Patients with primary cortisol producing adenomas have elevated cortisol levels and a low ACTH level. In addition, these patients should have a CT scan or MRI finding of an adrenal mass. Approximately 20% of patients with Cushing's syndrome are due to a cortisol-producing adenoma. The signs and symptoms of Cushing's syndrome include weight gain, hypertension, diabetes mellitus, and centripetal obesity. Other causes of Cushing's syndrome are aldosteronomas and adrenocortical carcinomas, although these are rare.

   This patient's adrenal mass is 3 cm in size. Adrenal cortical carcinoma should be suspected with adrenal masses greater than 6 cm. The risk of a 3-cm adrenal mass being a carcinoma is very low.

   Percutaneous biopsy of an adrenal mass is not commonly performed. One indication for a percutaneous biopsy is obtaining tissue diagnosis prior to initiating treatment on a patient who has adrenal metastasis on imaging. A biopsy should not be performed on patients suspected to have pheochromocytoma due to the possibility of precipitating a hypertensive crisis. As a rule, percutaneous biopsy has a minimal role in the diagnosis of an adrenal mass.

2. **B.** Pheochromocytoma evaluation is necessary in all patients with an adrenal mass, even if they have no signs or symptoms of tachycardia, severe hypertension, cardiac palpitations, arrhythmias, anxiety, and sweating. Plasma-free metanephrine and normetanephrine levels are sensitive markers for pheochromocytoma and are easier to obtain than a 24-hour urine collection. The plasma-free metanephrine and normetanephrine levels should be three to four times the normal in patients with pheochromocytoma.

   Some medications can falsely elevate plasma-free metanephrine and normetanephrine levels. These include MAOIs, tricyclic antidepressants, decongestants, amphetamines, and phenoxybenzamine. If possible, these medications should be discontinued prior to testing for pheochromocytoma.

   Pheochromocytomas are hypervascular and they have intense enhancement on the arterial phase of the CT scan. They also have a slow washout on delayed imaging. With a non-contrast CT scan, the density of pheochromocytoma is similar to that seen in muscle. They also represent a small percentage of all incidentalomas found on a CT scan, comprising 0% to 11%. Nonfunctioning adrenal adenomas are the most common incidentalomas found on CT scan examinations.

3. **B.** All patients with a diagnosis of pheochromocytoma should undergo alpha-adrenergic blockade. This should be initiated approximately 1 to 2 weeks before surgery. Alpha blockade should help with blood pressure control and control of intraoperative arrhythmias. After initiation of alpha blockade, beta-blockers can be used in patients with persistent tachycardia or hypertension. Some side effects of alpha blockers are fatigue, loose stools, dizziness, and somnolence.

During the surgery for pheochromocytoma, careful dissection of the adrenal gland must be performed due to the fact that tumor manipulation may cause a sudden release of catecholamines. This may result in a sharp increase in blood pressure and bleeding from the small vessels. Immediate cessation of manipulation of the adrenal gland will help normalize the blood pressure. Good communication with the anesthesiologist throughout the procedure is necessary.

Patients with an aldosterone-secreting adrenal tumor have hypokalemia. The aldosterone causes the distal renal tubules to increase sodium and water resorption and thereby increasing the potassium loss, resulting in hypokalemia. Hypokalemia is associated with increased risk of arrhythmias. Therefore, oral and intravenous supplementation should be given to correct the hypokalemia.

Patients with cortisol-producing tumors are hypercoagulable due to the hyperhomocysteinemia, increased clotting factors, impaired fibrinolysis, and abnormalities in von-Willebrand factor. Therefore, these patients should be considered for preoperative heparin injection to decrease the risk of venous thromboembolic events.

4. **D.** Adrenocortical carcinoma is not common and the frequency ranges from 1.2% to 12% of all incidentalomas found on CT scan. Carcinoma is rare for an adrenal mass size of less than 4 cm. Malignant transformation should be considered if a mass enlarges by 1 to 2 cm over 1 to 3 years. Since this patient has an adrenal mass of 3 cm, it can be followed by serial CT scans if the mass is nonfunctional. However, with increased use of CT scans and other imaging modalities, a greater number of adrenal masses are being discovered incidentally. However, with a mass greater than 4 cm, the risk of cancer is 10% and nearly doubles to 19% when the mass is greater than 6 cm in size. A mass greater than 8 cm has a 47% chance of being malignant. In addition to size of the mass, imaging characteristics can raise suspicion for cancer. These include Hounsfield Units >10 on CT scan or presence of signal on out of phase MR.

With a family history of medullary carcinoma of the thyroid, multiple endocrine neoplasia (MEN) syndrome must be considered. However, if the patient has a nonfunctioning adrenal adenoma and workup for pheochromocytoma is negative, there is no need to perform an adrenalectomy in a 3-cm adrenal mass.

Metastatic cancer presenting as a true adrenal incidentaloma is extremely rare. In a study by Lee et al., only 0.2% of patients had unknown primary cancer presenting as an adrenal mass. All of these patients had tumor sizes greater than or equal to 6 cm. Adrenal carcinomas may be isolated metastasis from other primary malignant neoplasms. When these lesions are isolated to the adrenal gland, surgical resection is beneficial for survival. With the advancements of laparoscopic surgery, it has been shown to be equivalent to open surgery for obtaining negative margins, local recurrence, disease-free survival, and overall survival.

In addition to the use of laparoscopic surgery in the resection of isolated metastasis to the adrenal gland, it can be safe and feasible for primary adrenocortical carcinomas. While there are some concerns about the use of laparoscopic surgery in large carcinomas due to the ability to obtain negative margins, it has been effectively used in small adrenocortical carcinomas. With proper training and experience, laparoscopic adrenalectomy has been shown to be safe and effective in carefully selected patients. Adrenocortical carcinoma is not an absolute contraindication to laparoscopic surgery.

Carcinomas of the adrenal gland have very poor prognosis. They have a high recurrence rate and often present late in the stage of disease. The estimated 5-year survival can range from 82% for stage I disease down to 13% for stage IV disease.

5. **A.** The anatomy of the right adrenal gland is different from the left in that the adrenal vein enters directly into the inferior vena cava (IVC). Therefore, during the operative approach, a plane is developed between the lateral aspect of the IVC and the medial border of the adrenal gland. The vein is double clipped or stapled with an Endo-GIA. On the left side, the adrenal vein drains into the left renal vein.

There is no clear literature on the use of laparoscopic adrenalectomy for adrenal carcinoma. Reviews have been done that show the laparoscopic approach to be equal to an open approach; and in a NSQIP review of over 600 patients, the laparoscopic approach was associated with shorter operations, shorter hospital stays, less transfusions, fewer reoperations, and less 30-day mortality. However, the surgeon has to be aware of the possibility of invasion to other structures. In cases of large adrenal cancers or invasion, an open approach may be advisable.

However, small lesions suspicious for carcinoma can be performed by the laparoscopic approach.

As the technique of laparoscopic adrenalectomy has grown in use, it is now considered a standard of care for small benign lesions. However, like laparoscopic cholecystectomy, there have not been randomized controlled trials comparing open to laparoscopic adrenalectomy.

There are two basic approaches to laparoscopic adrenalectomy: the transabdominal and the posterior retroperitoneal. The laparoscopic posterior retroperitoneal adrenalectomy has certain advantages over the standard transabdominal approach. It eliminates the need to retract the liver for the right side and the spleen for the left side. It also reduces the risk of injury to organs such as the liver and spleen. However, patient selection is important and it can be technically more demanding than the transabdominal approach.

6. A. There have been significant advances in minimally invasive and robotic surgery through the years. Laparoscopic adrenalectomy is now accepted as the treatment of choice in the surgical management of benign adrenal diseases. With the rise of robotic surgery, more and more general surgery procedures are utilizing the robot. Therefore, surgeons today need to be well informed on both robotic and laparoscopic approaches to various disease processes.

Robotic adrenalectomy has been shown to be safe. Review of the literature reveals that the conversion rates to open procedures are very low (as low as 2.5% to 3%). With increase in experience, the conversion rates go down. Blood loss is also very low with the use of the robot.

There is always some controversy with calculating the costs for robotic procedures. The SAGES guidelines for minimally invasive treatment of adrenal pathology concluded that there was an increased cost with the robot compared to laparoscopic procedures. Along with the high cost, the learning curve for the use of the robot in adrenal surgery is high. This learning curve does not only affect the surgeon, but it affects the entire surgical team. Often, the increased learning curve can place a barrier in instituting robotic adrenalectomy as an option for a patient.

The length of stay for patients after adrenalectomy is very similar between robotic and laparoscopic. Typically, patients were discharged after 1 to 2 days.

It is difficult to show a statistically significant difference in length of stay due to the advancements allowing for patients to be discharged faster from the hospital after surgical procedures.

BIBLIOGRAPHY

Abiven G, Coste J, Groussin L, et al. Clinical and biological features in the prognosis of adrenocortical cancer: poor outcome of cortisol-secreting tumors in a series of 202 consecutive patients. *J Clin Endocrinol Metab*. 2006;91: 2650–2655.

Bickenbach KA, Strong VE. Laparoscopic transabdominal lateral adrenalectomy. *J Surg Onco*. 2012;106:611–618.

Bittner JG, Brunt LM. Evaluation and management of adrenal incidentaloma. *J Surg Onco*. 2012;106:557–564.

Boland GW, Blake MA, Hahn PF, et al. Incidental adrenal lesions: principles, techniques, and algorithms for imaging characterization. *Radiology*. 2008;249:756–775.

Brunaud L, Bresler L, Ayav A, et al. Robotic-assisted adrenalectomy: what advantages compared to lateral transperitoneal laparoscopic adrenalectomy? *Am J Surg*. 2008;195: 433–438.

Brunt LM, Moley JF. Adrenal incidentaloma. *World J. Surg*. 2001;25:905–913.

Duh QY. Resecting isolated adrenal metastasis: why and how? *Ann Surg Oncol*. 2003;10:1138–1139.

Fassnacht M, Johanssen S, Quinkler M, et al. Limited prognostic value of the 2004 International Union Against Cancer staging classification for adrenocortical carcinoma: proposal for a revised TNM classification. *Cancer*. 2009;115: 243–250.

Greilsamer T, Nomine-Criqui C, Thy M, et al. Robotic-assisted unilateral adrenalectomy: risk factors for perioperative complications in 303 consecutive patients. *Surg Endosc*. 2019;33:802–810.

Huynh KT, Lee DY, Lau BJ, et al. Impact of laparoscopic adrenalectomy on overall survival in patients with nonmetastatic adrenocortical carcinoma. *J Am Coll Surg*. 2016;223(3): 485–492.

Kahramangil B, Berber E. Comparison of posterior retroperitoneal and transabdominal lateral approaches in robotic adrenalectomy: an analysis of 200 cases. *Surg Endosc*. 2018;32:1984–1989.

Kim SH, Brennan MF, Russo P, et al. The role of surgery in the treatment of clinically isolated adrenal metastasis. *Cancer*. 1998;82:389–394.

Lee J, El-Tamer M, Schifftner T, et al. Open and laparoscopic adrenalectomy: analysis of the National Surgical Quality Improvement Program. *J AM Coll Surg*. 2008;206(5): 953–959.

Lee JE, Evans DB, Hickey RC, et al. Unknown primary cancer presenting as an adrenal mass: frequency and implications for diagnostic evaluation of adrenal incidentalomas. *Surgery*. 1998;124:1115–1122.

Malayeri AA, Zaheer A, Fishman EK, et al. Adrenal masses: contemporary imaging characterization. *J Comput Assist Tomogr*. 2013;37:528–542.

Mansmann G, Lau J, Balk E, et al. The clinically inapparent adrenal mass: update in diagnosis and management. *Endocr Rev.* 2004;25:309–340.

Morino M, Beninca G, Giraudo G, et al. Robot-assisted vs laparoscopic adrenalectomy: a prospective randomized controlled trial. *Surg Endosc.* 2004;18:1742–1746.

Nordenstrom E, Westerdahl J, Hallgrimsson P, et al. A prospective study of 100 robotically assisted laparoscopic adrenalectomies. *J Robot Surg.* 2011;5:127–131.

Phitayakorn R, McHenry CR. Perioperative considerations in patients with adrenal tumors. *J Surg Onco.* 2012;106: 604–610.

Pineda-Solis K, Medina-Franco H. Robotic versus laparoscopic adrenalectomy: a comparative study in high-volume center. *Surg Endosc.* 2013;27:599–602.

Sarela AI, Murphy I, Coit DG, et al. Metastasis to the adrenal gland: the emerging role of laparoscopic surgery. *Ann Surg Oncol.* 2003;10:1191–1196.

Stefanidis D, Goldfarb M, Kercher KW, et al. SAGES guidelines for minimally invasive treatment of adrenal pathology. *Surg Endosc.* 2013;27:3960–3980.

Strong VE, Angelica MD, Tang L, et al. Laparoscopic adrenalectomy for isolated adrenal metastasis. *Ann Surg Oncol.* 2007;14(12):3392–3400.

Sturgeon C, Shen WT, C OH, et al. Risk assessment in 457 adrenal cortical carcinomas: how much does tumor size predict the likelihood of malignancy? *J Am Coll Surg.* 2006;202(3):423–430.

Taskin HE, Siperstein A, Mercan S, et al. Laparoscopic posterior retroperitoneal adrenalectomy. *J Surg Onco.* 2012;106:619–621.

Terzolo M, Stigliano A, Chiodini I, et al. AME position statement on adrenal incidentaloma. *Euro J Endocrinology.* 2011;164:851–870.

Vazquez BJ, Richards ML, Lohse CM, et al. Adrenalectomy improves outcomes of selected patients with metastatic carcinoma. *World J Surg.* 2012;36:1400–1405.

Winter JM, Talamini MA, Stanfield CL, et al. Thirty robotic adrenalectomies: a single institution's experience. *Surg Endosc.* 2006;20:119–124.

Yoo JY, McCoy KL, Carty SE, et al. Adrenal imaging features predict malignancy better than tumor size. *Ann Surg Oncol.* 2015;22:S721–S727.

50

Hyperparathyroidism

Jill Findlay, MD

A 30-year-old female is referred to your practice for evaluation of hypercalcemia by her primary care physician. A chemistry panel performed for her insurance a month ago shows an elevation of her serum calcium levels. Her primary care physician reordered the chemistry panel two days ago, which shows a persistent calcium elevation but her urinalysis and complete blood count (CBC) are also normal. He is concerned she may have primary hyperparathyroidism. The patient states she feels fine. Her past medical history is significant for a kidney stone a couple of years ago. Her physical exam is unremarkable.

1. **You decide to check the patient's parathyroid hormone level. If the patient has primary hyperparathyroidism, which of the following would be true?**

   A. Low ionized calcium
   B. Increased phosphate
   C. Decreased chloride
   D. Decreased alkaline phosphatase
   E. Normal parathyroid hormone (PTH) level

2. **The patient's parathyroid hormone (PTH) level and following 24-hour urinary collection for calcium and creatinine excretion confirm your suspicion of primary hyperparathyroidism. You obtain a sestamibi scan for preoperative planning that shows a likely adenoma of the right lower parathyroid gland. Your management of this patient would be:**

   A. Repeat observation and follow up
   B. Bilateral neck exploration with identification of all four parathyroid glands and subtotal resection of 3½ glands

   C. Bilateral neck exploration with identification of all four parathyroid glands and removal of the abnormal parathyroid adenoma
   D. Bilateral neck exploration with identification of all four parathyroid glands with total resection of all four glands and reimplantation of ½ a normal gland in the sternocleidomastoid muscle

3. **During your parathyroidectomy for the above patient, you are unable to locate the right lower parathyroid gland despite finding the other three normal-appearing glands. The next step would be:**

   A. Close up and repeat sestamibi scan
   B. Right thyroid lobectomy
   C. Explore the retroesophageal space.
   D. Perform a partial median sternotomy.
   E. Selective venous sampling for parathyroid hormone

4. **If the patient had opted for a minimally invasive approach, how is intraoperative PTH level monitoring used to help aid in confirmation of successfully parathyroidectomy?**

   A. Send the PTH level when the patient is in the post anesthesia care unit (PACU).
   B. Send the PTH level immediately after parathyroid gland is excised, if normal, can close and complete surgery, if still abnormal, continue search for additional abnormal parathyroids.
   C. Send the PTH level 10 minutes after parathyroid gland excision. If >50% drop from pre-incision PTH level, then can close and complete operation. If <50% drop, obtain additional level at 20 minutes, or continue the search for additional hyperfunctioning glands.

D. Send the PTH level 10 mins after parathyroid gland excision. If >90% drop from pre-incision PTH level, then can close and complete the operation. If <90% drop, continue the search for additional hyperfunctioning gland.

5. **Acute kidney injury (AKI) of agreeing to a parathyroidectomy after initial workup and evaluation, your patient has refused surgery since she feels she is asymptomatic. Three years later, she is brought into the emergency room, after multiple bouts of emesis and altered mental status. She is found to be severely dehydrated, with an AKI, and has a calcium level of 15 mg/dL. What is the next best step in the management of this patient?**

   A. IV Lasix
   B. Emergent parathyroidectomy
   C. Fluid bolus in the ER, discharge home, and schedule for elective parathyroidectomy
   D. Fluid resuscitation
   E. Bisphosphonates

6. **Which of the following patients would you recommend for a parathyroidectomy?**

   A. A 55-year-old female, otherwise healthy, with incidental finding of hypercalcemia on routine labs, confirmed on repeat labs to be .5 mg/dL above the upper limit of normal. Normal DEXA scan, normal kidney function, no history of psychiatric disease, and normal PTH level.
   B. A 75-year-old male, otherwise healthy, with incidental finding of hypercalcemia on routine labs, confirmed on repeat labs to be .5 mg/dL above the upper limit of normal. Normal DEXA scan, normal kidney function, no history of psychiatric disease, and normal PTH level.
   C. A 30-year-old male, otherwise healthy, with incidental finding of hypercalcemia on routine labs, confirmed on repeat labs to be 5 mg/dL above the upper limit of normal. Normal DEXA scan, normal kidney function, no history of psychiatric disease, and normal PTH level. Due to a family history of benign hypercalcemia, his urinary calcium was noted to be low.
   D. A 55-year-old female, with CKD 3 (GFR 50), with incidental finding of hypercalcemia on routine labs, confirmed on repeat labs to be .5 mg/dL above the upper limit of normal. DEXA Scan T score of −2.75, and evidence of old vertebral fractures on recent imaging.

7. **After performing a total thyroidectomy in a 55-year-old female, the patient develops Chvostek's sign and parasthesias on post-operative day one. She is started on calcium and vitamin D replacement therapy and discharged home with those medications as well as teriparatide shots (parathyroid hormone replacement therapy). After one year postsurgery, the patient still requires calcium and vitamin D replacements as well as teriparatide shots. The likely structure injured during the thyroidectomy was the:**

   A. Superior thyroid arteries
   B. Middle thyroid veins
   C. Recurrent laryngeal nerves
   D. Most of the time, the inferior and superior parathyroid arteries are derived from branches off of the inferior thyroid artery. Another common variant is the superior parathyroid arteries arising from the anastomosing branches of the superior and inferior thyroid arteries.
   E. Superior laryngeal nerves

ANSWERS

1. **E.** Hypercalcemia or high-normal serum calcium levels with normal or elevated parathyroid hormone levels confirm primary hyperparathyroidism. Elevated calcium levels should normally suppress PTH production. Other associated lab findings of primary hyperparathyroidism may include decreased serum phosphate levels and elevated levels of serum chloride, BUN, Cr, and alkaline phosphatase.

   Primary hyperparathyroidism is usually found by routine lab testing, and most patients are asymptomatic. If symptoms are present, they usually consist of history of renal calculi, bone pain, pathologic fractures, bone shaft tumors, muscle weakness, and depression/lethargy and body aches/pains.

2. **C.** A single parathyroid adenoma causes primary hyperparathyroidism in 80% to 85% of cases. The rest of the cases are caused by parathyroid gland hyperplasia (10%), double adenomas (4%), and parathyroid carcinoma (1%). Observation and medical management is not cost effective in the management of primary hyperparathyroidism. The resection of the 3½ parathyroid glands would be most applicable to parathyroid gland hyperplasia using clinical appearance and PTH-assay before and after resection to confirm appropriate removal. There is no need to remove 3½ glands.

   A more recent alternative to the traditional approach of bilateral neck exploration and four gland identification is the removal of the parathyroid adenoma using preoperative/intraoperative gamma-probe localization with or without the use of intraoperative PTH assay. This approach (minimally invasive radioguided parathyroidectomy or MIRP) relies on the adenoma being seen on the technetium-99m sestamibi (MIBI) scan, which it does about 80% to 90% of the time. If the MIBI scan is positive, then the long-term success rate of the MIRP (98%) is equivalent to conventional four gland identification with the benefits of a significantly decreased hospital stay and the possible avoidance of general anesthesia. However, this was not one of the options.

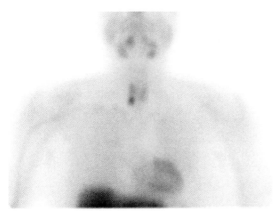

Sestamibi scan at 20 minutes' post-injection shows normal-appearing uptake in the thyroid gland and a nodular region of intense uptake in the inferior pole of the right lobe of the thyroid gland.

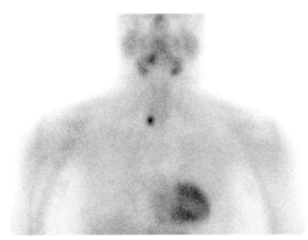

Sestamibi scan at 2 hours' post-injection shows normal washout of the thyroid with a persistent increased uptake in the region of the inferior pole of the right lobe of the thyroid gland, which is consistent with a parathyroid adenoma. (Images and descriptions courtesy of Andrew Mullins DO and John Yasmer MD)

3. **C.** Surgical excision of the parathyroid adenoma is curative of primary hyperparathyroidism in 90% to 97%. A missed parathyroid adenoma accounts for the majority of surgical treatment failures. Methods described to acquire the missing parathyroid gland via the transcervical incision include examining the retroesophageal space, the carotid sheath, the submandibular region, and the thymus gland. The most common location for a missing parathyroid adenoma is the retroesophageal space. Additional adjuncts include intraoperative ultrasound. Partial or complete thyroid lobectomy, bilateral internal jugular vein sampling of PTH to evaluate for which side of the neck the adenoma is on, and partial or complete median sternotomy are additional options to consider. If the parathyroid gland is still missing, a last approach is to ligate the inferior thyroid artery and its arterial branches on the side of the missing gland.

4. **C.** The Miami protocol was the first described, and has been well studied and validated. A PTH sample is collected pre-incision (prior to starting the operation) and pre-excision (prior to removing the gland). The PTH level is collected again 10 minutes after parathyroid gland excision, and if the PTH level drops >50% of the highest pre-excision level, the procedure is concluded without further gland exploration. If the level does not drop >50%, a repeat PTH level can be collected at 20 minutes post-gland excision, and again, if there is a drop >50% the pre-excision level, the procedure can be stopped. If after 20 minutes, the PTH level has failed to drop >50% pre-excision level, additional exploration should be pursued until additional glands are removed and the criteria is met, or until a complete bilateral exploration is performed. Use of this protocol has led to excellent long-term cure rates of 97% to 99%.

5. **D.** Hypercalcemic crisis is rare but can be deadly if left untreated. The goals of treatment include resuscitation, increasing renal calcium excretion, and treating the underlying cause of hypercalcemia. The first step in management of this patient is fluid resuscitation. Once adequately resuscitated, treatment can focus on decreasing calcium levels, usually first with furosemide to promote renal excretion of calcium and, if necessary, calcitonin, cinacalcet, or bisphosphonates may also be required. There is no great data to support the perfect timing of parathyroidectomy or precise calcium level to target prior to surgery, but

guidelines recommend expeditious parathyroidectomy after medical resuscitation.

6. D. Indications for parathyroidectomy for hyperparathyroidism include symptomatic hypercalcemia and asymptomatic hypercalcemia with at least one of the following: Calcium >1 mg/dL the upper limit of normal, Age <50, GFR <60, evidence of osteoporosis (T score <−2.5), evidence of vertebral fracture, hypercalciuria, 24-hour urine calcium >400 mg/day, nephrolithiasis or nephrocalcinosis on imaging. A contraindication to parathyroidectomy is familial hypercalcemic hypocalciuria. FHH is a very rare, autosomal dominant condition, which causes decreased excretion of calcium, causing the serum calcium to be elevated. This calcium level is "normal" for these patients, and they will therefore be asymptomatic, and will gain no benefit from parathyroidectomy.

BIBLIOGRAPHY

AACE/AAES Task Force on Primary Hyperparathyroidism. The American Association of Clinical Endocrinologists and the American Association of Endocrine Surgeons position statement on the diagnosis and management of primary hyperparathyroidism. *Endocr Pract.* 2005;11: 49–54.

Ahmad S, Kuragnati G, Steenkamp D. Hypercalcemic crisis: a clinical review. *Am J Med.* 2015;28(3):239–245.

Callender GG, Udelsman R. Surgery for primary hyperparathyroidism. *Cancer.* 2014;120(23):3602–3616.

Goldstein RA, Billheimer D, Martin WH, et al. Sestamibi scanning and minimally invasive radioguided parathyroidectomy without intraoperative parathyroid hormone measurement. *Ann Surg.* 2003 May; 237(5): 722–731.

Goldstein RE, Blevins L, Delbeke D, et al. Effect of minimally invasive radioguided parathyroidectomy on efficacy, length of stay, and costs in the management of primary hyperparathyroidism. *Ann Surg.* 2000;231:732–742.

Halsted WS, Evans HM. The parathyroid glandules: their blood supply, and their preservation in operation upon the thyroid gland. *Ann Surg.* 1907;46(4):489–506.

Heath DA, Heath EM. Conservative management of primary hyperparathyroidism. *J Bone Miner Res.* 1991;6:S117–S120.

Jaskowiak N, Norton JA, Alexander HR, et al. A prospective trial evaluating a standard approach to reoperation for missed parathyroid adenoma. *Ann Surg.* September 1996;224(3):308–320.

Udelsman R, Donovan PI. Remedial parathyroid surgery: changing trends in 130 consecutive cases. *Ann Surg.* September 2006;244(3):471–479.

Vaghaiwalla TM, Khan ZF, Lew JI. Review of intraoperative parathormone moniotoring with the Miami criterion: a 25-year experience. *World J Surg Proced.* 2016;6(1):1–7.

Wilhelm SM, Wang TS, Ruan DT, et al. The American Association of Endocrine Surgeons guidelines for definitive management of primary hyperparathyroidism. *JAMA Surgery.* 2016;151(10):959–968.

51

Thyroid Disease

Joy Sarkar

SCENARIO 1

A 43-year-old female is referred to your office by her primary care physician for evaluation of a left thyroid lesion. The primary care physician thought the left side of the neck felt fuller than the other and ordered an ultrasound of the neck and lab work. A lesion was seen on the ultrasound and her primary care physician referred her to general surgery for evaluation. The patient states that she feels perfectly well with no loss in weight or hot flashes. She has no family history of cancer or neck irradiation. After performing a thorough physical examination, you feel a fullness in her left neck corresponding with her left thyroid gland but no obvious discrete mass. Her lab work shows a normal chemistry panel and normal thyroid panel. The ultrasound reveals a 0.4-cm circular, smooth, solid, intracapsular lesion.

1. **What would be your next step in management for this lesion?**
   A. Fine-needle aspiration (FNA)
   B. Repeat lab work
   C. Observation
   D. Subtotal thyroidectomy

2. **What would be your next step if the lesion were 1.1 cm on imaging and palpable?**
   A. FNA
   B. Repeat lab work
   C. Follow-up with repeat ultrasound in 6 months
   D. Subtotal thyroidectomy

3. **What would be your treatment option if the 1.1-cm lesion showed suspicion for a papillary thyroid cancer on FNA and no lymphadenopathy on ultrasound?**
   A. Left thyroid lobectomy
   B. Left thyroidectomy with isthmusectomy
   C. Total thyroidectomy
   D. Total thyroidectomy with left modified radical neck dissection
   E. Total thyroidectomy with central neck dissection (CND)

4. **What is the recommended initial surgical approach if the 1.1-cm lesion was nondiagnostic on initial and repeat FNA, no lymphadenopathy is seen, and the patient desires a limited surgical procedure?**
   A. Repeat FNA again
   B. Left thyroid lobectomy
   C. Near-total thyroidectomy
   D. Total thyroidectomy

SCENARIO 2

A 23-year-old Pacific Islander female is referred to you for evaluation for a left neck mass. She rarely receives any medical care. She has noticed the neck mass for the past 6 months. The lump is increasing in size with time. She states that otherwise, she feels normal. On physical exam, she has a palpable lump on her left thyroid gland as well as left neck lymphadenopathy. She is very thin with long limbs and round, firm lumps in her lips.

5. **FNA of the thyroid nodule is performed and shows small, round cells in nests, with amyloid deposits in the stroma. Immunohistochemical staining is positive for calcitonin. The same findings are noted in FNA of a palpable left cervical lymph node. This cytology is most consistent with a diagnosis of:**

   A. Papillary thyroid cancer
   B. Metastatic neuroendocrine carcinoma
   C. Hurthle cell carcinoma
   D. Follicular thyroid cancer
   E. Medullary thyroid cancer (MTC)

6. **The patient tests positive for a RET proto-oncogene mutation. What potential abnormalities would you suspect and work up?**

   A. Papillary thyroid cancer
   B. Pituitary adenoma
   C. Pheochromocytoma
   D. Parathyroid hyperplasia
   E. Hirschsprung's disease

SCENARIO 3

A 37-year-old male presents to his primary care physician with a 2-month history of anxiety and palpitations. On examination, his heart rate is 114 bpm, and he is noted to have a symmetrically enlarged, nontender thyroid gland. A thyroid panel is drawn, and his serum TSH is <0.01 mU/L, while serum T_4 and T_3 are both elevated.

7. **Which of the following is true about the workup and diagnosis of this patient's condition?**

   A. The next best step in management is an ultrasound of the thyroid gland and FNA to rule out malignancy.
   B. Radioactive iodine uptake (RAIU) measurements will be useful in differentiating between Graves' disease and toxic multinodular goiter.
   C. Factitious ingestion of thyroid hormone can be distinguished from other causes of thyrotoxicosis by an elevated serum thyroglobulin.
   D. Elevated levels of thyroid-stimulating hormone receptor antibodies (TRAb) are characteristic of Graves' disease.
   E. The presence of anti-thyroid peroxidase (TPO) antibodies is diagnostic for Hashimoto's thyroiditis.

8. **The patient is found to have Graves' disease after the workup is completed; the treatment options are discussed with him and he elects to undergo thyroidectomy. Which of the following is the most appropriate preoperative preparation?**

   A. Lugol's solution
   B. Propanolol, methimazole (MMI), and Lugol's solution
   C. Propylthiouracil (PTU) and Lugol's solution
   D. Propanolol, PTU, and hydrocortisone
   E. Propanolol and MMI

ANSWERS

1. **C.** Thyroid nodules are common, with approximately 4% of the population having a palpable nodule and more than 50% having a nodule on ultrasound. Per 2015 et al., the majority of patients with asymptomatic, sonographically or cytologically benign thyroid nodules will not undergo any significant size increase or display cancer at 5 years. No FNA or surgery is required for this nodule per the American Thyroid Association (ATA) 2015 guidelines and repeating lab work is not indicated for this patient. The ATA in its 2015 guidelines recommends considering repeat ultrasound at 6 to 12 months for nodules with highly suspicious ultrasound patterns (hypoechoic, taller than wide) and 12 to 24 months for nodules with low to intermediate suspicion on ultrasound pattern (iso or hyperechoic, hypoechoic with smooth margins and no microcalcifications).

2. **A.** The ATA and the American Association of Clinical Endocrinologists (AACE) recommend biopsy if the nodules are >1 cm. The ATA recommends biopsy of subcentimeter nodules larger than 5 mm that are suspicious appearing on ultrasound (hypoechoic with microcalcifications) and individuals with a high-risk history (e.g., family history of papillary thyroid cancer, history of irradiation as a child or adolescent, prior hemithyroidectomy with discovery of thyroid cancer, and positron emission tomography [PET] positive thyroid nodules). The AACE recommends biopsy of nodules of any size for suspicious history (e.g., history of irradiation in childhood or adolescence, family history of thyroid cancer or MEN syndrome, previous thyroid surgery for cancer, or increased calcitonin levels) or suspicious ultrasound findings (e.g., hypoechogenicity, irregular borders, microcalcifications, and taller than wide, chaotic intranodular vascular images).

3. **C.** For patients with FNA biopsies showing thyroid cancer, the initial surgical procedure should be near-total or total thyroidectomy for lesions greater than 1 cm. Thyroid lobectomy may be considered for <1 cm, low risk, unifocal, intrathyroidal papillary carcinomas in patients with no history of prior head and neck irradiation and no evidence of cervical nodal metastases. While prophylactic CND is controversial for papillary thyroid cancer in the absence of clinically involved central lymph nodes, the ATA recommends thyroidectomy without prophylactic CND for small (T1 or T2) noninvasive papillary thyroid cancers and most follicular cancers. CND would be appropriate in MTC due to the high rate of metastasis to the central compartment lymph nodes. Modified radical neck dissection should be performed for biopsy-proven metastatic disease in the lateral neck; there is no role for prophylactic modified radical neck dissection in papillary thyroid cancer.

4. **B.** For indeterminate biopsies on FNA, such as follicular neoplasms or Hurthle cell neoplasms on pathology, the malignancy risk is approximately 20%. This risk increases with large tumors (>4 cm) and pathology findings consistent with cellular pleomorphism or other atypia and suspicion for papillary carcinoma. Other risk factors include family history of thyroid carcinoma and previous radiation exposure.

   Per the 2015 ATA guidelines, for patients with an isolated indeterminate solitary nodule, thyroid lobectomy is the recommended initial surgical approach. Total thyroidectomy is recommended for indeterminate nodules, which are large (>4 cm), show marked atypia present on biopsy, in patients with a family history of thyroid cancer, in patients with a history of radiation exposure, or for those with FNA biopsy results suspicious for papillary carcinoma.

5. **E.** MTC originates from the calcitonin-producing C cells of the thyroid; its morphology on FNA can vary, but generally shows neuroendocrine cells in nests, with amyloid deposits in the stroma. Immunohistochemical staining is usually positive for calcitonin and CEA. Papillary thyroid cancer is characterized by sheets of cells, and the cell nuclei demonstrate inclusions and grooves; psammoma bodies are also often seen. Follicular neoplasms and Hurthle cell carcinoma (a subtype of follicular neoplasm) are characterized by vascular or capsular invasion and therefore cannot be diagnosed as malignant or benign based on FNA; surgical excision is necessary. Hurthle cells are characterized by abundant granular cytoplasm and round nuclei. Distant metastasis to the thyroid gland is rare, and a metastatic neuroendocrine tumor would not be expected to stain positive for calcitonin.

6. **C.** The RET proto-oncogene is found to be mutated in patients with multiple endocrine neoplasia (MEN) 2A and MEN 2B syndromes, while the menin gene is mutated in patients with MEN 1 syndrome. The MEN 2B syndrome is characterized by MTC, pheochromocytomas, and mucosal neuromas as well as marfanoid appearance, and should be suspected in this patient due to her marfanoid appearance and neuromas in the setting of MTC. MEN 2A syndrome is characterized by MTC, pheochromocytomas, and parathyroid hyperplasia causing hyperparathyroidism as well as Hirschsprungs and cutaneous lichen amyloidosis. MEN 1 syndrome is characterized primarily by pituitary, pancreatic, and parathyroid tumors.

7. **D.** Hyperthyroidism is characterized by signs and symptoms of hypermetabolism, to include palpitations, weight loss, anxiety, diaphoresis, tachycardia, tremor, and goiter. There are multiple possible causes, including Graves' disease, toxic adenoma, multinodular goiter, autoimmune thyroiditis, and drug-induced thyrotoxicosis. In hyperthyroidism, serum TSH levels are subnormal, and total T_3 is elevated; free T_4 may be normal in mild hyperthyroidism or elevated in overt hyperthyroidism.

   Ultrasound and FNA are helpful in the initial assessment of thyroid nodules, but are less high-yield in the evaluation of a diffusely enlarged gland. FNA biopsy can be used to differentiate between various types of thyroiditis, such as Hashimoto's vs. lymphocytic thyroiditis, but would not be the first step in the workup, and malignancy would not be highest on the differential based on this presentation.

   RAIU measurements determine the percentage of administered radioactive iodine that is concentrated into thyroid tissue after a fixed interval. Both Graves' disease and toxic multinodular goiter would be associated with an elevated RAI uptake over the neck, while most types of thyroiditis as well as factitious ingestion of thyroid hormone are associated with near-absent uptake. In contrast, a technetium

(Tc-99m) pertechnetate scan produces images depicting the pattern of Tc-99m uptake, which may help to differentiate between Graves' disease (diffuse bilateral uptake), multinodular goiter (patchy bilateral uptake), toxic adenoma (focal uptake with suppressed activity in the remainder of the gland), and thyroiditis (near-absent uptake).

The presence of antibodies to thyroid antigens can identify an autoimmune etiology of thyroid dysfunction, for example, Graves' disease or Hashimoto's thyroiditis. TRAb are found in 90% of patients with Graves' disease, but in only about 10% of patients with Hashimoto's thyroiditis. TPO antibodies, also called antimicrosomal antibodies, are found in 90% to 95% of patients with Hashimoto's thyroiditis, but also in 80% of patients with Graves' disease; therefore, this is not a pathognomonic finding.

8. B. When surgery is chosen as the treatment method, patients should be rendered euthyroid prior to the procedure to avoid precipitating thyroid storm. Per the 2016 ATA guidelines, this is accomplished with the use of antithyroid drugs, with or without β-blockade. In the United States, the antithyroid drugs MMI and PTU are available. Both drugs decrease thyroid hormone synthesis, and PTU additionally blocks the peripheral conversion of T_4 to T_3. MMI should be used preferentially, except in the first trimester of pregnancy, thyroid storm, or intolerance to MMI, in which cases PTU should be used. The ATA also recommends that all patients with symptoms of thyrotoxicosis (in this patient's case, tachycardia) should be placed on a β-blocker. Preoperative iodine (KI, SSKI, or Lugol's solution) should be administered for 10 days before surgery, as it decreases thyroid blood flow, vascularity, and therefore intraoperative blood loss. Corticosteroids are not routinely used as preoperative preparation for thyroidectomy in the setting of hyperthyroidism, but are part of the treatment of thyroid storm, along with β-blockers, PTU, KI, cooling measures, and supportive care.

BIBLIOGRAPHY

Durante C, Costante G, Lucisano G, et al. The natural history of benign thyroid nodules. *JAMA*. 2015;313(9):926–935.

Fröhlich E, Wahl R. Thyroid autoimmunity: role of antithyroid antibodies in thyroid and extra-thyroidal diseases. *Front Immunology*. 2017;8:521.

Gharib H, Papini E, Baskin HJ, et al. American Association of Clinical Endocrinologists and associazione medici endocrinologi medical guidelines for clinical practice for the diagnosis and management of thyroid nodules. *Endocr Pract*. January–February 2006;12(1):63–102.

Haugen BR, Alexander EK, Bible KC, et al. 2015 American Thyroid Association management guidelines for adult patients with thyroid nodules and differentiated thyroid cancer: the American Thyroid Association guidelines task force on thyroid nodules and differentiated thyroid cancer. *Thyroid*. January 2016;26(1):1–133.

Levine RA. Current guidelines for the management of thyroid nodules. *Endocr Pract*. July–August 2012;18(4):596–599.

Raue F, Frank-Raue K. Genotype-phenotype relationship in multiple endocrine neoplasia type 2: implications for clinical management. *Hormones*. 2009;8(1):23–28.

Ross DS, Burch HB, Cooper DS, et al. 2016 American Thyroid Association guidelines for diagnosis and management of hyperthyroidism and other causes of thyrotoxicosis. *Thyroid*. 2016;26(10):1343–1421.

Thakker RV, Newey PJ, Walls GV, et al. Clinical practice guidelines for multiple endocrine neoplasia Type 1 (MEN1). *J Clin Endocrinol Metab*. September 2012;97(9):2990–3011.

52

Pancreatic Endocrine Tumors

Jigesh A. Shah, Omar Yusef Kudsi, and Kenneth J. Bogenberger

1. **The patient from the previous question denies any family history of multiple endocrine neoplasia (MEN). In regard to MEN syndromes, which of the following is correct?**

   A. The most common endocrinopathies in MEN-1 are pituitary adenomas, reaching 100% penetration by age 50.

   B. The most common endocrinopathy in MEN-2 is pheochromocytoma.

   C. MEN-2B includes medullary thyroid cancer and pheochromocytoma in all patients.

   D. Prophylactic thyroidectomy is not recommended in patients with a confirmed RET germ-line mutation and a discernable thyroid mass by ultrasound if the serum calcitonin levels are normal.

   E. During work up for a MEN, if a pheochromocytoma is detected, it should be resected prior to surgery on the thyroid.

2. **A 40-year-old male was found to have recurrent hypoglycemic symptoms with a plasma glucose level of 44 mg/dL and a C-peptide level of ≥200 pmol/L. He has relief of his symptoms with the administration of glucose. Further workup includes a positive 72-hour fast. In regard to pancreatic neuroendocrine tumors (PNETs), which of the following is true?**

   A. PNETs are common and 75% of cases are found in association with symptoms related to a specific hormone.

   B. With PNET lesions located in the body or tail of the pancreas, a distal pancreatectomy can be performed and even if the lesion is thought to be malignant, splenic preservation may still be attempted.

   C. Enucleation and formal resection of PNETs generally lead to equivalent outcomes for the management of small PNETs less than 2 cm.

   D. Most nonfunctional PNETs are benign, even if they have local invasion and regional lymph node involvement.

   E. Formal resection with appropriate lymphadenectomy is recommended for patients with insulinoma/gastrinoma smaller than 2 cm and other functional tumors such as VIPoma, somatostatinoma, and glucagonoma, which demonstrate no evidence of metastatic disease.

3. **You are evaluating a 50-year-old male with a history of recurrent duodenal ulcers located in the second portion of the duodenum. Further workup demonstrates that he is *H. pylori* negative and an upper endoscopy shows markedly hypertrophic gastric folds. Which of the following is true regarding his likely underlying diagnosis?**

   A. A fasting serum gastrin level of more than 1,000 pg/mL (normal is <100 pg/mL) is considered diagnostic for gastrinoma.

   B. Following intravenous secretin injection, gastrin suppression is diagnostic.

   C. The majority of gastrinomas are generally found within an area bound by the junction of the cystic and common bile duct, the junction of the duodenum and jejunum at the ligament of Treitz, and the junction of the neck and body of the pancreas.

   D. Gastrinomas are commonly found in locations such as the gallbladder, renal capsule, splenic hilum, mesentery, omentum, ovary, lymph nodes, and heart.

E. Medical treatment of Zollinger-Ellison Syndrome with proton pump inhibitors is very effective, eliminating any malignant potential, and can preclude the need for surgery.

4. **A 59-year-old male patient presents with diabetes, anemia, and a 30 pound weight loss. Recently, he started to develop a rash described as raised erythematous plaques that developed central bullae that sloughed, leaving necrotic centers and serous crusts. Serum glucagon levels are 1,100 pg/dL. A computerized tomography (CT) scan of the abdomen and pelvis demonstrated a 4 cm mass in the tail of the pancreas. Which of the following is true regarding his diagnosis?**

   A. Localization with CT and staging with somatostatin receptor scintigraphy are generally insufficient for obtaining a diagnosis.
   B. Necrolytic migratory erythema occurs in approximately 5% of these patients.
   C. Patients should be fully anticoagulated at the time of diagnosis and inferior vena cava filters should be considered preoperatively.
   D. These lesions are most commonly located in the head of the pancreas and are usually sensitive to chemotherapy.

5. **With regard to PNETs, which characteristic presentation is associated with poorest prognosis?**

   A. A symptomatic patient presenting with hypoglycemia and relief of symptoms with ingestion of glucose.
   B. A functional mass measuring 1.5 cm in size.
   C. A nonfunctioning pancreatic mass discovered after imaging for abdominal pain.
   D. Tumor pathology demonstrating low Ki-67 index on biopsy.

6. **Which is true regarding the diagnosis of PNETs?**

   A. CT scan is greater than 90% effective at localizing insulinomas, which tend to be large at presentation.
   B. Hepatic venous sampling is the gold standard for localizing functional tumors within the pancreas.
   C. Tumors are rarely metastatic.
   D. Nonfunctional tumors will not overexpress chromogranin A or somatostatin.
   E. Endoscopic ultrasound is 70% to 90% sensitive for localizing tumors within the pancreas.

ANSWERS

1. **E.** MEN-1 is manifested by hyperparathyroidism, pituitary adenomas, and PNETs. MEN-2A is manifested by medullary thyroid cancer in nearly all patients but pheochromocytoma develops in only 40% to 50% of patients.

   Hyperparathyroidism occurs in approximately 20% of patients. Medullary thyroid cancer (MTC) is typically the first presenting endocrine tumor manifesting between the age of 5 and 25 years. MEN-2B is relatively rare, accounting for less than 10% of the cases of familial medullary thyroid cancers. This syndrome includes medullary thyroid cancer in all patients and pheochromocytoma in approximately 50%. Affected patients also exhibit a marfanoid body habitus and enlarged lips, and have mucosal neuromas of the eyelids, lips, and tongue.

   MEN-2B is an aggressive form of MEN-2 in that MTC tends to present earlier than in MEN-2A or familial medullary thyroid carcinoma (FMTC), often during the first year of life. If a carrier state is identified in a preclinical setting, surgery should be done before the age of typical onset of cancer or metastasis. In a prophylactic setting, the procedure of choice is a total thyroidectomy. If the patient has an elevated calcitonin level, then a total thyroidectomy and central neck dissection should be done. The American Thyroid Association (ATA) has developed risk groups based on the specific mutation. Carriers with MEN-2B should have a thyroidectomy within the first year of life. Patients with MEN-2A are risk stratified based on their specific mutation. High-risk patients should have a thyroidectomy before the age of 5 and patients at moderate risk should have a thyroidectomy between the ages of 5 and 10 years.

2. **C.** PNETs are uncommon in the general population, accounting for only 3% to 5% of pancreatic malignancies, a majority of which are sporadic and functional. Several important factors must be considered when selecting the operative approach, including the tumor's functional status, involvement with contiguous structures, presence of metastatic disease, and whether the tumor is sporadic or associated with a genetic syndrome. Clinical symptoms and biochemical evidence of hormone excess determine the tumor's functional status. Preoperative evaluation by cross-sectional and functional (somatostatin) imaging combined with endoscopic ultrasound are used to localize the lesion and assess for local invasion,

lymph node involvement, and metastases to the liver and other organs. Endoscopic fine needle aspiration biopsy can confirm diagnosis and grade the tumor based on number of mitoses and Ki-67 index.

Accurate history and genetic testing can determine whether the tumor is sporadic or associated with a genetic syndrome and must be considered during preoperative decision making and planning for resection. The goal of surgery for primary PNETs is to resect the primary tumor and associated lymph nodes while preserving the maximal amount of pancreatic mass. The indications for surgery in patients with PNETs include systemic symptoms due to hormone over-production, local compressive symptoms due to mass effect, and prevention of malignant transformation or dissemination. Formal pancreatic resection with appropriate lymphadenectomy is recommended for patients with established known malignancy, including splenectomy when lesions are found within the tail of the pancreas. With insulinomas/gastrinomas larger than 2 cm and other functional tumors such as VIPoma, somatostatinoma, and glucagonoma with no evidence of metastatic disease, a formal resection is the preferred operative management strategy. For those lesions smaller than 2 cm, the survival of simple enucleation is similar to a formal resection.

3. A. Gastrinomas are associated with Zollinger-Ellison syndrome (atypical peptic ulcer disease, gastric hyperacidity, and hyper-secretion). Proton-pump inhibitors have no effect on the natural history of the disease. Most patients are male (~60%) and the average age at diagnosis is about 60 years. A fasting serum gastrin level of more than 1,000 pg/mL (10 times the upper limit of normal) is diagnostic of gastrinomas. Gastrinomas can be distinguished from these other conditions by virtue of its paradoxical effect on serum gastrin levels in response to a secretin infusion (secretin stimulation test). After baseline gastrin measurement, secretin is administered and gastrin levels are rechecked. An increase in gastrin levels of greater than 120 pg/mL over basal levels has 94% sensitivity and 100% specificity for gastrinoma. The majority of gastrinomas are generally found within the gastrinoma triangle, which is bound by the junction of the cystic and common bile duct, the junction of the second and third portion of the duodenum and the junction of the neck and body of the pancreas. Localization of gastrinomas is best performed with endoscopic ultrasonography and somatostatin-receptor scintigraphy. Because of the malignant potential of gastrinomas, medical treatment alone does not prevent progression of malignant disease and with the development of excellent pharmacologic therapy for the control of gastric acid hypersecretion, surgery for gastrinomas has shifted toward tumor localization and resection.

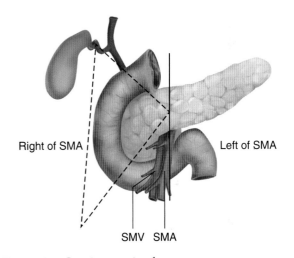

Right of SMA   Left of SMA

SMV SMA

Figure 52-1 Gastrinoma triangle.

Syndrome	Chromosome	Gene	Associated Pathology
MEN 1	Chromosome 11	MENIN	Parathyroid Hyperplasia (4-gland)
			Pancreatic Islet Cell Tumors (Gastrinoma)
			Pituitary Tumors (Prolactinoma)
MEN 2A	Chromosome 10	RET proto-oncogene	Parathyroid Hyperplasia (4-gland)
			Pheochromocytoma
			Medullary Thyroid Carcinoma
MEN 2B	Chromosome 10	RET proto-oncogene	Pheochromocytoma
			Medullary Thyroid Carcinoma
			Mucocutaneous Ganglioneuroma, Marfanoid Body Habitus

MEN—Multiple Endocrine Neoplasia; RET—Rearranged during Transfection.

4. C. Glucagonomas have been described as causing the 4 "D's": dermatitis, diabetes, depression, and deep vein thrombosis. Weight loss and a characteristic skin rash (necrolytic migratory erythema) are the most common presenting features, occurring in about 70% of patients, with other symptoms occurring less frequently at initial presentation. Necrolytic migratory erythema, which is an intensely pruritic rash that usually presents on the lower abdomen, perineum, perioral area, or lower extremities, may present before any other signs or symptoms and is pathognomonic for glucagonoma and is found in up to 70% of patients. Most glucagonoma patients have glucose intolerance and fasting serum glucagon levels between 1,000 and 5,000 pg/mL.

The initial management of a patient with a glucagonoma should focus on blocking and treating the metabolic effects of glucagon hypersecretion and preventing or treating venous thromboembolism. Octreotide and intravenous fluids should be administered. Additionally, due to their hypercoagulable state and predisposition to thromboembolic events, patients should be fully anticoagulated. Glucagonomas are most commonly located in the tail of the pancreas and surgical resection usually consists of a distal pancreatectomy along with a splenectomy. A cholecystectomy should be performed prophylactically at the time of the initial operation to eliminate the potential for gallstone-related complications, which are associated with octreotide therapy.

5. C. Nonfunctioning pancreatic masses tend to be metastatic at presentation. They are found

Tumor	Symptoms
Insulinoma	Hypoglycemia, Whipple's triad (symptoms of hypoglycemia, blood glucose <50 mg/dL, relief of symptoms with glucose)
VIPoma	Achlorhydria, hypokalemia, watery diarrhea
Glucagonoma	Necrolytic migratory erythema, stomatitis/glossitis, glucose intolerance, DVT
Somatostatinoma	Cholelithiasis, steatorrhea, hyperglycemia, achlorhydria

incidentally on axial imaging or present with nonspecific symptoms after becoming locally advanced. They most commonly present with abdominal pain but can also present with anorexia, weight loss, jaundice from biliary obstruction, and intra-abdominal hemorrhage. The incidence of metastasis approaches 85% in nonfunctioning tumors due to its delayed presentation. A patient presenting with Whipple's triad is diagnostic for an insulinoma. Insulinomas are most commonly small tumors with low potential for malignancy (<10%). A 1.5-cm tumor is a T1 tumor and not at increased risk of malignancy based on size. Ki-67 is an important histologic marker and important for grading. A high Ki-67 portends a worse prognosis.

6. D. Endoscopic ultrasound is sensitive in detecting small neuroendocrine tumors of the pancreas, and is an important diagnostic study for identifying lesions not seen on CT or MRI. Axial imaging with CT is usually the first diagnostic test obtained in these patients but is only 60% to 80% sensitive for detecting the primary tumor. Endoscopic ultrasound should be considered when a functional pancreatic mass is suspected in the absence of findings on CT or MRI. Hepatic venous sampling can be considered for identifying functional tumors within the pancreas if imaging is otherwise negative and you have a high suspicion for a pancreatic origin for a functional tumor. Use of venous sampling is rarely performed because it is invasive and requires access to advanced angiography capabilities within the hospital.

The rates of metastasis for neuroendocrine tumors of the pancreas vary based on histology; however, in general, rates are high. Up to 40% of tumors are nonfunctioning and are associated with high rates of metastasis attributable to late presentation of symptoms. Glucagonoma, VIPoma, and somatostatinoma are also strongly associated with malignancy. Chromogranin A and somatostatin are characteristically elevated in neuroendocrine tumors, including nonfunctional tumors. Chromogranin A is an important marker and can be used in follow up to monitor for recurrence. Somatostatin-based scans (Octreotide scan or Ga-68 DOTATE) are important imaging adjuncts and because of somatostatin overexpression in tumors, can help identify metastatic disease or an occult primary tumor.

BIBLIOGRAPHY

Brandi ML, Gagel RF, Angeli A, et al. Guidelines for diagnosis and therapy of MEN type 1 and 2. *J Clin Endocrinol Metab.* 2001;86:5658–5671.

Goldfinger SE. Zollinger-Ellison syndrome (gastrinoma): Clinical manifestations and diagnosis. http://www.uptodate.com/contents/zollinger-ellison-syndrome-gastrinoma-clinical-manifestations-and-diagnosis

Halfdanarson TR, Rubin J, Farnell MB, Grant CS, Petersen GM. Pancreatic endocrine neoplasms: epidemiology and prognosis of pancreatic endocrine tumors. *Endocr.-Relat. Cancer.* 2008;15(2):409–427.

Lou I, Chen H. The management of pancreatic islet cell tumors excluding gastrinomas. In: Cameron JL, Cameron A, eds. *Current Surgical Therapy.* Mosby Elsevier; 2017.

Norton JA, Fraker DL, Alexander HR, et al. Surgery increases survival in patients with gastrinoma. *Ann Surg.* 2006;44(3):410–419.

O'Riordain DS, O'Brien T, Crotty TB, et al. Multiple endocrine neoplasia type 2B: More than an endocrine disorder. *Surgery.* 1995;118:936–942.

Passaro E, Howard TJ, Sawicki MP, et al. The origin of sporadic gastrinomas within the gastrinoma triangle: a theory. *Arch Surg.* 1998;133(1):13–16.

Phan GQ, Yeo CJ, Hruban RH, et al. Surgical experience with pancreatic and peripancreatic neuroendocrine tumors: review of 125 patients. *J Gastrointest Surg.* 1998;2:473.

Pitt SC, Pitt HA, Baker MS, et al. Small pancreatic and periampullary neuroendocrine tumors: resect or enucleate? *J Gastrointest Surg.* 2009;13:1692.

Plockinger U, Rindi G, Arnold R, et al. Guidelines for the diagnosis and treatment of neuroendocrine gastrointestinal tumours. A consensus statement on behalf of the European Neuroendocrine Tumour Society (ENETS). *Neuroendocrinology.* 2004;80:394–424.

Stabile BE, Morrow DJ, Passaro EJr. The gastrinoma triangle: operative implications. *Am J Surg.* 1984;147:25–31.

Tamm EP, Kim EE, Ng CS. Imaging of neuroendocrine tumors. *Hematol Oncol Clin North Am.* 2007;21:409–432.

Wells SA, Asa SL, Dralle H, et al. Revised American Thyroid Association guidelines for the management of medullary thyroid carcinoma. *Thyroid.* 2015;25(6):567–610.

Wermers RA, Fatourechi V, Wynne AG, et al. The glucagonoma syndrome. Clinical and pathologic features in 27 patients. *Medicine.* 1996;75(2):53–63.

53

Salivary Gland Tumors

Maxwell Sirkin, William V. Rice, and Jayne Stevens

A 55-year-old Caucasian male is referred to your clinic for a palpable 2-cm mass located 2 to 3 cm anterior to his right tragus. He states that it has been present for about 9 months and has slowly been getting larger. He denies any pain, facial weakness or numbness, fevers, weight loss, fatigue, and dry mouth. He has no medical or surgical history and does not take any medications. On physical examination, you find a well-circumscribed, mobile, non-tender 2-cm mass, with no overlying skin changes. There is no lymphadenopathy and the rest of the exam is normal.

1. **Regarding the above patient, which of the following is the most likely diagnosis?**

   A. Mucoepidermoid carcinoma
   B. Adenoid cystic carcinoma
   C. Pleomorphic adenoma
   D. Papillary cystadenoma lymphomatosum
   E. Sjogren's syndrome-related glandular enlargement

2. **Which of the following studies is the next best step in the diagnostic workup?**

   A. Core needle biopsy
   B. Incisional biopsy
   C. Positron emission tomography/computed tomography (PET/CT) scan
   D. Fine needle aspiration (FNA)
   E. Ultrasound

3. **Which of the following factors would increase the concern for malignancy in a patient?**

   A. Loss of taste
   B. 2-cm size
   C. paresthesia

   D. Personal history of smoking
   E. Gustatory sweating

4. **Tissue and imaging studies reveal a pleomorphic adenoma that appears to be confined to the superficial parotid gland. What is the next best step?**

   A. Total parotidectomy
   B. Superficial parotidectomy, sparing the facial nerve
   C. Superficial parotidectomy, sacrificing any facial nerve that may be involved
   D. Enucleation of the mass, sparing nerve and normal glandular tissue
   E. Surveillance of the mass with serial CT scans

5. **Tissue and diagnostic studies instead reveal a high-grade mucoepidermoid carcinoma that is clearly deep to the facial nerve. What is the next best step?**

   A. Total parotidectomy with resection of any adjacent facial nerve and immediate interposition nerve graft
   B. Total parotidectomy with sparing of the facial nerve, followed with postoperative radiation
   C. Radiation and chemotherapy with post-treatment surveillance
   D. Radiation alone
   E. Superficial parotidectomy, sparing the facial nerve, followed with postoperative radiation

6. **During superficial parotidectomy, you are having difficulty identifying the main branch of the facial nerve. Which of the following is the most reliable method for main trunk identification?**

A. Dissection medial and inferior to the tragal pointer

B. Dissection 1-cm superior and deep to Erb's point

C. Identification of the marginal mandibular nerve

D. Dissection at the depth of the digastric muscle

E. Identification of the tympanomastoid suture line

ANSWERS

1. **C.** Most salivary gland tumors arise in the parotid gland (70%) with fewer being found in the submandibular gland (20%). The larger the gland, the more likely the tumor will be benign. In the parotid gland, 80% of tumors will be benign. Submandibular glands have a ratio of 50:50 and minor salivary glands have a ratio of 25:75 benign to malignant, respectively.

   It is important to realize that pleomorphic adenomas are the most common neoplasms in the parotid gland and account for 40% to 70% of cases. Though these tumors are benign, they are associated with malignant transformation over time, with 1.5% transforming in the first five years and 9.5% malignant transformation rate after 15 years. As such, they should be treated surgically. Mucoepidermoid carcinoma is the most common malignant tumor of the parotid gland. Adenoid cystic carcinomas are the most common malignant tumors of the submandibular and minor salivary glands. In the sublingual gland, adenoid cystic and mucoepidermoid carcinomas occur with similar frequencies and are the two most common neoplasms in this gland. Sjogren's syndrome is associated with diffuse glandular enlargement, and would not be the most likely diagnosis in this patient with a focal 2-cm mass.

2. **D.** This patient's signs and symptoms suggest a benign tumor; however, malignancy may be present. Therefore, tissue diagnosis is recommended prior to proceeding with surgical intervention, as the histopathology can impact surgical plan. The next best step for surgical planning and patient counselling would be to obtain tissue preoperatively with a fine needle aspiration. FNA has excellent sensitivity (92%), specificity (100%), and accuracy (98%). FNA with or without ultrasound guidance would be the initial study of choice. Core needle biopsy in the face and neck is more invasive and is usually not recommended due to the proximity of sensitive structures, though this has been described in the literature as a safe option in the parotid gland.

   Magnetic resonance imaging (MRI) and CT scans are being used more frequently to help assess for regional lymphadenopathy, extent/depth of tumor, and tumor location in relationship to other important structures. Ultrasound alone, without an FNA, will yield little additional value than what a CT, MRI, and FNA will provide and may be considered a waste of resources. While Warthin's tumors and several of the malignant neoplasms can demonstrate avidity, a PET/CT would not be indicated prior to establishing a malignant histology and also does not offer significant additional information in comparison with the aforementioned imaging options.

   Incisional biopsy of the tumor for tissue diagnosis is not appropriate due to concerns for tumor seeding, with the potential to turn a single lesion into multiple lesions and significantly complicate and worsen treatment options and outcomes.

3. **C.** Signs and symptoms of pain, rapid growth, facial nerve weakness, paresthesias, cervical lymphadenopathy, and fixation to underlying tissue are all concerning for malignancy. While tobacco use is associated with malignancy in many other head and neck cancers, it is not associated with malignancy in parotid masses. Conversely, a history of smoking suggests an etiology of a Warthin's tumor, which is the second most common parotid mass. This tumor is benign and occurs bilaterally in 6% of cases. It is seen almost exclusively in smokers and can be safely observed once the diagnosis is established with an FNA. Gustatory sweating is also known as Frey's syndrome. Frey's syndrome is a complication of parotid tumor surgery and is the result of necessary injury to the auriculotemporal nerve when resecting the parotid gland. The auriculotemporal nerve has parasympathetic fibers that originate from the inferior salivatory nucleus, and trigger secretion of saliva from the parotid gland. When these fibers are injured during parotidectomy and undergo healing, they can sometimes cross innervate with sympathetic nerve fibers that travel to the skin and sweat glands. The result is "gustatory sweating" or triggering of the sweat glands from signals in the auriculotemporal nerve, meant to trigger salivation in a gland that no longer exists or has had part of it removed.

4. **B.** Pleomorphic adenomas are more often present in the superficial parotid than the deep parotid tissue and typically respect the plane of the facial neve. Thus, superficial parotidectomy should be the first surgical intervention for most of these benign tumors. Pleomorphic adenomas do not invade into the nerve and all attempts should be made to identify and spare the facial nerve and its branches during the surgery. A total parotidectomy involves greater risk to the facial nerve and causes a more severe cosmetic defect, so would not be recommended for a superficial lobe tumor.

Enucleation of the tumor is not recommended as there is a higher risk for recurrence when this is performed. Surveillance of parotid gland tumors with serial radiographic examinations is appropriate for patients who refuse surgery or are poor surgical candidates, but surgery is preferable for most patients. Additionally, if serial imaging is obtained, ultrasound can be considered to minimize cost and radiation exposure.

5. **B.** In this patient, there is involvement of the deep lobe, which is an indication for total parotidectomy. Since the patient has no neurologic symptoms prior to the operation, if the nerve is not being visibly/directly invaded, all attempts should be made to preserve the facial nerve, with surgery followed by postoperative radiation. The sural nerve and greater auricular nerve are commonly used conduits for nerve grafting, should this become necessary. Nonsurgical management, preoperative chemotherapy, and radiation only of malignant salivary tumors are not currently recommended methods of treatment.

Malignant salivary tumors are staged according to size and degree of local invasion. They are also classified according to histological grade, which separates them into either high or low, based on the number of mucoid cells and epidermoid components. High-grade tumors indicate a more aggressive tumor and thus exhibit a worse prognosis. Ipsilateral elective neck dissection can be considered for high-grade histology, given higher rates of occult disease, though this is controversial. Therapeutic neck dissection is indicated in all cases of diagnosed regional metastasis. Indications for postoperative radiation include: high grade, extra-glandular involvement, peri-neural invasion, direct invasion of surrounding structures, dissection of tumor off the facial nerve, and metastatic disease.

6. **E.** The most reliable landmark for the facial nerve is the tympanomastoid suture, which as a bony landmark has a constant relationship and close proximity to the facial nerve. The tragal pointer, located on the deep medial aspect of the tragal cartilage, is another commonly used landmark. Identification of the digastric muscle is useful, as the main trunk is located anterior and superior to the muscle belly, at the same depth. If the location of the tumor makes direct identification of the main trunk challenging, an alternative method is retrograde dissection of a peripheral branch. The marginal mandibular branch is the most frequently utilized for this purpose, though the frontal branch also has a relatively reliable location and can be used as well for retrograde dissection. Erb's point describes the point at which the great auricular wraps around the lateral aspect of the sternocleidomastoid muscle and is a useful tool for identification of the spinal accessory nerve, not the facial nerve.

BIBLIOGRAPHY

Boukheris H, Curtis RE, Land CE, et al. Incidence of carcinoma of the major salivary glands according to the WHO classification, 1992 to 2006: a population-based study in the United States. *Cancer Epidemiol Biomarkers Prev.* 2009 Nov;18(11):2899–2906.

Gordon AB, Fiddian RV. Frey's syndrome after parotid surgery. *Am J Surg.* 1976;132(1):54–58.

Kaplan M, Abemayor E. Major salivary glands. In: Fu YS, Wenig BM, Abemayor E, et al., eds. *Head and Neck Pathology: With Clinical Correlations.* Churchill-Livingstone; 2001: 231.

Kim SY, Min C, Oh DJ, Choi HG. Tobacco smoking and alcohol consumption are related to benign parotid tumor: a nested case-control study using a National Health Screening Cohort. *Clin Exp Otorhinolaryngol.* 2019;12(4):412–419.

Lorenz RR, Couch ME, Burkey BB. Head and neck. In: Beauchamp DR, Townsend CM, Evers MB, et al., eds. *Sabiston Textbook of Surgery: The Biological Basis of Modern Surgical Practice.* 19th ed. Elsevier Saunders; 2012: 811–813.

Maiorano E, Lo Muzio L, Favia G, Piattelli A. Warthin's tumour: a study of 78 cases with emphasis on bilaterality, multifocality and association with other malignancies. *Oral Oncol.* 2002;38(1):35–40.

Miller MC, Moyer JS, Teknos TN. Head and neck. In: Mulholland MW, Lillemoe KD, Doherty GM, et al., eds. *Greenfield's Surgery: Scientific Principles & Practice.* 5th ed. Lippincott Williams & Wilkins; 2011: 615–617.

Rahbar R, Grimmer FJ, Vargas SO, et al. Mucoepidermoid carcinoma of the parotid gland in children: a 10-year experience. *Arch Otolaryngol Head Neck Surg.* 2006;132: 375–380.

Stewart CJ, MacKenzie K, McGarry GW, et al. Fine-needle aspiration cytology of salivary gland: a review of 341 cases. *Diagn Cytopathol.* 2000;22:139–146.

Wetmore SJ. Surgical landmarks for the facial nerve. *Otolaryngol Clin North Am.* 1991;24(3):505–530.

Witt RL. The significance of the margin in parotid surgery for pleomorphic adenoma. *Laryngoscope.* 2002;112: 2141–2154.

SECTION 3

Surgical Subspecialties

BARIATRIC SURGERY

54

Marginal Ulcers

Ryan Bram and Chan W. Park

A 50-year-old female presents to the emergency department complaining of sharp epigastric abdominal pain that has gotten worse over the last several days. It seems to happen right after she eats or drinks, and this morning it doubled her over. She has some nausea but denies vomiting. Past medical history is significant for hypertension, obstructive sleep apnea on continuous positive airway pressure (CPAP), hypercholesteremia, and type 2 diabetes. Her surgical history is significant for laparoscopic gastric bypass 1 year ago. She denies any drug use, but she drinks a glass of red wine most evenings to "help her heart." After much probing, she relates that even though she quit smoking prior to surgery, she resumed smoking about 6 months ago and is back up to one pack per day. She relates that at the time of her surgery, she weighed 345 lb with a body mass index (BMI) of 59 kg/m^2 and now has lost 120 lb with a BMI of 38.6 kg/m^2. She hasn't seen a bariatric surgeon since her 3-month postoperative visit, mostly because she is embarrassed that she started smoking again. She stopped taking her omeprazole when her prescription ran out months ago.

Vital signs are heart rate 115, blood pressure 97/62, respiratory rate 18, pulse oxygen 98% on the right atrium. Her exam is noted to have diffuse abdominal tenderness, significant tenderness in the epigastrium, with voluntary guarding. Bowel sounds are absent. Hemoccult testing is positive.

1. **Which of the following is a factor potentially contributing to this patient's current problem?**
   A. Hypercholesterolemia
   B. Active smoking
   C. Obstructive sleep apnea
   D. Increase in carbohydrate intake
   E. Age >50

2. **Which of the following is the most common complication (early or late) following laparoscopic gastric bypass?**
   A. Internal hernias
   B. Small bowel obstruction
   C. Marginal ulceration (anastomotic/gastrojejunal ulcer)
   D. Gastrojejunal leak

3. **Which of the following statements is true regarding marginal ulcer following gastric bypass?**
   A. Most marginal ulcers are asymptomatic.
   B. About one-third of patients with marginal ulcer formation smoke.
   C. Active *H. pylori* infection is an independent risk factor for ulcer perforation.
   D. Use of proton pump inhibitors (PPIs) is not protective of ulcer formation in the setting of nonsteroidal anti-inflammatory drugs (NSAID) use.
   E. Suture material or type of anastomosis performed does not relate to ulcer formation.

4. **Regarding the treatment of marginal ulcers (MUs) following gastric bypass,**
   A. the majority can be successfully managed medically.
   B. nearly half of patients will require revision of the gastrojejunostomy for persistent and/or recurrent ulcers.
   C. late MUs are self-limiting and rarely require treatment.

D. *H. pylori* infection preoperatively or persistence postoperatively increases perforation rates.

E. endoscopy is of limited value in the treatment of an MU.

5. **Which of the following is true regarding perforated MUs following gastric bypass?**

A. About 40% of patients with marginal ulceration will develop a perforation.

B. May be managed operatively (open or laparoscopically) with oversewing of the ulcer and omental patch.

C. Most commonly occurs after 18 months from surgery.

D. Develops in about 10% of all patients that undergo gastric bypass.

6. **Many bariatric patients have chronic joint pain, particularly of the knees, and psychiatric diseases. Which of the following medications should be avoided in a gastric bypass patient to prevent the formation of an MU?**

A. Acetaminophen

B. Paxil (paroxetine hydrochloride)

C. Tramadol

D. Lidocaine

E. Wellbutrin (bupropion)

7. **After undergoing an esophagogastroduodenoscopy (EGD), your patient is diagnosed with a marginal ulcer. She is started on omeprazole and Carafate and told to avoid acidic spicy food, alcohol, smoking, and appropriate medications. Eight weeks later, she presents to your clinic with continued epigastric pain and endoscopic evidence of an ulcer with a widely patent gastrojejunostomy (GJ) anastomosis. No foreign bodies or fistulae are seen. Which of the following options is a reasonable next step for the management of her MU?**

A. Total gastrectomy

B. Continued medical therapy

C. Repeat EGD in 1 month

D. Truncal vagotomy

E. Computed tomography (CT) abdomen/pelvis scan with PO contrast

ANSWERS

1. **B.** This patient most likely has a marginal ulcer, which, at a rate of about 5% after Roux-en-Y gastric bypass, is one of the more common complications. Risk factors associated with the development of marginal (gastrojejunal/anastomotic) ulcers include environmental (smoking and alcohol), medication (NSAIDs), anatomical (gastrogastric fistula or an enlarged gastric pouch), and technique (use of nonabsorbable sutures). There is no link associated with specific food types and ulcer formation. Other risk factors that are associated with a marginal ulcer (MU) are increased acid exposure via a gastrogastric fistula (not confirmed in this patient but more commonly seen with patients who have had an open gastric bypass versus laparoscopic), hypertension, and the use of nonabsorbable suture in the anastomosis and recent surgery.

2. **C.** MUs are a late complication of gastric bypass surgery. Along with GJ stricture they are one of the most common complications (early or late) of gastric bypass surgery. Reported rates of MUs range from 1–25%, with most series indicating 5% incidence. GJ stricture rates are reported between 3–27%. The incidence of internal hernia after gastric bypass is nearly nonexistent in the open gastric bypass, but after laparoscopic gastric bypass, it occurs in approximately 2.5% of patients. Small bowel obstruction is linked to internal hernia formation, and the rates are equivalent. Further recent high quality data shows internal hernias and therefore small bowel obstructions can be reduced by routine closure of mesenteric defects. GJ leaks are an early complication after gastric bypass. In the laparoscopic approach, rates are reported at about 1–1.8%.

3. **B.** Of patients presenting with an MU, more than 30% are found to be smoking at the time of diagnosis. Most MUs are symptomatic (72%). The most common symptoms after surgery that lead to the diagnosis of MU are pain (34%), dysphagia (17%), weight gain (13%), nausea and vomiting (8%), and gastrointestinal (GI) bleed (3%). Active *H. pylori* infection has not been determined to be an independent risk factor in the development of a perforated MU. There are data that suggest that in the setting of patients who must use NSAIDs following gastric bypass, PPIs are protective of MU formation. While there is still debate as to whether hand-sewn GJ versus stapled anastomosis is better in relation to postoperative outcomes, the data clearly relate that nonabsorbable suture material at the anastomosis has a high association with MU formation. Because of this fact, the use of a nonabsorbable suture at the GJ anastomosis has essentially ceased.

4. **A.** The treatment of an MU is largely medical. The standard of treatment is PPI therapy initiation/continuation and cytoprotective agents (i.e., sucralfate or Carafate). Additionally, the cessation of smoking and/or NSAID use is critical, as recurrence is high in patients who continue with these high-level risk factors. Studies report the incidence of surgical intervention for an MU to be 4–10%. This usually occurs in this subset of MUs for recalcitrant and/or recurrent ulcers. Continued smoking and NSAID use were found to be independent risk factors for continued nonhealing ulcers. Late ulcers (those occurring after 30 days) are rarely self-limiting. Csendes et al. did a prospective evaluation of patients and performed endoscopy at 1 month and at 1–2 years. They found a 12% rate of MU at 1 month. Many authors believe this to be part of the natural progression and healing process of the anastomosis within such a short time frame. Most clinicians advocate for PPI use in the immediate postoperative period because of this. Clinically apparent MUs are unlikely to heal without intervention (as mentioned earlier). Although the data are not completely clear about the role of *H. pylori* infection and ulcer formation, the risk of perforation of an MU is not increased by the presence of *H. pylori*. One study found that in patients that were *H. pylori*–positive and eradicated prior to surgery, the rate of MU after surgery with short-term PPI use was significantly reduced. Endoscopy should be part of the armamentarium of diagnosing and treating MUs.

5. **B.** Most ulcers become apparent within the first 12 months following surgery. Although they can develop beyond 18 months following surgery, this is not the most common time frame in which they are seen. The incidence of perforation in all patients undergoing laparoscopic gastric bypass is approximately 1% and the incidence of MUs on average is 5% (range 1–16%); therefore, the rate of perforation of MUs is 20%. Felix et al. in 2008 found that many cases could be managed laparoscopically. In their series, over 30% were managed by oversewing of the ulcer and utilizing an omental patch. Other series have confirmed similar treatment strategies utilizing the omental patch for MU perforation. It may be necessary or more appropriate to consider revising the GJ for an MU with bleeding, with or without perforation; recurrent ulceration, when a gastrogastric fistula is present; or when the pouch is greatly enlarged.

6. **B.** MUs or ulcers about the GJ anastomosis can be debilitating complications of bypass operations. In addition to pain, there is an associated risk of bleeding and, even worse, frank perforation. There are several other risk factors for their development beyond smoking and alcohol use. These include high doses of aspirin, persistent use of NSAIDs, and high doses of selective serotonin reuptake inhibitors (such as Paxil) can also contribute to marginal ulcer formation. The thought is that similar to peptic ulcer disease, the decreased production of endogenous prostaglandins decreases the protective mucus barrier that naturally coats the gastric lumen, thus making it more vulnerable to any acid it comes in contact with. Although a recent population-based study from Sweden remarked that short-term, low-dose use of these medications did not seem to significantly increase the risk for MU formation. Wellbutrin (bupropion) is an antidepressant, but it is not known to cause peptic ulcer disease.

7. **D.** After diagnosing a marginal ulcer the treatment consists of identifying the likely precipitating cause, for example, smoking or alcohol cession, stopping all NSAIDs, and avoiding spicy and acidic food, as well as considering screening for *H. pylori* if this was not done preoperatively. Additionally pharmacotherapy with a PPI/H2-blocker and oral suspension of Carafate for 4–6 weeks with endoscopic follow-up to determine resolution is recommended. If the patient is still having symptoms despite this and other causes such as *H. pylori*, suture or staple material, and gastrogastric fistula are ruled out, then surgical intervention by means of thoracoscopic truncal vagotomy is a possible option. In some case series, this procedure has been shown to be upward of 80% effective for reducing symptoms in recalcitrant marginal ulcers. The other answer choices are useful if there is still a aneed further diagnostic workup, but in this question, the proper workup has already been completed and intervention is needed.

BIBLIOGRAPHY

Azagury DE, Abu Dayyeh BK, Greenwalt IT, Thompson CC. Marginal ulceration after Roux-en-Y gastric bypass surgery: Characteristics, risk factors, treatment, and outcomes. *Endoscopy.* 2011;43(11):950–954.

Bhayani NH, Oyetunji TA, Chang DA, et al. Predictors of marginal ulcers after laparoscopic gastric Roux-en-Y gastric bypass. *J Surg Res.* 2012;177(2):224–227.

Bonanno A, Tieu B, Dewey E, et al. Thoracosocpic truncal vagotomy versus surgical revision of the gastrojejunal anastomosis for recalcitrant marginal ulcers. *Surg Endosc.* 2019;33(2):607–611.

Coblijn UK, Goucham AB, Lagarde SM, Kuiken SD, van Wagensveld BA. Development of ulcer disease after Roux-en-Y gastric bypass, incidence, risk factors, and patient presentation: a systematic review. *Obes Surg.* 2014;24(2):299–309.

Coblijn UK, Lagarde SM, de Castro SMM, Kuiken SD, van Wagensveld BA. Symptomatic marginal ulcer disease after Roux-en-Y gastric bypass: incidence, risk factors and management. *Obes Surg.* 2015;25:805–811.

Csendes A, Burgos AM, Altuve J, Bonacic S. Incidence of marginal ulcer 1 month and 1 to 2 years after gastric bypass: A prospective consecutive endoscopic evaluation of 442 patients with morbid obesity. *Obes Surg.* 2009;19:135–138.

D'Hondt MA, Pottel H, Devriendt D, Van Rooy F, Vansteenkiste F. Can a short course of prophylactic low-dose proton pump inhibitor therapy prevent stomal ulceration after laparoscopic Roux-en-Y gastric bypass? *Obes Surg.* 2010;20:595–599.

Eckhauser A, Tourquati A, Youssef Y, et al. Internal hernia: postoperative complication of Roux-en-Y gastric bypass surgery. *Am Surg.* 2006;72(7):581–584.

El-Hayek K, Timratana P, Shimizu H, Chand B. Marginal ulcer after Roux-en-Y gastric bypass: what have we really learned? *Surg Endosc.* 2012;26:2789–2796.

Felix EL, Kettelle J, Mobley E, Swartz D. Perforated marginal ulcers after laparoscopic gastric bypass. *Surg Endosc.* 2008;22:2128–2132.

Hunter J, Stahl RD, Kakade M et al. Effectvienss of thoacoscopic truncal Vagotomy in the treatment of marginal ulcers after laproscopic Roux-en-Y gastric bypass. *Am J Surg.* 2012;78(6):663–668.

Ibele AR, Bendewald FP, Mattar SG, McKenna DT. Incidence of gastrojejunostomy stricture in laparoscopic Roux-en-Y gastric bypass using an autologous fibrin sealant. *Obes Surg.* Published March 6, 2014.

Kalaiselvan R, Exarchos G, Hamza N, Ammori BJ. Incidence of perforated gastrojejunal anastomotic ulcers after laparoscopic gastric bypass for morbid obesity and role of laparoscopy in their management. *Surg Obes Relat Dis.* 2012;8(4):423–428.

Rasmussen JJ, Fuller, W, Ali MR. Marginal ulceration after laparoscopic gastric bypass: an analysis of predisposing factors in 260 patients. *Surg Endosc.* 2007;21:1090–1094.

Scheffel O, Daskalakis M, Weiner RA. Two important criteria for reducing the risk of postoperative ulcers at the gastrojejunostomy site after gastric bypass: patient compliance and type of gastric bypass. *Eur J Obes.* 2011;4:39–41.

Sverdén E, Mattsson F, Sondén A, et al. Risk factors for marginal ulcer after gastric bypass surgery for obesity. *Ann Surg.* 2016;263(4):733–737.

Yurcisin BM, DeMaria EJ. Management of leak in the bariatric gastric bypass patient: re-operate, drain, and feed distally. *J Gastrointest Surg.* 2009;13:1564–1566.

Wilson JA, Romagnuolo J, Byrne TK, et al. Predictors of endoscopic findings after Roux-en-Y gastric bypass. *Am J Gastroenterol.* 2006;101(10):2194–2199.

55

Bariatric Surgery—Bypass—Abdominal Pain

Theresa Jackson

A 37-year-old female presents to the emergency department. She complains of abdominal pain that awoke her from sleep that has been persistent over the last 3–4 hours. She cannot get comfortable and is experiencing nausea and some emesis. She relates that she has had similar episodes approximately 1–2 times per week over the past few months, but the pain is always self-limited. However, this time, the pain is the worst she has ever felt.

Her surgical history is significant for two C-sections about 4 and 6 years ago, a laparoscopic Roux-en-Y gastric bypass (RYGB) a little over 2 years ago, and an open appendectomy when she was 12. She denies any drug, alcohol, or tobacco use. She relates that at the time of her surgery she weighed 290 lb, with a body mass index (BMI) of 53 kg/m^2, and now has lost 155 lb, with a BMI of 24.7 kg/m^2. She has not seen a bariatric surgeon in over a year since she just moved here for her new job 11 months ago.

Vital signs are heart rate 102, blood pressure 138/67, respiration rate 20, pulse oxygen 99% on the right atrium. Her exam is noted to have diffuse, nonspecific tenderness most predominant in the upper mid-abdomen and without rebound or guarding. Bowel sounds are present.

1. **What is the most common late complication that may result in abdominal pain after a laparoscopic Roux-en-Y gastric bypass (LRYGB)?**

   A. Marginal ulcer (ulcer at the gastrojejunostomy anastomosis)

   B. Biliary disease (e.g., cholelithiasis, biliary dyskinesia)

   C. Internal hernia causing a small bowel obstruction

   D. Intussusception of the jejunojejunostomy (JJ)

2. **Which of the following is the most appropriate first diagnostic test for this patient?**

   A. Upper endoscopy (EGD)

   B. Right upper quadrant ultrasound

   C. Magnetic resonance cholangiopancreatography (MRCP)

   D. Computed tomography (CT) scan of the abdomen and pelvis

3. **Which of the following statements is true regarding internal hernias after laparoscopic gastric bypass?**

   A. Internal hernias after laparoscopic gastric bypass are more common than those seen with open gastric bypass.

   B. Small bowel obstruction after laparoscopic gastric bypass can be conservatively managed in about 80% of cases.

   C. Internal hernias should never be evaluated laparoscopically.

   D. Large defects, such as Petersen's defect, as seen with an ante-colic Roux limb, do not require definitive closure.

4. **A target sign is noted on CT with dilated small bowel proximal to the JJ anastomosis. You suspect the etiology of this finding is an intussusception at the JJ anastomosis. How should this patient be managed?**

   A. Nasogastric decompression and observation

   B. Reduction of the intussusception and pexy

C. Reduction of the intussusception with resection of the JJ anastomosis and reconstruction

D. Reversal of the Roux-en-Y gastric bypass

5. **The CT scan of the abdomen and pelvis was unremarkable. You subsequently perform an upper endoscopy and a marginal ulcer is noted. Which of the following statements are true pertaining to marginal ulcers?**

A. Marginal ulcers are found on the gastric mucosa adjacent to the gastrojejunal anastomosis.

B. Risk factors for marginal ulcers include spicy food and stress.

C. First-line management for marginal ulcers includes removing a nidus (such as suture) if found on endoscopy, eliminating risk factors, and medical therapy with proton pump inhibitors (PPIs) and sucralfate.

D. All marginal ulcers ultimately require operative revision of the gastrojejunal anastomosis.

6. **The CT of the abdomen and pelvis was normal. On laboratory workup, the patient was noted to have leukocytosis and elevated liver function tests (LFTs) and was subsequently diagnosed with choledocholithiasis. Which of the following statements is true regarding the management of biliary disease in a bariatric patient?**

A. Cholecystectomies should be performed routinely in all patients undergoing bariatric surgery.

B. Right upper quadrant (RUQ) ultrasounds are unable to diagnose acute cholecystitis in patients' status post-bypass due to anatomical challenges.

C. Patients who are status post sleeve gastrectomy cannot undergo an ERCP (endoscopic retrograde cholangiopancratography) to relieve biliary obstruction from choledocholithiasis.

D. Patients who are status post–gastric bypass may require a laparoscopic-assisted transgastric ERCP to relieve biliary obstruction.

7. **When evaluating a patient for intermittent abdominal pain in your office after laparoscopic gastric bypass,**

A. the patient should be offered psychological counseling because most pain after a laparoscopic gastric bypass is psychosomatic.

B. the patient should be referred to their primary care physician as chronic abdominal pain is not a bariatric problem.

C. a diagnostic laparoscopy should be considered.

D. the patient should be offered reversal of the RGYB.

ANSWERS

1. **B.** The differential diagnosis for abdominal pain after LRYGB is broad and includes, but is not limited to, internal hernias, marginal ulcers, intussusception, and biliary disease. Biliary disease, including cholelithiasis, is the most frequent late complication following gastric bypass with approximately one-third of patients developing de novo cholelithiasis.

That said, in patients with acute abdominal pain who are status post-LRYGB, physicians must have a high index of suspicion for an internal hernia or, in rarer circumstances, intussusception. These patients require operative intervention as conservative management can have catastrophic consequences. To complicate the diagnostic process, internal hernias, marginal ulcers, intussusception, and gallstone disease can all present with epigastric pain associated with nausea and emesis.

2. **D.** Episodic upper abdominal pain associated with nausea and emesis is indicative of an internal hernia. Diagnosis of an internal hernia is often dependent on CT. Several signs in CT have been described to assist in the diagnosis of an internal hernia with a "mesenteric swirl sign" in conjunction with a small bowel obstruction as the most sensitive and accurate marker for an internal hernia.

CT imaging can aid in the diagnosis of several complications status post–gastric bypass. CT is the study of choice in those patients following gastric bypass with severe acute or chronic abdominal pain of unknown origin. Findings include dilation of the biliopancreatic limb or a "target sign." Dilation of the biliopancreatic limb with gastric remnant distention is indicative of a pathologic problem at the JJ anastomosis. This could be due to an intussusception or a more distal obstruction in the common channel. A "target sign" identified in a patient status post–gastric bypass is pathognomonic for intussusception and immediate surgery is warranted.

If CT findings are negative, a stepwise approach to the workup of the bariatric patient must be conducted. This may include an upper endoscopy, RUQ ultrasound, or MRCP. An upper endoscopy is the gold standard for diagnosis of a marginal ulcer, whereas a RUQ ultrasound and an MRCP are best used to diagnosis acute cholecystitis and choledocholithiasis, respectively. Based on this patient's clinical presentation and history, these imaging tests are not the best first diagnostic test. However, after ruling out an internal hernia, each of these tests may be considered in the ongoing workup.

3. **A.** Internal hernias are a protrusion of a viscus through a peritoneal or mesenteric aperture. Internal hernias after gastric bypass have the potential to form in two or three potential spaces depending on technique. These include the mesocolic window if a retrocolic orientation is performed, as well as Petersen's defect and the mesomesenteric defect at the JJ anastomosis. During gastric bypass creation, all defects, such as Petersen's defect, should be closed to reduce the incidence of internal hernias.

Retrocolic and antecolic pathways of the Roux limb

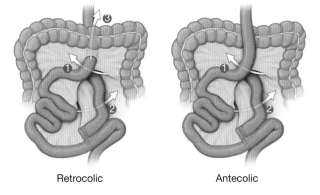

Retrocolic   Antecolic

Internal hernias after laparoscopic gastric bypass are more common than after open gastric bypass due to a reduction in adhesion formation. Adhesion formation acts to close down potential spaces created from anatomic reorientation. It should be noted that despite intraoperative closure of these defects, internal hernias may still form if the defects were improperly or incompletely closed. Additionally, the repair may be weakened by increased intra-abdominal pressure, such as during pregnancy or when significant weight loss occurs, causing a reduction in intra-abdominal fat leading to enlargement of these defects.

Small bowel obstruction after laparoscopic gastric bypass is rarely successfully managed conservatively, with most cases requiring operative intervention. A delay in getting to the operating room can lead to bowel ischemia and necrosis. Laparoscopic

evaluation of an internal hernia after laparoscopic gastric bypass is well documented and safe. The clinician's comfort with laparoscopy versus open surgery should be the defining factor regarding exploration as either can provide good outcomes. The key component to successful reduction of an internal hernia is defining the anatomy. It is recommended that a reduction of an internal hernia begin with identifying the ileocecal valve and following the bowel proximally. This will serve to both reduce the hernia on the appropriate side of the defect and will facilitate the identification of the anatomic landmarks of the JJ, biliopancreatic limb, and Roux limb.

4. **C.** Intussusception following gastric bypass typically occurs as retrograde (antiperistaltic) intussusception at the JJ. It is a rare finding with an incidence of less than 0.6%. Although small bowel intussusception in adults is typically due to a benign or malignant "lead point," this is not the case following gastric bypass. The etiology is thought to be due to motility disturbances resulting from the separation of the distal jejunum from the duodenal pacemaker. Similar to an internal hernia, intussusception results in abdominal pain associated with nausea and vomiting. This abdominal pain can be acute, intermittent, or chronic. The findings of a "target sign" on CT are pathognomonic for intussusception. Like an internal hernia, intussusception requires immediate surgery. Reduction alone results in an unacceptably high recurrence rate. Most recommend en bloc resection of the JJ with reconstruction. While reduction and enteropexy have been described, there is a statistically higher recurrence rate after plication/pexy without resection. Reversal of the gastric bypass and/or conversion to another procedure may be an option, but it is not the first-line management in patients with acute intussusception.

5. **C.** Marginal ulcers present following gastric bypass as epigastric pain associated with nausea and emesis. Rarely, they may present as a gastrointestinal hemorrhage or perforation. Their presentation is bimodal and can occur either early (less than 12 months) or late (more than 12 months) following surgery. The ulceration occurs on the jejunal side of the gastrojejunostomy due to insufficient protective mechanisms against gastric acid. Risk factors for marginal ulcers include foreign bodies such as sutures, nonsteroidal anti-inflammatory drugs (NSAIDs), and smoking. The gold standard for diagnosis is upper endoscopy

during which a nidus, if found, such as suture material or staples should be removed. First-line management for marginal ulcers is medical with the elimination of risk factors (smoking and NSAIDs), as well as sucralfate and a PPI. In very rare circumstances, if a marginal ulcer fails to resolve with medical therapy, reoperation with revision of the gastrojejunostomy anastomosis may be performed.

6. **D.** Both obesity and rapid weight loss are risk factors for the development of cholelithiasis. The incidence of de novo cholelithiasis following bariatric surgery occurs in approximately 33% of patients. In fact, cholelithiasis is the most common long-term complication following bariatric surgery. Nonetheless, only 6–16% will go on to develop symptomatic disease requiring cholecystectomy. Despite the high incidence of both asymptomatic and symptomatic biliary disease, a concomitant cholecystectomy at the time of bariatric surgery should not be offered as it portends higher rates of morbidity and mortality. Moreover, only about 8–10% of patients require a cholecystectomy after an RYGB.

In the general surgeon's armamentarium, management of biliary disease is commonplace. In general, the management of biliary disease for the bariatric patient is equivocal with some notable exceptions. Bariatric patients present in a typical fashion with postprandial RUQ or epigastric abdominal pain associated with nausea and emesis. An RUQ ultrasound remains the gold standard for diagnosis, and if choledocholithiasis is suspected, an MRCP can assist in making the diagnosis.

As with any patient, symptomatic cholelithiasis is managed with a cholecystectomy assuming the benefits outweigh the risks. For those with choledocholithiasis status post–gastric band or –gastric sleeve, management does not vary, with ERCP being the most frequent modality utilized. However, if a patient has undergone an RYGB, an ERCP is difficult, or in the case of duodenal switch, an ERCP is impossible due to altered anatomy. Common bile duct explorations may be performed. However, laparoscopic-assisted transgastric ERCP has been met with technical success and is advocated now by many.

7. **D.** Patients that present with abdominal pain after laparoscopic gastric bypass warrant a full evaluation due to the broad differential diagnosis. Pain is rarely a psychological source, and as such, an appropriate history should be taken followed by systematic workup. Workup should include, but not be limited

to, an EDG to rule out gastrojejunal ulcer or gastrogastric fistula, a CT scan to evaluate for an internal hernia or intussusception, a colonoscopy to assess for a colonic source, and an RUQ ultrasound, as well as a hepatobiliary iminodiacetic acid scan to eliminate gallstone disease or biliary dyskinesia as the culprit.

After a complete workup has been conducted, a diagnostic laparoscopy should be performed. Diagnostic laparoscopy is a safe and often therapeutic tool that detects pathologic findings in over half of post–bariatric surgery patients with chronic abdominal pain of unknown etiology. It should be noted that normal radiologic studies do not exclude the presence of an internal hernia or intussusception. Intermittent small bowel obstructions can occur in post-bariatric patients. As such, visual inspection of potential hernia spaces and the JJ is imperative.

BIBLIOGRAPHY

Aiolfi A, Asti E, Rausa E, Bernardi D, Bonitta G, Bonavina L. Trans-gastric ERCP after Roux-en-Y gastric bypass: systematic review and meta-analysis. *Obes Surg.* 2018;28(9): 2836–2843

Alsulaimy M, Punchai S, Ali FA, et al. The utility of diagnostic laparoscopy in post-bariatric surgery patients with chronic abdominal pain of unknown etiology. *Obes Surg.* 2017;27(8):1924–1928.

Blachar A, Federle MP. Internal hernia: an increasingly common cause of small bowel obstruction. *Semin Ultrasound CT MR.* 2002;23(2):174–183.

Carr WR, Mahawar KK, Balupuri S, Small PK. An evidence-based algorithm for the management of marginal ulcers following Roux-en-Y gastric bypass. *Obes Surg.* 2014;24(9):1520–1527.

Daellenbach L, Suter M. Jejunojejunal intussusception after Roux-en-Y gastric bypass: a review. *Obes Surg.* 2011;21(2):253–263.

Dilauro M, McInnes MD, Schieda N, et al. Internal hernia after laparoscopic Roux-en-Y gastric bypass: optimal CT signs for diagnosis and clinical decision making. *Radiology.* 2017;282(3):752–760.

Pineda O, Maydón HG, Amado M, et al. A prospective study of the conservative management of asymptomatic preoperative and postoperative gallbladder disease in bariatric surgery. *Obes Surg.* 2017;27(1):148–153.

Rasmussen JJ, Fuller W, Ali MR. Marginal ulceration after laparoscopic gastric bypass: an analysis of predisposing factors in 260 patients. *Surg Endosc.* 2007;21(7):1090–1094.

Stenberg E, Szabo E, Ågren G, et al. Closure of mesenteric defects in laparoscopic gastric bypass: a multicentre, randomised, parallel, open-label trial. *Lancet.* 2016;387(10026): 1397–1404.

Worni M, Guller U, Shah A, et al. Cholecystectomy concomitant with laparoscopic gastric bypass: a trend analysis of the nationwide inpatient sample from 2001 to 2008. *Obes Surg.* 2012;22(2):220–229.

56

Sleeve Gastrectomy Leaks

Brooke Pati

A 42-year-old female with a body mass index of 42 kg/m² and multiple comorbidities to include diabetes mellitus, hypertension, hyperlipidemia, and obstructive sleep apnea (OSA) has completed her preoperative evaluation for surgical management of her obesity and weight-related comorbidities. She uses continuous positive airway pressure (CPAP) nightly for her OSA. She is felt to be a good candidate for surgery, and she has opted for a sleeve gastrectomy (SG).

1. **Regarding the immediate postoperative management, which of the following is correct?**

    A. The use of CPAP is contraindicated for the first postoperative week.

    B. Sustained tachycardia is the most reliable indicator of a leak.

    C. The most likely cause of death after bariatric surgery is a myocardial infarction.

    D. This patient should have had an inferior vena cava (IVC) filter to prevent a pulmonary embolus.

    E. The leak rate from an SG is less than that of a Roux-en-Y gastric bypass (RYGB).

2. **Regarding intraoperative factors that affect staple line leaks after SG, which of the following is correct?**

    A. Staple line buttressing has decreased the incidence of staple line leak.

    B. Oversewing of the staple line has decreased the incidence of staple line leak.

    C. Performance of SG with a bougies <36ƒ decreases the likelihood of staple line leak.

    D. Treatment of the staple line with fibrin glue has decreased the staple line leak rate.

    E. Choice of staple height does not have an effect on staple line leak rates.

3. **The patient presents with fever, abdominal pain, and sustained tachycardia on postoperative day (POD) 4. Which of the following is correct?**

    A. A normal upper gastrointestinal (GI) contrast series rules out a staple line leak.

    B. Operative management of a staple line leak is more likely to be successful in this patient than in patients whose leaks present 10 days or more after the operation.

    C. If present, a drain amylase level is the same as the serum amylase level, this finding reliably rules out a staple line leak.

    D. A positive preoperative *Helicobacter pylori* test increased this patient's chance of having a staple line leak.

    E. Endoscopic therapies should be the first approach to gain control of a staple line leak.

4. **The patient undergoes operative repair of the staple line leak on POD 4. A closed suction drain is left. Which of the following is correct?**

    A. If this patient develops a gastrocutaneous fistula, endoscopic treatments should be discouraged unless the patient's condition is severe.

    B. The median time for staple line leaks to heal is less than 2 weeks.

    C. If an endoscopic stent is placed, the biggest problem that can occur is erosion.

D. If the patient develops a controlled gastrocutaneous fistula, drainage alone is still an acceptable option for treatment.

E. Chronic leaks/fistulae can be managed with late surgical therapy, such as Roux-en-Y anastomosis to the fistula site.

5. **Which of the following is correct regarding staple line leaks after SG?**

A. Leaks >10 days after the operation are more likely to occur after gastric bypass than SG.

B. Leaks most commonly occur in the distal third or antral staple lines.

C. Patients whose sleeves leak are treated by endoscopic stenting require parenteral nutrition.

D. Nonoperative management of leaks is unacceptable in any sleeve patient.

E. Patients with fistulae that fail to close may require conversion to a gastrectomy.

6. **On the morning of POD 1, the patient complains of abdominal pain radiating to the left shoulder that is not improved with oral or IV analgesics. She becomes febrile to 100.6°F and has a heart rate of 125 beats per minute. Both an upper GI series and a computed tomography (CT) scan with PO and IV contrast are negative for pathology. Her troponin level is 0.75, and her hematocrit is 30. Which of the following is the best course of action?**

A. Cardiology consult

B. Transfusion

C. Surgical exploration

D. Heparin bolus

E. Intubation

7. **Which of the following is correct regarding the role of intraoperative leak tests during SG?**

A. The use of air insufflation is the only method of detecting a staple line leak during SG.

B. Routine intraoperative leak tests during SG help prevent subsequent leaks.

C. The use of endoscopy to perform an intraoperative leak test during SG increases postoperative leaks compared to nonendoscopic methods.

D. Intraoperative leak testing is useful in cases with intraoperative complications, that is, staple line misfires.

ANSWERS

1. **B.** Sustained tachycardia greater than 120 is the most reliable indicator of a postoperative leak from bariatric surgery. Other complications that can lead to tachycardia, such as myocardial infarction, pulmonary embolism, bleeding, hypovolemia, and respiratory insufficiency, should also be ruled out, but unexplained and sustained tachycardia should prompt an intervention to find and treat a leak, which includes operative exploration. The leak rate of an SG (2.4%) is higher than that of an RYGB (0.8%).

CPAP is not contraindicated after an SG or an RYGB, and people who suffer from OSA should plan to use CPAP in the postoperative period. There are no data that suggest it increases the risk of a leak. Although people who have respiratory complication after bariatric surgery are at an increased risk of mortality, the most common cause of death after bariatric surgery is sepsis, followed by myocardial infarction, then a pulmonary embolism.

The recommended venous thromboembolic (VTE) prophylaxis for this patient is mechanical prophylaxis, ambulation on the night after surgery, and chemical prophylaxis with low-molecular-weight heparin or unfractionated heparin. There is no absolute indication for preoperative IVC filter placement, but it can be considered, along with mechanical and chemical prophylaxis in high-risk patients, especially if the risk of a VTE is higher than that of a filter-related complication.

2. **C.** Gastric leaks after SG are an important cause of morbidity and mortality. In a large published case series of open and laparoscopic cases, the reported incidence of gastric leaks is between 0.1–8.3% after RYGB and 0–7% after SG. Upper UGI series and CT scans with PO contrast have been noted to be unreliable. Management options are varied and dependent on the timing and clinical presentation of the leak. Immediate reoperation is the preferred course of action for the unstable patient, usually with prompt resuscitation, intravenous hydration and antibiotics, and surgical intervention with washout, irrigation of the abdominal cavity, wide drainage, and an attempt at suturing of the leak is the tissue condition allows it. Sound surgical judgment is imperative when deciding whether the tissues are amendable to

suturing or whether further intervention will only impose further damage.

At the same time, patients who remain hemodynamically stable, have a negative workup, and have persistent tachycardia >120 still require an operation. A leak that is allowed to persist will most likely lead to circulatory collapse, systemic inflammatory response syndrome, or sepsis. A negative exploration would be much better tolerated than any of those. Patients with persistent tachycardia should not be simply observed.

Even though the patient has an elevated troponin, this would not be surprising given the amount of tachycardia and any cardiac therapy would not treat the underlying cause. A CT scan with IV contrast with a pulmonary angiogram protocol should be done in this patient to rule out a pulmonary embolism (PE), and heparin should not be started unless a PE is determined or highly suspected. The indication for transfusion in a post-bariatric patient would be the same for any postoperative patient and with a hematocrit of 32, there is no indication for transfusion.

3. **B.** Staple line leaks after SG present challenging problems in terms of both diagnosis and management. Surgical treatment of staple line leaks that occur early (<10 days) the after operation are more likely to be successful than surgical treatment of late (>10 days) leaks. Although clinical signs can be subtle, upper GI series have been noted to be unreliable. Closed suction drain amylase has been suggested as a reasonable adjunct to clinical suspicion of a leak, but patients with leaks and normal drain amylase levels have been demonstrated. Therefore, a normal drain amylase or a negative upper GI should not prevent a surgeon from returning a patient to the OR if clinical suspicion for a leak remains.

Although preoperative detection and eradication of *H. pylori* infections have been advocated to reduce postoperative dyspepsia or ulceration, the presence of *H. pylori* does not appear to impact staple line leak rates. Although endoscopic therapies provide a useful adjunct in the treatment of gastric sleeve staple line leaks, they generally should not be used as the initial or primary therapy. Resuscitation, intravenous hydration and antibiotics, and either early surgical or interventional radiologic drainage of intra-abdominal fluid collections to control sepsis should be first-line therapies.

4. **E.** One of the largest reviews of staple line leaks after SG demonstrated that the median time for leak healing was 40 days (range 2–270). Endoluminal therapies for staple line leaks show a fairly high rate of success at resolving leaks and fistulas, with the main problem being stent migration. Although endoluminal therapies are useful adjuncts, standard fistula management with drainage is still an acceptable option, but it also mandates nutritional support. Chronic fistulae that develop can be successfully managed by late surgical therapy, such as bringing a Roux limb to the fistula site to control the drainage.

5. **E.** Late leaks (>10 days after initial surgery) are more likely to occur in SG patients than in gastric bypass patients. The majority (89%) of leaks occur in the proximal third of the stomach. Nonsurgical therapy is clearly an appropriate option in selected patients with leak, and endoluminal stenting has the specific advantage of allowing patients to take food by mouth. Total gastrectomy with esophagojejunostomy, conversion to gastric bypass, and lateral Roux-en-Y gastrojejunostomy all have been described as surgical therapy for sleeve fistulae that fail to heal.

6. **E.** Multiple intraoperative techniques have been employed and studied to attempt to reduce staple line leak rates after SG. Although there is some evidence that the use of buttressing material can reduce bleeding from the staple line, there are no conclusive data that staple line leak rates are reduced. Similarly, the choice of staple height and oversewing of the staple line did not show any benefit in reducing staple line leak.

The use of a bougie >40*f* in diameter has been shown to decrease the leak rate without a discernible impact on weight loss at up to 3 years compared to smaller bougies (<40*f*). The distance from pylorus where the staple line was begun also did not affect leak rates. Finally, treatment of the staple line with fibrin glue did not conclusively demonstrate any benefit in reducing staple line leak in gastric bypass patients, and few data exist to suggest it has any benefit in SG patients.

7. D. There are several methods of performing an intraoperative leak test, including air insufflation, endoscopy, and dyes, but there are no data to suggest any technique is superior or highly accurate. Although widely used, intraoperative leak tests have not been found to reduce the incidence of leak after SG. The American Society for Metabolic & Bariatric Surgery (ASMBS) states that intraoperative leak tests can identify otherwise undetectable areas of staple line disruption and have not been reported to prevent subsequent leaks. In cases with technical errors, such as staple line misfiring, multiple studies and an international expert panel consensus acknowledge the utility of intraoperative leak testing during these cases. Overall, the routine use of intraoperative leak tests during SG remains controversial as the ASMBS states that intraoperative leak tests should be used at the discretion of the surgeon.

REFERENCES

Aurora AR, Khaitan L, Saber AA. Sleeve gastrectomy and the risk of leak: a systematic analysis of 4,888 patients. *Surg Endosc.* 2011;26(6):1509–1515. doi:10.1007/s00464-011-2085-3

Bingham J, Kaufman J, Hata K, et al. A multicenter study of routine versus selective intraoperative leak testing for sleeve gastrectomy. *Surg Obes Relat Dis.* 2017;13(9): 1469–1475. doi:10.1016/j.soard.2017.05.022

Bingham J, Lallemand M, Barron M, et al. Routine intraoperative leak testing for sleeve gastrectomy: is the leak test full of hot air? *Am J Surg.* 2016;211(5):943–947. doi:10.1016/j.amjsurg.2016.02.002

Brethauer SA, and the American Society of Metabolic and Bariatric Surgery Clinical Issues Committee. ASMBS updated position statement on prophylactic measures to reduce the risk of venous thromboembolism in bariatric surgery. *SOARD.* 2013;9(4):493–497.

Burgos AM, Braghetto I, Csendes A, et al. Gastric leak after laparoscopic-sleeve gastrectomy for obesity. *Obes Surg.* 2009;19(12):1672–1677. doi:10.1007/s11695-009-9884-9

Casella G, Soricelli E, Rizzello M, et al. Nonsurgical treatment of staple line leaks after laparoscopic sleeve gastrectomy. *Obes Surg.* 2009 July;19(7):821–826.

Chen BI, Kiriakopoulos A, Tsakayannis D, Wachtel MS, Linos D, Frezza EE. Reinforcement does not necessarily reduce the rate of staple line leaks after sleeve gastrectomy. A review of the literature and clinical experiences. *Obes Surg.* 2009 Feb;19(2):166–172.

Gagner M, Hutchinson C, Rosenthal R. Fifth International Consensus Conference: current status of sleeve gastrectomy. *Surg Obes Relat Dis.* 2016;12(4):750–756. doi:10.1016/j.soard.2016.01.022

Gaspari A, Gentileschi P, Tacchino R, Basso N. The use of fibrin sealant to prevent major complications following laparoscopic gastric bypass: results of a multicenter, randomized trial. *Surg Endosc.* 2008 Nov;22(11):2492–2497.

Ghosh SK, Roy S, Chekan E, Fegelman EJ. A narrative of intraoperative staple line leaks and bleeds during bariatric surgery. *Obes Surg.* 2016;26(7):1601–1606. doi:10.1007/s11695-016-2177-1

Gupta PK, Gupta H, Kaushik M, et al. Predictors of pulmonary complications after bariatric surgery. *SOARD.* 2012;8(5):574–581.

Kim J, Azagury D, Eisenberg D, Demaria E, Campos GM. ASMBS position statement on prevention, detection, and treatment of gastrointestinal leak after gastric bypass and sleeve gastrectomy, including the roles of imaging, surgical exploration, and nonoperative management. *Surg Obes Relat Dis.* 2015;11(4):739–748. doi:10.1016/j.soard.2015.05.001

Maher JW, Bakhos W, Nahmias N, et al. Drain amylase levels are an adjunct in detection of gastrojejunostomy leaks after Roux-en-Y gastric bypass. *J Am Coll Surg.* 2009 May;208(5):881–884; discussion 885–886.

Mittermair R, Sucher R, Perathoner A, Wykypiel H. Routine upper gastrointestinal swallow studies after laparoscopic sleeve gastrectomy are unnecessary. *Am J Surg.* 2014;207(6):897–901. doi:10.1016/j.amjsurg.2013.06.015

Nelson DW, Blair KS, Martin MJ. Analysis of obesity-related outcomes and bariatric failure rates with the duodenal switch v gastric bypass for morbid obesity. *Arch Surg.* 2012;147(9):847–854.

Parikh MI, Issa R, McCrillis A, Saunders JK, Ude-Welcome A, Gagner M. Surgical strategies that may decrease leak after laparoscopic sleeve gastrectomy: a systematic review and meta-analysis of 9991 cases. *Ann Surg.* 2013;257(2): 231–237.

Rossetti G, Moccia F, Marra T, et al. Does helicobacter pylori infection have influence on outcome of laparoscopic sleeve gastrectomy for morbid obesity? *Int J Surg.* 2014;12(Suppl 1):S68–S71.

Sakran N, Goitein D, Raziel A, et al. Gastric leaks after sleeve gastrectomy: a multicenter experience with 2,834 patients. *Surg Endosc.* 2012;27(1):240–245. doi:10.1007/s00464-012-2426-x

Silecchia GI, Boru CE, Mouiel J, et al. Utility of routine versus selective upper gastrointestinal series to detect anastomotic leaks after laparoscopic gastric bypass. *Obes Surg.* 2011 Aug;21(8):1238–1242.

van de Vrande S, Himpens J, El Mourad H, Debaerdemaeker R, Leman G. Management of chronic proximal fistulas after sleeve gastrectomy by laparoscopic Roux-limb placement. *Surg Obes Relat Dis.* 2013 Nov–Dec;9(6):856–861.

57

Biliopancreatic Diversion with Duodenal Switch for Morbid Obesity

Christopher G. Yheulon

A 34-year-old morbidly obese female with a current body mass index (BMI) of 55 kg/m^2 is being evaluated for potential bariatric surgery. She has tried numerous diet and exercise programs, including a medically supervised program for 12 months, and has failed to maintain any significant weight loss. She has type 2 diabetes, gastroesophageal reflux disease (GERD), hypertension, and sleep apnea. She has had two prior C-sections and a laparoscopic cholecystectomy but no other surgeries. She has done independent research on the Internet and is interested in getting more information about the "switch" procedure.

1. **Which of the following statements about bariatric surgical procedures is correct?**

   A. True bariatric surgery achieves weight loss through restrictive and malabsorptive effects.
   B. The duodenal switch is the most malabsorptive of the currently performed bariatric procedures.
   C. The duodenal switch is the most restrictive of the currently performed procedures.
   D. Candidates for the duodenal switch must have a BMI greater than 55 kg/m^2.
   E. This patient's medical comorbidities disqualify her for bariatric surgery.

2. **The patient is confused about the anatomic difference between the duodenal switch and the gastric bypass. Which of the following statements is correct about the anatomy?**

   A. Both the duodenal switch and the gastric bypass involve the creation of a low-pressure gastric pouch.
   B. The duodenal switch involves preservation of the pylorus.
   C. The duodenal switch creates a shorter biliopancreatic limb.
   D. The alimentary limb is anastomosed to the stomach in both operations.
   E. The amount of malabsorption with the duodenal switch is primarily a function of the length of the biliopancreatic limb.

3. **The patient is interested in knowing about the potential benefits of surgery and whether she is a candidate for laparoscopic or open surgery. Which of the following statements are correct regarding the duodenal switch?**

   A. The patient is not a candidate for a laparoscopic approach due to her prior abdominal surgery.
   B. The surgery has a 50% chance of improving her diabetes after she has achieved significant weight loss.
   C. The surgery has a near 100% likelihood of curing her gastroesophageal reflux disease.
   D. She can expect to lose 40–50% of her excess body weight in the first year after surgery.
   E. The duodenal switch is associated with a >80% rate of resolution for her hypertension, sleep apnea, and diabetes at 1 year after surgery.

4. **The patient also wishes to know about the risks of surgery and common complications associated with the duodenal switch. Which of the following statements is correct?**

   A. There is no postoperative risk of an internal hernia after the duodenal switch procedure.

   B. Chronic diarrhea and steatorrhea may be a complication of this procedure.

   C. Protein and calorie malabsorption that requires parenteral nutrition or surgical revision only occurs in fewer than 1% of patients.

   D. Fat malabsorption may result in deficiencies of vitamins B6 and C.

   E. Symptoms of dumping syndrome after a duodenal switch are likely.

5. **The patient undergoes an uncomplicated laparoscopic duodenal switch procedure and is discharged home on postoperative day (POD) 3. On POD 5, she presents to the emergency department with worsening abdominal pain, distension, fevers, and emesis. She is febrile to 102.7°F, tachycardic to 125, tachypneic, and has a systolic blood pressure of 80. Her abdomen is diffusely tender. She states that she has had diarrhea for the past 3 days and has not been able to tolerate oral intake. Which of the following statements about the evaluation and management of this patient is correct?**

   A. Intravenous fluid resuscitation should not be given due to the concern for possible volume overload and pulmonary edema.

   B. A normal upper gastrointestinal (GI) series with oral contrast (swallow study) will rule out an abdominal source of pathology.

   C. An urgent computed tomography (CT) pulmonary angiogram scan must be obtained to rule out a pulmonary embolus.

   D. The patient requires emergent surgical exploration to identify the cause of her symptoms.

   E. The most likely cause of her symptoms is an internal hernia.

6. **What is the most common nonemergent indication for revision of a duodenal switch?**

   A. Malnutrition
   B. Diarrhea
   C. Abdominal pain
   D. Emesis
   E. Liver disease

7. **A patient in your clinic inquires about a single anastomosis duodenal ileal bypass with sleeve gastrectomy (SADI-S). When compared to standard duodenal switch, what does the data show for outcomes of SADI-S?**

   A. SADI-S has less weight loss and fewer malabsorptive side effects when compared to duodenal switch.

   B. SADI-S has less weight loss and similar malabsorptive side effects when compared to duodenal switch.

   C. SADI-S has less weight loss and more malabsorptive side effects when compared to duodenal switch.

   D. SADI-S has similar weight loss and fewer malabsorptive side effects when compared to duodenal switch.

   E. SADI-S has more weight loss and more malabsorptive side effects when compared to duodenal switch.

ANSWERS

1. **B.** All currently performed bariatric procedures achieve weight loss primarily through either restriction, malabsorption, both, or hormonal effects. Restriction is achieved by reducing the volume capacity of the stomach through a reduction in size or external compression. The sleeve gastrectomy and adjustable gastric band are the only endorsed restrictive procedures. Malabsorption is achieved through rerouting of the small intestine and digestive enzymes to decrease the length of intestine available for absorption. The duodenal switch (also known as the biliopancreatic diversion with duodenal switch) involves the longest length of bypassed intestine and thus is more malabsorptive than other procedures, such as the gastric bypass. Hormonal changes are less clear, but the changes in ghrelin and leptin, in particular, occur with the sleeve, the Roux-en-Y gastric bypass (RYGB), and the duodenal switch such that hunger is abated and meal satisfaction is increased. This also contributes to weight loss.

   The restrictive component of the duodenal switch involves the formation of a gastric sleeve, which achieves moderate restriction. Other procedures such as the gastric bypass and adjustable gastric band are more restrictive than the duodenal switch. Candidacy for a duodenal switch is the same as for any bariatric procedure (BMI >40 or >35 with obesity-related comorbidities), although most surgeons reserve this option for higher BMI patients. Medical comorbidities related to obesity are not contraindications to surgery, and improving or resolving these comorbidities is the primary goal of bariatric surgery.

2. **B.** The gastric bypass involves creating a small proximal gastric pouch that is highly restrictive, but because it does not include the pyloric sphincter, it is also considered a low-pressure pouch. In contrast, the duodenal switch involves creating a vertical sleeve gastrectomy (see Figure 57-1) and division of the duodenum just past the pylorus, resulting in a greater gastric capacity and less restriction than the gastric bypass. The duodenal switch operation preserves the pylorus and at least part of the antrum, which provides the advantage of controlled gastric emptying and avoidance of the "dumping syndrome" frequently seen with gastric bypass. However, the presence of a pyloric sphincter means that the sleeve portion of the duodenal switch is a high-pressure stomach. The duodenal switch results in more bypassed intestine than the gastric bypass and is the most malabsorptive bariatric procedure currently in use.

The final anatomy of the duodenal switch is as shown in Figure 57-1: The alimentary limb (AL, and analogous to the "Roux" limb in gastric bypass) is typically 150–200 cm long and the proximal end is anastomosed to the duodenum just past the pylorus. The biliopancreatic limb (BPL) is typically long and unmeasured. The small intestine distal to the junction of the AL and BPL is called the common channel or common limb (CL) and is typically 50–150 cm in length from the ileocecal valve. The amount of malabsorption is primarily a function of the length of the common channel, as this is where nutrients mix with the biliopancreatic digestive enzymes. A shorter common channel will result in greater malabsorption, and vice versa.

3. **E.** Among the currently performed bariatric procedures, the duodenal switch has been associated with the greatest absolute and relative weight loss (Figure 57-2), as well as the highest rates of improvement or resolution of obesity-related comorbidities. The duodenal switch can be performed as an open or a laparoscopic procedure, although it is arguably the most technically challenging bariatric procedure to perform laparoscopically. This patient would be an excellent candidate for laparoscopic surgery, and prior pelvis or laparoscopic abdominal surgery is not

Biliopancreatic diversion with duodenal switch

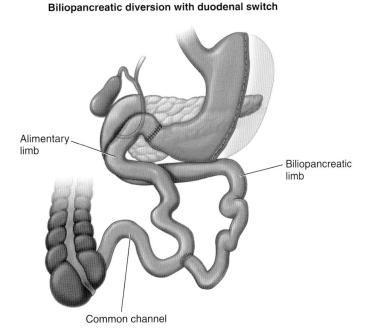

Figure 57-1 Diagram of the duodenal switch anatomy including the alimentary limb (AL), the biliopancreatic limb (BPL), and the common limb or common channel (CL). Reprinted with permission from Gagner et al. (2009).

RYGB Roux-en-Y gastric bypass
BPD/DS Biliopancreatic diversion with duodenal switch

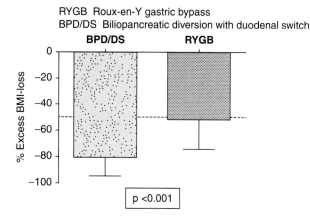

Figure 57-2 Average weight loss (percent BMI lost) at 4 years for duodenal switch (BPD/DS) versus gastric bypass (RYGB) patients in a prospective randomized study. Figure reproduced with permission from Hedberg et al. (2012).

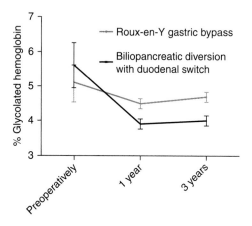

Figure 57-3 Average change in glycolated hemoglobin (HgBA1C) levels at 1 and 3 years postoperatively in a prospective randomized study of duodenal switch versus gastric bypass. Despite starting at a higher HgBA1C level at baseline, patients undergoing duodenal switch demonstrated lower levels at 1 and 3 years. Figure reproduced with permission Hedberg et al. (2012).

a contraindication to a laparoscopic approach. The duodenal switch has been reported to achieve an average 80% to 100% rate of improvement or resolution of type 2 diabetes and normalization of HgbA1C levels (Figure 57-3).

In addition, there is often a marked improvement in diabetes immediately after surgery, and this has been attributed to both the marked change in dietary intake as well as the bypass of digested food away from the duodenopancreatic complex. One caveat to the high rates of improvement of obesity-related comorbidities is that gastroesophageal reflux disease may not improve, or may even worsen, after converting the stomach to a sleeve gastrectomy configuration. The percentage of excess weight loss seen with the duodenal switch is typically in the 60–80% range at 1 year and has been shown to be superior to gastric bypass or sleeve gastrectomy alone in multiple series. Resolution rates of 80–100% for other weight-related comorbidities, including hypertension, sleep apnea, hyperlipidemia, and hypertriglyceridemia, have been demonstrated. The duodenal switch has also been shown to result in a superior reduction in cardiovascular risk profiles.

4. **B.** An internal hernia can occur following any surgery that involves division of the small intestine and then performance of an anastomosis and is one of the most feared late complications of the duodenal switch or gastric bypass. Any acute small bowel obstruction or chronic abdominal pain syndrome in these patients should prompt immediate evaluation for an internal hernia. The duodenal switch primarily affects absorption of fats and proteins, and the fat malabsorption may result in significant diarrhea and steatorrhea postoperatively. The duodenal switch carries the highest risk of protein/calorie malnutrition due to the high degree of malabsorption, with approximately 5% of patients requiring parenteral supplementation or surgical revision.

Dumping syndrome is thought to be due to the rapid passage of high-carbohydrate and high-osmolar nutrients directly into the jejunum and is commonly seen after gastric bypass surgery. This can cause immediate symptoms ("early" dumping) of abdominal pain, bloating, diarrhea, flushing, nausea, and emesis and then delayed symptoms ("late" dumping) of sweating, weakness, and dizziness due to hypoglycemia. Dumping syndrome is very uncommon after the duodenal switch as the pylorus is preserved and gastric emptying should be more controlled compared to the gastric bypass.

5. **D.** Bariatric surgical patients are at risk for a number of potential perioperative complications in the early postoperative period. These include surgical site infections, venous thrombosis, pulmonary embolus, anastomotic or staple line leaks, bleeding, iatrogenic bowel injury, and early postoperative bowel obstruction. This patient's presentation is extremely concerning due to her abnormal hemodynamics, abdominal pain, and fever. The primary concerns in a patient

presenting like this after a duodenal switch are for anastomotic leak, staple line leak (from the sleeve gastrectomy or the duodenal stump), or an iatrogenic bowel injury. Initial management should focus on resuscitation of the patient, identification of the source of the problem (if possible), and preparation for likely operative intervention. A normal "swallow" or upper GI study does not definitively rule out an anastomotic leak and does not evaluate the duodenal stump or the distal anastomosis.

Although a pulmonary embolus is possible, this patient's constellation of symptoms is much more consistent with an acute abdominal pathology, and intervention should not be delayed to obtain a CT scan for a less likely diagnosis. This patient most likely has a leak from a staple line or an anastomosis resulting in peritonitis and sepsis. Immediate surgical exploration, either open or laparoscopically, is indicated to identify and correct the source of the problem. If the patient presented with minimal symptoms and normal hemodynamics, then a thorough imaging evaluation would be indicated to identify or rule out a leak and to direct possible nonoperative management with the placement of an intraluminal stent. Although an internal hernia with incarcerated and compromised bowel is possible, these are typically seen much later in the postoperative period (months to years) after significant weight loss has occurred.

6. **A.** The most common reason for nonemergent revision of duodenal switch is malabsorption, followed by diarrhea (also considered a sequela of malabsorption). Surgical revision for this problem usually involves lengthening of the common channel to reduce the degree of malabsorption. The high degree of fat malabsorption affects the absorption of the fat-soluble vitamins (A, D, E, K), and these should either be routinely supplemented or closely monitored and selectively supplemented.

7. **D.** Retrospective studies following patients for up to 5 years after SADI-S show a percentage of excess weight loss (%EWL) of 87–98%. For comparison, 10-year data for standard duodenal switch shows a %EWL of 62–80%. However, small series have demonstrated that SADI-S have a lower incidence of diarrhea (0.8%) and malnutrition (0.8%), than standard DS (11.2% and 8%, respectively). These data are encouraging as SADI-S is a technically easier operation with only one anastomosis. However, longer-term data must still be analyzed to truly compare the two procedures. The SADI-S is now endorsed by the ASMBS.

BIBLIOGRAPHY

Aasheim ET, Bjorkman S, Sovik TT, et al. Vitamin status after bariatric surgery: a randomized study of gastric bypass and duodenal switch. *Am J Clin Nutr.* 2009;90:15–22.

Anderson B, Gill RS, de Gara CJ, et al. Biliopancreatic diversion: the effectiveness of duodenal switch and its limitations. *Gastroenterol Res Pract.* 2013;2013:974762.

Anthone GJ. Duodenal switch operation for morbid obesity. *Adv Surg.* 2004;38:293–309.

Banerjee A, Ding Y, Mikami DJ, et al. The role of dumping syndrome in weight loss after gastric bypass surgery. *Surg Endosc.* 2013;27:1573–1578.

Biertho L, Lebel S, Marceau S, et al. Laparoscopic sleeve gastrectomy: with or without duodenal switch? A consecutive series of 800 cases. *Dig Surg.* 2014;31:48–54.

Blachar A, Federle MP. Internal hernia: an increasingly common cause of small bowel obstruction. *Semin Ultrasound CT MR.* 2002;23:174–183.

Buchwald H, Kellogg TA, Leslie DB, et al. Duodenal switch operative mortality and morbidity are not impacted by body mass index. *Ann Surg.* 2008;248:541–548.

Causey MW, Fitzpatrick E, Carter P. Pressure tolerance of newly constructed staple lines in sleeve gastrectomy and duodenal switch. *Am J Surg.* 2013;205:571–574; discussion 574–575.

Chandler RC, Srinivas G, Chintapalli KN, et al. Imaging in bariatric surgery: a guide to postsurgical anatomy and common complications. *AJR Am J Roentgenol.* 2008;190:122–135.

Chiu CC. Randomized clinical trial of laparoscopic gastric bypass versus laparoscopic duodenal switch for superobesity. *Br J Surg.* 2010;97:160–166.

Comeau E, Gagner M, Inabnet WB, et al. Symptomatic internal hernias after laparoscopic bariatric surgery. *Surg Endosc.* 2005;19:34–39.

Dolan K, Hatzifotis M, Newbury L, et al. A clinical and nutritional comparison of biliopancreatic diversion with and without duodenal switch. *Ann Surg.* 2004;240:51–56.

Dorman RB, Rasmus NF, al-Haddad BJ, et al. Benefits and complications of the duodenal switch/biliopancreatic diversion compared to the Roux-en-Y gastric bypass. *Surgery.* 2012;152:758–765; discussion 765–767.

DuPree CE, Blair K, Steele SR, et al. Laparoscopic sleeve gastrectomy in patients with preexisting gastroesophageal reflux disease: a national analysis. *JAMA Surg.* 2014;149:328–334.

Elder KA, Wolfe BM. Bariatric surgery: a review of procedures and outcomes. 2007;132:2253–2271.

Ellison SR, Ellison SD. Bariatric surgery: a review of the available procedures and complications for the emergency physician. *J Emerg Med.* 2008;34:21–32.

Ferchak CV, Meneghini LF. Obesity, bariatric surgery and type 2 diabetes—a systematic review. *Diabetes Metab Res Rev.* 2004;20:438–445.

Frenken M, Cho EY, Karcz WK, et al. Improvement of type 2 diabetes mellitus in obese and non-obese patients after the duodenal switch operation. *J Obes*. 2011;2011:860169.

Gagner M, Boza C. Laparoscopic duodenal switch for morbid obesity. *Expert Rev Med Devices*. 2006;3:105–112.

Gagner M, Deitel M, Kalberer TL, et al. The Second International Consensus Summit for Sleeve Gastrectomy, March 19–21, 2009. *Surg Obes Relat Dis*. 2009;5:476–85.

Gagner M, Matteotti R. Laparoscopic biliopancreatic diversion with duodenal switch. *Surg Clin North Am*. 2005;85: 141–149; x–xi.

Hamoui N, Chock B, Anthone GJ, et al. Revision of the duodenal switch: indications, technique, and outcomes. *J Am Coll Surg*. 2007;204:603–608.

Hedberg J, Hedenstrom H, Karlsson FA, et al. Gastric emptying and postprandial PYY response after biliopancreatic diversion with duodenal switch. *Obes Surg*. 2011;21:609–615.

Hedberg J, Sundbom M. Superior weight loss and lower HbA1c 3 years after duodenal switch compared with Roux-en-Y gastric bypass—a randomized controlled trial. *Surg Obes Relat Dis*. 2012;8:338–343.

Hedberg J, Sundstrom J, Sundbom M. Duodenal switch versus Roux-en-Y gastric bypass for morbid obesity: systematic review and meta-analysis of weight results, diabetes resolution and early complications in single-centre comparisons. *Obes Rev*. 2014;15:555–563.

Hess DS, Conference ABSC. Biliopancreatic diversion with duodenal switch. *Surg Obes Relat Dis*. 2005;1:329–333.

Hess DS, Hess DW. Biliopancreatic diversion with a duodenal switch. *Obes Surg*. 1998;8:267–282.

Iqbal A, Miedema B, Ramaswamy A, et al. Long-term outcome after endoscopic stent therapy for complications after bariatric surgery. *Surg Endosc*. 2011;25:515–520.

Jacobsen HJ, Nergard BJ, Leifsson BG, et al. Management of suspected anastomotic leak after bariatric laparoscopic Roux-en-y gastric bypass. *Br J Surg*. 2014;101:417–423.

Kawkabani Marchini A, Denys A, Paroz A, et al. The four different types of internal hernia occurring after laparascopic Roux-en-Y gastric bypass performed for morbid obesity: are there any multidetector computed tomography (MDCT) features permitting their distinction? *Obes Surg*. 2011;21:506–516.

Kim J. American Society for Metabolic and Bariatric Surgery statement on single-anastomosis duodenal switch. *Surg Obes Relat Dis*. 2016;12(5):944–945.

Laurenius A, Olbers T, Naslund I, et al. Dumping syndrome following gastric bypass: validation of the dumping symptom rating scale. *Obes Surg*. 2013;23:740–755.

MacPherson BH. Iron absorption and the duodenal switch operation. *Obes Surg*. 1999;9:221–222.

McConnell DB, O'Rourke RW, Deveney CW. Common channel length predicts outcomes of biliopancreatic diversion alone and with the duodenal switch surgery. *Am J Surg*. 2005;189:536–540; discussion 540.

Mason RJ. Duodenal switch for morbid obesity: is it safe? *Adv Surg*. 2013;47:153–176.

Nelson D, Porta R, Blair K, et al. The duodenal switch for morbid obesity: modification of cardiovascular risk markers compared with standard bariatric surgeries. *Am J Surg*. 2012;203:603–608.

O'Brien PE, Hindle A, Brennan L, et al. Long-term outcomes after bariatric surgery: a systematic review and meta-analysis of weight loss at 10 or more years for all bariatric procedures and a single-centre review of 20-year outcomes after adjustable gastric banding. *Obes Surg*. 2019;29(1):3–14.

Prachand VN, Davee RT, Alverdy JC. Duodenal switch provides superior weight loss in the super-obese (BMI > or = 50 kg/m2) compared with gastric bypass. *Ann Surg*. 2006; 244:611–619.

Prachand VN, Ward M, Alverdy JC. Duodenal switch provides superior resolution of metabolic comorbidities independent of weight loss in the super-obese (BMI > or = 50 kg/m2) compared with gastric bypass. *J Gastrointest Surg*. 2010;14:211–220.

Ren CJ, Patterson E, Gagner M. Early results of laparoscopic biliopancreatic diversion with duodenal switch: a case series of 40 consecutive patients. *Obes Surg*. 2000;10:514–523; discussion 524.

Sovik TT, Aasheim ET, Taha O, et al. Weight loss, cardiovascular risk factors, and quality of life after gastric bypass and duodenal switch: a randomized trial. *Ann Intern Med*. 2011;155:281–291.

Strain GW, Gagner M, Inabnet WB, et al. Comparison of effects of gastric bypass and biliopancreatic diversion with duodenal switch on weight loss and body composition 1–2 years after surgery. *Surg Obes Relat Dis*. 2007;3: 31–36.

Sudan R, Jacobs DO. Biliopancreatic diversion with duodenal switch. *Surg Clin North Am*. 2011;91:1281–1293; ix.

Topart P, Becouarn G. The single anastomosis duodenal switch modifications: a review of the current literature on outcomes. *Surg Obes Relat Dis*. 2017;13(8):1306–1312.

Topart P, Becouarn G, Ritz P. Comparative early outcomes of three laparoscopic bariatric procedures: sleeve gastrectomy, Roux-en-Y gastric bypass, and biliopancreatic diversion with duodenal switch. *Surg Obes Relat Dis*. 2012;8:250–254.

Ukleja A, Stone RL. Medical and gastroenterologic management of the post-bariatric surgery patient. *J Clin Gastroenterol*. 2004;38:312–321.

Yimcharoen P, Heneghan HM, Tariq N, et al. Endoscopic stent management of leaks and anastomotic strictures after foregut surgery. *Surg Obes Relat Dis*. 2011;7:628–636.

58

Bariatric Surgery—Nutrition Complications

Brooke Pati

A 35-year-old female with a past medical history of hypertension, type II diabetes mellitus, and morbid obesity underwent a Roux-en-Y gastric bypass (RYGB) 9 months ago without complication. Preoperatively, the patient had screening laboratory tests and was found to have normal levels of vitamins A, C, D, E, K, thiamine, folate, and cobalamin and minerals iron, calcium, and copper. On her last visit office visit 3 months ago, no complications were noted, and weight loss was found to be appropriate. In the clinic today, the patient reports recent difficulty with concentration at work, increased fatigue, and shortness of breath walking up the stairs.

1. **What nutritional deficiency is most likely associated with the described presentation?**
   A. Vitamin D
   B. Folate
   C. Vitamin A
   D. Thiamine
   E. Iron

2. **What is the best screening test for detecting iron deficiency?**
   A. Serum iron concentration
   B. Hemoglobin
   C. Total iron-binding capacity
   D. Serum ferritin
   E. Transferrin

3. **What treatment regimen would have likely prevented this patient's symptoms?**
   A. Adequate intake of clear liquids (64 oz/day)
   B. Daily iron ferrous gluconate

   C. Daily multivitamin supplement with iron
   D. Monthly intravenous iron therapy
   E. Consumption of 2 g/kg of protein daily

4. **The patient responds to the previous therapy and her symptoms resolve. At her 2-year follow-up, she complains of an unsteady gait, worsening vision, and a poor appetite. Her daughter notes that she seems to be confused. She did not, for instance, obtain the nutrition labs that were ordered prior to this appointment. What is the next step in management?**
   A. A computed tomography (CT) scan of the brain
   B. Hydration and immediate administration of 100 mg of IV thiamine
   C. Neurologic exam
   D. Hydration and IV glucose followed by 100 mg of IV thiamine
   E. Oral thiamine only

ANSWERS

1. **E.** Iron deficiency anemia is one of the most common nutritional problems following bariatric surgery and results in hypochromic microcytic anemia. It is commonly seen in patients who have undergone RYGB secondary to the decrease in pH in the gastric pouch, which affects absorption in the duodenum and proximal jejunum. The symptoms of iron deficiency after gastric bypass are similar to those from other causes of iron deficiency and include fatigue, pallor, dyspnea on exertion, and difficulty with concentration.

Anemia from B6 (folate) or B12 deficiency is also common after RYGB and would have a similar presentation, but iron deficiency occurs more frequently. Thiamine deficiency is more likely to present with neurologic complaints and is more common in patients who have been vomiting. Vitamin A deficiency would present with visual complaints, particularly with vision in low lighting, and it is uncommon. Vitamin D deficiency is common but would present with symptoms of hypocalcemia, such as weakness, numbness, and possibly a fracture.

2. **D.** For the purpose of screening patients for iron deficiency anemia, serum ferritin is the best laboratory test available. It is a more specific and earlier indicator of iron body capacity and becomes abnormal prior to a decrease in serum iron concentration. Because ferritin is an acute-phase reactant, it can be elevated in patients with chronic inflammation or infection; therefore, obtaining a combination of tests (serum iron, serum transferrin, total iron-binding capacity, serum ferritin levels) is recommended for diagnosing iron deficiency.

3. **B.** The American Society for Metabolic & Bariatric Surgery (ASMBS) guidelines recommend that iron status should be monitored in all patients within the first 3 months after bariatric procedures, then every 3 to 6 months until 12 months, and then annually thereafter. Anemia is more evident in the menstruating female, and thus, prophylactic iron supplementation is shown to decrease the incidence of this presentation. Prophylactic treatment regimens include 150 to 200 mg of elemental iron daily with either oral ferrous sulfate, fumarate, or gluconate. Intravenous iron infusion, often with ferric gluconate or sucrose, may be needed in those patients with gastrointestinal toxicity or severe intolerance to oral iron supplements or refractory deficiency due to severe iron malabsorption after bariatric surgery. It is also not intended for continuous monthly use. Most patients undergo monthly IV therapy for 3 consecutive months only. Multivitamins with iron do not typically contain enough elemental iron to maintain adequate levels, and vitamin C in those products hinders the absorption of the iron.

4. This patient has evidence of thiamine deficiency and the first step in managing these patients is to do a thorough neurologic exam. Many of the findings can

be subtle to surgeons, but a failure to diagnose or a missed diagnosis of a neurologic defect can be devastating to the patient. Thiamine deficiency management requires prompt identification, hydration, and administration of IV thiamine only based on clinical grounds. Failure to treat thiamine deficiency can lead to permanent neurologic deficit and Wernicke's encephalopathy (WE). WE classically presents with symptoms of dementia, ataxia, and ocular problems. The recommended regimen is 500 of IV thiamine over 30 minutes three times a day for 2 consecutive days or intramuscular for 5 days in combination with other vitamins that include B12 and folate. It is important to administer glucose after thiamine deficiency and not before because it is known to worsen the WE symptoms. Oral thiamine will not be absorbed enough in the acute presentation that would be needed to prevent further neurologic deficit. A CT scan of the brain is important to rule out other causes of a neurologic deficit but is not immediately required.

BIBLIOGRAPHY

Brolin RE, Gorman JH, Gorman RC, et al. Prophylactic iron supplementation after Roux-en-Y gastric bypass: a prospective, double-blind, randomized study. *Arch Surg.* 1998;133:740.

Cook CC, Hallwood PM, Thomson AD. B vitamin deficiency and neuropsychiatric syndromes in alcohol misuse. *Alcohol Alcohol.* 1998;33:317.

Gehrer S, Kern B, Peters T, Christoffel-Courtin C, Peterli R. Fewer nutrient deficiencies after laparoscopic sleeve gastrectomy (LSG) than after laparoscopic Roux-Y-gastric bypass (LRYGB)—a prospective study. *Obes Surg.* 2010;20(4):447–453. doi:10.1007/s11695-009-0068-4

Goddard AF, James MW, McIntyre AS, Scott BB. Guidelines for the management of iron deficiency anaemia. *Gut.* 2011;60(10):1309–1316. doi:10.1136/gut.2010.228874

Love AL, Billett HH. Obesity, bariatric surgery, and iron deficiency: true, true, true and related. *Am J Hematol.* 2008;83(5):403.

Lupoli R, Lembo E, Saldalamacchia G, Avola CK, Angrisani L, Capaldo B. Bariatric surgery and long-term nutritional issues. *World J Diabetes.* 2017;8(11):464. doi:10.4239/wjd.v8.i11.464

Mechanick JI, Apovian C, Brethauer S, et al. Clinical practice guidelines for the perioperative nutrition, metabolic, and nonsurgical support of patients undergoing bariatric procedures—2019 update: cosponsored by American Association of Clinical Endocrinologists/American College of Endocrinology, The Obesity Society, American Society for Metabolic & Bariatric Surgery, Obesity Medicine Association, and American Society of Anesthesiologists. *Surg Obes Relat Dis.* 2020;16(2):175–247. doi:10.1016/j.soard.2019.10.025

Obinwanne KM, Fredrickson KA, Mathiason MA, et al. Incidence, treatment, and outcomes of iron deficiency after laparoscopic Roux-en-Y gastric bypass: a 10-year analysis. *J Am Coll Surg.* 2014;218:246.

Salgado W Jr, Modotti C, Nonino CB, Ceneviva R. Anemia and iron deficiency before and after bariatric surgery. *Surg Obes Relat Dis.* 2014;10:49.

Singh S, Kumar A. Wernicke encephalopathy after obesity surgery: a systematic review. *Neurology.* 2007;68:807.

Thomson AD, Ryle PR, Shaw GK. Ethanol, thiamine and brain damage. *Alcohol Alcohol.* 1983;18:27.

Wordem, RW, Allen HM. Wernicke's encephalopathy after gastric bypass that masqueraded as acute psychosis: a case report. *Curr Surg.* 2006;63(2):114–116.

59

Revisional Bariatric Surgery

Hussna Wakily

A 45-year-old female with a history of type 2 diabetes, hypertension, sleep apnea on continuous positive airway pressure CPAP, hyperlipidemia, and a body mass index (BMI) of 42 presents to clinic with failure to lose weight after having a laparoscopic adjustable gastric band placed 4 years ago. She has been compliant with diet and exercise but has not been able to lose weight with the band. She is interested in the Roux-en-Y gastric bypass (RYGB) and would like to know her options for revisional surgery.

1. **Which of the following is a candidate for bariatric surgery?**

   A. A 50-year-old female with a BMI of 37 with no comorbidities

   B. A 34-year-old male with a history of debilitating gastroesophageal reflux disease (GERD) and a BMI of 34

   C. A 19-year-old female with a history of type 1 diabetes and a BMI of 32

   D. A 48-year-old male with a history of hypertension, type 2 diabetes, hyperlipidemia, and a BMI of 33

   E. An 89-year-old male with a history of pulmonary embolus, pulmonary hypertension, and a BMI of 39

2. **In which scenario would a revisional weight loss surgery be most indicated?**

   A. A 45-year-old female with a history of a lap band, a current BMI of 44 kg/m^2, and has had poor compliance with diet and exercise

   B. A 38-year-old female with a history of lap band, persistent hypertension, a BMI of 39 kg/m^2, and compliance with nutrition and exercise

   C. An 87-year-old male with a history of RYGB, a current BMI of 43 kg/m^2, and who is an active smoker and drinks alcohol on weekends

   D. A 42-year-old male with a history of RYGB, a BMI of 32 kg/m^2, and an inability to lose more weight over the past 2 years

   E. A 25-year-old female with a sleeve gastrectomy, a BMI of 31 kg/m^2, and new onset reflux

3. **An upper gastrointestinal (UGI) series can be used as part of the preoperative workup to evaluate for revision surgery. What will a UGI series miss that will require a revision?**

   A. Prolapse or slippage of adjustable gastric band

   B. Marginal ulcers

   C. Anastomotic leaks

   D. Gastrogastric fistulae

4. **Patients who have revisional bariatric surgery for weight recidivism**

   A. have a higher risk of intraoperative and postoperative complications.

   B. have a predictable amount of weight loss.

   C. do not necessarily need a consultation with behavioral health and nutrition care providers.

   D. usually have an anatomical reason for the regain.

5. **What is the most common postoperative complication from revisional surgery?**

   A. Bleeding

   B. Leak

   C. Wound infection

   D. Ulcer

   E. Hernia

6. Which of the following is false? The answer should be B.

A. Doing the surgery in a single stage will increase the chance of an anastomotic leak.

B. Patients who have conversions to RYGB do much better with weight loss than do patients converted to a sleeve gastrectomy.

C. Patients should be expected to gain weight if a two-stage plan is done.

D. Surgeon experience with revisions is the most important factor regarding postoperative leaks.

E. Staple line reinforcement has been shown to decrease bleeding.

ANSWERS

1. D. Candidates for bariatric surgery are those with
1. BMI > 40 kg/m^2;
2. BMI > 35 kg/m^2 and at least one weight-related comorbidity, such as hypertension, hyperlipidemia, diabetes, sleep apnea, depression, arthritis, or pseudotumor cerebri; and
3. BMI >30 kg/m^2 with dysmetabolic syndrome X or difficult to control type 2 diabetes mellitus.

Patient D clearly meets these guidelines for bariatric surgery and represents the best candidate among these choices. Recent evidence and consensus opinion support the extension of bariatric candidacy in lower-BMI patients, particularly in patients with a BMI of 30–35 and type 2 diabetes.

The importance of considering weight-loss surgery is due to the widespread increase in obesity and associated comorbidities in the population. Many studies have shown that surgical therapy is more effective than medical intervention or supervised diet programs at achieving significant and sustained weight loss and resolving associated comorbidities.

These patients must undergo preoperative screening prior to surgery that entails psychiatric evaluation, nutritional counseling, and medical clearance. They must be educated very thoroughly on the realistic outcomes and the work involved in undergoing weight-loss surgery.

GERD is often associated with obesity and those patients with Class I obesity and who are surgical candidates for reflux disease still have very good results with anti-reflux surgery despite their obesity. Anti-reflux surgery, however, is not as successful in treating GERD in patients with a BMI >35 kg/m^2. Type

1 diabetes is not as successfully treated with bariatric surgery, but it may make the disease easier to control. However, surgery is still not recommended for patient C's level of obesity. Patient E is at high risk for surgery and would not see much long-term benefit due to his advanced age. Patients older than 70 are treated on an individual basis regardless of their BMI.

2. B. Revisions are necessary for complications of the initial bariatric procedure or for failure of weight loss and/or control of weight-related comorbidities. Surgery is considered a failure if the postoperative BMI remains >35 kg/m^2, less than 50% excess weight loss achieved, the presence of persistent or recurrence of comorbidities, and there is significant weight regain. Complications from the initial procedure that might require surgical revision can include strictures, ulceration, fistulae, dysphagia, severe reflux (especially after a sleeve gastrectomy), or nutritional deficiencies. These may require surgical revision, conversion to a different bariatric procedure, or, in severe cases, even reversal of the bariatric procedure. Those with Class I obesity from their first procedure, even with the inability to lose more weight, are not considered candidates for revision. The most common reason for a sleeve revision is due to reflux that is refractory to proton pump inhibition (PPI). Most post–sleeve gastrectomy reflux, however, responds to a PPI and diet modification. Those with severe, unresponsive reflux are candidates for revision, regardless of their BMI.

Identifying the source of the complication is critical to determining candidacy for revision and deciding on the type of revisional procedure. Anatomic complications can be based on the type of surgery. Common adjustable gastric band complications include band slippage or gastric prolapse through the band, band erosion, and pouch or esophageal dilation. In addition, the adjustable gastric band has the highest rate of failure of weight loss or requiring band revision or removal. Complications of RYGB include marginal ulcers, internal hernias, bowel obstructions, gastrogastric fistulas, steatorrhea, inadequate or excessive weight loss, and nutritional deficiencies. It is crucial to identify the cause of failure prior to considering revision.

Most sources of weight-loss failure are due to behavioral maladaptation or noncompliance. It is critical to have a standardized approach to the bariatric patient seeking revisional surgery, including complete evaluations of their understanding and compliance with the required diet and nutritional strategies to maximize the success of bariatric surgery. If this is the source of weight-loss failure, then behavioral adjustments may be more beneficial as opposed to undergoing revision surgery. Patients who are compliant are probably the best candidates in which to consider a revision. Therefore, identifying the source of the failure is key to considering who will benefit from revision surgery.

3. **B.** A thorough evaluation of the source of the failure is important to decide which surgery would be most beneficial, or if revisional surgery is indicated at all. A UGI series is usually used preoperatively to help clarify the anatomy of prior surgeries and identify the presence of complications. It can reliably help identify band slippage or prolapse, esophageal dilation, leaks, or fistulae. A band that has slipped or caused a prolapse must be removed because the prolapse can cause an incarceration of the stomach leading to a surgical emergency. A gastrogastric fistula may also be seen but not every fistula requires a revision. If the fistula is causing recurrent marginal ulcerations or weight regain, then the patient can then be considered for a revision. It must always be appreciated that a UGI series may not identify small leaks or fistulae, and many centers now perform a UGI study followed immediately by a CT scan. This approach significantly increases the sensitivity for identifying smaller leaks, fistulae, or other anatomic complications. Small leaks seen on UGI can be controlled by drainage, total parenteral nutrition, NPO status, or with the adjunct of a stent or clip place endoscopically. A UGI study typically lacks the resolution to identify subtle mucosal problems such as a marginal ulcer. The diagnosis of marginal ulceration typically requires direct luminal visualization with a flexible upper endoscopy.

4. **A.** Revisional surgery is significantly more complex than an initial bariatric procedure for multiple reasons, including the altered anatomy, the presence of significant adhesions or inflammatory changes, and the need for more complex surgical maneuvers and reconstructions. There have been several studies that have shown that patients who have undergone revision surgery have higher short- and long-term complication rates. These rates range from 13–50% depending on the type of revision involved, the most

common being wound infections or surgical site infections. Significantly longer operative times and greater blood loss have also been noted. The mortality rate, however, remains at less than 1%, similar to initial weight-loss surgeries, meaning revision can still be a viable option. The reported results of additional weight loss after revisional surgery are also significantly more variable than after an initial bariatric procedure.

There are multiple options for revision of a bariatric procedure, and the choice will depend on the current anatomy and the reason for the revisional procedure. There is also a significant current interest and developing technology in the field of endoluminal approaches to both primary and revisional bariatric surgery, most commonly to achieve a reduction in the size of the gastric pouch or to decrease the size of a dilated upper anastomosis to produce additional restriction. Weight-loss results are more variable and less predictable compared to primary bariatric surgery; multiple studies have shown acceptable success rates with weight loss after revisional surgeries.

Weight regain after a primary bariatric procedure can be multifactorial, but often it is due to poor lifestyle habits and not due to technical complications from the surgery. As such, all patients being considered for revision require consultation with behavioral health and nutritional services. Follow-up after surgery should be lifelong to help with long-term weight management control.

5. **C.** Revisional surgery has higher complication rates than primary surgery: 41% of revisions experienced complications compared to 15% for primary surgery. Complications include wound infections, which is the most common at 24%. In general, the scarred tissue planes and vascular supply, as well as the increased dissection, will lead to a more difficult procedure and higher complication rates. The leak rate is estimated at 10% and a transfusion rate around 7%. There tend to be more hernias after revision surgery, but this is mostly due to the need for an open procedure.

6. **B.** Complication rates for revisional surgery are generally higher, but this does not preclude the conversion of an adjustable gastric banding to a gastric as a single-stage procedure. The leak rate can vary widely, from 0–12.9%, which relies heavily on the surgeon's technique and experience. The most important

criteria for determining a leak rate will be based on using healthy tissue for the anastomosis, as well as making sure to avoid tissue ischemia. Reinforcement of the staple line has also been shown to benefit with bleeding but not with decreased leak rates.

For patients who undergo a two-stage procedure, the removal of the band will decrease restriction in the patient. So it is not unusual for patients to gain weight between the removal and the revision; however, it should not be expected, especially if the patient is complying with a healthy lifestyle. As weight loss is variable after a revision for weight regain, it is not clear if conversion to RYGB is better than a conversion to a sleeve gastrectomy.

BIBLIOGRAPHY

Buchs NC, Bucher P, Pugin F, et al. Value of performing routine postoperative liquid contrast swallow studies following robot-assisted Roux-en-Y gastric bypass. *Swiss Med Wkly*. 2012;142:w13556.

Buchwald H, Avidor Y, Braunwald E, et al. Bariatric surgery: a systematic review and meta-analysis. *JAMA*. 2004;292(14):1724–1737.

Frantzides CT, Alexander B, Frantzides AT. Laparoscopic revision of failed bariatric procedures. *JSLS*. 2019;23(1): e2018.00074. doi:10.4293/JSLS.2018.00074

Fulton C, Sheppard C, Birch D, Karmali S, de Gara C. A comparison of revisional and primary bariatric surgery. *Can J Surg*. 2017;60(3):205–211. doi:10.1503/cjs.006116

Gastrointestinal Surgery for Severe Obesity. NIH Consensus Development Conference. *Nutrition* 1996;12(6):397–404.

Griffith PS, Birch DW, Sharma AM, et al. Managing complications associated with laparoscopic Roux-en-Y gastric bypass for morbid obesity. *Can J Surg*. October 2012;55(5):329–336.

Inabnet WB 3rd, Belle SH, Bessler M, et al. Comparison of 30-day outcomes after non-lapband primary and revisional bariatric surgical procedures from the Longitudinal Assessment of Bariatric Surgery study. *Surg Obes Relat Dis*. 2010;6(1):22–30.

Karmali S, Brar B, Shi X, et al. Weight recidivism postbariatric surgery: a systematic review. *Obes Surg*. 2013;23(11):1922–1933.

Mikami D, Needleman B, Narula V, et al. Natural orifice surgery: initial us experience utilizing the StomaphyX device to reduce gastric pouches after Roux-en-Y gastric bypass. *Surg Endosc*. 2010;24(1):223–228.

Nesset EM, Kendrick ML, Houghton SG, et al. A two-decade spectrum of revisional bariatric surgery at a tertiary referral center. *Surg Obes Relat Dis*. 2007;3(1):25–30.

Sjöström L. Lifestyle, diabetes, and cardiovascular risk factors 10 years after bariatric surgery. *N Engl J Med*. 2004;351(26):2683–2693.

Tran TT, Pauli E, Lyn-Sue JR, et al. Revisional weight loss surgery after failed laparoscopic gastric banding: an institutional experience. *Surg Endosc*. 2013;27(11):4087–4093.

Unick JL, Beavers D, Bond DS, et al. The long-term effectiveness of a lifestyle intervention in severely obese individuals. *Am J Med*. 2013;126(3):236–242.

Zhang L, Tan WH, Chang R, Eagon JC. Perioperative risk and complications of revisional bariatric surgery compared to primary RYGB. *Surg Endosc*. 2015 Jun;29(6):1316–1320.

60

Adjustable Gastric Band Complications

Ryan Bram and Chan W. Park

A 40-year-old female presents to the emergency department with acute onset of intractable nausea and vomiting with intolerance to food intake. She has a prior history of a laparoscopic adjustable gastric band (LAGB) placement several years ago. A surgical consultation is requested, and her medical/surgical history is significant for type 2 diabetes, obstructive sleep apnea, and gastroesophageal reflux disease (GERD). Physical examination demonstrates vital signs within normal limits and a benign exam, without evidence of peritonitis. The patient is admitted for further evaluation and kept NPO with IV fluids. A swallow study was performed, the results of which are shown.

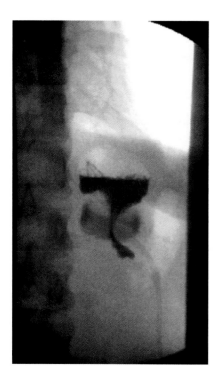

1. **The radiology study shown demonstrates**
   A. gastric prolapse
   B. gastric dilation
   C. esophageal failure
   D. inferior vena cava (IVC) inclusion in the band
   E. gastric erosion

2. **Which of the following is the most common complication of LAGB placement?**
   A. Gastric prolapse
   B. Tubing/access port problems
   C. Esophageal dilation
   D. IVC inclusion in the band
   E. Gastric erosion

3. **Which of the following strategies could have the greatest impact on preventing this complication?**
   A. Small portion sizes
   B. A rebuckling procedure
   C. Pars flaccida technique
   D. Remove all fluid from the band
   E. Gastropexy

4. **If this patient has had good weight-loss results and reports satisfaction with her gastric band, what is the ideal treatment for this complication?**
   A. "Unbuckling," reduction, and "rebuckling" procedure
   B. Removal with plans to perform an alternative weight-loss procedure
   C. Removal of all fluid in band port
   D. Band deflation and begin proton pump inhibitor
   E. Perform an esophagogastroduodenoscopy (EGD) and then remove band if indicated

5. **If the swallow study showed a diffusely dilated esophagus and pouch with impaired passage of contrast past the lower esophageal sphincter (LES). Which of the following tests should be ordered next, and what results do you expect?**

A. Upright chest x-ray; free air under the diaphragm

B. Thick and thin blood smears and polymerase chain reaction test; intracellular *Trypanosome cruzi* parasite and DNA

C. Esophageal manometry; impaired peristalsis with increased resting LES pressures

D. EGD; erosion of gastric band into the fundus

E. 24-hr pH probe testing; DeMeester score of 10.5

6. **If this patient presented with pain, warmth, and redness at her port site, without any evidence of a drainable subcutaneous abscess, what would be the best next step in management?**

A. Oral antibiotic treatment only

B. Localized exploration only

C. Endoscopy

D. Removal of the port and adjacent tubing only

E. Removal of band, along with the entirety of tubing and port

ANSWERS

1. A. Band prolapse occurs when part of the stomach herniates under the band. Gastric prolapse symptoms include dysphagia, worsening GERD, nausea/emesis, and food intolerance. Patients are at increased risk for gastric prolapse if they have emesis immediately postoperative, which can dislodge sutures that were placed using the gastroplexy technique to avoid this complication. A contrast or upper gastrointestinal (GI) study is used to make the diagnosis. The study will likely show contrast pooling in the prolapsed stomach with the band in a horizontal position for an anterior prolapse (as is the case in the earlier scenario) or in a vertical position for a posterior prolapse. If the gastric wall remains prolapsed, it can become strangulated and may result in gastric incarceration.

2. A. In a review of 2,283 patients, a total of 238 (8.5%) patients experienced a complication after placement of a LAGB. The most frequent was proximal pouch dilation and gastric prolapse (4.2%). The incidence of gastric prolapse has decreased since changing from the perigastric technique to the pars flaccida technique and adding a gastrogastric suture or gastropexy

technique. Tubing/access port problems were next at 1.2%, as well as explantation. Erosion into the gastric lumen was the least frequent in this study at 0.5%. Including IVC into the band can result in an intraabdominal or intrathoracic emergency and is a rare complication but has been reported and described.

3. E. Restricting the patient to small portion sizes will prevent gastric dilation, which can lead to gastric prolapse, but this is not the most effective method in preventing this complication. Educating patients on the importance of portion size does play a large role in their postoperative weight-loss success. An unbuckling, reduction, and rebuckling procedure is performed by some surgeons to fix a gastric prolapse; however, recurrence is common with this procedure. Removing fluid from the port to a "zero"-fill volume is the initial treatment for gastric prolapse and will not necessarily prevent gastric prolapse, nor would it assist in weight loss with "zero" fill. Performing a pars flaccida technique has been shown to decrease the incidence of gastric prolapse when compared to the older perigastric technique; however, placing gastrogastric sutures or performing a gastropexy is currently considered the most effective technique.

4. B. The unbuckling, reduction, and rebuckling procedure is used by some surgeons as a technique to repair gastric prolapse; however, recurrence rate has been found to be quite high. Removing all fluid in the band port would be considered the nonoperative management for gastric prolapse. The patient may be able to consume food more easily when fluid is removed completely from the band. Removing all fluid in the band port would be the treatment of choice for gastric pouch dilation, for which the band would be in normal position on the barium swallow if this was the diagnosis. Deflating the band and beginning a proton pump inhibitor would be the recommended treatment for a patient experiencing an exacerbation of GERD symptoms after band placement and may ultimately need conversion to a laparoscopic Roux-en-Y gastric bypass.

An EGD would be indicated to rule out the presence of a gastric erosion, and if one is seen, then removal of the band and repair of the erosion is indicated. Gastric prolapse can result in a surgical emergency if strangulation or incarceration occurs. If the patient is hemodynamically stable, then an elective procedure can be performed. This patient would benefit from band removal initially to prevent the incarceration and plan for a future weight-loss surgery if desired by the patient.

5. C. This question describes the rare but impairing issue of pseudoachalasia due to LAGB. As with true or primary achalasia, pseudoachalasia presents with symptoms of dysphagia, dyspepsia, and food intolerance. The underlying pathophysiology is not known, but it has been suggested that it is the mechanical obstruction caused by the band that increases gastric pouch and esophageal pressures, leading to increased LES pressures and altered esophageal peristalsis. Patients presenting with these symptoms should undergo barium swallow and esophageal manometry to help further characterize these symptoms. Barium swallow could show a diffusely enlarged dilated esophagus, dilated gastric pouch, or decreased lower esophageal diameter. Manometry findings are varied but have been reported to show increased LES resting and relaxation pressures and decreased number for peristaltic waveforms. Treatment involves loosening the band and repeating an esophagram in 6 weeks or removal of the lap band. Unfortunately, in most case series, symptoms only responded to band removal, although most patients experience a complete reversal of their symptoms afterward.

6. C. This question describes a port site infection. The foreign body can become primarily infected, but an infection secondary to a gastric erosion must be ruled out. As such, endoscopy is warranted in this patient. If there is no erosion and if there is no obvious drainable abscess, there is little use for surgical intervention as oral antibiotics alone are usually enough to treat these infections. If an abscess is present, then as a tenant of surgery, it should be drained although in this question this is not the case. If the PO antibiotics are not effective, it is reasonable to attempt IV formulations and broaden coverage. If concern remains, then the port should be temporarily removed until the pain and erythema resolve. It should be noted that in contrast to early port site infections, late infections are usually due to band erosion, are not usually amenable to antibiotics, and often require band removal. Band erosions should be treated with removal of the entire band system, including the tubing and the port along with repair of the erosion. This can be done endoscopically, laparoscopically, or via an open technique.

BIBLIOGRAPHY

Aarts E, Koehestanine P, Dogan K, et al. Revisional surgery after failed gastric banding: results of one-stage conversion to RYYGB in 195 patients. *Surg Obes Relat Dis.* 2014;10(6):1077–1083.

Altieri MS, Yang J, Telem DA, et al. Lap band outcomes from 19,221 patients across centers and over a decade within the state of New York. *Surg Endosc.* 2016;30(5):1725–1732.

Coblijn, UK, Verveld, CJ, van Wagensveld, BA, et al. Laparoscopic Roux-en-Y gastric bypass or laparoscopic sleeve gastrectomy as revisional procedure after adjustable gastric band—a systematic review. *Obes Surg.* 2013;23:1899–1914.

Cobourn C, Chapman MA, Ali A, Amrhein J. Five-year weight loss experience of outpatients receiving laparoscopic adjustable gastric band surgery. *Obes Surg.* 2013;23(7):903–910. doi:10.1007/s11695-013-0881-7

Eid I, Birch DW, Sherman V, Karmali S. Complications associated with adjustable gastric banding for morbid obesity: a surgeon's guide. *Can J Surg.* 2011;54(1):2011.

Fielding GA. Should the lap band be removed to treat pseudoachalasia? *Gastroenterol Hepatol (N Y).* 2013;9(7):471–473.

Lipka S, Katz S. Reversible pseudoachalasia in a patient with laparoscopic adjustable gastric banding. *Gastroenterol Hepatol (N Y).* 2013;9(7):469–471.

Quon MG, Jean MC. Pseudo-achalasia following laparoscopic adjustable gastric band (Lap-band©). *Proceedings of UCLA Health.* 2018;22.

Schirmer B, Schauer PR. The surgical management of obesity. In: Brunicardi FC, Andersen DK, Billiar TR, Dunn DL, Hunter JG, Matthews JB, et al. eds. *Schwartz's Principles of Surgery.* 9e. 2010. http://accesssurgery.mhmedical.com/content.aspx?

Snow J, Severson PA. Complications of adjustable gastric banding. *Surg Clin North Am.* 2011;91(6):1249–1264.

te Riele WW, van Santvoort HC, Boerma D, et al. Rebanding for slippage after gastric banding: should we do it? *Obes Surg.* 2014;24:588–593.

Walker G. Devine formula for ideal body weight. MDCalc. March 3, 2014. http://www.mdcalc.com/ideal-body-weight/

PEDIATRIC SURGERY

61

Pediatric Head and Neck Masses

Justin C. Scheidt and Margaret E. Gallagher

A 4-year-old girl is brought in to see her primary care provider (PCP) by her parents. They have noticed a small mass on the anterior portion of her neck, but recently started noticing that it was spontaneously draining and has become erythematous and painful. Her PCP has the girl stick out her tongue and notices that the mass moves with tongue protrusion. The physician then refers the child to surgery.

1. What is the most appropriate treatment for this mass?

A. Surgical resection of the cyst
B. Resection of the thyroglossal duct and complete hyoid bone resection
C. Removal of the cyst en bloc, excising a core of tissue around the tract to the base of the tongue, and including the central 1/3rd of the hyoid bone
D. Surgical resection of the cyst via a total thyroidectomy

2. What is the most appropriate treatment for an infected thyroglossal duct cyst?

A. Incision and drainage followed by resection after resolution of the infection
B. Aspiration followed by resection after resolution of the infection
C. Sistrunk procedure at the time of presentation
D. Antibiotics with resection after the infection resolves

3. Regarding branchial cleft cysts, which of the following statements is correct?

A. The first branchial cleft extends to the auditory canal, placing both the facial nerve and the parotid at risk for injury.
B. Type I cysts are the most common, accounting for 80% to 90% of all lesions.
C. When a child presents with an infected branchial cleft cyst, it is imperative to perform resection immediately.
D. Cysts located on the anterior border of the sternocleidomastoid muscle are type II branchial cleft cyst.

4. Which of the following statements is true regarding lymphatic malformations?

A. Lymphatic malformations do not present with airway compromise.
B. Ninety percent of lymphatic malformations are apparent at birth and diagnosed during prenatal ultrasound.
C. Fine needle aspiration (FNA) is necessary to confirm the diagnosis of a lymphatic malformation prior to resection.
D. Given that lymphatic malformations are benign, radical resection should never be performed.

5. What is the most common childhood malignancy presenting as a head or neck mass in children over the age of 5?

A. Thyroid carcinoma
B. Lymphoma
C. Rhabdomyosarcoma
D. Neuroblastoma
E. Melanoma

6. **Which of the following is true regarding treatment for torticollis?**

    A. Division of the sternocleidomastoid muscle is only indicated if the infant has plagiocephaly or hemihypoplasia.

    B. Botulinum toxin injection should be the first treatment, ideally preventing the infant from needing to undergo physical therapy.

    C. Physical therapy, with passive range of motion and neck-stretching, is the primary treatment modality.

    D. Ocular imbalance causing torticollis will be fixed by corrective lenses.

7. **For infantile hemangiomas, which of the following is false?**

    A. This lesion often starts small before rapidly enlarging and peaking at about 6 months of age.

    B. The mainstay of treatment is expectant management.

    C. In cases requiring treatment, surgery is more beneficial than medical management.

    D. Lesions near eyes, lips, or over cartilage such as the nose or ears should be considered for early intervention.

ANSWERS

1. **C.** This is a thyroglossal duct cyst and the diagnosis can be made by this patient's physical exam alone. Thyroglossal duct cysts are found typically in the midline of the neck. These are the second most common congenital pediatric neck masses, though the most common midline anomaly. Although classically described as midline, up to 40% may lie just lateral to the midline. These cysts, based on their embryological descent, are found to have a tract extending from the hyoid bone up to the base of the tongue. The normal thyroglossal duct involutes by the 8th fetal week, with remnants leading to cyst formation or ectopic thyroid tissue anywhere along the tract. Approximately 60% of these cysts lie adjacent to the hyoid bone, 24% lie above, and 13% lie below the hyoid bone. Cysts may also present intralingually, with 2% occurring at the base of the tongue. Intralingual thyroglossal duct cysts may place an infant at risk for airway obstruction. Surgery involves removal of the cyst, its tract, and the middle 1/3 of the hyoid bone, which is called the Sistrunk procedure. Removal of the hyoid is necessary to prevent recurrence.

This procedure was first described in 1920, and Sistrunk described the importance of an en bloc dissection, excising a core of tissue around the tract, which is necessary, given the possible existence of multiple tracts. Recurrence rates are less than 10% and usually related to incomplete excision or intraoperative rupture. There is a possible association between preoperative infection and risk of recurrence, though not confirmed in recent analyses. These congenital lesions have the potential for malignant transformation, with papillary adenocarcinoma found in up to 10% of adults presenting with a thyroglossal duct cyst. Papillary carcinoma can arise in adulthood from the dysgenetic ectopic thyroid tissue and is reason to perform complete excision of the lesion in a child with a thyroglossal duct cyst or sinus. Though these cysts, similarly to branchial cleft cysts, often present with an acute infection during childhood, up to 40% present after the age of 20. Dermoid cysts are also often found midline on the neck, potentially being confused with a thyroglossal duct cyst. However, they are not associated with the thyroid and will not move when the patient swallows or with protrusion of the tongue, as opposed to a thyroglossal duct cyst. It is recommended that the presence of normal thyroid tissue outside of the thyroglossal duct cyst is confirmed prior to excision. Ectopic thyroid tissue is identified in surgical specimens in approximately 25% to 35% of cases, though it is actually rare that this is the child's only thyroid tissue.

2. **D.** Thyroglossal duct cysts lie deep to the strap muscles but can involve the skin if they rupture, get infected, or undergo an incision and drainage. An incision and drainage should be avoided as it can lead to a thyroglossal duct fistula and persistent drainage.

It is important that branchial cleft cysts and thyroglossal duct cysts be excised after the acute infection has been cleared in order to prevent recurrence. The initial treatment of an infected congenital neck lesion is antibiotics and not surgery. If absolutely needed, an aspiration could be performed, but the goal is to avoid an incision and drainage. Surgery should be 6 to 8 weeks later, and the entire tract, to include the skin punctum if present, needs to be removed as recurrent infections are common with incomplete excision.

Congenital lesions may present while acutely infected and, prior to operative intervention, their close relationships to major nerves and vessels needs to be understood. Injury to the parotid gland and facial nerve may occur from recurrent infection of a type I branchial cleft cyst, or from a complication of an incision and draining. Infections of the third and fourth branchial cleft cysts are rare and more challenging to diagnose and treat, which may require barium swallow and laryngoscopy to identify. Suppurative thyroiditis may be due to an infected third or fourth arch sinus. Type III and IV cysts may cause airway edema and difficulty swallowing, which can often be controlled by controlling the acute infection.

3. **A.** The differential diagnosis of a lateral neck mass is extensive and includes branchial cleft remnants, lymphatic malformation, dermoid cyst, hemangioma, lymphadenitis, torticollis, neurofibroma, lipoma, benign enlarged lymph nodes, or metastatic malignancy to the cervical lymph nodes. Branchial cleft cysts are the most common congenital neck lesion, accounting for approximately 20% to 30% of all pediatric neck masses. Sinuses, fistulas, and remnants are usually noticed at birth or early in life, opposed to branchial cleft cysts, which are more likely to present later in childhood. There are six paired branchial arches, containing ectodermal, mesodermal, and endodermal components.

Understanding the relationships of these arch components is helpful to conceptualize and categorize congenital neck masses. The dorsal portion of the first cleft becomes the external auditory canal. Given this tract's location, it places the facial nerve at risk for injury during resection. Type I cysts can present as parotid masses and an ultrasound and magnetic resonance imaging (MRI) are important to assess facial nerve involvement. Type II is the most common abnormality, with 90% to 95% of cases. The opening is found along the anterior border of the sternocleidomastoid muscle (SCM) in the middle to lower third, and may be bilateral in 10% of cases. Sinus tracts of second branchial anomalies pass between the external and internal carotid arteries, entering the lateral wall of the pharynx at the tonsillar fossa. Anomalies of the third cleft are extremely rare but can also be found along the anterior border of the SCM. However, they are usually lower in the neck and pass lateral to the carotid bifurcation rather than through it. A typical presentation of a third branchial cleft anomaly in an older child is an abscess nearby or within the left thyroid lobe.

Figure 61-1 demonstrates the relationships between the first, second, and third branchial cysts and fistulas.

4. **D.** Lymphatic malformations, previously referred to as cystic hygromas or lymphangiomas, are commonly located in the head and neck. However, they can be found anywhere in the soft tissues of the face or oral cavity, with other locations, including the axilla, chest, extremities, retroperitoneum, or perineum. These are vascular malformations, occurring in 1 out of every 2,000 to 4,000 births. They occur due to sequestrations of lymphatic tissue that don't communicate with the normal lymphatic system. Ninety percent of these lesions appear before the age of 2, with 50% to 65% appearing at birth. These lesions are more commonly located on the left side of the neck and if large enough, may be noted on prenatal ultrasound. When diagnosed prenatally, a fetal echocardiogram should be obtained due to the risk of cardiac failure and fetal demise due to a high-flow lesion. Serial ultrasounds are obtained to assess for polyhydramnios or the development of hydrops.

The majority of lymphatic malformations are asymptomatic, though large lesions can invade the

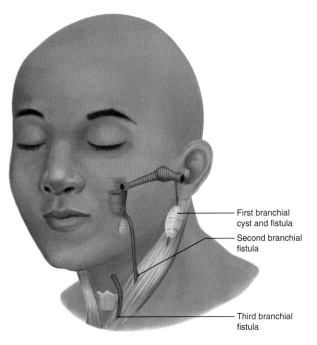

Figure 61-1 A child with a cleft cyst and remnants of the first three branchial systems. Note the important relation to the sternocleidomastoid muscle and fistula's origin. (Reprinted with permission from Welch, Randolph, Ravitch, et al.)

floor of the mouth and cause upper airway obstruction. When they involve the tongue or the mediastinum, they may result in airway compromise, dysphagia, or failure to thrive. FNA should not be used to diagnose a lymphatic malformation due to the possibility of hemorrhage into the lesion and subsequent rapid expansion, causing airway compromise. The only indication for aspiration of the lymphatic malformation is if there is a need to emergently decompress the cyst to relieve airway obstruction. Spontaneous hemorrhage within the mass may also occur, causing rapid enlargement with swelling and ecchymosis. Hemorrhage predisposes the child for infection and antibiotics should be started. Complete excision may be difficult without involving vital structures, so multiple debulking procedures may be performed. Computed tomography (CT) scan with intravenous contrast or magnetic resonance angiography can be used when planning for resection to evaluate the extension from one body space to another and delineate associated vital structures. Radical resection is not indicated. Sclerotherapy has also been studied and is an option particularly in macrocystic lesions. Picinabil (OK-432), bleomycin, doxycycline, acetic acid, alcohol, and hypertonic saline have all been used as sclerosing agents. There is a small possibility of spontaneous regression in low-stage macrocystic lymphatic malformations, so observation and monitoring may also be an option in some of these patients.

5. **B.** Malignancies of the head and neck account for approximately 12% of pediatric malignancies, with an increasing incidence. Head and neck malignancies are more common in 15 to 18 year olds, followed by age group <4 years. Females aged 11 to 18 are most likely to have thyroid carcinoma. However, lymphoma is the number one cause of a malignant head or neck mass, with up to 80% of pediatric patients with Hodgkin's disease having cervical lymph node involvement. Though non-Hodgkin's lymphoma is more common in the younger pediatric population, it is less likely to have cervical lymph node involvement. Rhabdomyosarcoma is the most common pediatric solid tumor in the head or neck and typically causes symptoms through localized compression or infiltration.

In children under the age of 5, neuroblastoma is the most common solid tumor. Neuroblastoma occurs anywhere along the sympathetic chain and may present with Horner syndrome. On imaging, calcifications will be evident. Melanoma should also be on the differential of either a primary tumor in the head and neck or as a cause for a malignant lymph node. Lastly, teratomas are a rare and usually benign tumor in children, of which only 0.47% to 6% present in the head and neck. Though rare, they are important to be aware of, given that the majority of those in the neck present at birth with respiratory distress. Despite being a benign disease, head and neck teratomas carry a 12.5% to 23% risk of intrauterine or neonatal death. If a cervical teratoma is diagnosed prenatally and there is polyhydramnios, indicating compression of the esophagus, then an EXIT procedure should be considered in order to secure an airway.

6. **C.** Torticollis occurs from fibrosis and shortening of the SCM and has an incidence as high as 16% in the newborn population. This fibrosis and shortening causes a "mass" in the muscle that causes the infant to turn his face toward the contralateral side and tilt the head toward the ipsilateral shoulder. In children who can walk, they may compensate for their torticollis by elevating one shoulder to keep their head and eyes level. Facial and cranial asymmetries can result from the abnormal positioning of the child's head if the torticollis is not treated. When the infant's head is turned toward the contralateral side, the contralateral occiput presses against the bed when they are supine, and flattening of the occiput then leads to secondary flattening of the ipsilateral forehead, referred to as plagiocephaly. As the torticollis resolves, the plagiocephaly also typically resolves.

The only indication to operate, by dividing the muscle, is facial hemihypoplasia. Here, the ipsilateral side of the face grows more slowly than the normal side, causing progressive asymmetry. Persistent symptoms after 1 year of conservative treatment may also be a possible indication for surgery. The etiology of torticollis is usually from trauma, though there are other possible etiologies such as ocular imbalance, cervical hemivertebrae, posterior fossa tumors, deep cervical infections, or atlanto-occipital subluxation. An ocular imbalance is usually due to superior oblique palsy, which is corrected surgically. Congenital muscular torticollis is thought to be due to fetal head descent or abnormal fetal positioning during the third trimester. Trauma during delivery is another potential cause. Treatment for torticollis is primarily physical therapy with passive range of motion and neck-stretching exercises. If torticollis persists after 6 months of physical therapy, then additional workup needs to be pursued, assessing for other potential causes such as a congenital vertebral malformation, or ocular imbalance. Botulinum toxin (botox) can also be used to assist in treatment. The botox enhances the effectiveness of stretching on the affected side, potentially making physical therapy more beneficial. However, if physical therapy is started before 3 months of age, studies show up to 100% success rates.

7. C. Infantile hemangiomas are benign vascular tumors that typically appear shortly after birth and undergo rapid expansion and peak in size around 6 months of age, with growth continuing up through the first year of life. The natural course of infantile hemangiomas is for them to involute and resolve, over the next few years, even up to age 7. Most of these lesions can be managed expectantly, with observation and reassurance. Sixty percent of infantile hemangiomas are located on the head and neck. They can also occur in the airway, causing stridor and need for treatment. Considerations for interventions are based on location and lasting effects. Permanent tissue loss can result from ulceration of a hemangioma involving the eyelid, tip of the nose, lip, or ear. While in the expansion phase, the lesions may damage cartilage and thus leave lasting disfigurement. Periorbital lesions can damage the cornea resulting in astigmatism or cause an amblyopia by blocking the visual axis. Those on the lips may impair feeding. In those cases in which treatment is required, the first-line medication is propranolol; its actions appear to decrease blood flow to the lesion, block angiogenesis, and allow for apoptosis. Due to the response and side-effect profile of propranolol, there is a minimal role for surgery.

BIBLIOGRAPHY

Albright JT, Topham AK, Reilly JS. Pediatric head and neck malignancies: U.S. incidence and trends over two decades. *Arch Otolaryngol Head Neck Surg.* 2002;128(6): 655–659.

Allard RH. The thyroglossal cyst. *Head Neck Surg.* 1982;5(2): 134–146.

Alexander VRC, Manjaly JG, Pepper CM, et al. Head and neck teratomas in children: A series of 23 cases at great ormond street hospital. *Int J Pediatr Otorhinolaryngol.* 2015;79(12):2008–2014.

Armstrong D, Pickrell K, Fetter B, Pitts W. Torticollis: an analysis of 271 cases. *Plast Reconstr Surg.* 1965;35: 14–25.

Badawy, MK. Pediatric neck masses. *Clin Pediatr Emerg Med.* 2010;11(2):73–80.

Chen A, Otto KJ. Head and neck surgery and oncology. Differential diagnosis of neck masses. In: Haughey BH, Robbins KT, eds. *Otolaryngology: Head & Neck Surgery.* 5th ed. Mosby Elsevier; 2003: 1636–1642.

Choi DK, Schmidt ML. Chemotherapy in children with head and neck cancers. *Oral Maxillofacial Surg Clin N Am.* 2016;28:127–138.

Davies K, Hamilton D. Investigation and management of the neck lump. *Head and Neck.* 2018;36(10):569–577.

Demirbilek S, Atayurt HF. Congenital muscular torticollis and sternomastoid tumor: results of nonoperative treatment. *J Pediatr Surg.* 1999;34(4):549–551.

Emil E. *Clinical pediatric surgery: a case-based interactive approach.* CRC Press; 2020:3–46.

Finn MC, Glowacki J, Mulliken JB. Congenital vascular lesions: clinical application of a new classification. *J Pediatr Surg.* 1983;18(6):894–900.

Geddes G, Butterly MM, Patel SM, Marra S. Pediatric neck masses. *Pediatr Rev.* 2013;34(3):115–124; quiz 125.

Goins MR, Beasley MS. Pediatric neck masses. *Oral Maxillofac Surg Clin North Am.* 2012;24(3):457–468.

Hutson JM, Beasley SW. The neck. *The surgical examination of children.* 2nd ed. Springer; 2013: 101–121.

Kekunnaya R, Isenberg SJ. Effect of strabismus surgery on torticollis caused by congenital superior oblique palsy in young children. *Indian J Ophthalmol.* 2014;62(3): 322–326.

Kuint J, Horowitz Z, Kugel C, Toper L, Birenbaum E, Linder N. Laryngeal obstruction caused by lingual thyroglossal duct cyst presenting at birth. *Am J Perinatol.* 1997;14(6):353–356.

Kuo AA, Tritasavit S, Graham JM Jr. Congenital muscular torticollis and positional plagiocephaly. *Pediatr Rev.* 2014; 35(2):79–87; quiz 87.

Lillehei C. Chapter 59. Neck cysts and sinuses. In: Coran AG, Adzick NS, Krummel TM, Laberge J, Shamberger RC, Caldamone AA, eds. *Pediatric Surgery.* 7th ed. Elsevier; 2012: 753–761.

Mulliken JB, Fishman SJ, Burrows PE. Vascular anomalies. *Curr Probl Surg.* 2000;37(8):517–584.

Oldham KT, Aiken JJ. Pediatric head and neck. In: Mulholland MW, Lillemoe KD, Doherty GM, Maier RV, Simeone DM, Upchurch GR, eds. *Greenfield's Surgery: Scientific Principles and Practice.* 5th ed. Lippincott Williams & Wilkins; 2011: 1843–1853.

Perkins JA, Manning SC, Tempero RM, et al. Lymphatic malformations: review of current treatment. *Otolaryngol Head Neck Surg.* 2010;142(6):795–803, 803.e1.

Sirinivasan J, Wells L, Ravenscroft J. Management of infantile haemangioma. *Pediatrics and Child Health.* 2019;29(2): 59–65.

Sistrunk WE. The surgical treatment of cysts of the thyroglossal tract. *Ann Surg*. 1920;71(2):121–122.

Stellwagen L, Hubbard E, Chambers C, Jones KL. Torticollis, facial asymmetry and plagiocephaly in normal newborns. *Arch Dis Child*. 2008;93(10):827–831.

Welch KJ, Randolph JG, Ravitch MM, et al. eds. *Pediatric Surgery*. 4th ed. Year Book Medical; 1986: 543.

Woo RK, Albanese CT. Pediatric surgery. In: Norton JA, Barie PS, Bollinger RR, et al., eds. *Surgery: Basic Science and Clinical Evidence*. 2nd ed. Springer; 2008: 649–696.

62

Pyloric Stenosis

Justin C. Scheidt and Margaret E. Gallagher

A 1-month-old Caucasian boy is brought to his primary care provider (PCP) by his parents due to difficulty feeding. This is their first child and they are very concerned. The child has been bottle-fed since birth and almost every time he eats, he has a bout of emesis. They state the emesis has gotten worse; it has remained non-bilious, but become increasingly projectile. The parents have tried changing formulas, and tried reflux medication, but without relief.

On exam, the infant's vitals are normal for his age, and he is afebrile. He is well-appearing, though small for his age. The PCP attempts to do an abdominal exam and thinks he feels a mass in his right upper quadrant, but the infant begins to cry, making the exam more difficult.

1. **What is the most appropriate method for diagnosis of infantile hypertrophic pyloric stenosis (HPS)?**
   A. Endoscopy
   B. Upper gastrointestinal contrast study (UGI)
   C. Physical exam
   D. Ultrasound

2. **What is the usual acid–base dysfunction associated with this condition?**
   A. Hyperchloremic, hyperkalemic metabolic alkalosis with alkalotic urine
   B. Hypochloremic, hypokalemic metabolic alkalosis with alkalotic urine
   C. Hyperchloremic, hypokalemic metabolic acidosis with alkalotic urine
   D. Hypochloremic, hypokalemic metabolic alkalosis with aciduria
   E. Hypochloremic, hyperkalemic metabolic alkalosis with aciduria

3. **Which of the following clinical presentations is most consistent with hypertrophic pyloric stenosis?**
   A. A 6-week-old infant vomits shortly after every feeding, but does not appear perturbed. The patient's mother states that the vomit runs down his bib.
   B. A 6-week-old infant vomits after every meal, but then appears hungry and tries to feed again. The parents state that the vomit has the same appearance as the feeds, looks like old formula or breast milk.
   C. A 6-week-old infant vomits after every meal; the parents state that the vomit appears a yellow/green color and their infant is not interested in continued feeds.

4. **When is an adequate pyloromyotomy achieved?**
   A. When the submucosa bulges into the myotomy site and both edges of the divided pyloric muscle are freely mobile.
   B. Division through the outer longitudinal muscle followed by division through 2/3 of the inner circular muscle. Approximately 1/3 of the circular muscle should remain intact.
   C. Longitudinal incision through the pyloric sphincter followed by a transverse closure.
   D. When you can pass an appropriately sized bougie, based on the patient's weight, through the pylorus without any resistance.

5. **What is thought to be the pathogenesis of this syndrome?**

   A. Congenital abnormality
   B. A deficiency in neuronal nitric oxide
   C. Bottle/formula feeding
   D. Increased testosterone levels in the infant

6. **What is the most common complication to occur with this operation?**

   A. Development of an incisional hernia
   B. Intraoperative perforation
   C. Incomplete pyloromyotomy
   D. Wound infection

7. **If the patient continues to vomit on postoperative day 2, which of the following is most likely to be true?**

   A. This is not unexpected for the postoperative course.
   B. The infant likely has an incomplete pyloromyotomy, and an upper gastrointestinal (GI) study should be performed to confirm the diagnosis.
   C. The infant likely has recurrent hypertrophy, and an upper GI study should be performed to confirm the diagnosis.
   D. This is concerning for a mucosal perforation.

ANSWERS

1. **D.** Infantile hypertrophic pyloric stenosis (HPS) is most common in Caucasian first-born males. The differential diagnosis of non-bilious vomiting in an infant includes gastroenteritis, food allergies, gastroesophageal reflux, pyloric duplication, antral web, or increased intracranial pressure. Though a definitive diagnosis can be made in 75% of infants with pyloric stenosis by careful physical examination, it is becoming a lost skill and is technically difficult in cases presenting early. If the stomach is distended, aspiration with a nasogastric tube may assist in successful palpation of "the olive," or the enlarged pylorus on physical exam. However, ultrasound (US) has now become not only the most common initial imaging technique for diagnosis, but the gold standard. The specificity and sensitivity of US reaches 98% and 100%, respectively.

   There continues to be some debate over the exact pathological pyloric measurements. Typically, a muscle thickness of >4.0 mm and a pyloric channel length >15 mm is consistent with the diagnosis. However, when infants present younger than 22 days, a 3.5 mm thickness may be a more useful or a more accurate cut-off point. A muscle thickness measuring between 3.0 and 4.0 mm may be considered borderline and require repeat US a few days later and after rehydration if the clinical suspicion remains high. Figure 62-1 shows that the gallbladder is an important anatomic landmark when looking for the pylorus. The most common reason for inability to visualize the pylorus is gastric overdistention, which displaces the pylorus dorsally.

2. **D.** Infants, if they present with electrolyte abnormalities, present with hypochloremic, hypokalemic, metabolic alkalosis, and paradoxical aciduria. These infants have gastric acid loss from emesis, renal loss of potassium, and renal retention of bicarbonate resulting in alkalosis. In an effort to retain chloride and potassium, the exchange of hydrogen ions in the urine for chloride and potassium, causing an aciduria. It is important to correct their abnormalities, specifically dropping bicarbonate levels to less than 30 mEq/L prior to going to the operating room in order to avoid intraoperative and postoperative apnea. The chloride level should be corrected to at least 90 to 95 mEq/L. An initial bolus of 20 mL/kg of normal saline should be given. Various intravenous fluid regimens have been described in the literature but after a fluid bolus, typically a 5% dextrose in 0.45 normal saline should then be given at one and a half to two times maintenance rate. Then 20 mEq of

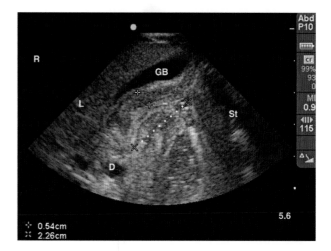

Figure 62-1 Surgeon-performed US of IHPS. The muscle thickness (5.4 mm) and channel length (22.6 mm) are measured. GB indicates gallbladder; St = stomach; L = liver; D = duodenum. Reprinted from Copeland, Cosper, McMahon et al.

potassium should be added into the fluid only after the baby is having adequate urine output. Indirect hyperbilirubinemia also occurs in a small percentage of infants with HPS. However, this invariably resolves postoperatively, so further evaluation at presentation is unnecessary. It is important to note that the majority (88%) of infants now present with normal laboratory values, and earlier diagnosis has led to fewer infants with electrolyte abnormalities.

3. **B.** The infant with hypertrophic pyloric stenosis can often be described as the hungry vomiter, since the infant is not able to ingest a full feed, they may be hungry shortly after vomiting and often their weight may plateau or decrease. The other key point in this story is that the vomit appears just like the feeds he experienced. Option A described the "happy vomiter"; this infant may vomit but there are no concerning signs without evidence of projection, the vomit is non-bilious, and the infant is otherwise meeting milestones. This infant described likely has gastroesophageal reflux. The last option describes an infant that is having bilious vomiting. This is more concerning and alludes to pathology beyond the pylorus such as malrotation or volvulus.

4. **A.** The Ramstedt pyloromyotomy remains the operation of choice, whether open or laparoscopic. An adequate pyloromyotomy is achieved when the submucosa bulges into the myotomy site and the edges of the pyloric muscle are freely mobile. Figure 62-2

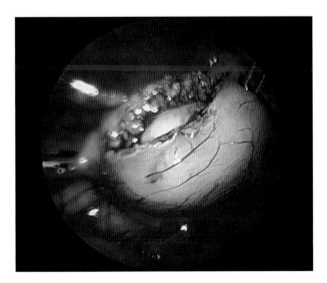

Figure 62-2 Intraoperative photograph of a completed pyloromyotomy. The submucosa can be seen in the depths of the myotomy.

demonstrates an adequate pyloromyotomy, with visualization of bulging submucosa.

5. **B.** The exact etiology of HPS is unknown and is thought to be multifactorial. The relative contributions of genetic and environmental factors and how they interact to cause the pylorus to hypertrophy during early infancy is unknown. Though environmental factors are associated with HPS, the most commonly accepted pathogenesis is decreased neuronal nitric oxide. Nitric oxide is a mediator of relaxation in the digestive tract. It is thought that the lack of nitric oxide synthase in the pyloric tissue causes pylorospasm and subsequent hypertrophy. This has been demonstrated in pyloric biopsies. Almost all patients with pyloric stenosis are not born with a hypertrophic pylorus. Though familial aggregation studies and twin reports point to a genetic involvement in the etiology of HPS, the exact heritability remains unclear. Males are affected four to five times more than females, but there is no clear explanation for this difference. No differences in testosterone levels between HPS patients and age-matched controls were found in a study of umbilical cord blood testing, and X-linked transmission patterns have not been shown to explain why HPS occurs more in males. Breastfeeding has been indicated as a potentially protective factor but bottle-feeding is not a direct cause or etiology of HPS.

6. **B.** The most common intraoperative complication is perforation. A distal perforation can be prevented by not carrying the distal part of the myotomy past the pyloric vein of Mayo. The incidence of duodenal perforation when pyloromyotomy was performed by general surgeons was found to be almost four times that of pediatric surgeons (relative risk 3.65; 95% CI 1.43–9.32). However, when adjusted for surgical volume, this was not significant. In a large series of 1,777 infants, only 4 required repeat surgery because of an incomplete pyloromyotomy. General surgeons have an overall higher complication rate when compared to pediatric surgeons (4.18% vs. 2.58%), though not statistically significant.

There was a small (0.87%) but statistically significant increase in the incidence of incomplete pyloromyotomy in the laparoscopic versus open group. In order to avoid an incomplete pyloromyotomy, an incision length of 2 cm should be used. In a randomized control trial, 200 patients underwent laparoscopic versus open pyloromyotomy. Two patients in the laparoscopic group and four patients in the open group had postoperative wound infections, not statistically significant.

7. A. Postoperative emesis is expected and is not a complication. More than 90% of patients in a series of 778 vomited for 1 to 3 days after surgery, and this is considered to be normal postoperatively. There has been no evidence to suggest that preoperative placement of an nasogastric tube has any effect on PO tolerance or length of stay. The vomiting is thought to be secondary to gastroesophageal reflux, discoordination of gastric peristalsis, pyloric edema, or gastric atony. However, if frequent vomiting persists past 7 days, then an incomplete myotomy or a perforation needs to be considered. A UGI should be performed and would demonstrate a gastric outlet obstruction to confirm the diagnosis. Another less common etiology would be a duodenal leak leading to extrinsic compression, which may also be diagnosed by UGI. Recurrent pyloric stenosis appears when the original symptoms of vomiting have resolved and the patient has regained weight, imaging will confirm hypertrophy of the pylorus, which should have regressed if a successful pyloromyotomy was performed, though this process may take up to 5 months.

BIBLIOGRAPHY

Boneti C, McVay MR, Kokoska ER, Jackson RJ, Smith SD. Ultrasound used as a diagnostic tool used by surgeons in Pyloric Stenosis. *J Pediatr Surg.* 2008;43:87–91.

Copeland DR, Cosper GH, McMahon LE, et al. Return of the surgeon in the diagnosis of pyloric stenosis. *J Pediatr Surg.* 2009;44(6):1189–1192; discussion 1192.

Ein SH, Masiakos PT, Ein A. The ins and outs of pyloromyotomy: what we have learned in 35 years. *Pediatr Surg Int.* 2014;30(5):467–480.

Emil S. *Clinical Pediatric Surgery: A Case-Based Interactive Approach.* CRC Press; 2020: 249–256.

Flageole HH, Pemberton J. Post-operative impact of nasogastric tubes on length of stay in infants with Pyloric Stenosis (POINTS). *J Pediatr Surg.* 2015;50:1681–1685.

Hall NJ, Simon E, Seims A, et al. Risk of incomplete pyloromyotomy and mucosal perforation in open and laparoscopic pyloromyotomy. *J Pediatr Surg.* 2014;49(7):1083–1086.

Jacobs C, Johnson K, Kahn FA, Mustafa MM. Life-threatening electrolyte abnormalities in pyloric stenosis. *J Pediatr Surg Case Reports.* 2019;43:16–18.

Kamata M, Cartabuke RS, Tobias JD. Perioperative care of infants with pyloric stenosis. *Paediatr Anaesth.* 2012;25(12):1193–1206.

Krogh C, Biggar RJ, Fischer TK, Lindholm M, Wohlfahrt J, Melbye M. Bottle-feeding and the risk of pyloric stenosis. *Pediatrics.* 2012;130(4):e943–e949.

Langer JC, To T. Does pediatric surgical specialty training affect outcome after ramstedt pyloromyotomy? A population-based study. *Pediatrics.* 2004;113(5):1342–1347.

Leaphart CL, Borland K, Kane TD, Hackam DJ. Hypertrophic pyloric stenosis in newborns younger than 21 days: Remodeling the path of surgical intervention. *J Pediatr Surg.* 2008;43(6):998–1001.

McAteer JP, Ledbetter DJ, Goldin AB. Role of bottle feeding in the etiology of hypertrophic pyloric stenosis. *JAMA Pediatr.* 2013;167(12):1143–1149.

Niedzielski J, Kobielski A, Sokal J, Krakos M. Accuracy of sonographic criteria in the decision for surgical treatment in infantile hypertrophic pyloric stenosis. *Arch Med Sci.* 2011;7(3):508–511.

Nsar A, Ein SH, Connolly B. Recurrent Pyloric Stenosis to Dilate or Operate? A Preliminary Report. *J Pediatr Surg.* 2008; 43: E17–E20.

Ostlie DJ, Woodall CE, Wade KR, et al. An effective pyloromyotomy length in infants undergoing laparoscopic pyloromyotomy. *Surgery.* 2004;136(4):827–832.

Peters B, Oomen MW, Bakx R, Benninga MA. Advances in infantile hypertrophic pyloric stenosis. *Expert Rev Gastroenterol Hepatol.* 2014;8(5):533–541.

Ross AR, Johnson PRV. Infantile hypertrophic pyloric stenosis. *Surgery.* 2019;37(11):620–622.

Sato TT, Oldham KT. Chapter 107. Pediatric abdomen. In: Mulholland MW, Lillemoe KD, Doherty GM, Maier RV, Simeone DM, Upchurch GR, eds. *Greenfield's Surgery: Scientific Principles and Practice.* 5th ed. Lippincott Williams & Wilkins; 2011: 1885–1946.

Schwartz MZ. Chapter 78. hypertrophic pyloric stenosis. In: Coran AG, Caldamone A, Adzick NS, Krummel TM, Laberge J, Shamberger R, eds. *Pediatric Surgery.* 7th ed. Elsevier; 2012: 1021–1028.

St Peter SD, Holcomb GW, Calkins CM, et al. Open versus laparoscopic pyloromyotomy for pyloric stenosis: a prospective, randomized trial. *Ann Surg.* 2006;244(3): 363–370.

Tutay GJ, Capraro G, Spirko B, Garb J, Smithline H. Electrolyte profile of pediatric patients with hypertrophic pyloric stenosis. *Pediatr Emerg Care.* 2013;29(4):465–468.

Vanderwinden JM, Mailleux P, Schiffmann SN, Vanderhaeghen JJ, De Laet MH. Nitric oxide synthase activity in infantile hypertrophic pyloric stenosis. *N Engl J Med.* 1992;327(8):511–515.

Ward E, Easley D, Pohl J. Previously unsuspected infantile hypertrophic pyloric stenosis diagnosed by endoscopy. *Dig Dis Sci.* 2008;53(4):946–948.

63

Hirschsprung's Disease

Benjamin Tabak

1. A newborn male infant has difficulty feeding the first day of life. This progresses to abdominal distension and bilious vomiting. The following plain X-ray is obtained on the second day of life.

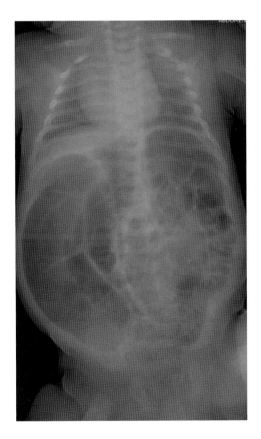

The differential diagnosis includes which of the following?
   A. Situs inversus
   B. Pyloric stenosis
   C. Cystic fibrosis
   D. Duodenal atresia
   E. Intestinal malrotation

2. The following contrast enema is obtained:

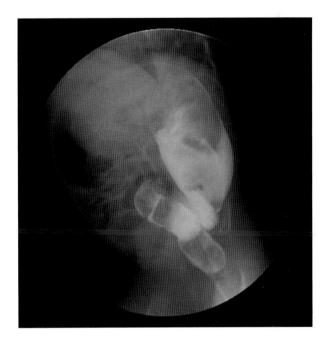

This diagnosis:
   A. Requires tissue biopsy
   B. Requires surgery prior to resumption of oral feeds
   C. Is not associated with chromosomal anomalies
   D. Typically has a family history of similar problems on the father's side
   E. Is cured with surgery

3. **Technical considerations of the corrective surgery for Hirschprung's disease include:**

   A. Taking multiple biopsies to determine exactly when the first few ganglion cells are seen, in order to resect as little colon as possible
   B. Resection from the level of the dentate line to the ganglionated intestine
   C. Routinely performing a protective colostomy or ileostomy
   D. A tension-free anastomosis

4. **A 5-year-old patient who underwent a pull through for Hirschprung's as a newborn and did well for years, now presents with a 6-month history of abdominal distension and fecal incontinence. The most likely diagnosis is:**

   A. Sphincter injury at the time of surgery
   B. Transition zone pull through at the time of surgery
   C. Hirschprung's associated enterocolitis
   D. Constipation
   E. Anastomotic stricture

5. **A 6-month-old patient with Down's syndrome and Hirschprung's disease underwent a leveling colostomy (at the level of normal ganglionated bowel) shortly after birth, followed by pull-through one month ago. He presents now with fever, lethargy, abdominal distension, and bilious vomiting. Plain films reveal no free air, but multiple dilated loops of bowel. Rectal exam results in an explosive output of bloody stained, foul smelling stool. Which of the following is required for the management of this patient?**

   A. Computed tomography (CT) scan to evaluate for intrabdominal abscess
   B. Immediate surgical intervention for a revision of the pull-through
   C. Lavage of saline through the anus
   D. Blood transfusion
   E. Nasogastric decompression

6. **A newborn infant is taken to surgery for operative management of Hirschprung's disease. A preoperative contrast enema is suggestive of a transition zone in the mid-sigmoid colon. Which of the following is correct?**

   A. A Swenson procedure entails stapling ganglionic to aganglionic bowel to augment the size of the neorectum.

   B. A Soave procedure leaves behind a muscular cuff of aganglionic colon.
   C. A Duhamel procedure involves removal of the entire aganglionic colon.
   D. A pull-through dissection begins at the dentate line.
   E. A purely transanal approach would be inappropriate in this patient.

ANSWERS

1. **C.** The film is consistent with a distal intestinal obstruction. The differential diagnosis for this in the newborn period includes cystic fibrosis, incarcerated inguinal hernia, small left colon syndrome, meconium ileus, meconium plug syndrome, Hirschprung's disease, imperforate anus, and ileal or colonic atresia. In a stable patient without peritonitis, the evaluation begins with a good physical examination. Patients with imperforate anus or hernias should be diagnosed readily at this time. Patients with Hirschprung's disease will often have explosive output of stool following rectal exam. The next diagnostic test should be a contrast enema with either isotonic or mildly hypertonic water-soluble contrast. This is typically therapeutic and diagnostic for small left colon syndrome, meconium plug, and meconium ileus.

   It is often (75%) diagnostic of Hirschprung's disease with correct identification of the transition zone. Findings of a microcolon without obstruction are very consistent with an ileal atresia. Plain film findings of malrotation can be normal, consistent with an ileus, or a proximal obstruction. Duodenal atresia on a plain film classically presents with a "double bubble" sign that shows air in the duodenum and stomach. Pyloric stenosis would most likely look normal on plain film.

2. **A.** The enema is consistent with a diagnosis of Hirschprung's disease with a transition zone in the rectosigmoid area. While contrast enema is accurate approximately 75% of the time, tissue diagnosis or anorectal manometry are the only ways to definitively make the diagnosis. Anorectal manometry is not practical in the newborn period, but is a useful study in older children or adults. A suction rectal biopsy at the bedside can sample the submucosa in an infant and does not require anesthesia or sedation. Hirschprung's disease is due to arrest of the

caudal descent of ganglion cells, which coordinate intestinal relaxation. Aganglionic bowel does not relax properly to allow propagation of intestinal contents and thus causes a functional obstruction. The biopsy should sample the submucosa 1 to 2 cm above the dentate line.

Findings of a lack of ganglion cells and nerve trunk hypertrophy are diagnostic. If H&E staining is inconclusive, "increased acetylcholinesterase" staining and "absent Calretinin" staining may help to confirm the diagnosis of Hirschsprung's disease.

Patients with transition zones in the rectosigmoid can usually be temporized by rectal irrigations, which allows for delayed surgical correction at several months of age, although surgery in the newborn period is also an acceptable treatment strategy. Most cases of Hirschprung's disease are sporadic, although some are familial. Several genes have been implicated, most notably the ret proto-oncogene. Hirschprung's has a strong association with Down's syndrome, Waadenburg-Shah, and others. Even patients who have successful surgeries have a high likelihood of fecal soiling (60%) and constipation requiring chronic laxative use (30%) in the long term. Surgery essentially converts the disease to ultrashort segment Hirschsprung's while taking away the rectal reservoir.

Ganglion cells on rectal biopsy specimens may occasionally be described by a pathologist as present, but "immature." This is common in babies who are severely premature and has also been described in term babies. These immature cells may be pathological and lead to functional obstruction. However, this functional obstruction may improve with time. Some case series have reported identifying normal "mature" ganglion cells in the same children when the biopsy was repeated at an older age.

3. **D.** Multiple intraoperative biopsies are required, but in order to avoid pull-through of the transition zone (where the bowel transitions from ganglionated to aganglionated), a level where plentiful ganglion cells are seen and nerve trunk hypertrophy is not present is the goal. Some authors advocate resection up to 10 to 12 cm above this level to more definitively ensure normal bowel is pulled through. It is critical to begin the dissection at least 0.5 to 1.0 cm above the dentate line in a newborn or 1.0 to 2.0 cm in an older child to preserve the anal canal and allow future continence. A protective ileostomy or colostomy is not typically done unless there is a technical concern about the anastomosis. The surgical principles of performing a tension-free, well-vascularized anastomosis should always be followed.

4. **D.** Persistent obstructive symptoms following a pull-through are not uncommon and all of the answers listed are possibilities. However, a patient that has done well for years and suddenly presents with distension and fecal soiling is likely to be constipated. Thirty to 85% of patients with Hirschsprung's disease will have constipation following pull-through that may require chronic laxatives, and 60% to 75% will have intermittent fecal soiling. Fecal soiling tends to become worse during periods of severe constipation. These patients are best evaluated with a physical exam and a plain X-ray. If these are consistent with constipation, then a clean out with enemas or oral laxatives can be initiated and incontinence will likely improve. Persistent obstruction after appropriate management or no significant improvement after pull-through should be evaluated with contrast enema, exam under anesthesia, and repeat rectal biopsy.

5. **C.** This patient has Hirschsprung's associated enterocolitis (HEC). Risk factors for this condition are Down's syndrome, diagnosis after 1 week of life, anatomic obstruction, and a history of previous HEC. Obstruction can be a result of an anastomotic stricture, swelling of the anastomosis in the early postop period and transition zone pull-through. However, HEC can also occur in the absence of these complications. This is one of the most feared complications of Hirschsprung's, as if treatment is not initiated quickly, patients may become severely ill and die. The etiology is bacterial translocation through the wall of the colon, presumably due to an ineffective mucosal barrier in the colon. Treatment involves fluid resuscitation, antibiotics, nutritional support, and most importantly, rectal irrigations. This is done transanally with warm saline. Unlike an enema, a catheter is used to evacuate stool and gas, while gently irrigating stool out of the colon. In severe cases, colostomy may be required. Patients can present with HEC both before and up to 2 years after pull-through. This clinical presentation is much more consistent with enterocolitis than an abscess. A CT scan is not typically utilized to evaluate for intra-abdominal abscess in infants. The lack of intra-abdominal fat makes

it difficult to discern an abscess cavity from a fluid filled loop of bowel. If imaging is needed to evaluate for this, ultrasound is typically a better study. Neither blood transfusion nor nasogastric decompression is required for treatment, but they may be utilized.

6. B. Several different approaches have been described for the treatment of Hirschsprung's disease.

The "Swenson" procedure is the most simple in concept. It involves the removal of the entire aganglionic colon, with an end-to-end anastomosis 0.5 cm to 1.5 cm above the dentate line. It is important to not perform any pull-through anastomosis directly to the dentate line, or below it. This is associated with a loss of sensation, an inability to detect fullness in the rectum, or the inability to discern between gas and stool, all of which may result in long-term problems with fecal incontinence.

The "Soave" procedure was designed to avoid the risk of injury to important pelvic structures (deep pelvic nerves, vagina, prostate, vas deferens, seminal vesicles, etc.), which may be inherent to removal of the entire aganglionic colon as described by Swenson. Instead, a "cuff" of aganglionic colon is left in situ. A submucosal endorectal dissection is performed for several centimeters proximal to the dentate line, and the ganglionated colon is pulled through the aganglionic rectal "cuff." The Soave cuff does not usually cause long-term problems, but recurrent enterocolitis, constipation, or failure to thrive can indicate a functional obstruction from the cuff. Reoperation with cuff resection may be required for those patients.

The "Duhamel" procedure has the benefit of providing a larger reservoir for holding stool, compared to the Swenson or Soave procedures. This may be of particular benefit for long-segment Hirschsprung disease, wherein the entire colon and possibly some of the small intestine must be removed. The native rectum, which is aganglionic, is left in situ, but the remainder of the aganglionic colon is removed. A linear stapler is then used to merge the walls of the native rectum and the pull-through segment. This procedure is similar in concept to the "J-pouch" that general surgeons may be more accustomed to performing in adult patients.

While all three of the aforementioned approaches were originally described using an abdominal approach, there is now a "purely transanal" approach, which does not require any abdominal incisions. The rectosigmoid colon, and sometimes even the

entire colon, can be mobilized from this transanal approach. For a more proximal transition point, laparoscopic assistance is often utilized. Some studies have demonstrated this technique to be faster, and associated with less postoperative pain, earlier feeding, and earlier discharge than the abdominal approaches. However, a surgeon must be prepared to enter the abdomen if the mobilization is inadequate for a higher-than-expected transition zone, which occurs in 8% to 10% of children who appear to have short-segment disease on contrast enema.

BIBLIOGRAPHY

Brady AC, Saito JM, Lukas K, et al. Suction rectal biopsy yields adequate tissue in children. *J Pediatr Surg*. 2016;51(6): 966–969.

Burki T, Kiho L, Scheimberg I, et al. Neonatal functional intestinal obstruction and the presence of severely immature ganglion cells on rectal biopsy: 6 year experience. *Pediatr Surg Int*. 2011;27(5):487–490.

DeLaTorre L, Langer JC. Transanal pull-through for Hirschsprung disease: technique, controversies, pearls, pitfalls and an organized approach to the management of postoperative obstructive symptoms. *Sem Ped Surg*. 2010;19:96–106.

Dickie BH, Webb KM, Eradi B, Levitt MA. The problematic Soave cuff in Hirschsprung disease: manifestations and treatment. *J Pediatr Surg*. 2014;49(1):77–81.

Engum SA, Grosfeld JL. Long-term results of treatment of Hirschsprung's disease. *Sem Ped Surg*. 2004;13;273–285.

Haricharan RN, Georgeson KE. Hirschprung disease. *Sem Ped Surg*. 2008;17:266–275.

Holcomb GW, Murphy JP, St. Peter S. *Ashcraft's Pediatric Surgery*. 7th ed. Elsevier; 2020.

Kapur RP, Kennedy AJ. Transition Zone pull through: surgical pathology considerations. *Sem Ped Surg*. 2012;21:291–301.

Kim AC, Langer JC, Pastor AC, et al. Endorectal pull-through for Hirschsprung's disease-a multicenter, long-term comparison of results: transanal vs transabdominal approach. *J Pediatr Surg*. 2010;45(6):1213–1220.

Langer JC. Hirschsprung's disease. In: Oldham KT, Colombani PM, Foglia RP, Skinner MA, eds. *Principles and Practice of Pediatric Surgery*. 2nd ed. Lippincott Williams and Wilkins; 2005: 1347–1364.

Levitt MA, Dickie BA, Pena A. Evaluation of the patient with Hirschprung disease who is not doing well after a pull through procedure. *Sem Ped Surg*. 2010;19:146–153.

Mundt E, Bates MD. Genetics of Hirschprung disease and anorectal malformations. *Sem Ped Surg*. 2010;19:101–117.

Mychaliska GB. Introduction to neonatal intestinal obstructions. In: Oldham KT, Colombani PM, Foglia RP, Skinner MA, eds. *Principles and Practice of Pediatric Surgery*. 2nd ed. Lippincott Williams and Wilkins; 2005: 1222–1226.

Rintala RJ, Pakarinen MP. Long-term outcomes of Hirschsprungs's disease. *Sem Ped Surg*. 2012;21:336–343.

Vieten D, Spicer R. Enterocolitis following Hirschsprung's disease. *Sem Ped Surg*. 2004;13:263–272.

64

Omphacele/Gastrochsis

Benjamin Tabak

1. **A fetus has been diagnosed on prenatal ultrasound with gastroschisis. The obstetrician caring for the mother has called and asked for surgical recommendations. Which of the following would be appropriate advice?**

   A. The baby should be delivered at 40 weeks' gestational age.

   B. The baby should be delivered by Caesarean section (C-section).

   C. The baby should only be delivered at a tertiary care center.

   D. The baby should be intubated prior to attempting reduction of abdominal contents.

   E. The baby should have a central venous catheter placed in the delivery room.

2. **A baby is born with gastroschisis. During exploration of the exposed abdominal contents, several conditions may be present. Which of the following would be appropriate management?**

   A. If an intra-abdominal testicle is identified, an orchiopexy should be performed.

   B. If an eviscerated ovary is performed, an oophoropexy should be performed.

   C. If a Meckel's diverticulum is identified, a diverticulectomy should be performed.

   D. If intestinal malrotation is identified, a Ladd's procedure should be performed.

   E. If a colonic atresia is identified, a colostomy or resection should be performed.

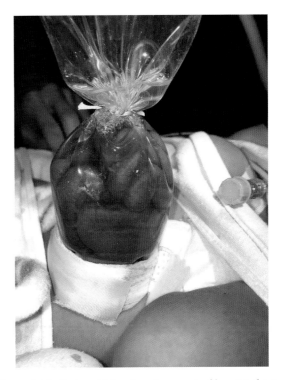

Figure 64-1 Gastroschisis, after placement of herniated intestines into a silicone silo bag.

3. **Abdominal closure for babies born with gastroschisis or omphalocele often results in intra-abdominal hypertension. Which of the following would qualify as abdominal compartment syndrome and mandate immediate reopening of the fascia?**

A. Decreased urine output
B. Peak inspiratory pressure greater than 20 cm H$_2$O
C. Intravesical pressure greater than 20 mmHg
D. Abdominal wall erythema
E. Differential cyanosis

4. **Which of the following best helps to distinguish between omphalocele and gastroschisis?**

   A. In gastroschisis, the liver is commonly herniated.
   B. In gastroschisis, a covering sac is present.
   C. In gastroschisis, associated anomalies are common.
   D. In omphalocele, the abdominal wall defect is to the right of the umbilicus.
   E. For omphalocele, the incidence and prevalence rates have remained stable in the United States.

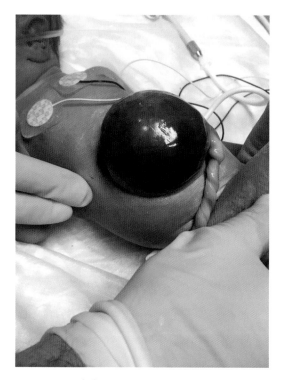

Figure 64-2 Omphalocele with herniating liver, contained by an intact amnion-lined sac.

5. **Which of the following best helps to describe the difference in management of omphalocele and gastroschisis?**

   A. For gastroschisis, an echocardiogram should be performed after birth.
   B. For gastroschisis, the bowels should be covered with saline-soaked gauze after birth.
   C. For omphalocele, feedings can usually be initiated earlier.
   D. For omphalocele, urgent surgical intervention is usually indicated.
   E. For omphalocele, aggressive fluid resuscitation is usually required.

6. **Omphalocele is associated with many syndromes, including the Pentalogy of Cantrell. Which of the following is a component of the Pentalogy of Cantrell?**

   A. Coloboma
   B. Gigantism
   C. Ectopic cordis
   D. Genital hypoplasia
   E. Ear anomalies

7. **Which of the following is the most reasonable strategy for the surgical treatment of these congenital abdominal wall defects?**

   A. Delayed staged closure for treatment for an omphalocele of the cord
   B. Scarification treatment for a ruptured omphalocele
   C. Sutureless closure of closed gastroschisis
   D. Immediate primary closure of a giant omphalocele
   E. Amnion inversion of a giant omphalocele

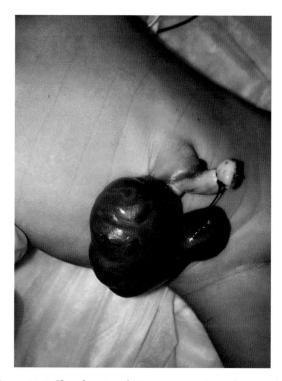

Figure 64-3 Closed gastroschisis – a rare variant of gastroschisis in which the abdominal wall defect closes in utero, causing incarceration of eviscerated bowel.

ANSWERS

1. C. Pregnancies complicated by gastroschisis have a 3% to 6% risk of intrauterine demise, which is seven-fold higher than for the general population. Several studies have suggested that planned early delivery may reduce the complications associated with gastroschisis, including stillbirth, without increasing the risks associated with premature delivery. The mean age of spontaneous labor in pregnancies that are affected by gastroschisis is between 36 and 37 weeks' gestation. Many institutions recommend a planned induction for gastroschisis babies if the mothers have not gone into spontaneous labor by this time. The mode of delivery is less controversial than the timing. Vaginal delivery is preferred, as there has been no proven benefit to C-section. Delivery outside of a tertiary referral center is associated with a longer time to fascial closure and more complications. Immediate endotracheal intubation for gastroschisis babies is not mandatory unless there is a respiratory indication to do so. A central venous catheter is generally required for the administration of intravenous fluids and total parenteral nutrition, but this is usually achieved via peripherally inserted central catheter (PICC) insertion in the neonatal intensive care unit, after the patient has been transferred from the delivery room and stabilized.

2. E. Cryptorchidism (undescended testicle) is commonly associated with gastroschisis. In one study of 24 such babies, all had an initial watch-and-wait approach without any attempt at orchidopexy during gastroschisis closure. Those with extra-abdominal testes at birth had the testicle repositioned in the abdomen before gastroschisis closure. A high rate of spontaneous migration (54.8%) during the first year of life was noted and greater than 90% of the testes were viable at follow-up. Ovaries encountered during gastroschisis closure should similarly be repositioned into the abdominal cavity, without sutures. The intestines in gastroschisis babies tend to be matted and any unnecessary additional surgery should be avoided, including a diverticulectomy. While malrotation (or non-rotation) occurs in nearly every gastroschisis patient, volvulus is considered rare due to adhesions. The Ladd's bands classically associated with congenital malrotation are generally absent in babies born with gastroschisis. Five to 25% of gastroschisis babies have an associated intestinal atresia. The management strategy traditionally applied involves abdominal closure, followed by another operation 4 to 8 weeks later to repair the atresia, due to the fear of anastomotic complications. However, a recent study found that early intestinal operations in patients with gastroschisis and intestinal atresia are not associated with increased complications, and allow patients to receive and tolerate enteral feeding earlier. When gastroschisis is associated with a colonic atresia, particularly in association with a competent ileocecal valve, the nonoperative management may result in massive colonic dilation, necrosis, and perforation. Those complications may be avoided by performing a diverting colostomy or resection and anastomosis at the time of abdominal wall closure.

3. E. Abdominal wall closure for babies with congenital abdominal wall defects is often performed under tension, as the lack of organs inside the abdomen during fetal development precludes the growth of adequate abdominal domain. Fascial closure should generally be deferred if the peak inspiratory pressure is persistently greater than 24 cm H_2O and the fraction of inspired oxygen (FiO_2) is persistently greater than 50%. Intra-abdominal pressure (IAP), which can be estimated with a Foley catheter, greater than 20 mmHg is also suggestive of intra-abdominal hypertension. Abdominal compartment syndrome occurs with resultant end organ compromise, as would be suggested by a lack of urine output. However, it is not uncommon for these indicators to be present for brief periods after abdominal closure, and respond to noninvasive measures, including improved sedation, improved pain control, and fluid resuscitation. Additionally, the splanchnic perfusion pressure (IAP subtracted from mean arterial pressure) may be a better predictor than IAP alone. Abdominal wall erythema is generally an ominous sign in neonates, as it can be reflective of underlying bowel ischemia, but is commonly seen in gastroschisis babies after abdominal wall closure, and may not necessarily be indicative of abdominal compartment syndrome. Differential cyanosis is the bluish, cyanotic appearance of the lower extremities, and its presence suggests impaired venous return. Immediate reopening of the fascia is required to relieve this phenomenon, or if any of the above indicators of abdominal compartment syndrome do not respond to the aforementioned interventions.

4. E. There are several defining characteristics that help to distinguish between omphalocele and gastroschisis. "Omphalocele" is an abdominal wall defect at the umbilicus. A sac present, and the umbilical cord inserts onto the sac. Both the liver and bowel can be herniated. Associated anomalies are common (~50%). Fetuses with omphalocele have a relatively high rate of demise due to stillbirths and late miscarriages. As opposed to gastroschisis, the incidence and prevalence of omphalocele has remained stable in the United States. "Gastroschisis" is an abdominal wall defect to the right of midline. The exposed viscera are not covered by a sac, which makes surgical intervention urgent. The liver is generally not herniated. Associated anomalies are relatively uncommon (~10%). There has been a significant worldwide increase in the incidence of gastroschisis in all maternal age groups over the past two decades.

5. C. There are several defining characteristics that help to distinguish between the management of omphalocele and gastroschisis. In omphalocele, it is important to quickly assess for associated anomalies. All neonates with omphalocele should get an echocardiogram, as congenital heart disease is the most common associated anomaly. As the viscera are protected by the sac, there is usually no need for urgent surgical intervention. The sac itself can be covered with saline-soaked gauze or another dressing to prevent fluid losses. However, the fluid losses are less severe than in gastroschisis, where the abdominal contents are exposed to air. There is usually no intestinal dysmotility associated with omphalocele, as the bowels have not been exposed to amniotic fluid or air. Feedings can therefore usually be initiated earlier.

6. C. Fetal central and epigastric omphaloceles may be different entities: central omphaloceles are more strongly associated with abnormal karyotype (69%) than are epigastric omphaloceles (12.5%). Epigastric omphaloceles may be associated with the Pentalogy of Cantrell—an association of midline defects, which includes omphalocele, anterior diaphgragmatic defect, bifid sternum, pericardiac defect, and intracardiac anomalies. The most severe expression of the Pentalogy of Cantrell presents with ectopia cordia—a severe condition in which the heart is outside of the thoracic cavity.

7. E. The entities listed are variants of omphaloceles and gastroschises. "Omphalocele of the cord" refers to very small omphaloceles that are less than 1.5 cm in diameter. Assuming there are no major associated anomalies prohibiting general anesthesia, these defects are usually repaired shortly after birth with excision of the small sac and primary closure of the skin and fascia. Occasionally, there will be an omphalomesenteric duct remnant that needs to be excised. Delivery room staff need to be aware of this anomaly, as the bowel in the small sac may be unrecognized and injured with application of the standard umbilical cord clamp. A "ruptured omphalocele" refers to an omphalocele in which the sac has ruptured. This scenario requires urgent surgical intervention, as the abdominal contents are exposed. A "closed gastroschisis" refers to an unusual condition in which the fascia and skin have closed almost completely around the exposed bowel and mesentery. The abdominal wall defect must be extended for the bowel to be replaced into the abdominal cavity. A "sutureless closure" refers to the closure of an abdomen with gastroschisis without the use of sutures. The bowels are reduced and umbilical cord is used to "plug" the abdominal wall defect, as adhesive strips are placed over top. "Scarification" refers to the application of agents to the intact amniotic sac of an omphalocele to induce eschar formation. This is a common strategy for "giant omphaloceles" (>5 cm), which are not amenable to primary closure in the neonatal period, particularly those associated with other major congenital anomalies. "Amnion inversion" refers to a technique in which the amniotic sac of an omphalocele is kept intact, and serially inverted into the abdominal cavity over time, prior to final excision and fascial closure. This has been described for the treatment of giant omphaloceles.

BIBLIOGRAPHY

Abdel-Latif ME, Bolisetty S, Abeywardana S, Lui K; Australian and New Zealand Neonatal Network. Mode of delivery and neonatal survival of infants with gastroschisis in Australia and New Zealand. *J Pediatr Surg.* 2008;43(9):1685–1690.

Alshehri A, Emil S, Laberge JM, Skarsgard E; Canadian Pediatric Surgery Network. Outcomes of early versus late intestinal operations in patients with gastroschisis and intestinal atresia: results from a prospective national database. *J Pediatr Surg.* 2013;48(10):2022–2026.

Brantberg A, Blaas HG, Haugen SE, Eik-Nes SH. Characteristics and outcome of 90 cases of fetal omphalocele. *Ultrasound Obstet Gynecol.* 2005;26(5):527–537.

de Lorimier AA, Adzick NS, Harrison MR. Amnion inversion in the treatment of giant omphalocele. *J Pediatr Surg.* 1991;26(7):804–807.

Gelas T, Gorduza D, Devonec S, et al. Scheduled preterm delivery for gastroschisis improves postoperative outcome. *Pediatr Surg Int.* 2008;24(9):1023–1029.

Haxhija EQ, Schalamon J, Höllwarth ME. Management of isolated and associated colonic atresia. *Pediatr Surg Int.* 2011;27(4):411–416.

Hill SJ, Durham MM. Management of cryptorchidism and gastroschisis. *J Pediatr Surg.* 2011;46(9):1798–1803.

Lap CCMM, Brizot ML, Pistorius LR, et al. Outcome of isolated gastroschisis; an international study, systematic review and metaanalysis. *Early Hum Dev.* 2016;103: 209–218.

Marshall J, Salemi JL, Tanner JP, et al. Prevalence, correlates, and outcomes of omphalocele in the United States, 1995–2005. *Obstet Gynecol.* 2015;126:284–293.

McGuigan RM, Mullenix PS, Vegunta R, Pearl RH, Sawin R, Azarow KS. Splanchnic perfusion pressure: a better predictor of safe primary closure than intraabdominal pressure in neonatal gastroschisis. *J Pediatr Surg.* 2006;41(5): 901–904.

Nasr A, Langer JC; Canadian Paediatric Surgery Network. Influence of location of delivery on outcome in neonates with gastroschisis. *J Pediatr Surg.* 2012;47(11): 2022–2025.

South AP, Stutey KM, Meinzen-Derr J. Metaanalysis of the prevalence of intrauterine fetal death in gastroschisis. *Am J Obstet Gynecol.* 2013;209(2):96–106.

OB/GYN

65

Ovarian Masses

Samantha Carson, Elise Barker, and Charles S. Dietrich III

A 52-year-old post-menopausal female presents with abdominal bloating and urinary frequency over the last several weeks. She denies abdominal or pelvic pain but confirms mild constipation with reported bowel movements every 3 days. She has had no vaginal or rectal bleeding. Her past medical and surgical history is significant for mild hypertension and a prior Cesarean delivery. Her mother was diagnosed with breast cancer at age 45.

On examination, her vital signs are unremarkable. Normal bowel sounds are noted and the abdomen is mildly distended. No abdominal pain is elicited and there are no palpable masses. On pelvic exam, a nodular fixed mass is noted in the left adnexal region. Rectal exam is unremarkable. Laboratory assessment shows a normal CEA, but her CA125 level is elevated at 430 U/mL.

1. **What is the BEST initial imaging study for a patient with a suspected ovarian mass?**

    A. Abdominal X-rays
    B. Transvaginal ultrasound (TVUS)
    C. Computerized tomography (CT) scan
    D. Magnetic resonance imaging (MRI)
    E. Positron emission tomography-computed tomography (PET-CT)

2. **Which of the following confers the HIGHEST risk for lifetime development of ovarian cancer?**

    A. BRCA1 mutation
    B. BRCA2 mutation
    C. Lynch syndrome

    D. Li Fraumeni syndrome
    E. Mother affected with ovarian cancer

3. **For the aforementioned patient, what is the BEST management strategy?**

    A. Observation
    B. Percutaneous core biopsy of the adnexal mass
    C. Surgical exploration with staging and cytoreduction
    D. Neoadjuvant chemotherapy
    E. Palliative care

4. **Which of the following procedures is included in the surgical management of an apparent early-stage ovarian malignancy?**

    A. Splenectomy
    B. Diaphragmatic stripping
    C. Cholecystectomy
    D. Pelvic and para-aortic lymph node sampling
    E. Distal pancreatectomy

5. **Which of the following adjuvant chemotherapy options is MOST COMMONLY used for the initial treatment of an epithelial ovarian cancer?**

    A. Intravenous (IV) cyclophosphamide and cisplatin
    B. Intravenous (IV) paclitaxel and cisplatin
    C. Intravenous (IV) paclitaxel and carboplatin
    D. Intraperitoneal (IP) chemotherapy with paclitaxel and cisplatin
    E. Olaparib

A 13-year-old gravida 0 presents to the Emergency Department with sudden onset, severe, right lower quadrant pain while at soccer practice earlier this afternoon. She endorses nausea and one episode of emesis. She denies fevers, diarrhea, and recent sexual activity. Her last menstrual period was approximately two weeks ago. Her past medical and past surgical history is unremarkable.

The patient's vital signs are within normal limits. Physical examination is notable for a distended abdomen, with severe tenderness to palpation in the right lower quadrant. Rebound and guarding are also present. A urine hCG is negative and her white blood cell count and hematocrit are within normal limits.

6. **What is the appropriate initial imaging study for this patient?**

   A. Abdominal X-ray
   B. CT scan of the abdomen/pelvis
   C. Abdominal ultrasound
   D. MRI pelvis

Transabdominal ultrasound of the patient reveals a normal appearing appendix and left ovary. The right ovary appears enlarged and edematous with reduced Doppler flow. There is an 8-cm heterogeneous appearing right ovarian cyst with internal debris. Ovarian torsion is suspected and the patient is scheduled for diagnostic laparoscopy. Intraoperatively, the right ovary appears dusky, enlarged, and torsion is present.

7. **What is the appropriate intraoperative management of this patient's ovarian torsion?**

   A. Detorsion
   B. Detorsion and ovarian cystectomy
   C. Right unilateral oophorectomy
   D. Right unilateral salpingo-oophorectomy

ANSWERS

1. **B.** The best initial imaging study for evaluating an ovarian mass is TVUS. Morphologic characteristics, volume of the mass, and assessment of vascular resistance through color Doppler assists in differentiating benign from malignant ovarian processes. The addition of abdominal ultrasound is important in delineating larger ovarian and uterine masses extending outside the pelvis. The sensitivity of TVUS with color Doppler is approximately 92% to 99% for identification of malignant tumors of the ovary. Findings on the ultrasound suggest a malignant process include

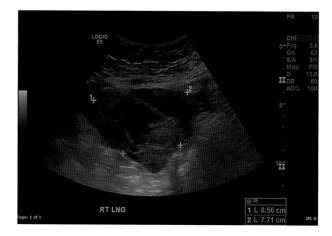

Figure 65-1 A TVUS of an ovarian high-grade serous carcinoma demonstrating a complex mass with solid and cystic regions.

complex masses with solid and cystic components, internal or external nodular excrescences, and surrounding pelvic ascites (Figure 65-1). Although there is no universal test or combination of tests that are recommended for ovarian cancer screening, there is data to support the use of the "morphology index" (based on tumor characteristics and volume) derived from TVUS findings to better risk stratify the ovarian abnormality as benign versus malignant.

Plain film X-rays are not very useful in the evaluation of ovarian masses as they are typically composed of fluid and soft tissue; however, a plain film may reveal incidental calcifications, one of the hallmark findings in ovarian teratomas. CT performance differentiating the soft tissue structures within the ovary is also limited. CT is most useful if malignancy is suspected to evaluate for metastatic disease in the preoperative planning phase. PET-CT has poor sensitivity and specificity for adnexal masses and is expensive. It is utilized most commonly in patients with a known ovarian malignancy following treatment to evaluate for recurrence.

MRI is reserved for indeterminate ultrasound findings. Recently, an Ovarian-Adnexal Reporting Data System Magnetic (O-RADS) MRI score (ranging from 1 to 5) was designed to provide the positive likelihood ratio for malignant neoplasm. A score of 4 or greater was associated with malignancy with a sensitivity of 93.5% and a specificity of 96.6%. A lesion with a score of 3 has the positive likelihood ratio of malignant tumor of 0.27. These patients may benefit from conservative management with continued close surveillance. A score of 2 or lower indicates a benign mass.

2. **A.** Obtaining a thorough, and accurate, family history is mandatory in evaluating the patient with a suspicious adnexal mass. In the United States, The average women's lifetime risk for developing ovarian cancer is 1.2%. However, in a meta-analysis published in 1998, the lifetime relative risk of developing ovarian cancer with one affected first-degree relative was 3.1 (95% CI 2.6–3.7), conferring a 5% lifetime risk. If more than one relative was affected, the estimated relative risk increased to 11.7 (95% CI 5.3–25.9) (approximate 20% lifetime risk).

Overall, approximately 24% of women diagnosed with epithelial ovarian, peritoneal, or fallopian tube carcinoma are found to have germline mutations in 12 different genes. As such, genetic testing is now recommended for all high-grade epithelial ovarian cancer patients. BRCA1 or BRCA2 mutations account for the majority of findings (18% of all ovarian cancers). Other genes less commonly affected include BARD1, BRIP1, CHEK2, MRE11A, MSH6, NBN, PALB2, RAD50, RAD51C, and TP53.

BRCA1 and 2 are tumor suppressor genes coding for a protein involved in the repair of double-stranded DNA breaks. Patients with BRCA1 mutations have a lifetime ovarian cancer risk of approximately 40% to 53%, while BRCA2 penetrance is 20% to 30%. Hereditary Non-Polyposis Colorectal Cancer (HNPCC), or Lynch Syndrome, results from a defect in mismatch repair (MMR) genes. These patients carry a very high risk of developing colon and endometrial cancer, as well as additional risk for other extracolonic malignancies. Ovarian cancer risk varies based on the actual genetic defect: MLH1/MSH2: 4–24%; MSH6: 1–11%; PMS2: 6%. Other familial syndromes, such as Li-Fraumeni (TP53 mutation) and Peutz-Jeghers (STK11 mutation) also carry increased risks of developing ovarian cancer.

3. **C.** The menopausal patient described has findings concerning for an ovarian malignancy based on her constitutional symptoms, the appearance of her adnexal mass and her elevated CA-125 level. In 2021, an estimated 21,410 new ovarian cancer cases will occur in the United States, and there will be an estimated 13,770 deaths. Ovarian cancer is the fifth-leading cause for

cancer deaths among women. While symptoms occur in women with ovarian malignancies, they are often vague and nonspecific. Unfortunately, almost 80% of patients at time of diagnosis are found to have disease spread beyond the ovaries. Persistent symptoms that should prompt evaluation of the ovaries include pelvic pain, changes in bowel habits, bloating, and urinary frequency. The overall 5-year survival for all patients diagnosed with ovarian cancer is currently around 49%.

The American College of Obstetricians and Gynecologists (ACOG) and Society of Gynecologic Oncology (SGO) recommend referral of the menopausal patient with an adnexal mass to a gynecologic oncologist if any of the following is found: any elevation in the CA-125, associated ascites, the mass is fixed or nodular, evidence of metastatic disease is noted, or if familial risk is determined. In the premenopausal patient with an adnexal mass, referral should occur for CA-125 >200 U/mL, ascites, evidence of metastatic disease, or hereditary risk.

Surgical exploration is recommended for this patient to establish her diagnosis. If malignancy is found on frozen diagnosis, then staging and cytoreductive surgery can be immediately performed. Observation has significant risk for delay in diagnosis and is not recommended. Percutaneous biopsy of an ovarian mass should only be undertaken after careful consideration of the risks and benefits. Biopsy can result in peritoneal tumor seeding and is often inaccurate, with sensitivity for malignancy detection ranging from 25% to 82%.

Neoadjuvant chemotherapy is another option for patients who have had a confirmation of ovarian cancer by paracentesis or other biopsy. Patients with comorbid conditions making them poor surgical candidates or those with bulky upper abdominal or stage IV disease may benefit most from this approach. Recent trials have shown that neoadjuvant chemotherapy offers a significant improvement in optimal cytoreduction at interval surgery, diminished surgical morbidity, and similar progression-free and overall survival rates in Stage IIIC and IV ovarian cancer. Palliative care is usually reserved for patients with progressive or recurrent disease unresponsive to therapy or for those with significant comorbidities.

4. **D.** If an ovarian malignancy is confirmed on intraoperative assessment, accurate staging is paramount to determine the extent of the disease and

appropriate adjuvant treatments. Upstaging of an apparent malignancy confined to the ovary ranges from 22% to 50% when formal staging procedures are performed. Formal staging of a suspected early stage ovarian cancer usually includes the following: removal of the affected ovary; removal of the uterus and contralateral ovary (if fertility is not desired); careful evaluation of all peritoneal surfaces with biopsy of any suspicious areas; peritoneal washings for cytologic evaluation; complete omentectomy; random peritoneal sampling from the right hemidiaphragm, paracolic gutters, pelvic sidewalls, bladder, and posterior cul-de-sac; and removal of pelvic and para-aortic lymph nodes. Lymphadenectomy probably is the most important and technically challenging component of adequate staging. In a review by Powless et al., 13% of apparent early stage ovarian cancers were found to have positive nodes. While still recommended, several investigators have questioned the utility of omentectomy and random peritoneal biopsies when no gross disease is visible. In their reviews, upstaging based on omentectomy occurred in less than 4% of patients. Similarly, less than 5% of patients were found to have microscopic disease on random peritoneal biopsies.

The ACTION trial confirmed the importance of adequate staging. In this study, patients with Stage IA to IIA ovarian epithelial carcinoma were randomized after surgery to observation or adjuvant chemotherapy. Groups were further stratified into optimal versus non-optimal staging categories. In a recent long-term analysis, overall survival was improved in patients with optimal surgical staging, even among those receiving adjuvant chemotherapy (HR = 1.89, p = 0.05). Considerable debate is ongoing regarding the route of surgical staging. Historically, laparotomy was felt to offer the best exposure for full evaluation of all peritoneal surfaces, and this approach is still standard today. With advances in minimally invasive surgery over the past decade, many investigators have concluded that operative outcomes with a laparoscopic approach are comparable to those seen with laparotomy.

When an advanced ovarian malignancy is present, the extent of surgical cytoreduction directly correlates with overall survival. The theoretic benefits of cytoreduction include improved patient comfort, increased tumor perfusion, increased tumor growth fraction, and improved immunologic response. Removal of all individual tumor implants to <1 cm is currently considered an optimal cytoreduction. However, the definition of optimal cytoreduction is rapidly changing, and most gynecologic oncologists now consider reduction to microscopic disease to be the goal. In a review of several Gynecologic Oncology Groups (GOG) studies, patients with Stage IIIC disease (later stage disease) had an overall survival of 71.9 months when cytoreduction to microscopic disease was achieved versus 42.4 months when disease was reduced to less than 1 cm. Achieving an optimal cytoreductive status often requires bowel resection and extensive upper abdominal procedures such as diaphragmatic stripping, splenectomy, and distal pancreatectomy.

5. C. Adjuvant chemotherapy is recommended for almost all epithelial ovarian cancers following surgical staging and tumor cytoreduction. Platinum-based treatment has remained the cornerstone of therapy since the 1970s. The current standard incorporates paclitaxel with carboplatin delivered intravenously every 3 weeks for six to eight cycles. It emerged in 2003 based on its excellent toxicity profile and trend toward improved overall survival when compared to older platinum-based regimens. Nearly 75% of patients with advanced disease will achieve remission. Unfortunately, recurrences are likely, usually occurring within two years of primary therapy, and are rarely curable. Intense efforts are ongoing to discover novel treatment options.

Intraperitoneal (IP) chemotherapy has long interested gynecologic oncologists as a strategy for dose intensification. However, due to the challenges in delivery and increased toxicities, this route of administration has not been readily adopted. In 2006, GOG 172 demonstrated one of the largest survival advantages for any ovarian cancer study ever published. In this trial, a 16-month overall survival advantage was found for an IP regimen (Day 1, intravenous paclitaxel; Day 2, intraperitoneal cisplatin; Day 8, intraperitoneal paclitaxel) when compared to intravenous paclitaxel and cisplatin every 3 weeks. Toxicities were significantly increased in the IP group. Most patients only completed 4/6 cycles and had a significant reduction in quality of life during treatment. A primary criticism of GOG 172 focused around the IP treatment arm being a dose-dense regimen that was compared to an inadequate control group. In response, GOG 252 was conducted with a modified GOG 172 IP regimen in an attempt to reduce toxicity and was compared to a control group treated with IV dose-dense weekly paclitaxel and carboplatin. Bevacizumab was added to all arms, which may have clouded the results. This study did not show any improvement in progression-free survival or overall survival with IP treatment. Despite this negative study, the IP debate continues, and a heightened interest in heated intraperitoneal chemotherapy (HIPEC) at the time of cytoreductive surgery is emerging as new strategy in ovarian cancer.

Significant efforts are focusing on targeted therapies in the treatment of ovarian cancer. Bevacizumab, a monoclonal antibody that prevents angiogenesis by inhibiting vascular endothelial growth factor (VEGF), has received considerable attention for its activity in a number of solid tumors. Several studies using bevacizumab in combination with cytotoxic chemotherapy have demonstrated a progression-free survival advantage in ovarian cancer; however, an overall survival advantage with bevacizumab has remained elusive to date. Considerable excitement has emerged with poly (ADP-ribose) polymerase (PARP) inhibitors. PARP inhibitors prevent repair of single-strand DNA breaks. In patients with defects in homologous recombination repair (i.e., BRCA1 or 2 mutations), accumulation of DNA damage and cell death occurs. While PARP inhibitors have been researched in both the upfront and recurrent settings, a maintenance strategy after completing primary chemotherapy holds the most promise. In the SOLO1 trial, maintenance olaparib in BRCA1/2 patients led to a 70% reduction in the risk of disease progression when compared to placebo.

6. **C.** Ultrasound is the most appropriate initial imaging study for an adolescent female with abdominal or pelvic pain, and it is preferred for evaluating pelvic pathology. It prevents the pediatric patient from receiving unnecessary radiation and is cost effective. Ultrasound can evaluate for many possible etiologies of pain including appendicitis, pregnancy, ruptured ovarian cyst and ovarian torsion. Transvaginal sonography is usually not necessary in the adolescent female and should be avoided if the ovaries can be visualized abdominally.

This patient's clinical presentation is suspicious for ovarian torsion. The estimated incidence of ovarian torsion among females 1 to 20 years old is 4.9/100,000, with a mean age of 14.5 years. Sudden onset pelvic pain is the most common presenting symptom. Adnexal torsion also usually occurs with waves of nausea and vomiting. Low-grade fevers and leucocytosis may also be present.

Ovarian torsion is a clinical diagnosis; however, ultrasound may aid making the diagnosis. The sensitivity of ultrasound for diagnosing ovarian torsion ranges from 46% to 75%. Diminished or absent blood flow is suggestive but not necessary to make the diagnosis. The ovary has a dual blood supply and normal Doppler flow may be present even in the setting of ovarian torsion. Therefore, direct visualization of a torsed ovary at the time of surgery is required to confirm the diagnosis. In a patient with acute pelvic pain and an adnexal mass, a presumptive diagnosis of ovarian torsion can be made after excluding appendicitis, tubo-ovarian abscess and ectopic pregnancy. Once the diagnosis is suspected, surgery should proceed expeditiously in order to preserve viable ovarian tissue.

7. **B.** Intraoperative management of ovarian torsion in the pre-menopausal patient should prioritize ovarian conservation to optimize reproductive potential and to maintain hormonal production. The gross appearance of the ovary does not correlate with ovarian viability or function. Therefore, detorsion and ovarian cystectomy is recommended. Oophoropexy to the pelvic sidewall or round ligament is sometimes performed to decrease the risk for future recurrences. Over 90% of females treated with detorsion were found to have functioning follicles 8 to 10 weeks after surgery, and many cases of successful pregnancy after detorsion have been reported. Despite this recommendation, salpingo-oophorectomy at the time of surgery for ovarian torsion is still common. A recent examination of pediatric patients in the National Inpatient Sample (NIS) demonstrated that 15% of patients underwent detorsion, 6% underwent detorsion with oophoropexy, and 78% underwent oophorectomy. A main factor cited to justify salpingo-oophorectomy is the theoretical risk of detorsion releasing thromboemboli, which could result in pulmonary embolism; however, there has never been a documented case of this in the literature. Another reason proposed for performing oophorectomy instead of detorsion is the risk for malignancy, but this risk is low and is mitigated if the patient is followed closely after surgery. In a systemic review of the literature performed in 2018, the rate of malignancy detected in resected ovaries in the

pediatric population ranged from 0.4% to 5%. This low incidence does not justify oophorectomy in the pediatric population.

BIBLIOGRAPHY

American College of Obstetricians and Gynecologists. ACOG Practice Bulletin. Management of adnexal masses. *Obstet Gynecol.* 2007;110(1):201–214.

Andrews L, Mutch D. Hereditary ovarian cancer and risk reduction. *Best Pract Res Clin Obstet Gynecol.* 2017;41: 31–48.

Anthoulakis C, Nikoloudis N. Pelvic MRI as the "gold standard" in the subsequent evaluation of ultrasound-indeterminate adnexal lesions: a systematic review. *Gynecol Oncol.* 2014;132(3):661–668.

Armstrong DK, Bundy B, Wenzel L, et al. Intraperitoneal cisplatin and paclitaxel in ovarian cancer. *N Engl J Med.* 2006;354(1):34–43.

Burger RA, Brady MF, Bookman MA, et al. Incorporation of bevacizumab in the primary treatment of ovarian cancer. *N Engl J Med.* 2011;365(26):2473–2483.

Colombo KM, Scambia G, Kim BG, et al. Maintenance olaparib in patients with newly diagnosed advanced ovarian cancer. *N Engl J Med.* 2018;379:2495–2505.

Dasgupta R, Renaud E, Goldin AB, et al. Ovarian torsion in pediatric and adolescent patients: a systematic review. *J Pediatr Surg.* 2018;53(7):1387–1391.

DePriest PD, Varner E, Powell J, et al. The efficacy of a sonographic morphology index in identifying ovarian cancer: a multi-institutional investigation. *Gynecol Oncol.* 1994;55(2):174–178.

Grabowski JP, Harter P, Buhrmann C, et al. Re-operation outcome in patients referred to a gynecologic oncology center with presumed ovarian cancer FIGO I-IIIA after substandard initial surgery. *Surg Oncol.* 2012;21:31–35.

Harris RD, Javitt MC, Glanc P, et al. ACR Appropriateness Criteria* clinically suspected adnexal mass. *Ultrasound Q.* 2013;29(1):79–86.

Kehoe S, Hook J, Nankivell M, et al. Chemotherapy or upfront surgery for newly diagnosed advanced ovarian cancer: Results from the MRC CHORUS trial. *J Clin Oncol. (Meeting Abstracts.)* 2013;31(15 suppl):5500.

Lee JY, Kim HS, Chung HH, et al. The role of omentectomy and random peritoneal biopsies as part of comprehensive surgical staging in apparent early-stage epithelial ovarian cancer. *Ann Surg Oncol.* 2014;21(8):2762–2766.

National Comprehensive Cancer Network. Genetic/familial high-risk assessment: colorectal (version 1.2014). http://www.nccn.org/professionals/physician_gls/pdf/genetics_colon.pdf.

Ozols RF, Bundy BN, Greer BE, et al. Phase III trial of carboplatin and paclitaxel compared with cisplatin and paclitaxel in patients with optimally resected stage III ovarian cancer: a Gynecologic Oncology Group study. *J Clin Oncol.* 2003;21(17):3194–3200.

Park HJ, Kim DW, Yim GW, et al. Staging laparoscopy for the management of early-stage ovarian cancer: a metaanalysis. *Am J Obstet Gynecol.* 2013;209:58e1–58e8.

Perren TJ, Swart AM, Pfisterer J, et al. A phase 3 trial of bevacizumab in ovarian cancer. *N Engl J Med.* 2011;365(26): 2484–2496.

Powless CA, Aletti GD, Bakkum-Gamez JN, et al. Risk factors for lymph node metastasis in apparent early-stage epithelial ovarian cancer: implications for surgical staging. *Gynecol Oncol.* 2011;122(3):536–540.

Powless CA, Bakkum-Gamez JN, Aletti GD, et al. Random peritoneal biopsies have limited value in staging of apparent early stage epithelial ovarian cancer after thorough exploration. *Gynecol Oncol.* 2009;115(1):86–89.

Ramus SJ, Gayther SA. The contribution of BRCA1 and BRCA2 to ovarian cancer. *Mol Oncol.* 2009;3(2):138–150.

Rossi BV, Ference EH, Zurakowski D, et al. The clinical presentation and surgical management of adnexal torsion in the pediatric and adolescent population. *J Pediatr Adolesc Gynecol.* 2012;25(2):109–113.

Siegal R, Miller KD, Jemal A. Cancer statistics, 2020. *CA Cancer J Clin.* 2020;70:7–30.

Sola R, Wormer BA, Walters AL, Heniford BT, Schulman AM. National trends in the surgical treatment of ovarian torsion in children: an analysis of 2041 pediatric patients utilizing the nationwide inpatient sample. *Am. Surg.* 2015 Sep 1;81(9):844–848.

Stratton JF, Pharoah P, Smith SK, et al. A systematic review and meta-analysis of family history and risk of ovarian cancer. *Br J Obstet Gynaecol.* 1998;105(5):493–499.

Thomassin-Naggara I, Aubert E, Rockall A, et al. Adnexal masses: development and preliminary validation of an MR imaging scoring system. *Radiology.* 2013;267(2):432–443.

Thomassin-Naggara I, Poncelet E, Jalaguier-Coudray A, et al. Ovarian-Adnexal Reporting Data System Magnetic Resonance Imaging (O-RADS MRI) score for risk stratification of sonographically indeterminate adnexal masses. *JAMA Network Open.* 2020;3(1):e1919896.

Trimbos B, Timmers P, Pecorelli S, et al. Surgical staging and treatment of early ovarian cancer: long-term analysis from a randomized trial. *J Natl Cancer Inst.* 2010;102:982–987.

Vergote I, Tropé CG, Amant F, et al. Neoadjuvant chemotherapy or primary surgery in stage IIIC or IV ovarian cancer. *N Engl J Med.* 2010;363(10):943–953.

Winter WE, Maxwell GL, Tian C, et al. Prognostic factors for stage III epithelial ovarian cancer: a Gynecologic Oncology Group study. *J Clin Oncol.* 2007;25(24):3621–3627.

Young R, Decker D, Wharton JT. Staging laparotomy in early ovarian cancer. *JAMA.* 1983;250:3072–3076.

Ectopic Pregnancy

Charles S. Dietrich III, Bradford P. Whitcomb, Jordan Kopf, and Alan P. Gehrich

A 24-year-old female presents to the emergency department with worsening right pelvic pain over the past 12 hours associated with vaginal spotting. She denies fevers and chills and has had no nausea or vomiting. Her bowel movements have been regular, and she denies any urinary symptoms. She is sexually active and not using contraception. Her last menstrual period was 7 weeks prior to presentation. Past medical and surgical history is remarkable only for a chlamydial infection 2 years ago.

Her vital signs show a temperature of 98.6°F with a heart rate of 101 and blood pressure of 95/55. Focused examination shows mild abdominal distention with right lower quadrant tenderness to deep palpation. No peritoneal signs are elicited. Her pelvic exam reveals a small amount of bleeding from a closed cervical os. There is no cervical motion tenderness, but exquisite tenderness with a slight fullness is appreciated in the right adnexal region.

Laboratory assessment is notable for a positive urine β-hCG test with a follow-up quantitative β-hCG of 2,200 mIU/mL. Her white blood count is 6.5 × 109/L, hemoglobin 9.8 g/dL, hematocrit 29.2%, and platelets are 230 × 109/L. Renal and liver function tests are within normal limits.

1. What is the BEST initial imaging modality for this patient?

A. Transvaginal ultrasound (TVUS)
B. Transabdominal ultrasound
C. Computerized tomography (CT) scan
D. Magnetic resonance imaging (MRI)
E. Abdominal X-ray

2. Which single quantitative β-hCG level can discriminate an ectopic from an intrauterine pregnancy (viable or nonviable) when there are confirmatory findings of an intrauterine pregnancy on ultrasound?

A. 500 mIU/mL
B. 1,000 mIU/mL
C. 2,000 mIU/mL
D. 3,000 mIU/mL
E. There is no such single β-hCG value.

3. Ectopic pregnancies can be managed by methotrexate therapy. Which of the following factors is a CONTRAINDICATION to the medical management of an ectopic pregnancy with methotrexate?

A. Absence of cardiac activity within the ectopic pregnancy on ultrasonography
B. Absence of pelvic pain
C. A β-hCG level of 4,500 mIU/mL
D. Hemodynamically stable patient
E. A patient with unreliable follow-up

4. In a patient demonstrating evidence of a ruptured ectopic pregnancy with hemodynamic instability, which is the BEST management option for an ectopic pregnancy in the distal fallopian tube?

A. Expectant management
B. Methotrexate
C. Salpingostomy
D. Salpingectomy
E. Salpingo-oophorectomy

5. **Once an ectopic pregnancy has been diagnosed, what is the risk for an ectopic implantation in a subsequent pregnancy?**

    A. 1%
    B. 10%
    C. 20%
    D. 50%
    E. 75%

6. **Which is the BEST option to distinguish between an abnormal intrauterine pregnancy and an ectopic pregnancy in a woman with a pregnancy of unknown location and abnormally rising β-hCG levels?**

    A. Trial of methotrexate therapy
    B. Hysteroscopy
    C. Sampling of the endometrial lining
    D. Serial pelvic ultrasounds to assess for free fluid in the posterior cul-de-sac
    E. Laparoscopy to assess fallopian tubes

7. **Gynecologists use β-hCG levels to determine the viability of a pregnancy before the gestation can be seen on ultrasound. In this patient, what is considered a NORMAL rise with a current β-hCG level measuring 2,200 mIU/mL?**

    A. 20% in 24 hours
    B. 20% in 48 hours
    C. 50% in 72 hours
    D. 40% in 48 hours
    E. 30% in 72 hours

8. **When counseling patients, which of the following risk factors confers the HIGHEST risk for ectopic pregnancy?**

    A. Prior cesarean delivery
    B. Previous elective pregnancy termination
    C. Age greater than 30 years
    D. Past history of pelvic inflammatory disease
    E. Present use of an intrauterine device (IUD)

9. **At which gestational age is an ectopic pregnancy most likely to become symptomatic?**

    A. 2–4 weeks
    B. 4–5 weeks
    C. 6–9 weeks
    D. 11–12 weeks
    E. >12 weeks

ANSWERS

1. **A.** Ectopic pregnancies account for 1.3% to 2.4% of pregnancy in the general population and 2% to 5% among patients utilizing assisted reproductive technology. The prevalence of ectopic pregnancy among women presenting to an emergency department with pain and vaginal bleeding in the first trimester of pregnancy is as high as 18%. Ectopic pregnancies, at any gestational age, account for 9% of pregnancy-related deaths, and the risk of maternal death increases with increasing gestational age of the ectopic. With improved ultrasound resolution, allowing for earlier identification of ectopic pregnancies, the maternal case-fatality rate has dropped to 3.8 deaths per 10,000 ectopic pregnancies in countries with advanced medical systems. Although risk factors such as prior ectopic pregnancy, prior pelvic infections, previous surgeries, and smoking increase risk, approximately half of all women who are diagnosed with ectopic pregnancy do not have a known risk factor.

   When a female patient presents with pain and bleeding in early pregnancy, the leading diagnoses on the differential include: a viable intrauterine pregnancy (VIP), a nonviable intrauterine pregnancy, or an ectopic pregnancy. TVUS, along with serum beta human chorionic gonadotropin (β-hCG) measurements, has become the cornerstone in the evaluation of early-pregnancy complications. Early pregnancy development tends to follow a predictable path first documented by normally rising β-hCG levels in the pre-discriminatory phase of gestation, followed by documentation of the pregnancy via TVUS. On TVUS, a gestational sac in the endometrial cavity of the uterus can typically be visualized at 5 weeks of gestational age as measured from the first day of the last menstrual period. The yolk sac appears at approximately 5½ weeks' gestation. The embryo can generally be visualized adjacent to the yolk sac at approximately 6 weeks' gestation. With a VIP, the fetal heartbeat can be appreciated once the embryo is clearly defined by TVUS. Any deviation from this sequence of TVUS findings raises concerns for an abnormal intrauterine gestation. TVUS can also accurately assess pregnancies outside the uterus in the fallopian tubes or on the ovaries.

   Findings on TVUS suggestive of an ectopic pregnancy include, the absence of an intrauterine pregnancy based on β-HCG levels or gestational age, identification of an adnexal mass adjacent to the uterus and medial to the ovary, and heterogeneous pelvic fluid as evidence of hemoperitoneum (Figures 66-1 and 66-2). While transabdominal ultrasonography can identify an intrauterine pregnancy, this modality lacks the penetration to accurately assess the adnexa. Imaging studies with ionizing radiation should be avoided in early pregnancy as ionizing radiation can have deterministic effects on the rapidly dividing cells of the embryo and placenta. Furthermore, modalities such as CT scan, abdominal X-rays, and MRI have lower sensitivity and specificity than real-time ultrasound in the evaluation of ectopic pregnancies.

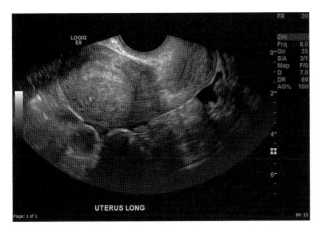

Figure 66-1 TVUS image of the uterus demonstrating a thin endometrial lining with no intrauterine gestational sac.

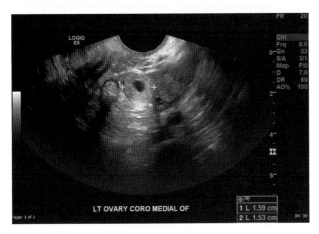

Figure 66-2 TVUS image demonstrating an ectopic mass adjacent to the left ovary (OV).

2. **E.** Pregnancy of Unknown Location (PUL) is a term used to describe a patient with a positive pregnancy test, but in whom a TVUS is unable to diagnose an intrauterine or ectopic gestation. With PUL, utilization of serial β-hCG measurements are the diagnostic tools of choice. β-hCG levels, can however, overlap for the three most common diagnoses in patients with first-trimester bleeding: VIPs, nonviable intrauterine pregnancies, and ectopic gestations. A single β-HCG value, therefore, cannot be used to reliably differentiate between these possibilities despite intensive research efforts to determine a discriminatory level. The discriminatory level is based on a β-hCG level above which components of a normally developing intrauterine pregnancy should be visible on ultrasound.

As the discriminatory capabilities of TVUS have improved, investigators reported an increasing accuracy in documenting intrauterine gestations with β-hCG levels between 1,000 to 2,000 mIU/mL. However, follow-up studies have questioned the accuracy of these assessments as a small percentage of IUP cannot be visually confirmed on TVUS at β-hCG levels below 2,000 mIU/mL. Several studies have also documented the appearance of viable (IUP) where the gestational sac was not initially seen on TVUS with β-hCG levels above 2,000 mIU/mL. Even higher levels of β-hCG are problematic, as multiple gestations produce higher levels of β-hCG at every stage of early embryological development and therefore do not have the same discriminatory levels of β-hCG as singleton pregnancies. Using the same β-hCG discriminatory level would significantly increase the risk of erroneously diagnosing an ectopic pregnancy in a patient with a viable single IUP. With increasing utilization of assisted reproductive technologies, multiple gestations are more commonly seen in modern-day obstetric practices. Although a β-hCG value of 3,500 mIU/mL and higher should allow visualization of an IUP, a single β-hCG measurement cannot definitively diagnose viability or location of an early pregnancy. Therefore, in an asymptomatic patient with a PUL, serial β-hCG measurements are recommended before diagnosing an ectopic pregnancy and initiating treatment.

3. **E.** Once an ectopic pregnancy has been confirmed by TVUS, four treatment options, two surgical and two nonsurgical, are available. The two nonsurgical options are expectant management and medical

treatment with methotrexate (MTX). The surgical options include salpingostomy and salpingectomy. The treating physician must take multiple factors into consideration when determining the best course of action. Although not a defensible in modern practice (this is unclear) expectant management can be considered in a patient with an ectopic pregnancy that is resolving on its own. MTX is the very commonly utilized for treatment; however, a patient must be able to reliably follow-up with her provider. The success of MTX therapy is determined by the effect on the β-hCG levels. After methotrexate is given, β-hCG levels are trended until their level reaches zero, to ensure medical treatment has been effective. MTX therapy avoids surgery but has risks of failure with potential catastrophic results. A systematic review by Menon et al. depicts failure rate of 14.3% or higher with MTX when pretreatment β-hCG levels are higher than 5,000 mIU/mL compared with failure rate of 3.7% with β-hCG levels <5,000 mIU/mL. High initial β-hCG concentration is therefore a relative contraindication not an absolute contraindication. Patients with elevated initial β-hCG concentrations need to be counseled that failure of MTX therapy is greater and that they may require repeat dosing. Other predictors of MTX treatment failure are the presence of an advanced or rapidly growing gestation. This is evidenced by the presence of fetal cardiac activity and a rapidly increasing β-hCG concentration defined at greater than 50% increase in 48 hours. Failure or delay in treatment can lead to rupture of the ectopic with acute and massive bleeding.

MTX is an antimetabolite that inhibits dihydrofolate reductase, thereby blocking DNA synthesis, repair, and cell replication. Rapidly proliferating tissues, such as trophoblastic cells in ectopic pregnancies, are severely affected, leading to apoptosis. Its use in treating ectopic pregnancies was first reported in 1982 and has become the mainstay of nonsurgical treatment for ectopic pregnancy in the United States over the past 25 years. Success rates with MTX range from 63% to 97%, depending on the size of the ectopic. The most commonly utilized treatment regimen involves a single-dose regimen of 50 mg/m^2, injected intramuscularly on Day 1. Serial β-hCG levels are trended, and a minimum of 15% decrease must be documented between Day 4 and Day 7. A second dose can be administered for rising or plateaued values on Day 7.

Before initiating MTX therapy, the treating physician must assess the health status of the patient and carefully weigh the risks and benefits of treatment. MTX has adverse effects on all tissues with high cell turnover rate, which includes bone marrow, the gastrointestinal tract, and respiratory epithelium. Intestinal mucositis, GI bleeding, and peptic ulcers are known adverse effects of MTX. Although cases of fatal mucosal necrosis in patients undergoing MTX therapy is rare, particularly with single dose regimens, this therapy is contraindicated in patients with active peptic ulcer disease. MTX is also directly toxic to the liver and the kidneys, as it is concentrated in hepatocytes and is cleared from the body by renal excretion. Renal and liver function tests are part of the pretreatment evaluation conducted prior to MTX therapy. A creatinine level of 2.5 mg/dl is consistent with moderate to severe renal disease, and is an absolute contraindication as a single dose of MTX in a patient with renal compromise can lead to death or severe complications. Liver disease can also slow metabolism of MTX and lead to bone marrow suppression and skin or mucosal disorders. The exact amount of MTX excreted into breast milk remains unknown, therefore breastfeeding is contraindicated when receiving MTX therapy. It is suggested that following one dose of MTX, women who are breastfeeding should pump and discard breast milk for at least 24 hours before resuming breastfeeding. MTX use may also lead to worsening anemia, secondary to its effect on bone marrow and it is contraindicated with moderate or severe anemia. In females, moderate anemia is classified as hemoglobin levels of 8–10.9 g/dl and severe anemia as levels less than 8 g/dl. Other contraindications to MTX therapy include embryonic cardiac activity, ectopic pregnancy greater than 4 cm in size as imaged on TVUS, and the refusal of the patient to accept blood transfusions.

4. **D.** Advanced ectopic pregnancies can rupture with life-threatening consequences for the patient. Patients with ruptured or impending ruptured ectopic can present with hemodynamic instability, hemoperitoneum, and severe lower or generalized abdominal pain. Surgical management is required when a patient is exhibiting any of these signs or symptoms. Surgical management may also be necessary if medical management fails or if a patient has a contraindication to MTX usage. β-hCG levels are not generally helpful in these cases, as management is dictated by the patient's hemodynamic status.

The fallopian tube is the most common location of ectopic implantation accounting for more than 90% of cases. Implantation can also be seen in the abdomen (1%), cervix (1%), ovary (1% to 3%) and cesarean scar (1% to 3%). Ectopic implantation in locations other than the fallopian tube often leads to delayed diagnosis, which result in greater morbidity. Ninety-seven percent of ectopic pregnancies in the fallopian tube are located in the distal portion. Heterotopic pregnancies, defined as synchronous ectopic and intrauterine pregnancies, are increasing in incidence secondary to assisted reproductive technologies. The incidence of heterotopic pregnancies has been estimated to be 1 in 30,000 pregnancies. More recent data indicates a much higher rate at 1 in 7,000 due to assisted reproductive technologies.

Surgical options for managing an ectopic in the distal fallopian tube include conservative salpingostomy (removal of the ectopic pregnancy while leaving the affected fallopian tube in situ) versus salpingectomy (removal of part or all of the affected fallopian tube). Both procedures are commonly performed via a laparoscopic approach. Laparotomy is reserved for severely unstable patients in which a 5 to 10 minutes' delay is contraindicated. During a salpingostomy, a linear incision is made over the anti-mesenteric portion of the tube, which contains the ectopic pregnancy. The ectopic is removed from the tube with gentle traction. Hydrodissection can be used to assist in separating the ectopic tissue from the walls of the fallopian tube. Small bleeding sites are generally controlled with monopolar energy. The tubal incision site is not sutured and is left to heal by secondary intention, as suturing of the wound is not found to improve tubal function.

The decision to pursue a salpingostomy versus salpingectomy is made clinically and often intraoperatively with consideration given to the amount of bleeding and extent of fallopian tube damage. This decision is also guided by the patient's desire for future fertility. In patients demonstrating hemodynamic instability and evidence of severe fallopian tube damage as in the above scenario, salpingectomy is preferred. Salpingectomy also has nearly 100% efficacy rate in treating an ectopic pregnancy and controlling bleeding. Salpingectomy is performed when the patient has a healthy-appearing contralateral fallopian tube. Salpingostomy should be reserved in hemodynamically stable patients who desire future fertility and have evidence of damage to the contralateral fallopian tube. If a salpingostomy has been performed, serial β-hCG levels are obtained to ensure definitive treatment of the ectopic trophoblastic tissue. If β-HCG remains elevated following surgical excision, the patient is diagnosed with a persistent ectopic, which results from trophoblastic tissue that has remained within the fallopian tube or has implanted on outside the fallopian tube on peritoneal surfaces. A persistent ectopic can be effectively treated with MTX.

5. **C.** Prior ectopic pregnancy is a strong risk factor for recurrent ectopic pregnancy, with a recurrence rate of 5% to 25%, or up to 10 times the risk in the general population. Some reports have concluded salpingostomy is an independent risk factor for recurrence, yet the DEMETER randomized trial and a systematic review found no statistically significant difference in the rate of IUP versus repeat ectopic pregnancy in patients that underwent salpingostomy compared to salpingectomy. Other known risk factors for ectopic pregnancy include age greater than 35, smoking, tubal surgery or tubal damage, prior pelvic infection, pregnancy with an IUD, and pregnancy conceived by assisted reproduction.

6. **C.** When the possibility of a normally progressing intrauterine gestation has been reasonably excluded, but the location of pregnancy has not been confirmed, sampling of the endometrial lining can be utilized to distinguish an abnormal early intrauterine pregnancy from an ectopic pregnancy. The identification of intrauterine chorionic villi on histology reliably confirms an intrauterine pregnancy and effectively rules out an ectopic pregnancy. If chorionic villi are not found, the likelihood of an ectopic pregnancy is markedly increased. Today, some sources suggest determining pregnancy location by endometrial sampling prior to MTX therapy in order to avoid unnecessary exposure to MTX. Others argue against this, stating that this could increase the risk of tubal rupture secondary to delay in treatment. Hysteroscopy is an incorrect choice, as this procedure is not used for ectopic pregnancy diagnosis. Increased cul-de-sac fluid identified on TVUS can be a finding associated with ectopic pregnancy; however, this is nonspecific and cannot be used to definitively diagnose ectopic pregnancy. Laparoscopy is a diagnostic option but not utilized commonly due to the high sensitivity and specificity of modern ultrasound.

7. **D.** As pointed out in the answer to question 2, a single β-hCG value cannot reliably define the viability of a gestation. In the presence of nondiagnostic studies on ultrasound, the likelihood of a viable pregnancy decreases as the β-hCG level increases. Guidelines suggest serial measurements of serum β-hCG every 48 hours to determine viability of early intrauterine pregnancies. The minimum expected rate of increase at 48 hours is 49% for an initial β-hCG of less than 1,500, 40% for an initial β-hCG level of 1,500 to 3,000 mIU/mL and 33% for an initial β-hCG level greater than 3,000 mIU/mL. This patient is found to have β-hCG level of 2,200 mIU/mL; therefore, an increase of at least 40% should be expected in 48 hours. Research shows that a slower rate of increase defines either an abnormal intrauterine gestation or an ectopic pregnancy. Serial β-hCG values must be used in combination with clinical judgment to assess pregnancy. Patients who have falling β-hCG levels over serial measurements and do not develop symptoms consistent with an ectopic pregnancy are likely experiencing a miscarriage. To ensure complete resolution of the abnormal pregnancy, the provider should follow weekly β-hCG levels until β-hCG becomes undetectable.

8. **D.** Pelvic inflammatory disease is an infectious disease of the female genital tract, which can lead to significant inflammation and scar formation. PID is most commonly caused by a gonorrheal or chlamydial infection found in sexually active females after the bacteria has ascended from the cervix through the uterus and fallopian tubes and has spread into the pelvic cavity. According to one cohort study, tubal occlusion is found in 12.8% of patients with a history of one PID infection and in 75% of patients after three or more infections. Abdominal surgeries can increase the risk of ectopic pregnancy; however, Cesarean sections have not been shown to increase the risk. Age greater than 35 is also associated with a slightly increased risk of ectopic pregnancy due to compromised age-related ciliary function within the fallopian tube. This leads to delayed transport of the fertilized egg and subsequent implantation onto the fallopian tube mucosa. Overall, women with an IUD have a lower risk of ectopic pregnancy than women not using any form of contraception, as IUDs are very effective in preventing pregnancy. However if a pregnancy is diagnosed in a patient with an IUD, her risk of having an ectopic pregnancy is >50%.

Contraindications for Methotrexate to Treat Ectopic Pregnancy
GI bleeding and peptic ulcer disease
Breastfeeding
Creatinine level > 2.5 mg/dl
Hemoglobin < 8.0 g/dl
Embryonic cardiac activity
Ectopic pregnancy > 4 cm
Patient's refusal to accept blood transfusions
Patient does not have reliable follow up

9. **C.** The vast majority of patients develop symptoms of ectopic pregnancy between 6 and 9 weeks' gestation. These symptoms include unilateral pelvic pain or vaginal bleeding. The challenge is that as up to 1/3 of women with normal pregnancies will experience vaginal bleeding or pain early in their pregnancy. Ectopic pregnancies can mimic a multitude of other gastrointestinal, urinary, and gynecological processes. The most common diagnoses with similar findings include appendicitis, enlarging or ruptured ovarian cysts, ovarian torsion, spontaneous abortions, urolithiasis, or urinary tract infections.

BIBLIOGRAPHY

ACOG Practice Bulletin No. 193. *Tubal ectopic pregnancy, obstetrics & gynecology*. March 2018;131(2): e65–e77.

Backman T, Rauramo I, Huhtala S, Koskenvuo M. Pregnancy during the use of levonorgestrel intrauterine system. *Am J Obstet Gynecol*. 2004;190:50–54.

Barnhart KT, Franasiak JM. ACOG practice bulletin number 183. Tubal ectopic pregnancy. March 2018. https://www.acog.org/clinical/clinical-guidance/practice-bulletin/articles/2018/03/tubal-ectopic-pregnancy

Barnhart KT, Guo W, Cary MS, et al. Differences in serum human chorionic gonadotropin rise in early pregnancy by race and value at presentation. *Obstet Gynecol*. 2016;128(3):504–511.

Barnhart KT, Sammel MD, Gracia CR, Chittams J, Hummel AC, Shaunik A. Risk factors for ectopic pregnancy in women with symptomatic first-trimester pregnancies. *Fertil Steril*. 2006;86:36–43.

Barnhart KT, Sammel MD, Rinaudo PF, et al. Symptomatic patients with an early viable intrauterine pregnancy: hCG curves redefined. *Obstet Gynecol*. 2004;104(1):50–55.

Benson CB, Doubilet PM, Peters HE, Frates MC. Intrauterine fluid with ectopic pregnancy: a reappraisal. *J Ultrasound Med*. 2013;32:389–393.

Bouyer J, Coste J, Fernandez H, Pouly JL, Job-Spira NN. Sites of ectopic pregnancy: a 10 year population based study of 1800 cases. *Hum Reprod*. 2002;17(2):3224–3230.

Capmas P, Bouyer J, Fernandez H. Treatment of ectopic pregnancies in 2014: new answers to some old questions. *Fertil Steril*. 2014;101(3):615–620.

Crochet JR, Bastian LA, Chireau MV. Does this woman have an ectopic pregnancy? The rational clinical examination systematic review. *JAMA*. 2013;309(16):1722–1729.

Curran Mark A. Beta HCG doubling time calculator. Perinatology.com, http://perinatology.com/calculators/beta hCG.htm

Doubilet PM, Benson CB. Further evidence against the reliability of the human chorionic gonadotropin discriminatory level. *J Ultrasound Med*. 2011;30:1637–1642.

Doubilet PM, Benson CB, Bourne T, Blaivas M. Diagnostic criteria for nonviable pregnancy early in the first trimester. *N Engl J Med*. 2013;369:1443–1451.

Fernandez H, Capmas P, Lucot JP, et al. Fertility after ectopic pregnancy: the DEMETER randomized trial. *Hum Reprod*. 2013;28:1247–1253.

Gershenson DM, Lentz GM, Valea FA, Lobo RA. *Comprehensive Gynecology*. Elservier; 2012.

Govindarajan MJ, Rajan R. Heterotopic pregnancy in natural conception. *J Hum Reprod Sci*. 2008;1(1):37–38.

Huang C-C, Huang C-C, Lin S-Y, et al. Association of pelvic inflammatory disease (PID) with ectopic pregnancy and preterm labor in Taiwan: a nationwide population-based retrospective cohort study. *PloS One*. 2019;14:8e0219351.

Kulak D, Weiss G, Morelli SS. Advanced extrauterine pregnancy. *Operative Obstetrics*. 4th ed. CRC Press; 2017:199–209.

Lipscomb GH, Stovall TG, Ling FW. Nonsurgical treatment of ectopic pregnancy. *N Engl J Med*. 2000;343:1325–1329.

Menon S, Colins J, Barhart KT. Establishing a human chorionic gonadotropic cutoff to guide methotrexate treatment of ectopic pregnancy: a systematic review. *Fertil Steril*. 2007;87: 481–484.

Mummert T, Gnugnoli DM. Ectopic pregnancy. [Updated 2019 Oct 11]. In: StatPearls [Internet]. https://www.ncbi.nlm.niih.gov/books/NBK539860/

Panelli DM, Phillips CH, Brady PC. Incidence, diagnosis and management of tubal and nontubal ectopic pregnancies: a review. *Fertil Res Pract*. 2015;1:15.

Pereira N, Bender JL, Hancock K, et al. Routine monitoring of liver function tests after single or double dose methotrexate treatment for ectopic pregnancies. *J Minim Invasive Gynecol*. 2015;104(3):e349–e350.

Pereira PP, Cabar FR, Gomez UT, Francisco RPV. "Pregnancy of unknown location." *Clinics (Sao Paulo, Brazil)*. 2019;74: e1111.

Shaw JL, Oliver E, Lee KF, et al. Cotinine exposure increases Fallopian tube PROKR1 expression via nicotinic AChRalpha-7: a potential mechanism explaining the link between smoking and tubal ectopic pregnancy. *Am J Pathol*. 2010;177:2509–2515.

Sivalingam VN, Duncan WC, Kirk E, Shephard LA, Horne AW. Diagnosis and management of ectopic pregnancy. *J Fam Plann Reprod Health Care*. 2011;37(4):231–240.

Tanaka T, Hayashi H, Kutsuzawa T, et al. Treatment of interstitial ectopic pregnancy with methotrexate: report of a successful case. *Fertil Steril*. 1982;37:851–852.

Taran F, Kagan K, Hübner M, et al. The diagnosis and treatment of ectopic pregnancy. *Dtsch Arztebl Int*. 2015;112(41): 693–703.

Tulandi Togas. Ectopic pregnancy: Clinical manifestations and diagnosis. UpToDate. https://www.uptodate.com/contents/ectopic-pregnancy-clinical-manifestations-and-diagnosis

Stovall TG, Ling FW. Ectopic pregnancy: diagnostic and therapeutic algorithms minimizing surgical intervention. *J Reprod Med*. 1993;38:807–812.

67

Pelvic Inflammatory Disease

Nicholas S. Pyskir, and Alan P. Gehrich

A 24-year-old gravida 0 Caucasian female with no significant medical or surgical history presents to the emergency room with complaints of acute onset right lower quadrant pain increasing over the preceding 24 hours. She also endorses fevers, nausea, and vomiting. Her social history is notable for marijuana use 4 to 5 days per week, but she denies regular alcohol consumption or smoking. She is sexually active in a monogamous relationship with her boyfriend for 2 years, and states that her partner consistently uses condoms during intercourse. She had been using oral contraceptives since 18 years of age, but 16 days ago, while menstruating, she had a levonorgestrel intrauterine device placed by her primary care physician.

Her vital signs show a temperature of 100.8°F, blood pressure 113/67, with respirations 18 and pulse 85. Pertinent positives on physical exam include tenderness in the right lower quadrant with voluntary guarding but no rebound and hypoactive bowel sounds. Pelvic exam reproduces exquisite right pelvic tenderness with a poorly defined pelvic mass. Laboratory evaluation includes a negative pregnancy test, a white blood count (WBC) of 15,000, hemoglobin and hematocrit of 13 and 39, respectively, and a platelet count of 350,000. She has normal renal and liver function tests. A computerized tomography (CT) scan shows an inflammatory mass in the right lower quadrant and pelvis.

1. **Which of the following bacteria is the MOST COMMON inciting organism in the development of acute pelvic inflammatory disease (PID)?**

   A. *Staphylococcus aureus*
   B. *Gonorrhea*
   C. *Escherichia Coli*
   D. *Peptostreptococcus sp.*
   E. *Bacteroides sp.*

2. **Which of the following elements INCREASES a patient's risk for PID?**

   A. Age > 25
   B. History of bacterial vaginosis
   C. Use of intrauterine device for more than 1 year
   D. Prolonged use of oral contraceptives
   E. Recent placement of levonorgestrel intrauterine device

3. **Which diagnostic radiologic study has the HIGHEST sensitivity and specificity in evaluating a pelvic abscess?**

   A. CT of the abdomen and pelvis with contrast
   B. Transabdominal ultrasound (TAUS)
   C. Transvaginal ultrasound (TVUS)
   D. Acute abdominal series
   E. Magnetic resonance imaging (MRI) of the abdomen and pelvis with contrast

4. **Hospitalization for PID is advocated in select groups of patients. Which of the following IS a criteria for inpatient management of PID?**

   A. Purulent cervical discharge
   B. Pelvic pain
   C. Presence of a tubo-ovarian abscess (TOA)
   D. Known allergic reaction to cephalosporins
   E. Cervical motion tenderness on exam

5. **For the aforementioned patient, imaging documents a right adnexal cystic structure 5 cm in greatest diameter consistent with an abscess. She is**

admitted for treatment. Which of the following is the MOST appropriate initial treatment option for this patient?

A. Operative laparoscopy with drainage of the abscess with intravenous cefotetan, and metronidazole

B. Intravenous cefoxitin plus doxycycline and metronidazole

C. Intravenous clindamycin and gentamicin

D. Intravenous ampicillin-sulbactam

E. CT-guided drainage with intravenous cefoxitin and doxycycline

6. **Further treatment is dependent on the patient's response to therapy. Which of the following statements is CORRECT?**

A. Sepsis is not commonly associated with a ruptured TOA and does not require surgical intervention.

B. *Bacteroides* is the most frequent cause of Gram-negative sepsis associated with TOA.

C. Antibiotics should be switched from parenteral to oral route of administration only after 72 hours of clinical improvement.

D. If this patient does not respond to intravenous antibiotics, a hysterectomy with bilateral salpingo-oophorectomy is required for cure of a TOA.

E. The most common sequelae of TOA are infertility, ectopic pregnancy, and chronic pelvic pain.

ANSWERS

1. **B.** Pelvic inflammatory disease (PID) is a polymicrobial infection that causes inflammation of the upper genital tract, including endometritis, salpingitis, pelvic peritonitis, and, in severe cases, formation of a TOA. PID is diagnosed in more than 1 million women annually in the United States. In 2013, the self-reported prevalence rate among women age 15 to 44 years was 4 percent, with most cases occurring in women under 25 years of age. Many women can experience PID without manifesting acute symptoms, making the true incidence difficult to determine.

The primary etiology of PID is an ascending infection via the vagina and cervix, but direct extension from inflammatory gastrointestinal disease (e.g., a ruptured appendiceal or diverticular abscesses) is another, albeit far less common, etiology. The general surgeon can be consulted in cases involving an

infectious process of the bowel such as diverticulitis or appendicitis, or when an extirpative surgery is being considered with severe pelvic adhesive disease involving the bowel. The general surgeon's expertise may also be required in the surgical drainage of a TOA, or to assist in managing a patient suffering from life-threatening sepsis arising from a suspected TOA.

The microbial epidemiology is diverse, but between one third and one half of all cases are associated with an acute *N. gonorrhoea* or *C. trachomatis* infection. The most common single inciting organism leading to acute PID is *N. gonorrhoea*, which causes a direct inflammatory response in the upper genital tract. All patients with a diagnosis of PID should be tested for *N. gonorrhoea* and *C. trachomatis*, as well as HIV. Endocervical testing for these organisms may be negative, even in cases with evidence of upper genital tract infection. Research has also identified *Mycoplasma genitalium* as a possible etiology. More than half of all cases of PID are not directly associated with an acute sexually transmitted infection (STI) and are caused by enteric Gram-negative rods, anaerobes, or other ascending vaginal or perianal flora. Common isolates from a TOA abscess cavity include *E. coli*, *Bacteroides*, *Peptostreptococcus*, and *Streptococcus* species.

2. **E.** Risk factors for the development of PID include a previous history of STI or PID, smoking, vaginal douching, and genital tract instrumentation that violates the cervical barrier. Risk factors for STI include younger age, multiple or non-monogamous sexual partners, and inconsistent use of barrier contraceptives. Barrier methods, which include condoms and diaphragms, and oral contraceptives decrease the risk and severity of PID. In this patient, age and recent sexual activity are unlikely contributors to the development of PID, given her monogamous relationship and consistent use of barrier methods during intercourse. There is no direct association between drug use and PID.

The patient in the aforementioned scenario had a recent placement of an IUD. A small but significant percentage of PID cases are thought to be related to instrumentation that penetrates the cervical mucous barrier. In addition to IUD insertion, procedures placing a patient at risk for PID include dilation and curettage, hysteroscopy, hysterosalpingograms, and chromopertubation. Patients are at increased risk for PID for approximately 3 weeks following the procedure, although the absolute risk remains low. Aseptic technique is critical in the prevention of iatrogenic cases of PID. Prolonged use of intrauterine devices is not associated with increased risk, and the levonogestrel intrauterine device theoretically becomes protective as it increases the viscosity of the cervical mucous. Removal of an intrauterine device as part of the management of PID is controversial and potentially unnecessary. In cases of PID in which a TOA is not present, an IUD can be left in place at the discretion of the provider if the patient does not otherwise want it removed. Removal of the IUD may be considered if there is no response to the initial 48 to 72 hours of antibiotic therapy.

3. **A.** PID is a clinical diagnosis for which radiologic imaging is not required. Clinical criteria required to make the diagnosis include the presence of uterine tenderness, adnexal tenderness, *or* cervical motion tenderness in the absence of other likely etiologies. These criteria emphasize a low threshold for the diagnosis of PID and were established to promote aggressive early treatment of PID. If there is no other source of illness, the patient with pelvic or lower abdominal pain and any one of these findings should be presumptively treated for PID. The CDC offers several other criteria to enhance the specificity of the minimum clinical criteria. These include an oral temperature greater than 101°F (38.3°C), abnormal cervical mucopurulent discharge or cervical friability, abundant WBCs on saline microscopy of vaginal discharge, elevated erythrocyte sedimentation rate, elevated C-reactive protein, and confirmed diagnosis of infection with *N. gonorrhoea* or *C. trachomatis*. Other classic symptoms associated with PID include abdominal pain, abnormal discharge, inter-menstrual or post-coital bleeding, urinary urgency, low back pain, nausea, and vomiting. Interestingly, PID patients more commonly present during menstruation or immediately following. This may be correlated with compromised endocervical barriers associated with the menstrual cycle.

A TOA is an inflammatory pelvic mass documented on exam or imaging such as in the above patient. It can be unilateral or bilateral involving the fallopian tube, which is typically dilated, and ovary with extension of severe inflammatory disease to the nearby bowel and uterus. Symptoms of TOA can be indistinguishable from acute salpingitis and appendicitis. A TOA can often be difficult

to distinguish from a peri-appendiceal abscess on imaging. TOAs generally manifest with symptoms to include abdominal and pelvic pain (>90%), fever (50%), vaginal discharge (28%), nausea (26%), and abnormal vaginal bleeding (21%).

Imaging studies are not required to make the diagnosis of PID but can provide important information to guide management of the patient diagnosed with PID. TVUS is considered the first-line imaging modality for gynecologic pathology because it provides excellent imaging of the cervix, uterus, fallopian tubes, and ovaries; is less expensive than other modalities; and does not expose the patient to radiation. The disadvantage of this form of imaging is reliance on the technical skill of the ultrasonographer. TAUS is inferior to TVUS because the low-frequency ultrasound waves needed for deep penetration result in lower spatial resolution of the image. The close proximity of the transvaginal probe to the tissues being examined allows use of higher frequency ultrasound, improving spatial resolution.

CT scan of the abdomen and pelvis, with contrast, is the second option for imaging in cases of suspected PID and is preferred in cases in which the diagnosis is uncertain or a skilled ultrasound technician is not available. It is also preferred in cases in which there is a known abdominal malignancy or gastrointestinal pathology such as appendicitis or diverticulitis. In the scenario detailed earlier, the patient would have likely undergone an initial TVUS followed by a CT scan particularly if the ultrasound was inconclusive. The CT scan has higher sensitivity to detect a TOA (78% to 100% versus 75% to 82%) and improved specificity (100% versus 91%) as compared to ultrasound. MRI and X-ray have limited utility in the evaluation of acute pelvic pain or suspected infection.

4. **C.** After diagnosis, the initial management decision is whether the patient requires hospitalization with intravenous antibiotics. In conjunction, a decision will be made whether the patient requires surgical intervention. The decision for inpatient management is based on clinical judgment, but certain populations should be considered strong candidates for admission. These include all severely ill patients as well as patients in which a surgical emergency (e.g., appendicitis) cannot be excluded. All pregnant patients, patients who have been unable to tolerate or are otherwise unresponsive to an oral antibiotic

Table 67-1 CANDIDATES FOR INPATIENT MANAGEMENT OF PELVIC INFLAMMATORY DISEASE AND TUBO-OVARIAN ABSCESS

Surgical emergencies (e.g., appendicitis) cannot be excluded;
Tubo-ovarian abscess;
Pregnancy;
Severe illness, nausea and vomiting, or high fever;
Unable to follow or tolerate an outpatient oral regimen; or
Poor clinical response to oral antimicrobial therapy.

Source: Centers for Disease Control and Prevention. Sexually transmitted diseases: treatment guidelines. *MMWR Morb Mortal Wkly Rep* 2015; 64:3.

regimen, and patients who are identified with TOA or suspected should also be admitted for inpatient management (Table 67-1).

Early broad-spectrum antibiotic therapy is the cornerstone of PID management and is essential to limit scarring of reproductive organs and other long-term sequelae of the disease. CDC guidelines emphasize prompt initiation of empiric antibiotic protocols that cover Gram-positive, Gram-negative, and anaerobic bacteria. Cephalosporins and doxycycline are used in parenteral therapy, with the addition of clindamycin or metronidazole for additional anaerobic coverage in the patient in whom a TOA is identified or suspected. An alternative regimen of clindamycin and gentamicin can be used for patients with severe penicillin allergies (Table 67-2). A 2017 Cochrane Review that considered the antibiotic regimens contained in the CDC guidelines found "no conclusive evidence that one treatment was safer or more effective than any other for the cure of PID."

All patients should complete a full 14-day course of antibiotics following a diagnosis with PID. Discharge on oral antibiotics can be considered after 24 to 48 hours of clinical improvement, including resolution of nausea and vomiting, fevers, and severe pain. These patients should be discharged with a doxycycline to complete the full 14-day course, with clindamycin or metronidazole added for anaerobic coverage in patients with concern for TOA. TOA is not in itself an indication for continued hospitalization, and a stable patient who has otherwise responded to therapy can be discharged on an oral regimen with precautions. Many of these patients

Table 67-2 INPATIENT PARENTERAL ANTIBIOTIC REGIMENS FOR TREATMENT OF PELVIC INFLAMMATORY DISEASE AND TUBO-OVARIAN ABSCESS

Recommended Regimen:
Cefotetan 2 g IV every 12 hours PLUS Doxycycline[a] 100 mg orally or IV every 12 hours (add Metronidazole 500 mg orally twice a day or clindamycin 450 mg four times a day for TOA)
OR
Cefoxitin 2 g IV every 6 hours PLUS Doxycycline[a] 100 mg orally or IV every 12 hours (add Metronidazole 500 mg orally twice a day or clindamycin 450 mg four times a day for TOA)
OR
Clindamycin 900 mg IV every 9 hours PLUS Gentamicin loading dose IV or IM (2mg/kg), followed by a maintenance dose (1.5 mg/kg) every 8 hours. Single daily dosing (3-5 mg/kg) can be substituted. Add Metronidazole 500 mg orally twice a day or clindamycin 450 mg four times a day for TOA
Alternate Regimen:
Ampicillin/Sulbactam 3 g IV every 6 hours PLUS Doxycycline[a] 100 mg orally or IV every 12 hours (add Metronidazole 500 mg orally twice a day or clindamycin 450 mg four times a day for TOA)

[a]Oral therapy is preferred where possible to avoid phlebitis associated with parenteral doxycycline.

Source: Centers for Disease Control and Prevention. Sexually transmitted diseases: treatment guidelines. *MMWR Morb Mortal Wkly Rep* 2015; 64:3.

will still require surgery, but a 2- to 3-month delay after treatment can reduce the challenges of surgical management.

In appropriately selected patients, PID can be managed on an outpatient basis without admission. Data suggests that oral and parental antibiotic regimens have similar efficacy in mild and even moderate disease. Sexual partners in the 60 days prior to presentation should be treated even if asymptomatic. Where local laws and healthcare regulations allow, it is appropriate to provide expedited partner therapy or referral for these individuals. Patients who are treated on an outpatient basis should be advised to abstain from intercourse until both the patient and their partners are asymptomatic and have completed the appropriate antibiotic regimens.

The CDC guidelines for outpatient therapy are outlined in Table 67-3. Oral cephalosporins have not been studied in the setting of PID. Though cephalosporins are the preferred antibiotic regimen due to emerging strains of fluoroquinolone-resistant *N. gonorrhoea*, an allergic reaction to these medications is not in itself a reason for admission. In select patients, outpatient fluroquinolone regimens are appropriate. Metronidazole is added for additional coverage of BV and anaerobes.

Table 67-3 OUTPATIENT INTRAMUSCULAR/ ORAL ANTIBIOTIC REGIMENS FOR TREATMENT OF PELVIC INFLAMMATORY DISEASE AND TUBO-OVARIAN ABSCESS

Recommended Regimen:
Ceftriaxone 250 mg IM in a single dose PLUS Doxycycline 100 mg orally or IV every 12 hours (add Metronidazole 500 mg orally twice a day for TOA)
OR
Cefoxitin 2 g 2 g IM in a single dose and Probenecid, 1 g orally, administered concurrently in a single dose PLUS Doxycycline 100 mg orally or IV every 12 hours (add Metronidazole 500 mg orally twice a day for TOA)
OR
Other parenteral third-generation cephalosporin (e.g., ceftizoxime or cefotaxime) PLUS Doxycycline 100 mg orally or IV every 12 hours (add Metronidazole 500 mg orally twice a day for TOA)
Alternate Regimen[a]:
Levofloxacin 500 mg orally once daily for 14 days OR
Ofloxacin 400 mg twice daily for 14 days OR
Moxifloxacin 400 mg orally once daily for 14 days AND
Metronidazole 500 mg orally twice a day for 14 days

[a]When using a fluoroquinolone based regimen, the CDC recommends that the patient be tested for gonorrhea. In positive patients, susceptibility testing should guide antibiotic therapy. For quinolone-resistant *N. gonorrhoeae* (QRNG), or if antimicrobial susceptibility cannot be assessed (e.g., if only NAAT testing is available), consultation with an infectious-disease specialist is recommended.

Source: Centers for Disease Control and Prevention. Sexually transmitted diseases: treatment guidelines. *MMWR Morb Mortal Wkly Rep* 2015; 64:3.

5. **B.** Appropriate treatment for TOA is dependent on many factors. At a minimum, all patients with TOA require admission and treatment with appropriately selected intravenous antibiotics. Recommended regimens are earlier discussed in detail (see Table 67-3). A cephalosporin with doxycycline is the recommended antibiotic therapy for PID, with clindamycin or metronidazole added in cases of known or suspected TOA. Clindamycin and metronidazole maximize anaerobic coverage and exhibit superior penetration of and activity within abscess cavities in animal models.

The least correct option listed involves the use of ampicillin-sulbactam. Due to the high rates of resistance of *E. coli*, ampicillin-sulbactam is no longer recommended as a single agent for the treatment of community acquired intra-abdominal infections. In addition, ampicillin-sulbactam provides minimal coverage for chlamydial infections. It remains available as one component of an alternative parenteral regimen, but at a minimum should be combined with doxycycline to cover for chlamydia. Drainage of the abscess via laparoscopy or interventional radiology would be considered if the TOA at admission is >8 cm, if patient is severely septic or not responding appropriately to intravenous antibiotics.

6. **E.** All patients with PID, with or without TOA, should receive antibiotics, but the timing and selection of other interventions in the setting of a TOA is highly dependent on the patient's clinical status. When a ruptured TOA is suspected based on findings of an acute abdomen or septic shock, prompt surgical intervention is required as antibiotics alone are ineffective in preventing severe morbidity and mortality in this clinical scenario. *E. coli* is the most common isolate in women with ruptured TOAs and a frequent cause of Gram-negative sepsis. In cases where fertility is desired, the surgeon must tread a careful line between sparing the uterus and ovaries and resecting infected tissue (to include the ovaries and fallopian tubes). Severe cases will necessitate complete extirpation with hysterectomy and bilateral salpingo-oophorectomy. The post-menopausal patient with a TOA should be consented for total abdominal hysterectomy with bilateral salpingo-oophorectomy due to the strong association with either gynecologic or intestinal malignancy. Hysterectomy with bilateral salpingo-oophorectomy has the least risk of recurrence of TOA but also the highest surgical morbidity.

If the patient does not require urgent surgery in the presence of a TOA, the team can proceed with 48 to 72 hours of antibiotics with or without drainage. Larger case series have shown that antimicrobial therapy alone is effective in up to 70% of all TOAs. In several of these studies, abscess size was predictive of treatment success with antibiotics alone. Reed et al. showed that 35% of abscesses 7 to 9 cm in size required surgery as compared to almost 60% of abscess >9 cm. DeWitt et al. showed that abscesses >8 cm more often required drainage or surgery. It is reasonable to observe the effect of IV antibiotic therapy without immediate surgery in women who are not developing signs of sepsis and whose abscess is 8 cm or less in diameter.

Retrospective studies suggest that drainage followed by antibiotics may improve outcomes compared to antibiotics alone. Data comparing drainage with surgical management is limited. Drainage may allow the provider to further tailor antibiotic therapy by isolating the bacteria from the abscess and avoid the risks of general anesthesia and surgery but may be less effective for complex abscesses and require additional time for complete resolution of the infection. When drainage is indicated, options include a percutaneous approach by interventional radiology or a surgical approach via either a laparoscopic or open procedure. Pelvic abscesses have been drained using ultrasound or CT guidance with a transabdominal, transgluteal, transrectal, or transvaginal approaches depending on the location of the abscess with success rates of 77.8% to 100%.

Many patients will demonstrate an excellent response to antibiotics, drainage, or both. Surgical management may be necessary in the future for ongoing pelvic pain or infertility, but in the otherwise improving patient, a 2- to 3-month delay between antibiotic treatment and surgery offers several advantages. Firstly, surgery may not become necessary for the asymptomatic patient without fertility concerns. Secondly, this delay will reduce tissue edema and friability and significantly increase the surgeons' ability to preserve the ovaries in cases where surgery is eventually performed. Thirdly, the long-term sequelae of PID, including infertility and chronic pelvic pain attributed to pelvic adhesive disease, do not appear to be made worse by this conservative approach.

BIBLIOGRAPHY

American College of Obstetricians and Gynecologists. Long-acting reversible contraception: implants and intrauterine devices. Practice Bulletin No. 121. *Obstet Gynecol.* 2011;118:184–196.

Birgisson NE, Zhao Q, Secura GM, Madden T, Peipert JF. Positive testing for *Neisseria gonorrhoeae* and *Chlamydia trachomatis* and the risk of pelvic inflammatory disease in IUD users. *J Womens Health (Larchmt).* 2015;24:354–359.

Boardman LA, Peipert JF, Brody JM, Cooper AS, Sung J. Endovaginal sonography for the diagnosis of upper genital tract infection. *Obstet Gynecol.* 1997;90(1):54–57.

Chappell CA, Wiesenfeld HC. Pathogenesis, diagnosis, and management of severe pelvic inflammatory disease and tuboovarian abscess. *Clin Obstet Gynecol.* 2012;55(4):893–903.

CDC. U.S. selected practice recommendations for contraceptive use, 2013: Adapted from the World Health Organization selected practice recommendations for contraceptive use, 2nd edition. *MMWR Recomm Rep.* 2013;62(No. RR-05):1–46.

Centers for Disease Control and Prevention. Sexually transmitted diseases: treatment guidelines. *Morb Mortal Wkly Rep.* 2015;64:3.

Dewitt J, Reining A, Allsworth JE, Peipert JF. Tuboovarian abscesses: s size associated with duration of hospitalization and complications? *Obstet Gynecol Int.* 2010;2010: 847041.

Gaitan H, Angel E, Diaz R, Parada A, Sanchez L, Vargas C. Accuracy of five different diagnostic techniques in mild-to-moderate pelvic inflammatory disease. *Infect Dis Obstet Gynecol.* 2002;10(4):171–180.

Granberg S, Gjelland K, Ekerhovd E. The management of pelvic abscess. *Best Pract Res Clin Obstet Gynaecol.* 2009;23(5):667–678.

Grimes DA. Intrauterine device and upper-genital-tract infection. *The Lancet.* 2000;356(9234):1013–1019.

Horrow MM. Ultrasound of pelvic inflammatory disease. *Ultrasound Q.* 2004;20(4):171–179.

Hiller N, Sella T, Lev-Sagi A, Fields S, Lieberman S. Computed tomographic features of tuboovarian abscess. *J Reprod Med.* 2005;50(3):203–208.

Jaiyeoba O, Soper DE. A practical approach to the diagnosis of pelvic inflammatory disease. *Infect Dis Obstet Gynecol.* 2011;2011: 753037.

Joiner KA, Lowe BR, Dzink JL, Bartlett JG. Antibiotic levels in infected and sterile subcutaneous abscesses in mice. *J Infect Dis.* 1981;143(3):487–494.

Kreisel K, Torrone E, Bernstein K, et al. Prevalence of pelvic inflammatory disease in sexually experienced women of reproductive age—United States, 2013–2014. *Morb Mortal Wkly Rep.* 2017;66(3):80.

Landers DV, Sweet RL. Tubo-ovarian abscess: contemporary approach to management. *Rev Infect Dis.* 1983;5(5):876–884.

Latimer RL, et al. Clinical features and therapeutic response in women meeting criteria for presumptive treatment for pelvic inflammatory disease associated with mycoplasma genitalium. *Sex Transm Dis.* 2019;46(2):73–79.

Leichliter JS, Chandra A., Aral SO. Correlates of self-reported pelvic inflammatory disease treatment in sexually experienced reproductive aged women in the United States, 1995 and 2006–2010. *Sex Transm Dis.* 2013;40(5):413.

Llata E, Braxton J, Trivedi S, Pathela P, Torrone L. Treatment practices of pelvic inflammatory disease at selected STD clinics: STD surveillance network, 2015–2017 [16R]. *Obstetrics & Gynecology.* May 2019; 33:195S.

McNeeley SG, Hendrix SL, Mazzoni MM, Kmak DC, Ransom SB. Medically sound, cost-effective treatment for pelvic inflammatory disease and tuboovarian abscess. *Am J Obstet Gynecol.* 1998;178(6):1272–1278.

Mingeot-Leclercq MP, Glupczynski Y, Tulkens PM. Aminoglycosides: activity and resistance. *Antimicrob Agents Chemother.* 1999;43(4):727–737.

Patton DL, Moore DE, Spadoni LR, Soules MR, Halbert SA, Wang SP. A comparison of the fallopian tube's response to overt and silent salpingitis. *Obstet Gynecol.* 1989;73(4):622–630.

Reed SD, Landers DV, Sweet RL. Antibiotic treatment of tuboovarian abscess: comparison of broad-spectrum beta-lactam agents versus clindamycin-containing regimens. *Am J Obstet Gynecol.* 1991;164(6 Pt 1):1556–1561; discussion 1561–1562.

Savaris RF, Fuhrich DG, Duarte RV, Franik S, Ross J. Antibiotic therapy for pelvic inflammatory disease. *Cochrane Database Syst Rev.* 2017;4:CD010285.

Solomkin JS, Mazuski JE, Bradley JS, et al. Diagnosis and management of complicated intra-abdominal infection in adults and children: guidelines by the surgical infection society and the infectious diseases society of America. *Surg Infect (Larchmt).* 2010;11(1):79–109.

Soper DE. Early recognition of serious infections in obstetrics and gynecology. *Clin Obstet Gynecol.* 2012;55(4):858–863.

Soper DE. Pelvic inflammatory disease. *Obstet Gynecol.* 2010;116(2 Pt 1):419–428.

Sutton MY, Sternberg M, Zaidi A, St Louis ME, Markowitz LE. Trends in pelvic inflammatory disease hospital discharges and ambulatory visits, united states, 1985–2001. *Sex Transm Dis.* 2005;32(12):778–784.

Tepper NK, Steenland MW, Gaffield ME, Marchbanks PA, Curtis KM. Retention of intrauterine devices in women who acquire pelvic inflammatory disease: a systematic review. *Contraception.* 2013;87(5):655–660.

Walker CK, Wiesenfeld HC. Antibiotic therapy for acute pelvic inflammatory disease: the 2006 CDC Sexually Transmitted Diseases Treatment Guidelines. *Clin Infect Dis.* 2007;28(Supp 1):S29–S36.

68

Endometriosis

Lindsey A. Choi and Alan P. Gehrich

A 26-year-old gravida 0 with a history of chronic pelvic pain presents to the emergency room with acute onset right lower quadrant pain over the course of the preceding 12 hours. The gynecology team has taken the patient to the operating room for a diagnostic laparoscopy with the pre-operative diagnosis of a ruptured ovarian cyst. They find evidence of severe endometriosis with a large right-sided endometrioma involving the appendix. The endometrioma and ovary are fixed to the right pelvic side wall and posterior uterus. Endometriosis has completely obliterated the posterior cul-de-sac with thick adhesions between the recto-sigmoid colon and the uterus. The gynecology service has requested assistance from general surgery to extricate the ovary and perform an appendectomy.

1. **Which of the following is the MOST common symptom for endometriosis?**

    A. Dyschezia
    B. Dyspareunia
    C. Infertility
    D. Dysmenorrhea
    E. Hematochezia

2. **The MOST common site of intestinal endometriosis is:**

    A. Rectum and sigmoid
    B. Appendix
    C. Cecum
    D. Small bowel

3. **Which of the following DECREASES the risk for endometriosis?**

    A. Early menarche
    B. Short menstrual cycles
    C. Nulliparity
    D. Formula feeding
    E. Regular exercise

4. **Which of the following statements is TRUE concerning the laparoscopic evaluation of endometriosis?**

    A. Endometriosis presents with a uniform type of lesion.
    B. The number and size of the lesions directly correlate with patient symptoms.
    C. Endometriosis is commonly found outside of the pelvis.
    D. Deep endometriotic lesions can become retroperitonealized and be difficult to appreciate laparoscopically.
    E. Endometriosis is not associated with infertility.

5. **A right oophorectomy and an appendectomy are performed in the aforementioned patient. If this patient has persistent pain postoperatively consistent with endometriosis, which of the following therapies would be MOST appropriate?**

    A. GnRH (gonadotropin releasing hormone) agonist therapy
    B. Oral combined contraceptive therapy
    C. Depo medroxy-progesterone acetate (DMPA) intramuscular injection therapy
    D. Left oophorectomy
    E. Non-steroidal anti-inflammatory therapy

6. **With endometriosis involving the recto-vaginal septum or bowel, which of the following statements is CORRECT?**

   A. Colonoscopy or rigid proctoscopy is of high yield in diagnosing bowel endometriosis.

   B. Transvaginal ultrasound has <50% sensitivity and specificity in diagnosing recto-vaginal endometriosis.

   C. Gross endometriotic lesions along the appendix and small bowel are common.

   D. Rectal endoscopic ultrasonography is used first-line for diagnosis of rectovaginal endometriosis.

   E. Pain outcomes with bowel resection of endometriosis are similar to those with rectal nodule excision without bowel resection.

7. **Which of the following is the BEST treatment option with an incidentally discovered 6-cm endometrioma involving the right ovary during a laparoscopic appendectomy in a nulliparous 35-year-old female desiring fertility?**

   A. Simple drainage and coagulation of the cyst wall
   B. Cyst wall excision
   C. Unilateral oophorectomy
   D. Bilateral oophorectomy with hysterectomy
   E. Complete appendectomy, and defer for outpatient management.

ANSWERS

1. **D.** The differential diagnosis for acute as well as chronic pelvic pain is broad involving the gynecological, urological, gastrointestinal, musculoskeletal, psychological, and neurological systems. Most commonly the general surgeon is consulted in cases of acute pelvic pain in which a gastrointestinal diagnosis such as appendicitis, diverticulitis, or hernia is entertained. However, as in the aforementioned scenario, the general surgeon may also be consulted to assist in the surgical treatment of advanced endometriosis in which bowel adhesiolysis is required.

   Endometriosis affects 6% to 10% of reproductive-aged women. The most common presentations include dysmenorrhea (79%), generalized pelvic pain (69%), and dyspareunia (45%). Bowel symptoms such as constipation, diarrhea, dyschezia, and tenesmus are present in up to 36% of patients with severe endometriosis. Hematochezia originating from endometriosis is rare.

2. **A.** Endometriosis is defined as hormonally responsive endometrial tissue found outside of the uterus. It is found most commonly on the ovary, uterine serosa, in the posterior cul-de-sac along the uterosacral ligaments, and in the ovarian fossae, but can be found throughout the peritoneal cavity. The leading theory on the pathophysiologic mechanism of endometriosis is retrograde menstruation. During menses, the endometrial lining is shed and expelled into the peritoneal cavity through the fallopian tubes. The endometrial tissues implant on the peritoneal surfaces. Other theories include hematogenous or lymphatic spread, is are supported by cases of lesions documented in the thorax presenting as catamenial pneumothorax and those found in central nervous system. These viable ectopic endometrial glands have hormonally sensitive stroma that continue to grow, shed, and bleed under the influence of the ovarian hormones. Rectovaginal or intestinal involvement is an estimated to be present in 5% to 12% of women with endometriosis. Intestinal endometriosis involves the rectum and sigmoid colon in 76% of cases, the appendix in 18%, and the cecum in 5%. Small bowel is rarely involved.

3. **E.** Risk factors for developing endometriosis include any characteristics that contribute to the increased frequency or duration of menstrual cycles. Based on the theory of retrograde, the greater the volume and duration of menstrual flow, the greater the risk of implantation of endometrial glands on peritoneal surfaces in the abdomen. Women with early age of menarche (occurring before 11 years of age), late onset menopause (>51 years of age), and shorter menstrual cycles (less 21 days between cycles) have an increased absolute number of menstrual cycles during their reproductive years. This is associated with increased frequency of endometrial shedding and, in turn, elevates a woman's lifetime risk for developing endometriosis. Hormonal contraception and pregnancy suppress the development of endometriosis. Nulliparous women not using hormonal contraception are therefore at increased risk compared to their multiparous cohorts or those using hormonal contraception. Similarly, breastfeeding suppresses cyclic hormone production by the ovary often leading to amenorrhea and thereby supressing the cycling of endometriosis lesions. Lastly, regular exercise of more than 4 hours per week has been associated with a reduced risk of developing endometriosis.

4. D. Laparoscopy with biopsy of visually identified endometriotic lesions is considered the "gold standard" for the diagnosis of endometriosis. The definitive diagnosis of endometriosis can only be made by histological evaluation. Three histologic subtypes of endometriotic lesions are found in the peritoneal cavity: superficial lesions, deep infiltrative lesions (DIE), and endometriomas. Endometriotic lesions are highly variable in size, texture, and color. Endometriosis can present as fibrotic scar tissue, hemorrhagic or clear vesicles, flat yellow-brown lesions, or the classic raised reddish-blue islands, which are typically found on the peritoneal lining of the pelvis. Although visual inspection by an experienced surgeon can have sensitivity of 94% to 97% and specificity of 77% to 85%, histopathologic confirmation remains the standard for diagnosis. Interestingly, neither the severity nor location of disease correlates directly with the severity of symptoms.

Superficial lesions can cause pain symptoms, however are rarely associated with adhesions. In contrast, deep infiltrative endometriosis lesions invade into neighboring tissue leading to significant pelvic adhesive disease, which can involve bladder and bowel such as depicted in the above scenario. Painful defecation and severe dyspareunia are the most predictable symptoms of deeply infiltrating endometriosis. In rare cases, this invasion is transmural leading to endometriosis in the lumen of the bladder or bowel with associated cyclic hematuria, dysuria, hematochezia, or dyschezia. Endometriotic lesions, particularly DIE, can also become reperitonealized making it difficult to appreciate the extent of the lesions when observing them laparoscopically. An endometrioma is a cystic mass arising from ectopic endometrial tissue implanted on the ovary. This can be superficial or deeply invasive into the ovarian stroma. It contains thick brown or tan fluid often referred to as a "chocolate cyst."

Endometriosis is a significant contributor to female infertility. Thirty-eight percent of infertile women have endometriosis. Endometriosis causes chronic inflammation in the female pelvis, and this inflammation in theory can disrupt many of the normal processes of reproduction. The chronic inflammation is thought to directly damage spermatic DNA reducing sperm function. The same inflammatory cytokines induce oxidative stress and DNA damage in the oocyte. In advanced disease, endometrioma formation can replace normal ovarian stroma and epithelium compromising normal ovulation. Pelvic adhesive disease resulting from chronic inflammation can result in anatomic abnormalities including tubal dysfunction.

5. C. Endometriosis can be treated both medically and surgically. A patient's desire for future fertility and the magnitude of her symptoms will help determine the primary mode of therapy. Medical therapy is either analgesic or hormonal. While there is no clear evidence that nonsteroidal anti-inflammatory medications improve pain associated with endometriosis, their use is considered a reasonable first-line therapy in appropriately selected patients. Given the extent of disease in this patient, NSAIDs would not be the most appropriate option. High-quality research has clearly documented that hormonal treatment options are effective in suppressing endometriosis-associated pain, including progestins, androgens, and GnRH agonists. Progestins can be seen in all forms of hormonal contraceptives such as birth control pills, patches, rings, injectable or implantable progestins, or the levonorgestrel intrauterine device. Although combined oral contraceptives are a reasonable choice in this patient, oral norethindrone acetate and subcutaneous DMPA are the only progestins approved by the FDA for endometriosis associated pain. These modalities prevent the cyclic stimulation of endometriosis tissue by inhibiting ovulation and supressing the paracrine effect of estrogen.

Second-line therapy for this patient involves gonadotropin releasing hormone (GnRH) agonist (Leuprolide) or antagonist (Elagolix), which eliminate the effects of the pulsatile GnRH signals from the hypothalamus on the pituitary. This process suppresses gonadotropin secretion from the pituitary, which, in turn, markedly decreases production of gonadal steroids by the ovary. A randomized, controlled double-blind clinical trial has shown that an empiric 3-month course of GnRH agonist significantly reduces dysmenorrhea, pelvic pain and pelvic tenderness for women that fail initial treatment with NSAIDS and hormonal contraception. Significant side effects include climacteric symptoms of hot flushes, night sweats, and vaginal dryness. Bone mineral density is adversely affected and osteopenia can result in long-term therapy if the patient does not receive concomitant add-back hormonal (either estrogen or progesterone) supplementation. GnRH agonists are approved for 6 months of continuous use for the indication of pelvic pain, and this therapy can be extended for an additional 6 months with add-back. Add-back therapy with oral norethindrone or combined oral contraceptives is used to minimize the hypoestrogenic side effects of the GnRH agonists to include bone loss.

If symptoms persist despite medical therapy in patients with suspected endometriosis, a diagnostic laparoscopy can be offered to confirm the diagnosis. The goal of surgery is to extirpate as much of the endometriosis as possible while re-establishing normal pelvic anatomy. The risks and benefits of aggressive surgical treatment for endometriosis need to be carefully weighed. Most patients with chronic pelvic pain secondary to endometriosis who wish to maintain their ovarian function benefit from postoperative hormonal suppression. For patients who have completed child-bearing and desire definitive management of endometriosis, the complete removal of all endometriosis lesions, uterus, and ovaries can be considered. A left oophorectomy would not be a recommended option in this patient desiring future fertility.

6. **E.** The general surgeon will most likely be involved in endometriosis surgery with bowel involvement as depicted in the aforementioned scenario. Gross endometriotic lesions along the appendix are rare but if found should prompt appendectomy. Preoperative radiographic evaluation for rectovaginal endometriosis is not routinely performed in clinical practice, however is sensitive in detecting these lesions. Based on a meta-analysis of 19 studies involving 2639 patients, transvaginal ultrasound (TVUS) has a sensitivity of 91% and specificity of 97% for rectovaginal endometriosis. It is typically used first-line for imaging purposes. Magnetic resonance imaging (MRI) is typically reserved for women who are suspected to have disease in the rectovaginal septum that is not detected on physical examination or TVUS. The sensitivity and specificity for MRI is similar to that for TVUS. Sigmoidoscopy and colonoscopy are of low value in diagnosing rectovaginal endometriosis as endometriotic lesions may invade through the serosa into the muscularis, but rarely into the bowel lumen. If bowel lumen invasion is suspected, a rectal endoscopic ultrasonography (REU) can be used to determine the lesion's depth of infiltration or distance from anal junction. While an REU has similar sensitivity (91% to 96%) and specificity (97% to 100%) to

TVUS, it is typically not used first-line for diagnosis as it is more uncomfortable and can require sedation.

Decision on the type of surgery for deeply invasive recto-vaginal endometriosis should be decided on a case-by-case basis. With superficial lesions (no bowel wall involvement), surgical treatment is limited to bowel shaving. With deeper lesions involving the bowel wall, discoid resection or segmental bowel resection with anastomosis is necessary. Discoid and segmental resection have been shown to completely relieve pain and decrease the rate of repeat surgery for endometriosis compared to shaving in retrospective studies. Postoperative complications are more likely with bowel resection, but the literature is sparse in this arena.

7. **B.** Endometriomas are accumulations of ectopic endometrial tissue on the ovary and have characteristic ultrasound findings. If a large endometrioma (>4 centimeters) is incidentally discovered in a patient without a surgically confirmed diagnosis of endometriosis, surgical removal is recommended. Endometriomas have similar characteristics to malignant ovarian masses including a complex appearance on transvaginal ultrasound and an elevated CA-125. Histological diagnosis via a surgical specimen is essential to rule out malignancy.

The management of an incidentally found endometrioma otherwise depends on the patient's fertility desires. Simple drainage and fulguration of endometriomas are associated with high recurrence rates. In patients desiring fertility, complete excision of the cyst wall is the best management option. This procedure is associated with lower recurrence rates, lower symptoms of endometriosis, and higher pregnancy rates when compared to simple drainage. For patients undergoing in-vitro fertilization, cystectomy can also improve access to follicles during oocyte retrieval and improve ovarian response to ovulation induction. However, the patient should be counseled that extensive ovarian surgery can comprise ovarian function and significantly diminish ovarian reserve. If a cyst wall excision is not possible or if the ovary has been consumed by endometriosis on gross examination, proceeding with a unilateral oophorectomy is a reasonable option. The treatment of patients has to be individualized based on the amount of disease and the patient's fertility desires. Bilateral oophorectomy with or without hysterectomy is reserved for women who no longer desire child bearing.

BIBLIOGRAPHY

Afors K, Centini G, Fernandes R, et al. Segmental and discoid resection are preferential to bowel shaving for medium-term symptomatic relief in patients with bowel endometriosis. *J Minim Invasive Gynecol.* 2016;23(7):1123–1129.

Bazot M, Bornier C, Dubernard G, et al. Accuracy of magnetic resonance imaging and rectal endoscopic sonography for the prediction of location of deep pelvic endometriosis. *Hum Reprod.* 2007;22(5):1457.

Bazot M, Lafont C, Rouzier R, et al. Diagnostic accuracy of physical examination, transvaginal sonography, rectal endoscopic sonography, and magnetic resonance imaging to diagnose deep infiltrating endometriosis. *Fertil Steril.* 2009;92(6):1825.

Benschop L, Farquhar C, van der Poel N, Heineman MJ. Interventions for women with endometrioma prior to assisted reproductive technology. *Cochrane Database Syst Rev.* 2010;(11):CD008571.

Berker B, Hsu THS, Lee KL, Nezhat C, Nezhat F, Nezhat C. Section 10.3 laparoscopic treatment of endometriosis. In: Nezhat C, Nezhat F, Nezhat C, eds. *Nezhat's Operative Gynecologic Laparoscopy and Hysteroscopy.* 3rd ed. Cambridge University Press; 2008:263–303.

Bourdel N, Comptour A, Bouchet P, et al. Long-term evaluation of painful symptoms and fertility after surgery for large rectovaginal endometriosis nodule: a retrospective study. *Acta Obstet Gynecol Scand.* 2018;97(2):158.

Chapron C, Vercellini P, Barakat H, Vieira M, Dubuisson JB. Management of ovarian endometriomas. *Hum Reprod Update.* 2002;8:591–597.

Cramer DW, Missmer SA. The epidemiology of endometriosis. *Ann N Y Acad Sci.* 2002;955:11–22;34–36, 396–406.

Duepree HJ, Senagore AJ, Delaney CP, Marcello PW, Brady KM, Falcone T. Laparoscopic resection of deep pelvic endometriosis with rectosigmoid involvement. *J Am Coll Surg.* 2002;195(6):754–758.

Falcone T, Lebovic DI. Clinical management of endometriosis. *Obstet Gynecol.* 2011;118(3):691–705.

Garcia-Velasco JA, Somigliana E. Management of endometriomas in women requiring IVF: to touch or not to touch. *Hum Reprod.* 2009;24:496–501.

Giudice LC, Kao LC. Endometriosis. *Lancet.* 2004;364(9447):1789–1799.

Guerriero S, Ajossa S, Orozco R, et al. Accuracy of transvaginal ultrasound for diagnosis of deep endometriosis in the rectosigmoid: systematic review and meta-analysis. *Ultrasound Obstet Gynecol.* 2016 Mar;47(3):281–289.

Leone Roberti Maggiore U, Scala C, Venturini PL, Remorgida V, Ferrero S. Endometriotic ovarian cysts do not negatively affect the rate of spontaneous ovulation. *Hum Reprod.* 2015;30(2):299–307.

Ling FW. Randomized controlled trial of depot leuprolide in patients with chronic pelvic pain and clinically suspected endometriosis. *Obstet Gynecol.* 1999;93:51–58.

Missmer SA, Hankinson SE, Spiegelman D, et al. Reproductive history and endometriosis among premenopausal women. *Obste Gynecol.* 2004;104:965–974.

Raffi F, Metwally M, Amer S. The impact of excision of ovarian endometrioma on ovarian reserve: a systematic review and meta-analysis. *J Clin Endocrinol Metab.* 2012;97(9):3146–3154.

Roman H, Vassilieff M, Gourcerol G, et al. Surgical management of deep infiltrating endometriosis of the rectum: Pleading for a symptom-guided approach. *Hum Reprod.* 2011;26(2):274–281.

Signorello LB, Harlow BL, Cramer DW, Spiegelman D, Hill JA. Epidemiologic determinants of endometriosis: a hospital-based case-control study. *Ann Epidemiol.* 1997;7:267–741.

Sinaii N, Plumb K, Cotton L, et al. Differences in characteristics among 1000 women with endometriosis based on extent of disease. *Fertil Steril.* 2008;89(3):538–545.

Thomassin I, Bazot M, Detchev R, et al. Symptoms before and after surgical removal of colorectal endometriosis that are assessed by magnetic resonance imaging and rectal endoscopic sonography. *Am J Obstet Gynecol.* 2004;190(5):1264.

Walter AJ, Hentz JG, Magtibay PM, Cornella JL, Magrina JF. Endometriosis: correlation between histologic and visual findings at laparoscopy. *Am J Obstet Gynecol.* 2001;184(7):1407–1411; discussion 1411–1413.

Wolthuis AM, Tomassetti C. Multidisciplinary laparoscopic treatment for bowel endometriosis. *Best Pract Res Clin Gastroenterol.* 2014;28(1):53–67.

ORTHOPEDIC SURGERY

69

Back Pain/Sciatica

Rachel Cuenca and Erin Swan

A 53-year-old female presents to the emergency room with the acute onset of left leg pain while walking her dog. The patient insists there is no history of recent trauma. The pain starts in the left buttock and radiates down the left leg to the posterior calf and foot. The patient also describes some numbness in the left calf and mild plantar-flexion weakness. She gives a past medical history of well-controlled hypertension and does not smoke cigarettes. After the emergency room, physician provides some pain relief in the form of narcotics, a consult to the surgical team is made.

1. **Which of the following would alert the physician of a more emergent disease process?**

    A. Urinary incontinence with saddle anesthesia
    B. Steroid use in the past for similar symptoms
    C. Poor response to narcotics
    D. Marijuana use
    E. A history of trauma

2. **After the history and physical examination are completed, what should the initial imaging be in the emergency room?**

    A. Magnetic resonance imaging (MRI) of the lumbar spine without gadolinium in the emergency room
    B. Computerized tomography scan (CT) without contrast of the lumbar spine
    C. CT myelogram of the lumbar spine
    D. No imaging in the acute setting in the absence of signs of cancer, fracture, or cauda equina syndrome
    E. Plain PA and lateral X-ray of the lumbar spine

3. **The patient is seen in clinic 2 weeks after the initial presentation to the emergency room. She continues to have severe pain in the left leg with a positive straight leg raise and a decreased ankle jerk. An MRI has been completed, which shows a disc herniation at L5-S1 impinging on the left S1 nerve root. What is the next best step in management of the patient?**

    A. A discectomy at L5-S1
    B. Continued rest for a total of 6 weeks
    C. Strict bed rest for 1 to 2 more weeks
    D. Steroids to reduce the inflammation around the nerve root
    E. Antidepressant therapy

4. **Which of the following facts concerning the anatomy and prevalence of lumbar herniated discs is true?**

    A. L4-5 and L5-S1 account for about 50% of herniated lumbar discs.
    B. The nerve root involved in a typical lateral recess herniated disc between L4 and L5 is the nerve L4.
    C. The nerve root involved in an extreme lateral herniated disc between L4 and L5 is the nerve L5.
    D. Cauda equina syndrome from a herniated lumbar disc accounts for only 1% to 2% of lumbar disc surgeries.
    E. Herniated lumbar discs in the pediatric age group are quite common but infrequently require surgery.

5. **The patient undergoes an uneventful micro-discectomy for her L5-S1 herniated disc. After surgery, her strength is noted to be intact in bilateral lower extremities throughout all muscle groups. The night of surgery, the patient complains of severe back pain, new weakness in her left plantar-flexion, and urinary retention. What is the most likely cause of these new symptoms?**

   A. Reherniation of a disc fragment at the operative level
   B. Inflammation of the nerve root from surgery
   C. Spinal epidural hematoma
   D. Damage of the nerve root from retraction at the time of surgery
   E. Unintended durotomy causing arachnoiditis

6. **If this patient's neurologic symptoms had been caused by anterior subluxation of L5 on S1 rather than a herniated disc, what would be the most likely radiograph finding that would explain this condition?**

   A. A defect in the pars articularis
   B. A tear in the anterior longitudinal ligament
   C. A fracture of the vertebral body
   D. A spinous process fracture
   E. A pathologic lesion

7. **What is the most common location of a degenerative spondylolisthesis?**

   A. C1-C2
   B. C8-T1
   C. T12-L1
   D. L4-L5
   E. L5-S1

ANSWERS

1. **A.** This is an extremely important question in evaluating a patient with back pain and radiculopathy. The physician must know the "red flag" symptoms that would alert him or her as to a more severe process. Acute onset of urinary or bladder and bowel incontinence with saddle anesthesia refers to cauda equina syndrome (CES). Though there is controversy as to whether the patient should go to surgery within 24 or 48 hours, it remains a surgically urgent case. Current steroid use could put a patient at risk for both an infectious or a minor traumatic process but a remote history of its use does not. Similarly, immunosuppression puts the patient at risk for an infectious process such as osteomyelitis or an epidural abscess. Narcotics are often used for this problem but NSAIDS and steroids are useful if patients don't respond to narcotics. IV drug use would also put the patient at high risk for an epidural abscess or osteomyelitis but marijuana use would not. A history of trauma may help explain the sudden onset of symptoms; however, it does not necessarily impact the diagnosis or treatment of sciatic pain.

2. **D.** This can be a difficult answer to arrive at for surgeons. In most cases, patients come to the clinic with a diagnosis and imaging already included with them. When the patient first comes to the ER on symptom onset, the correct answer is *No imaging in the first month of symptoms.* This remains true only in the absence of the "red flag" symptoms discussed as these red flags aid the physician in ruling out cancer, infection, spinal fracture, and cauda equina syndrome. Some red flags that should tip off a surgeon to a possible malignancy are a history of cancer (the most predictive), age over 50, unexplained weight loss, and a failure to improve after 1 month. Possible malignancies include primary tumors such as osteoblastoma, osteosarcoma, and lymphoproliferative tumors and metastatic bone disease from lung, thyroid, prostate, kidney, and colon cancer among others. If pain persists, MRI is generally the imaging modality of choice performed without gadolinium. In patients with a contraindication for an MRI (pacemakers, etc.), a CT myelogram can provide adequate visualization.

3. **B.** The patient in the question stem is only 2 weeks out from onset of pain. Barring a neurologic deficit or signs of cauda equina syndrome, patients are given time to recover from the herniation. Over 85% of herniated disc patients will improve without surgical intervention in approximately 6 weeks. Bed rest is an option for 2 to 3 days maximum in patients with radicular complaints, as more time can be harmful for recovery. Additionally, antidepressants are more indicated for chronic back pain and oral steroids have not been shown to improve symptoms. There is also a role for physical therapy in improving back pain.

4. **D.** This question addresses the prevalence and anatomy of herniated discs in the lumbar spine. L4-5 and L5-S1 account for over 90% of herniated lumbar discs. When examining the lumbar spine, the nerve root that exits between L4 and L5 is the L4 root. Most discs herniate into the lateral recess,

which is medial to the exiting nerve root. In this way, the disc impinges on the nerve root "on deck" (see Figure 69-1).

An L4-5 disc herniation in the lateral recess would cause pain in an L5 distribution. An extreme lateral disc at L4-5, on the other hand, would impinge on the exiting nerve root, L4. It is important to realize that cauda equina syndrome is uncommon accounting for only 1% to 2% of all herniated disc surgeries. Also, herniated lumbar discs in the pediatric age group are quite rare.

5. **C.** When performing or providing care for a patient who underwent a discectomy, it is extremely important to perform thorough neurologic tests. Complications associated with a discectomy can include a reherniation of the disc (up to 4% over 10 years), temporary worsening of motor function (1% to 8% of patients[3]), and unintended durotomy (0% to 14% of cases). All of these may be a cause of temporary worsening neurologic function; however, any new neurologic deficit in a patient following surgery should be assumed to be a spinal epidural hematoma until proven otherwise. The workup should include an immediate MRI and return to the operating room. Long-term complications of microdiscectomy are uncommon and are often related to reherniation or instability in the spinal segment. These complications can present with recurrence of the patient's leg pain, pain in the back or buttocks, and weakness/numbness in the distribution of the compressed nerve root.

6. **A.** Anterior displacement of one vertebra on another is called spondylolisthesis. When this is caused by a defect in the pars articularis, it is called adult isthmic spondylolisthesis (Figure 69-2). The presence of a pars defect is called spondylolysis, which is usually caused by microtrauma over a period of time. Spondylolysis is thus more common in sports that involve repetitive hyperextension (e.g., gymnasts, weightlifters, and football linemen). This condition is present in 4% to

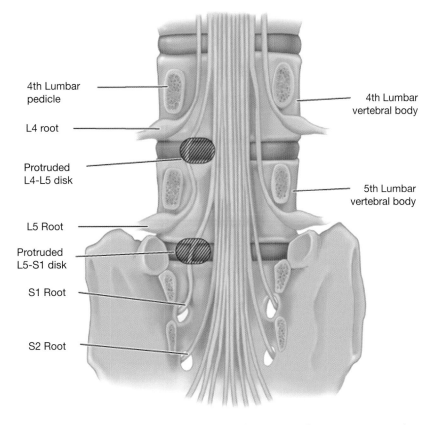

Figure 69-1 Anatomy of the lower lumbar and upper sacral nerve roots. Note that an L4/5 herniated disc most commonly affects the transversing L5 nerve root, as most disc herniations occur in the lateral recess. A far lateral L4/5 disc herniation would affect the exiting L4 nerve root.

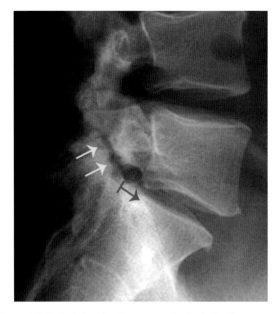

Figure 69-2 A defect in the pars articularis (yellow arrows) causing anterior subluxation of L5 on S1 (red arrow).

6% of the population, but the majority of these defects are asymptomatic. Therefore, it is not alarming to see a pars defect on a patient, and no further treatment or workup is indicated if they are asymptomatic. Patients only start becoming symptomatic when spondylolisthesis occurs, and only 5% of patients with spondylolysis develop spondylolisthesis. Eighty-two percent of cases of adult isthmic spondylolisthesis occur at the L5-S1 level and 11% occur at L4-L5. When it occurs at L5-S1, the symptoms manifest as radicular symptoms caused by compression on the exiting L5 nerve root at the L5-S1 foramen. Patients will present with axial back pain, weakness with ankle dorsiflexion and of the extensor hallucis longus (EHL), and paresthesias in the first webspace and on the top of the foot. Just as in disc herniation, the majority of these can be treated nonoperatively with NSAIDs, activity modification, and physical therapy. Patients who are indicated for surgery have failed 6 months of nonoperative treatment and continue to have persistent and incapacitating pain, have a progressive neurologic deficit, have progression of the vertebral slip, or develop cauda equina syndrome.

7. **D.** Degenerative spondylolisthesis is lumbar spondylolisthesis without a defect in the pars. The absence of a pars defect is what differentiates it from adult isthmic spondylolisthesis. Also differentiating it from isthmic spondylolisthesis is that it is five times more common at the L4/5 level than other levels. The L5 nerve root is

affected in degenerative spondylolisthesis by the degenerative slip causing central and lateral recess stenosis. The L4 nerve root is also affected due to compression of the foramen. L4 radiculopathy manifests as difficult with knee extension as well as sensory deficits on the lateral thigh, anterior knee, and medial leg.

BIBLIOGRAPHY

Allen C, Glasziou P, Del Mar C. Bed rest: a potentially harmful treatment needing more careful evaluation. *Lancet.* October 9, 1999;354(9186):1229–1233.

Chau AM, Xu LL, Pelzer NR, Gragnaniello C. Timing of surgical intervention in cauda equina syndrome: A systematic critical review. *World Neurosurg.* March–April 2014;81(3-4):640–650.

Davis RA. A long-term outcome analysis of 984 surgically treated herniated lumbar discs. *J Neurosurg.* March 1994;80(3):415–421.

Deyo RA, Rainville J, Kent DL. What can the history and physical examination tell us about low back pain? *JAMA.* August 12, 1992;268(6):760–765.

Downie A, Williams CM, Henschke N, et al. Red flags to screen for malignancy and fracture in patients with low back pain: systematic review. *BMJ.* 2013;347:f7095.

Ebersold MJ, Quast LM, Bianco AJ, Jr. Results of lumbar discectomy in the pediatric patient. *J Neurosurg.* November 1987;67(5):643–647.

Evans N, McCarthy M. Management of symptomatic degenerative low-grade lumbar spondylolisthesis. *EFORT Open Reviews.* 2018;3(12):620–631.

Fager CA. Observations on spontaneous recovery from intervertebral disc herniation. *Surg Neurol.* October 1994;42(4):282–286.

Graves JM, Fulton-Kehoe D, Jarvik JG, Franklin GM. Early imaging for acute low back pain: one-year health and disability outcomes among Washington State workers. *Spine.* August 15, 2012;37(18):1617–1627.

Greenberg MS, ed. *Handbook of Neurosurgery.* 7th ed. Thieme Medical Publishers; 2010.

Henschke N, Maher CG, Ostelo RW, de Vet HC, Macaskill P, Irwig L. Red flags to screen for malignancy in patients with low-back pain. *Cochrane Database Syst Rev.* 2013;2:CD008686.

Hodges SD, Humphreys SC, Eck JC, Covington LA. Management of incidental durotomy without mandatory bed rest. A retrospective review of 20 cases. *Spine.* October 1, 1999;24(19):2062–2204.

Jones TR, Rao RD. Adult isthmic spondylolisthesis. *J Am Acad Orthop Surg.* 2009;17(10): 609-617.

Matz PG, Meagher RH, Lamer T, et al. Guideline summary review: an evidence-based clinical guideline for the diagnosis and treatment of degenerative lumbar spondylolisthesis. *Spine J.* 2015;16(3):439–448.

Webster BS, Bauer AZ, Choi Y, Cifuentes M, Pransky GS. Iatrogenic consequences of early magnetic resonance imaging in acute, work-related, disabling low back pain. *Spine.* 2013;38(22):1939–1946.

70

Calcaneus Fractures

Rachel Cuenca and Erin Swan

A 27-year-old professional painter sustained a fall from a 15-foot scaffold while on the job. By his report, he landed on both feet in a standing position and had immediate severe foot and leg pain and was unable to ambulate. His primary survey was unremarkable and his secondary survey is normal except for the examination of his right foot. He presents to the emergency department with a swollen and deformed right foot and complains of severe pain at rest and with any palpation or manipulation of the foot. Radiographs of the right foot are shown.

1. **What other associated injury is described from this type of mechanism and associated with the presence of this injury?**

   A. Closed head injury
   B. Hollow viscous injury
   C. Pelvic fracture
   D. Lumbar spine fracture
   E. Concomitant foot fractures

2. **Anteroposterior, lateral, and oblique radiographs are performed and reveal a displaced calcaneus fracture. What other imaging modality should be ordered to further delineate the injury?**

   A. Non-contrast magnetic resonance imaging (MRI)
   B. Weight-bearing foot films
   C. Non-contrast computerized tomography (CT) scan with reconstructions
   D. Triple-phase bone scan
   E. Ultrasound

3. **Several hours have gone by while awaiting further workup and disposition of the patient and you**

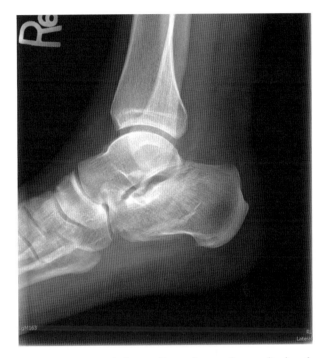

Figure 70-1 Lateral foot radiograph revealing a displaced, intra-articular calcaneus fracture with depression of the posterior facet. Radiographs courtesy of MAJ Justin Fowler.

notice that the skin overlying the Achilles tendon is becoming dark and appears to be tented by the fracture. **What is the next most appropriate course of action?**

   A. Emergent closed reduction in the emergency room
   B. Emergent surgical reduction and stabilization
   C. Splint and strict elevation
   D. CT angiography of the lower extremity
   E. Emergent compartment pressure check of the foot

4. What is the preferred treatment for a displaced, intra-articular fracture of this bone in a young, active patient?

A. Well-padded splint with conversion to a short leg cast

B. Closed reduction and casting

C. Percutaneous screw fixation

D. Emergent open reduction internal fixation

E. Delayed open reduction internal fixation

5. Which of the following is predictive of a better outcome after open reduction and internal fixation of a displaced, intra-articular fracture of this type?

A. Female gender

B. Significant articular impaction

C. Workers compensation

D. Age >50

E. Heavy laborer

6. The patient subsequently undergoes operative fixation as shown in Figure 70-2. Postoperatively in the recovery room, he presents with an isolated, fixed flexed great toe. What is the most likely etiology of this finding?

A. Plantar nerve palsy

B. Missed foot compartment syndrome

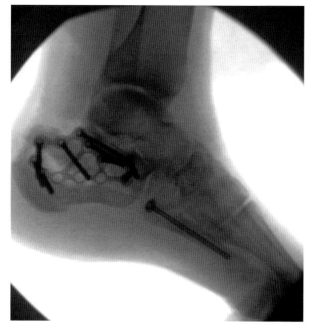

Figure 70-2 Lateral foot radiograph that shows a calcaneus fracture with a lateral plate and screws.

C. Use of a lateral extensile approach to the calcaneus

D. Traumatic arthritis

E. Use of screws in the sustentaculum tali that are too long

7. What is the most common complication associated with open reduction internal fixation of calcaneus fractures?

A. Subtalar arthritis

B. Wound infection or dehiscence

C. Malunion

D. Compartment syndrome

E. Deep peroneal nerve palsy

ANSWERS

1. D. This patient has a calcaneus fracture. The associated injuries, specifically lumbar spine injuries, have been historically reported in up to 50% of patients. The most common mechanism of injury for calcaneus fractures has been a fall from a height with the patient initially striking the ground with their feet in a standing or semi-standing position. This results in the calcaneus fracture, but also the transmission of impact forces up the spine, with the lumbar region bearing most of the burden. As motor vehicle collisions have become an increasingly prevalent mechanism, newer data has suggested that roughly 10% of patients with calcaneus fracture will have a concomitant lumbar spine injury and approximately 25% have other additional lower extremity injuries. The other injuries listed can occur with any significant trauma mechanism but are all less commonly associated with calcaneus and other fractures of the foot. Any patient with this type of mechanism should be suspected of having a lumbar spine fracture until proven otherwise, and the optimal diagnostic study is a dedicated CT scan of the lumbar spine.

2. C. Initial diagnosis of a calcaneus fracture can be readily made with conventional plain X-rays of the foot (Figure 70-1). The simplest broad classification of calcaneus fractures is based on whether there is articular involvement, with 75% of fractures being intra-articular, and approximately 25% being extra-articular. Although the initial diagnosis can often be made with standard X-rays, a high-quality CT of the hindfoot is the definitive imaging modality of choice for diagnosis, classification, and operative planning. The CT scan should be performed with 2- to 3-mm

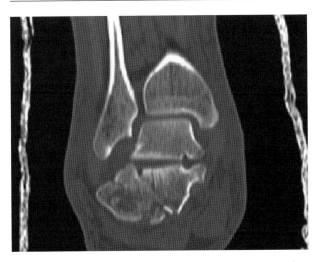

Figure 70-3 Coronal CT scan showing the articular involvement of this impacted calcaneus fracture.

interval slices in the sagittal, axial, and 30° semi-coronal planes (Figure 70-3). This imaging modality allows for accurate characterization of the fracture pattern and facilitates planning for the patient's definitive treatment. A CT scan is useful in assessing the amount and location of joint impaction, lateral wall blowout, involvement of calcaneocuboid joint, and the number of primary fracture lines in the posterior facet. An MRI has little additional utility compared to a high-quality CT scan for diagnosing, characterizing, or directing treatment plans for calcaneus fractures. Similarly, additional X-rays including weight-bearing films will not provide sufficient anatomic details, and will also likely be poorly tolerated by the patient with a calcaneus fracture. There is no role for ultrasonography in acute fractures.

3. **B.** Displaced avulsion fractures of the posterior tuberosity with impending skin necrosis require immediate reduction to prevent full-thickness skin loss over the posterior ankle and Achilles tendon. Emergent orthopaedic surgical consultation should be obtained as closed reduction typically is not adequate to remove tension from the skin. This is typically treated as an orthopaedic emergency and usually requires surgical reduction and stabilization in the operating room in an acute fashion.

The ankle can be splinted in plantar-flexion in an attempt to take pressure off the overlying skin while awaiting surgical consultation. Placement of a splint will not provide any benefit, and in fact could produce additional pressure necrosis on the area if not fitted well or if there is additional swelling after the splint is placed. CT angiography is only useful if there is a suspicion of a concomitant vascular injury in the fractured extremity, and has no role in the evaluation of foot fractures with a normal vascular exam. Emergent compartment pressures are indicated if there is suspicion of a compartment syndrome, but in this scenario, the primary problem is the displaced fracture and not an elevated compartment pressure.

4. **E.** Intra-articular displacement of the calcaneus has been shown to lead to subtalar arthrosis, subfibular impingement, difficulty with shoe wear, hindfoot stiffness, and limited function. If the articular surface is amenable to reconstruction in a young, healthy patient, then surgical fixation should be attempted. The status of the soft tissue envelope dictates the timing of surgical intervention. Traditionally, delayed fixation through a lateral approach has been the mainstay treatment for these fractures. These patients will typically have a significant amount of swelling, bruising, and soft tissue edema of the foot, which can result in poor wound healing if surgery is performed during the acute phase. Open reduction and internal fixation is typically delayed to allow this soft tissue swelling to subside and mitigate the risk of surgical site complications, poor wound healing, soft tissue loss, and hardware infections.

5. **A.** A prospective, randomized, controlled trial of nonoperatively treated versus operatively treated calcaneus fractures from four Canadian trauma centers revealed that certain patient demographics were predictive of better versus worse outcomes after treatment of displaced intra-articular calcaneus fractures. Women treated with operative fixation had significantly higher quality of life scores than women who were managed nonoperatively. The study also showed that heavy laborers, workers compensation cases, older age, higher degree of articular comminution, and smoking are all predictors of worse outcomes after operative fixation. The exact reason for this gender disparity remains unknown, but these factors should be taken into consideration when planning a management strategy and in counseling the patient regarding the risks versus benefits of operative versus non-operative management.

6. **E.** The flexor hallucis longus (FHL) runs along the medial aspect of the hindfoot, medial to the

posterior fact of the calcaneus and just under the sustentaculum tali (constant fragment). This tendon can be injured with poor drilling technique used during open reduction internal fixation of a calcaneus fracture using a lateral plate. Too long of a screw can catch the tendon and tether it there. FHL injury presents with the great toe in a fixed, flexed position.

7. **B.** Wound complications occur in 10% to 25% of patients with calcaneus fractures. Smokers, diabetics, and patients with open injuries are all at increased risk of wound complications. Furthermore, 21% of patients with tongue-type fractures have some degree of skin compromise. Delayed presentation puts patients at an increased risk of developing wound complications, which highlights the importance of prompt treatment of these injuries. If wound breakdown does occur, the first step to treat this complication is to immobilize the patient's injured extremity.

BIBLIOGRAPHY

Benirschke SK, Kramer PA. Wound healing complications in closed and open calcaneal fractures. *J Orthop Trauma.* 2004;18(1):1–6.

Buckley R, Tough S, McCormack R, et al. Operative compared with non-operative treatment of displaced intra-articular calcaneal fractures: a prospective, randomized, controlled multicenter trial. *J Bone Joint Surg Am.* 2002;84(10):1733–1744.

Buckley RE, Tough S. Displaced intra-articular calcaneal fractures. *J Am Acad Orthop Surg.* 2004;12(3):172–178.

Cave EF. Fracture of the oscalcis—the problem in general. *Clin Orthop Relat Res.* 1963;30:64–66.

Folk JW, Starr AJ, Early JS. Early wound complications of operative treatment of calcaneus fractures: analysis of 190 fractures. *J Orthop Trauma.* 1999;13(5):369–372.

Gardner MJ, Nork SE, Barei DP, Kramer PA, Sangeorzan BJ, Benirschke SK. Secondary soft tissue compromise in tongue-type calcaneus fractures. *J Orthop Trauma.* 2008;22(7):439–445.

Gilmer PW, Herzenberg J, Frank JL, Silverman P, Martinez S, Goldner JL. Computerized tomographic analysis of acute calcaneal fractures. *Foot Ankle.* February 1986;6(4):184–193.

Koski A, Kuokkanen H, Tukiainen E. Postoperative wound complications after internal fixation of closed calcaneal fractures: a retrospective analysis of 126 consecutive patients with 148 fractures. *Scand J Surg.* 2005;94(3):243–245.

Protheroe K. Avulsion fractures of the calcaneus. *J Bone Joint Surg Br.* 1969;51(1):118–122.

Sanders RW, Clare MP. Fractures of the calcaneus. In: Mann RA, ed. *Surgery of the Foot and Ankle.* Mosby; 2007:2017–2075.

71

Shoulder Trauma

Rachel Cuenca and Erin Swan

A 24-year-old male presents as an acute trauma after injury in a motorcycle crash. On initial presentation, he is a GCS 11 (E3V3M5). Because of severe pain and labored breathing, he is intubated and sedated. During your secondary survey, you note the patient has significant edema, swelling, and abrasions about the right shoulder girdle.

1. **What potentially devastating diagnosis is characterized by lateral displacement of the scapula?**

    A. Pnuemothorax
    B. Multiple rib fractures
    C. Scapulothoracic dissociation
    D. Shoulder dislocation
    E. Sternoclavicular dislocation

2. **What study is best to further investigate and diagnose the suspected injury in Question 1?**

    A. Ventilation–perfusion (V–Q) scan
    B. External rotation anterior-posterior (AP) shoulder X-ray
    C. Axillary X-ray
    D. Internal rotation AP shoulder X-ray
    E. Chest X-ray

3. **While reviewing a chest computerized tomography (CT) obtained as part of the initial workup, you note a displaced right scapular fracture. What additional injuries are most commonly associated with scapular fractures?**

    A. Pulmonary injury
    B. Head Injury

    C. Femur fracture
    D. Arterial injury
    E. Brachial plexus injury

4. **Upon further clinical evaluation, you note that the patient has a prominence along the anterior aspect of his shoulder and a sulcus adjacent to the posterior acromion. He is still not following commands, but examination with gentle range of motion demonstrates limitations in internal rotation and abduction. What is your next step in management?**

    A. Attempt a closed reduction.
    B. Obtain a chest CT.
    C. Schedule an outpatient magnetic resonance image (MRI).
    D. Obtain orthogonal X-rays.
    E. Diagnosis should be made based on physical exam.

5. **What is the most common neurovascular injury associated with an anterior shoulder dislocation?**

    A. Musculocutaneous nerve
    B. Axillary nerve
    C. Axillary vein
    D. Subclavian artery
    E. Radial nerve

6. **The patient's shoulder is reduced acutely. Post-reduction X-rays demonstrate no fracture. What is the next step in management?**

    A. Urgent operative fixation of suspected labral tear
    B. Operative fixation once patient has been extubated and is stable from his other injuries

C. Physical therapy with early range of motion and strengthening

D. Strict immobilization of the shoulder using a figure-of-eight brace

E. NSAID use and observation

7. **A 65-year-old sustains the same injury, which was reduced without complication. He continues to have significant weakness post-reduction. What imaging study should be obtained next and for which diagnosis?**

A. Magnetic resonance imaging (MRI) of the shoulder to evaluate the rotator cuff

B. MRI of the shoulder to evaluate the labrum

C. Electomyography to evaluate for axillary nerve palsy

D. CT of the shoulder to evaluate the glenoid

E. CT of the shoulder to assess for an occult fracture

ANSWERS

1. C. Scapulothoracic dissociation results from complete disruption of the scapulothoracic articulation with associated lateral translation of the scapula without associated partial or complete amputation of the soft tissue, with the overlying skin typically intact. This is considered a flail extremity. Scapulothoracic dissociation typically results from a high energy, traction force to the upper extremity. Motorcycle accidents are the most commonly described mechanism for this injury. Considered analogous to a closed forequarter amputation, it is associated with a myriad of concomitant injuries including: dislocation of the acromioclavicular and sternoclavicular joints, clavicle fracture, vascular injury to the subclavian and axillary vessels, brachial plexus injuries, and complete or partial disruption of the surrounding musculature.

The clinician must maintain a high index of suspicion as patients are often obtunded, sedated, or intubated during initial evaluation, preventing a complete neurological examination. Additionally, because these injuries are associated with a high-energy mechanism and severe and potentially life-threatening concomitant injuries, scapulothoracic dissociation can be missed or overlooked without appropriate and complete evaluation. Typically these patients will have significant swelling and edema of the entire shoulder girdle from neck to axilla from underlying hematoma. Evaluation and comparison of pulses of the upper extremity should be promptly performed, and if absent or uneven, further studies, including arterial pressure indexes, and if abnormal (<0.9), arteriogram should be obtained.

With the low incidence of injury, outcomes studies are limited. However, previous studies have suggested a mortality rate of roughly 20% (3 of 15 patients), though the true rate is likely higher as a result of death from associated injuries in these patients. Associated neurovascular injury is extremely common, with neurologic injury in 94% of patients and vascular injury in 88%. In addition to a mortality rate between 10% and 20%, outcomes are universally poor with 52% rate of flail extremity and early amputation rate of 21%. Early recognition of scapulothoracic injury, and likely associated neurovascular injury, is paramount as diagnosis guides treatment and affects long-term outcomes.

2. E. See Figure 71-1. The diagnosis of scapulothoracic dissociation can be made based on a non-rotated chest X-ray. Lateral displacement of the scapula is pathognomonic. Comparison of the scapular position can be made with the contralateral side, and differences and asymmetry noted. The amount of scapular lateralization, or scapular-index, can be measured. The distance from the sternal notch or midline of the spine to the glenoid or medial border of the scapula can be measured and compared with the contralateral side. The injured side measurement is divided by the non-injured side measurement. The normal scapular-index is about 1.09, and in one of the largest series, the ratio in patients with a scapulothoracic dissociation averaged 1.29.

3. A. In a review of 58 scapula fractures as a result of blunt trauma, Thompson et al. found a high rate of concomitant injury to the ipsilateral lung, chest wall, and chest contents. Fifty-three percent of patients had a pulmonary contusion, 53% rib fractures, and 26.8% clavicle fractures. Neurovascular injury was not uncommon, with an incidence of brachial plexus injury of 12.5% and a 10.7% incidence of subclavian, brachial, or axillary artery injury.

Baldwin et al. controlled for injury severity score in order to determine if commonly associated injuries with scapula fractures were simply a result of an increased injury severity score. They showed the following injuries had increased frequency in patients

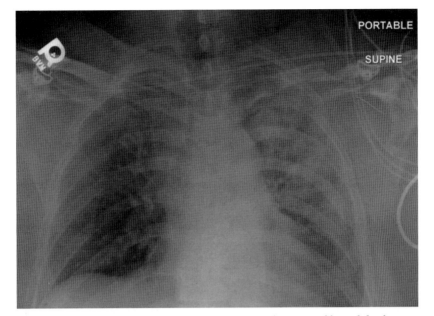

Figure 71-1 A chest X-ray demonstrating scapulothoracic dissociation with increased lateral displacement of the left scapula as compared to the right

with a scapula fracture compared to those without: rib fractures, pneumothorax, lung injury, ipsilateral extremity injury, and spine injury.

A scapula fracture, with a high energy blunt mechanism of injury, should alert the clinician to the possibility of additional injury to the ipsilateral lung, chest wall, shoulder girdle, and surrounding neurovascular structures.

4. **D.** Based on the clinical exam findings present, the patient has a suspected shoulder dislocation. Anterior shoulder dislocations are by far the most common, accounting for approximately 98% of all glenohumeral dislocations. The typical mechanism for an anterior dislocation is with the arm in an abducted and externally rotated position. Posterior dislocations are relatively rare, and result from axial load to an adducted, flexed, and internally shoulder, and can also be associated with electrical shocks or seizures.

An acutely dislocated shoulder is typically very painful. The patient with an anterior dislocation will typically hold the arm in slight abduction and range of motion will be limited secondary to pain.

Radiographs are an essential part of the initial assessment, ensuring appropriate diagnosis, including the direction of dislocation, presence of associated fractures, and potential blocks to reduction.

The standard shoulder trauma series must include orthogonal X-rays including a true AP, axillary lateral, and scapular Y view. Obtaining only a single view of the shoulder can lead to missed injury and inaccurate diagnosis. CT can help aid in diagnosis if appropriate imaging cannot be obtained.

After appropriate diagnosis is made, a reduction can be performed. There are several classic methods for relocation, including the Kocher, traction-counter traction, and Stimson and Milch to name a few. Newer studies and techniques focus on limiting pre-medication. Recent meta-analysis have shown equivalent effectiveness using an intra-articular lidocaine injection instead of intravenous analgesia and sedation for manual acute closed reduction of anterior shoulder dislocation with decreased risk of post-procedure complications.

5. **B.** The axillary nerve (C5, C6) is a direct continuation of the posterior cord of the brachial plexus. Because it is tethered, anterior and posterior, to the glenohumeral joint with limited excursion, it is susceptible to injury from shoulder dislocation. In a study of 105 patients with acute primary anterior shoulder dislocations, 21% of patients (22/107) were found to have a nerve injury, the most common ($n = 13$) involving injury to the axillary nerve. The authors of this study note that the incidence of nerve injury may have been

underestimated as it was diagnosed by clinical examination alone, not with electrophysiologic testing.

In a prospective study of 101 consecutive patients with anterior shoulder dislocation or humeral neck fracture, de Laat et al. found electrophysiologic evidence of nerve injury in 45% of patients. The axillary nerve was most commonly injured (37%) followed by the suprascapular nerve (29%) and the musculocutaneous nerve (22%).

Initial diagnosis of a nerve injury can be difficult secondary to pain. The axillary nerve innervates the deltoid and teres minor muscles. If the patient's shoulder is dislocated, however, they will have significant pain and obtaining a reliable motor exam may be difficult. Instead, evaluate the patient for paresthesias. The axillary nerve provides sensation to the lateral aspect of the shoulder (the deltoid patch); test this area for paresthesias and compare it to the sensation of the patient's uninjured lateral shoulder. Detailed initial exam and assessment, additional follow-up for repeat examination, or electrophysiologic testing, can help detect injury early, and potentially prevent long-term poor functional outcome.

6. **C.** Traumatic dislocations should be reduced urgently. In first-time dislocators, patients can be treated nonoperatively with physical therapy to work on strengthening of the shoulder's dynamic stabilizers. Patients should be given a sling for comfort but need to engage in early range of motion to prevent stiffness of the shoulder. If the patient has recurrent dislocations after their traumatic event, a referral to follow-up with an orthopedic surgeon should be placed and a CT scan should be obtained to assess for glenoid bone loss and Hill Sachs defects.

7. **A.** Following shoulder dislocations, elderly patients should be evaluated for rotator cuff tears with MRI. In patients over the age of 80, rotator cuff tears have been found to occur in up to 80% of patients who sustain a shoulder dislocation. Untreated tears may cause persistent pain, weakness, dysfunction, instability, and lead to degenerative changes. An MRI is useful to not only diagnose the tear, but to evaluate for fatty degeneration and retraction of the rotator cuff to determine if it is repairable or not. Surgical repair of these acute rotator cuff tears in the elderly have been shown to provide improved pain relief and higher patient satisfaction as compared to nonoperative management.

BIBLIOGRAPHY

Baldwin KD, Ohman-Strickland P, Mehta S, et al. Scapula fractures: a marker for concomitant injury? A retrospective review of data in the National Trauma Database. *J Trauma*. 2008;65:430–435.

Brucker PU, Gruen GS, Kaufmann RA. Scapulothoracic dissociation: evaluation and management. *Injury*. 2005;36:1147–1155.

Damschen DD, Cogbill TH, Siegel MJ. Scapulothoracic dissociation caused by blunt trauma. *J Trauma*. 1997;42:537–540.

de Laat EA, Visser CP, Coene LN, et al. Nerve lesions in primary shoulder dislocations and humeral neck fractures. A prospective clinical and EMG study. *J Bone Joint Surg Br*. 1994;76:381–383.

Eachempati KK, Dua A, Malhotra R, et al. The external rotation method for reduction of acute anterior dislocations and fracture-dislocations of the shoulder. *J Bone Joint Surg Am*. 2004;86-A:2431–2434.

Ebraheim NA, An HS, Jackson WT, et al. Scapulothoracic dissociation. *J Bone Joint Surg Am*. 1988;70:428–432.

Flanagin BA, Leslie MP. Scapulothoracic dissociation. *Orthop Clin North Am*. 2013;44:1–7.

Gombera MM, Sekiya JK. Rotator cuff tear and glenohumeral instability: a systematic review. *Clin Orthop Relat Res*. 2014;472(8):2448–2456.

Jiang N, Hu YJ, Zhang KR, et al. Intra-articular lidocaine versus intravenous analgesia and sedation for manual closed reduction of acute anterior shoulder dislocation: an updated meta-analysis. *J Clin Anesth*. 2014;26:350–359.

Izquierdo R, Van Thiel GS, Trenhaile S, Provencher MT, & Romeo A. (2021). Chapter 6: Management Decisions for Acute Versus Chronic Shoulder Instability. In Orthopaedic knowledge update: Shoulder and elbow (5th ed., pp. 75-83). S.l.: WOLTERS KLUWER.

Kelbel JM, Jardon OM, Huurman WW. Scapulothoracic dissociation. A case report. *Clin Orthop Relat Res*. 1986;210–214.

Nagi ON, Dhillon MS. Traumatic scapulothoracic dissociation. A case report. *Arch Orthop Trauma Surg*. 1992;111:348–349.

Oreck SL, Burgess A, Levine AM. Traumatic lateral displacement of the scapula: a radiographic sign of neurovascular disruption. *J Bone Joint Surg Am*. 1984;66:758–763.

Robinson CM, Aderinto J. Posterior shoulder dislocations and fracture-dislocations. *J Bone Joint Surg Am*. 2005;87:639–650.

Rockwood CA, ed. *The Shoulder*. Saunders Elsevier; 2009.

Rubin SA, Gray RL, Green WR. The scapular "Y": a diagnostic aid in shoulder trauma. *Radiology*. 1974;110:725–726.

te Slaa RL, Wijffels MP, Brand R, Marti RK. The prognosis following acute primary glenohumeral dislocation. *J Bone Joint Surg Br*. 2004;86:58–64.

Thompson DA, Flynn TC, Miller PW, et al. The significance of scapular fractures. *J Trauma*. 1985;25:974–977.

Wolf BR, Dunn WR, Wright RW. Indications for repair of full-thickness rotator cuff tears. *Am J Sports Med*. 2007;35(6):1007–1016.

Zelle BA, Pape HC, Gerich TG, et al. Functional outcome following scapulothoracic dissociation. *J Bone Joint Surg Am*. 2004;86(1):2–8.

72

Pediatric Trauma

Rachel Cuenca and Erin Swan

You are called to a trauma code in the emergency room to evaluate a 6-year-old female who was restrained in the back seat of a car when it lost control and went over an embankment. When you arrive, the child is conscious and breathing spontaneously. Initial vitals are stable and she is following commands. The child is in significant pain, but is able to communicate to you that her right elbow and left leg hurt.

1. **With regard to pediatric trauma patients, compared to adult trauma patients, the former have a:**
   A. Small head-to-body ratio
   B. Larger total blood volume
   C. Decreased capacity for plastic deformation
   D. Increased baseline metabolic rate combined with a larger physiologic reserve
   E. Smaller surface area to body volume

2. **After your initial assessment you begin to order labs and imaging. In consideration of cervical spine evaluation, you make the following decision:**
   A. Cervical spine radiographs are not indicated but lumbar spine radiographs are, because lumbar spine injuries are more common in children.
   B. Cervical spine radiographs are indicated because she may have lost consciousness.
   C. Cervical spine radiographs are not indicated because children are unlikely to sustain injury to the cervical spine as a result of their unique osseous anatomy.
   D. Cervical spine radiographs are indicated as a result of potential distracting injuries of her left leg and right elbow.

   E. Cervical spine radiographs are not indicated, but a magnetic resonance imaging (MRI) of her cervical and thoracolumbar spine is.

3. **Upon further evaluation of her right elbow, you notice an obvious deformity. What is your initial step in management of this potential injury?**
   A. Obtain labs to rule out infection.
   B. Obtain a computerized tomography (CT) scan to evaluate potential fracture.
   C. Perform a careful neurovascular examination.
   D. Perform a closed reduction, and then obtain X-rays.
   E. Provide sedation to allow evaluation of stability and range of motion.

4. **She is unable to extend her wrist or fingers, and X-rays of the elbow and forearm are obtained (Figures 72-1 and 72-2). What nerve has most likely been affected?**
   A. Axillary nerve
   B. Musculocutaneous nerve
   C. Median nerve
   D. Radial nerve
   E. Ulnar nerve

5. **In the trauma bay, peripheral IV access is not able to be obtained after multiple attempts and the pateint's blood pressure is 110/70. Which of the following is the most appropriate method to obtain vascular access in this patient?**
   A. Placement of an intraosseous infusion device
   B. Peripherally inserted central catheter (PICC) placement in the uninjured extremity

C. Femoral venous cutdown

D. Subclavian central line placement

E. Continue attempts at obtaining peripheral IV access

6. **Radiographs of the left femur demonstrate a displaced midshaft fracture. How would the workup of this femur fracture differ, if the child was a non-ambulatory 11 months old, injured as a result of a fall?**

A. Obtain labs to rule out infection.

B. Obtain a CT scan to further evaluate the fracture.

C. Obtain inlet and outlet pelvic X-rays.

D. The child would need to be evaluated for possible non-accidental trauma.

E. The workup would be unchanged.

7. **What fractures would be concerning for non-accidental trauma?**

A. Rib fractures

B. Distal radius and ulna fractures

C. Supracondylar humerus fracture

D. Spiral tibia shaft fracture

E. Proximal metadiaphyseal tibia fracture

ANSWERS

1. D. There are many important differences in the anatomy, physiology, mechanism, and characteristics of injuries that make pediatric trauma unique. The proportions of a child's body are different from those of an adult, predisposing to certain injuries. Children have a *large* head-to-body ratio; the younger the child the more disproportionate the ratio. Their relatively larger heads predispose them to head, neck, and upper cervical spine injuries.

Pediatric bone growth and development is incomplete, with bone more deformable and able to fracture with (relatively) less force. These characteristics can lead to internal organ damage without apparent injury or fracture of the thoracic rib cage. Additionally, the immature cage leaves the spleen and liver exposed and vulnerable to injury.

Children have a smaller total blood volume (80 mL/kg) than adults. As a result, equivalent or small-volume blood loss can have more significant physiologic consequences, with hypovolemia developing more rapidly. Additionally, because of a higher baseline metabolic rate and increased physiologic reserve, the apparent hemodynamic response to trauma may

be minimal. Additionally, children have a more minimal metabolic response to trauma, and hypotension is often a late sign of shock in these patients. They are also more prone to hypothermia because of an increased ratio of body surface area to volume.

2. D. The pediatric spine, especially in children under 8 years old, has many important anatomic and biomechanical differences that predispose it to cervical injury. As previously stated, children have a larger head-to-neck ratio. Additionally, in early childhood, the fulcrum of flexion is at the C2–C3 level, compared to C5–C6 by age 11. This too, predisposes to upper cervical spine injury. Pediatric cervical spine trauma may present as fracture, fracture with subluxation, subluxation alone (without fracture), or spinal cord injury without radiographic abnormality (SCIWORA). The incidence of SCIWORA and isolated soft tissue injury alone are more common in children <9 years old. As a result of these, and other, complicating factors, the assessment and clearance of pediatric patients with potential spine injuries is challenging. Incomplete and inaccurate assessment can result in missed cervical spine injuries while prolonged can be associated with significant morbidity.

Lee et al. developed a multidisciplinary approach to pediatric cervical spine injury evaluation and clearance. The authors use the presence of any of the following as a reason for immobilization and radiographic evaluation: child is unconscious or inconsolable; mechanism of injury suggestive of possible cervical spine injury (motor vehicle crash, fall from height, pedestrian struck, etc.), neck pain or focal neck tenderness; presence of a distracting injury; abnormal neurologic exam findings or history of transient neurologic symptoms that suggest c-spine injury; physical signs of neck trauma; significant trauma to head and or face; or an unreliable exam secondary to substance abuse. In short, in the multiply injured patient, a cervical spine is presumed present and must be ruled out by physical exam and radiographic evaluation.

3. C. Pediatric elbow injuries present a challenge to the treating physician because diagnosis, physical examination, radiographic evaluation and interpretation, and surgical treatment can all be difficult. Additionally, complications, both acute and chronic, are not uncommon. Unfortunately, while fractures around the elbow can be difficult, they are also quite common. Elbow injuries in children occur more commonly than in adults, and account for approximately 30% of all extremity fractures in patients age 0 to 7 years. Injuries to the upper extremity account for 65% of all fractures and dislocations in children, with fractures of the distal end and forearm being most common, followed by fractures and dislocations of the elbow. Of all pediatric elbow fractures, supracondylar fractures are the most common.

While physical examination in the uncooperative child with a swollen elbow can be challenging, it is absolutely essential, and should be the first step in treatment. The two most important aspects of the exam are the neurovascular assessment and the presence of any soft tissue injury. Examination and documentation of neurovascular status must be completed prior to any reduction, and following any reduction maneuver, to assess for any interval change. For supracondylar distal humerus fractures specifically, neurologic injury is relatively common, ranging from 10% to 18%.

Supracondylar humerus fractures requiring fixation were previously thought to be a surgical emergency. However, there has been a shift in thinking that those fractures without vascular compromise, severe soft tissue swelling, or pressure on the skin can wait (i.e., wait until morning) until an OR team familiar with this operation is available. Again, this decision hinges and underlines the importance of accurate and complete physical examination. However, these patients must be splinted and admitted for observation with continued neurovascular checks until surgery can safely be performed.

4. **D.** This patient has sustained a radial head dislocation with a proximal ulna fracture (also known as a Monteggia fracture). She is now unable to extend her wrist or fingers, which is indicative of a posterior interosseous nerve (PIN) palsy. The posterior interosseous nerve is the motor branch of the radial nerve. It winds around the radial neck then travels within the substance of the posterior compartment of the forearm. The PIN innervates the common extensors (extensor carpi radialis brevis, extensor digitorum communis, extensor digiti minimi, and extensor carpi ulnaris) as well as the deep extensors (supinator, abductor pollicis longus, extensor pollicus brevis, extensor pollicus longus, and extensor indicis proprius). The PIN is injured in 10% of acute Monteggia fractures. This palsy almost always resolves spontaneously. The injury is treated by closed reduction of the ulna fracture and radial head dislocation with long arm casting. Typically, the radial head will reduce spontaneously with reduction of the ulna and restoration of ulnar length Figures 72-1 and 72-2.

5. **A.** Intraosseous (IO) infusion is the most appropriate method of obtaining venous access in a normotensive pediatric trauma patient who is unable to obtain a peripheral IV line. Intraosseous lines can be rapidly and easily inserted, have low complication rates, and are safe to use with resuscitation medications. Guy et al. evaluated intraosseous line indications, insertion sites, complications, and outcomes in 27 pediatric trauma patients. They reported minimal IO-related complications, and high success of obtaining peripheral access with this technique. They concluded that IO infusion is a rapid, safe, and simple method of obtaining short-term vascular access in both critically ill and injured children when venous access is not rapidly obtainable. Orlowski et al. performed an animal study to determine the comparative pharmacokinetics of six emergency drugs administered through different routes (central intravenous, PIV, and IO) in randomized sequence. The authors found that the IO route of administration was comparable with the central and peripheral intravenous routes for all of the emergency drugs and solutions studied, and that it is a clinically feasible

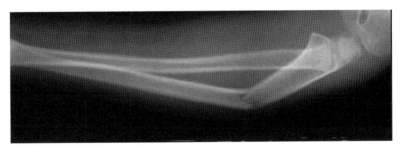

Figure 72-1 Lateral X-ray of the forearm demonstrates a dorsally angulated proximal ulna fracture with a posteriorly dislocated radial head.

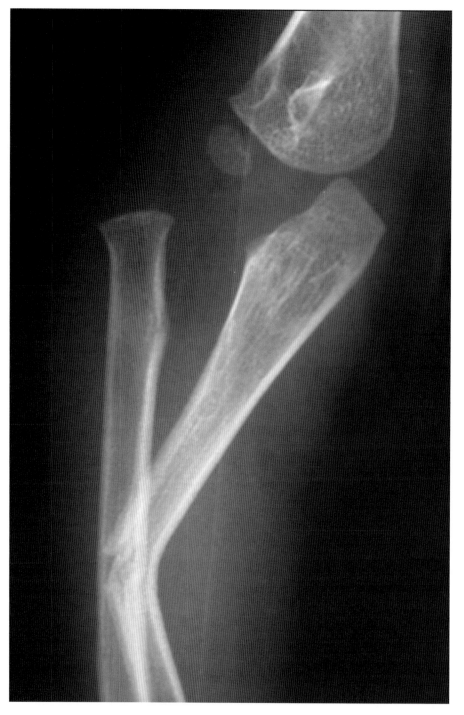

Figure 72-2 AP X-ray of the elbow demonstrates a proximal ulna fracture with a laterally dislocated radial head.

alternative when intravenous access will be critically delayed.

6. **D.** Pediatric diaphyseal femur fracture rates continue to increase, accounting for 1.4% to 1.7% of all pediatric fractures. They are the most common reason for hospitalization in a pediatric patient with orthopedic injury. Treatment of these fractures is largely dependent on patient age: infants, 6 months to 5 years, 5 to 11 years, and patients age 11 to skeletal maturity. The child in our example would likely be treated operatively with flexible intramedullary nails.

The treating physician of a non-ambulatory child <36 months old with a femur fracture has to consider, and rule out, non-accidental trauma as the cause of injury, according to the Academy of Orthopedic

Surgeons clinical guidelines. The recommendation is based on Level II studies, which reported that 14% of femur fractures were the result of child abuse in children aged 0 to 1 year, and 12% in patients aged 0 to 3 years. This evaluation should include a complete history and physical, direct communication with the child's pediatrician or physician, and if available, consultation with a child protective services team. Additionally, a selective skeletal survey should be ordered if felt appropriate by the treating physician.

The true incidence of child abuse and related fractures is likely underestimated as a result of underreporting. The consequences of missing a case of abuse can result in serious complications, including continued abuse or death.

7. A. Rib fractures, especially posteromedial, are concerning for child abuse. Other fracture patterns that are red flags for child abuse are long bone fractures in a non-ambulatory child, scapula fractures, sternal fractures spinous process fractures, and classic metaphyseal fractures are indicative of torsional/traction-shearing strain when an infant's extremity is pulled or twisted violently (corner fractures and bucket handle fractures). With long bone fractures in child abuse, humerus fractures are seen more commonly than tibia, which is more common than femur. The most common presenting lesion overall, however, is a skin lesion.

Distal radius and ulna fractures as well as supracondylar humerus fractures are common injuries in children from falling onto an outstretched arm. Spiral tibial shaft fractures are common in children due to low-energy twisting or falls. Proximal tibia metaphyseal fractures are caused by an impact injury, such as being "double bounced" on a trampoline or going down a slid in the lap of an adult with legs extended.

BIBLIOGRAPHY

Beutel BG. Monteggia fractures in pediatric and adult populations. *Orthopedics*. 2012;35(2):138–144.

Cheng JC, Lam TP, Shen WY. Closed reduction and percutaneous pinning for type III displaced supracondylar fractures of the humerus in children. *J Orthop Trauma*. 1995;9:511–515.

d'Amato C. Pediatric spinal trauma: injuries in very young children. *Clin Orthop Relat Res*. 2005;(432):34–40.

Dormans JP, Squillante R, Sharf H. Acute neurovascular complications with supracondylar humerus fractures in children. *J Hand Surg Am*. 1995;20:1–4.

Eleraky MA, Theodore N, Adams M, et al. Pediatric cervical spine injuries: report of 102 cases and review of the literature. *J Neurosurg*. 2000;92:12–17.

Foran I, Upasani VV, Wallace CD, et al. Acute pediatric monteggia fractures: a conservative approach to stabilization. *J Pediatr Orthop*. 2017;37(6):e335–e3341.

Green NE, Van Zeeland N. Fractures and dislocations about the elbow. In: Green N, Swiontkowski MF, eds. *Skeletal Trauma in Children*. 4th ed. Elsevier; 2009:207–282.

Guy J, Kaley K, Zuspan SJ. Use of intraosseous infusion in the pediatric trauma patient. *J Pediatr Surg*. 1993;28(2):158–161.

Hanlon CR, Estes WL Jr. Fractures in childhood: a statistical analysis. *Am J Surg*. 1954;87:312–323.

Hinton RY, Lincoln A, Crockett MM, et al. Fractures of the femoral shaft in children. Incidence, mechanisms, and sociodemographic risk factors. *J Bone Joint Surg Am*. 1999;81:500–509.

Jones TM, Anderson PA, Noonan KJ. Pediatric cervical spine trauma. *J Am Acad Orthop Surg*. 2011;19:600–611.

Kocher MS, Sink EL, Blasier RD, et al. Treatment of pediatric diaphyseal femur fractures. *J Am Acad Orthop Surg*. 2009;17:718–725.

Lee SL, Sena M, Greenholz SK, et al. A multidisciplinary approach to the development of a cervical spine clearance protocol: process, rationale, and initial results. *J Pediatr Surg*. 2003;38:358–362; discussion 358–362.

Lichtenberg RP. A study of 2,532 fractures in children. *Am J Surg*. 1954;87:330–338.

McCartney D, Hinton A, Heinrich SD. Operative stabilization of pediatric femur fractures. *Orthop Clin North Am*. 1994;25:635–650.

Mohseni S, Talving P, Branco BC, et al. Effect of age on cervical spine injury in pediatric population: a National Trauma Data Bank review. *J Pediatr Surg*. 2011;46:1771–1776.

Orlowski JP, Porembka DT, Gallagher JM, Lockrem JD, VanLente F. Comparison study of intraosseous, central intravenous, and peripheral intravenous infusions of emergency drugs. *Am J Dis Child*. 1990;144(1):112–117.

Osenbach RK, Menezes AH. Pediatric spinal cord and vertebral column injury. *Neurosurgery*. 1992;30:385–390.

Otsuka NY, Kasser JR. Supracondylar fractures of the humerus in children. *J Am Acad Orthop Surg*. 1997;5:19–26.

Rewers A, Hedegaard H, Lezotte D, et al. Childhood femur fractures, associated injuries, and sociodemographic risk factors: a population-based study. *Pediatrics*. 2005;115:e543–e552.

Sahlin Y. Occurrence of fractures in a defined population: a 1-year study. *Injury*. 1990;21:158–160.

Sink EL, Hyman JE, Matheny T, Gerogopoulos G, Kleinman P. Child abuse: the role of the orthopaedic surgeon in nonaccidental trauma. *Clin. Orthop. Relat. Res.* 2011;469(3):790–797.

Skaggs DL. Elbow fractures in children: diagnosis and management. *J Am Acad Orthop Surg*. 1997;5:303–312.

Weisman DS, Frick SL. Ch 44: Problematic pediatric fractures. In: Schmidt A, Teague D eds. *Textbook Orthopaedic Knowledge Update: Trauma 4*. 1st ed. American Academy of Orthopaedic Surgeons; 2010:579–587.

Wilber JH, Thompson GH, Son-Hing J. The multiply injured child. In: Green N, Swiontkowski MF, eds. *Skeletal Trauma in Children*. 4th ed. Elsevier; 2009:57–83.

73

Knee Injuries

Rachel Cuenca and Erin Swan

A 27-year-old healthy male is transported to the emergency department after a motor vehicle crash. He was a restrained driver in a head on collision with another car and was reportedly traveling about 25 mph. His vehicle's airbag deployed and the driver denies a loss of consciousness. The responding medics report he was responsive at the scene and complained of isolated right knee pain with numbness and tingling to his right lower extremity below the knee. A head to toe assessment by the on call trauma team in the emergency department confirms injury is localized to the right lower extremity. Physical examination reveals significant soft tissue swelling around the right knee with deformity but soft and supple leg muscular compartments, a 2-cm bleeding laceration along the anterolateral aspect of the knee, and diffuse numbness of the right foot and lateral leg. Both the dorsalis pedis and posterior tibial pulses are palpable but noticeably weaker compared to his contralateral extremity. His motor examination reveals significant weakness with foot and great toe dorsiflexion but the exam is limited due to pain.

1. **After applying a saline-soaked dressing and ace wrap to the wound, initial management should include which of the following?**

   A. A computerized tomography (CT) scan of his head, abdomen, pelvis, and CT angiography of the right lower extremity

   B. Immediate right leg compartment pressure testing

   C. Immediate portable X-rays of his right hip, knee, and lower extremity

   D. Admit for observation, antibiotics, and serial examinations

   E. Transport to the OR for irrigation, exploration, debridement of the open wound, and other procedures as indicated

2. **Anteroposterior and lateral radiographs are obtained and shown in Figure 73-1. X-rays of the hip, femur, and below the knee are normal. Regarding the neurovascular status of the right lower extremity, which of the following should be the next step in management?**

   A. Immediately transport to the OR for open reduction and vascular repair.

   B. Obtain immediate vascular studies including an angiography.

   C. Conscious sedation followed by closed reduction and reassessment of distal pulses and neurologic exam.

   D. Operative washout of the wound and knee joint reduction followed by ice, elevation, and observation of neurovascular status.

   E. Immediately referral to orthopedic surgery.

3. **Regarding vascular injury associated with knee dislocations, which of the following statements is true?**

   A. The incidence of injury to the popliteal artery is low (<2%).

   B. Vascular repair can be delayed up to 24 hours, after which amputation rates dramatically increase.

   C. Physical exam alone is sufficient in detecting all vascular injuries after knee dislocation.

   D. After reduction and return of pulses, serial examinations at least every 4 to 6 hours for a

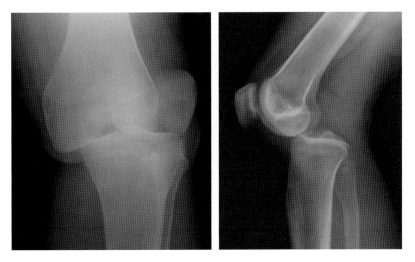

Figure 73-1 AP and Lateral x-rays of a knee demonstrating a knee dislocation

minimum of 48 hours are necessary to monitor for late-developing complications.

E. Easily palpable pulses rule out an arterial injury.

4. **Assuming injury to the popliteal artery is confirmed preoperatively, which statement regarding surgical management is correct?**

A. Vascular repair should be completed followed by splinting.

B. Ligament repair or reconstruction is indicated prior to vascular repair.

C. Vascular repair and management of the open wound should be completed followed by bracing and outpatient rehabilitation of the ligamentous knee injury.

D. Only vascular repair and management of the open wound is needed.

E. Vascular repair and knee reconstruction should occur simultaneously.

5. **Regarding neurovascular injuries associated with knee dislocations, which of the following statements is correct?**

A. The incidence of neurovascular compromise increases proportionately with increasing energy of injury.

B. Delayed recognition of an associated vascular injury significantly increases the chance of poor functional outcomes or limb loss.

C. Neurovascular injury is unlikely in low-energy injuries.

D. The most common neurologic injury associated with knee dislocation is a tibial nerve injury.

E. Neurovascular injuries are more common in non-obese patients.

A 62-year-old female is transported to the emergency department due to injuries incurred as a restrained front seat passenger in a roll-over motor vehicle accident. She has a past medical history significant for type 2 diabetes, hypertension, hyperlipidemia, and hypothyroidism. During the trauma assessment, she is noted to have a pneumothorax, multiple facial contusions, and a closed injury to her right knee. Focused examination of the knee reveals severe soft tissue swelling, mild blistering of the skin over the anterior portion of her knee but no open wounds, and significant diffuse pain with active and passive motion. Her distal neurovascular exam is intact. X-rays of the knee reveal a displaced tibial plateau fracture.

6. **Management of her knee injury should include which of the following?**

A. Urgent surgical treatment with open reduction and internal fixation

B. Urgent definitive surgical treatment with external fixation

C. Long leg casting until bony union

D. Splint versus external fixation until soft tissue swelling resolves followed by open reduction and internal fixation

E. Splint versus knee immobilizer until soft tissue swelling resolves followed by use of a bone stimulator, functional bracing, and physical therapy

7. **Which of the following is the most likely concomitant knee injury?**

    A. Meniscus tear
    B. Ligament tear
    C. Osteochondral or chondral injury to the articular surface
    D. Knee capsule tear

8. **Which of the following factors most strongly predicts an increased risk of leg compartment syndrome in this patient?**

    A. Severity of soft tissue swelling
    B. Integrity of the knee joint capsule
    C. Time since injury
    D. Amount of displacement of the tibial fracture
    E. Tourniquet time during surgery

A 19-year-old male patient presents to the emergency department after sustaining a left knee injury earlier that day playing basketball. He reports a similar injury to this knee a year previously, after which he has had frequent episodes of his knee giving way. Physical examination reveals an effusion and soft tissue swelling about the knee. He has pain but is able to fully flex and extend the knee. X-ray examination of the knee is normal but a magnetic resonance imaging (MRI) scan obtained the next day reveals a complete tear of the anterior cruciate ligament (ACL).

9. **Which of the following physical examination tests is most reliable at diagnosing an ACL tear?**
    A. Anterior drawer test
    B. Lachman test
    C. Pivot shift test
    D. McMurray test
    E. Apley compression test

10. **What is the most likely associated injury with an acute ACL tear?**

    A. Medial collateral ligament tear
    B. Medial meniscus tear
    C. Lateral meniscus tear
    D. Medial patellofemoral ligament tear
    E. Medial joint impaction fracture (bone contusion)

11. **Which of the following should be included in initial management of this patient?**

    A. Narcotic medication for pain control
    B. Urgent reconstructive knee surgery
    C. Referral to physical therapy

    D. Knee immobilization in a brace until swelling is resolved
    E. Referral for a well-fitted ACL brace

12. **Which of the following is the most likely complication of ACL reconstructive surgery?**

    A. Stiffness
    B. Intra-articular infection
    C. Deep venous thrombosis (DVT)
    D. Iatrogenic neurovascular injury
    E. Graft failure

A 64-year-old female presents to the emergency department after falling forward onto her knees. She reports having her right leg caught behind her when she fell onto her right knee, and now has significant pain and edema of her knee. X-rays demonstrate a transverse patella fracture, as demonstrated in Figure 73-2.

13. **Based on this fracture pattern, what physical exam maneuver would you expect this patient to be unable to perform?**

    A. Straight leg raise
    B. Flexion of the knee against resistance
    C. Dorsiflexion of the ankle
    D. Plantarflexion of the ankle
    E. Flexion of the hip

14. **What is the next best step in treatment?**

    A. Long-leg cast and continued non-operative treatment
    B. Hinged knee brace and continued non-operative treatment
    C. Partial patellectomy
    D. Total patellectomy
    E. Open reduction internal fixation

ANSWERS

1. C. The patient has clinical evidence of a knee dislocation. After evaluation and stabilization of the patient, radiographs should be obtained to confirm the diagnosis. Radiographs should not unnecessarily delay the reduction of the knee. Given up to 50% of knee dislocations can undergo a spontaneous reduction prior to radiographs, normal radiographs do not rule out a history of a knee dislocation. Rim fractures, joint asymmetry, avulsion fractures, and mild subluxation of the tibiofemoral joint may be the only radiographic finding. An MRI of the knee

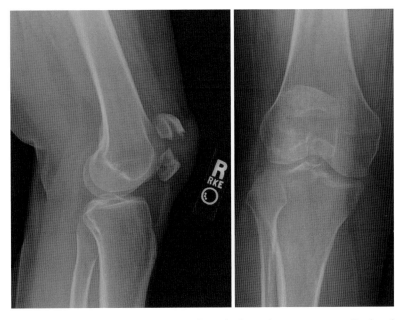

Figure 73-2 Lateral and AP X-rays of a right knee demonstrating a displaced transverse patella fracture.

can be obtained on an elective basis once the patient is acutely stabilized and is the diagnostic imaging modality of choice. The question stem states this is an isolated injury making option A incorrect. Compartment syndrome in a knee dislocation is not uncommon and may be secondary to the initial trauma, hemorrhage, or reperfusion of an ischemic limb.

Option B, a low threshold to measure compartment pressures, is appropriate; however, obtaining radiographs and attempting reduction of the knee are the more appropriate next steps in management. The patient needs further workup before options D or E would be applicable.

2. **C.** The images in Figure 73-1 reveal a posteromedial knee dislocation without obvious fractures. Once a knee dislocation is identified, emergent closed reduction with sedation should be attempted. The reduction maneuver depends on the direction of dislocation and generally involves gentle traction-countertraction. The reduction should be performed as atraumatically as possible with sedation (if needed to avoid further damage). Occasionally the injuries cannot be reduced in a closed fashion. In a posterolateral dislocation, the medial femoral condyle buttonholes through the joint capsule or the medial collateral ligament, causing a puckering of the skin and preventing a closed reduction. If closed reduction fails, the patient is indicated for emergent

surgical reduction. Options A, B, and D are incorrect because a closed reduction has not been attempted. After reduction, the injured knee is frequently unstable and should be placed into a long leg splint (above the knee splint) in approximately 20 degrees of flexion to prevent posterior subluxation of the tibia. A circumferential splint/cast should be avoided to help prevent compartment syndrome. Post-reduction radiographs should be obtained to confirm adequate reduction. After reduction, the vascular assessment should be repeated. Option E, referral to an orthopedic surgeon, is recommended for a knee dislocation; however, reduction should not be needlessly delayed while waiting for a consultation.

3. **D.** Vascular injuries associated with fractures/dislocations are relatively uncommon, but there is a strong association with posterior knee dislocations and popliteal artery/vein injuries. Option A, the rate of popliteal artery injury, has been reported to range from 14% to 65%. Multiple algorithms have been published for assessment of the vascular status of the lower extremity in the incidence of suspected knee dislocation. Initially, a physical exam should be performed assessing both posterior tibial and dorsalis pedis pulses in comparison to the contralateral extremity. Options C and E, normal pulses, do not "rule out" a vascular injury. In the presence of "hard signs" of ischemia (cool, pulseless, obviously

dysvascular extremity) vascular surgery consultation should be obtained immediately. However, when a patient presents with "soft signs" of ischemia (asymmetric pulses and/or warmth), further assessment is warranted. Measurement of the ankle-brachial index (ABI) can augment the physical exam. An ABI >/= 0.9 is reassuring that there is no clinically significant vascular injury. However, choice D is correct because delayed thrombus is a continued risk, making reassessment every 4 to 6 hours important. If the ABI is abnormal, further studies are indicated. Either an arterial ultrasound, which is technician dependent and may not always be available, or CT angiography versus conventional angiography should be completed. Emergent vascular repair is indicated if a significant injury is identified, with the (B) amputation rate as high as 86% in cases where vascular repair was delayed greater than 8 hours.

4. **E.** If a vascular injury is identified both vascular and orthopedic surgery should be urgently consulted. The key to this question is that both teams will need to work simultaneously in stabilizing and restoring blood flow to the lower extremity. Options A and C are incorrect because vascular repair without stabilizing the leg will likely fail. Option B is incorrect because restoring vascular flow to the leg is the first priority and should be done within 8 hours and option D is incorrect because reconstructive knee surgery will be needed to protect the vascular repair and regain functional range of motion in the short term as well as to prevent long-term knee instability.

5. **B.** Multiple series have demonstrated that suboptimal functional outcomes and even amputation can result when there is delayed recognition of an associated injury to the popliteal vessels, and all knee dislocations should be assumed to have a vascular injury until it has been ruled out. Several studies have also demonstrated an increased incidence of these injuries among obese patients versus nonobese. Options A and C are incorrect because in a review of low energy dislocations, 41% were found to have a vascular injury. This is comparable to the vascular injury rates of cohorts with combined (low and high energy and high energy injuries). The most commonly injured nerve in a knee dislocation is the peroneal nerve, not the (D) tibial nerve. Neurologic injury occurs in 16% to 40% of knee dislocations. Less than 50% of patients with peroneal nerve injuries have nerve recovery.

6. **D.** Displaced tibial plateau fractures greater than 0.5 to 1 cm are managed with operative reduction and fixation (options C and E). Protected mobilization can be used for fractures that are non- to minimally displaced with a stable ligamentous exam. High-energy injuries can lead to severe injury to the overlying soft tissue as demonstrated by swelling and fracture blisters. Bicondylar fractures, fracture-dislocations, and shaft dissociated fractures have worse soft tissue injury. Definitive surgical reduction and treatment should be delayed in high-energy injuries until the soft tissue envelope allows (option A). In high energy trauma, it may take 8 to 21 days for the swelling to subside and skin conditions to improve. Interval treatment can range from a well applied splint to *temporary* spanning external fixation. The goal is to maintain length and alignment until definitive fixation can be preformed and post-reduction radiographs should be obtained. Rarely are closed injuries treated definitively with external fixation, making option B incorrect. Traction radiographs and post reduction CT scan can be helpful in evaluation and planning of treatment. Even with staged management of these fractures, infection rates still range from 8.4% to 18%.

7. **B.** Regarding option A, meniscal tears occur in up to 50% of plateau fractures, but ligamentous injuries can occur in up to 77% of fractures. Options C and D are incorrect because capsular tears and chondral injury can both be present as part of the injury pattern but are less common. Segond fractures (avulsion fracture off the lateral tibia that is pathopneumonic for an ACL tear), reverse. Segond fractures (avulsion fracture off the medial tibia that indicates an MCL avulsion), anteromedial tibial margin fractures, and semimembranosus tendon insertion site fractures are all evidence of ligamentous or tendon injuries associated with tibial plateau fractures.

8. **D.** The rate of compartment syndrome in tibial plateau fractures is 10% to 15%. Presenting symptoms include pain out of proportion to injury, swelling, pain on passive stretching, pallor, absence of pulses, hyperesthesia, and motor weakness. The external physical appearance can be unreliable (option A) and the presenting symptoms of pain out of proportion to injury, pain on passive stretching, pallor, absence of pulses, hyperesthesia, and motor weakness should be used to evaluate. If the patient is obtunded and such exam findings are unable to be assessed, the compartment pressures should be measured. The

amount of displacement (correct option D) as well as a higher Shatzker or OA/OTA classification are associated with increased risk of compartment syndrome. Repeat examination of the leg for compartment syndrome should be continued at regular intervals because it can occur 24 hours or more after injury (option C).

Table 73-1 Schatzker Classification of Tibial Plateau Fractures

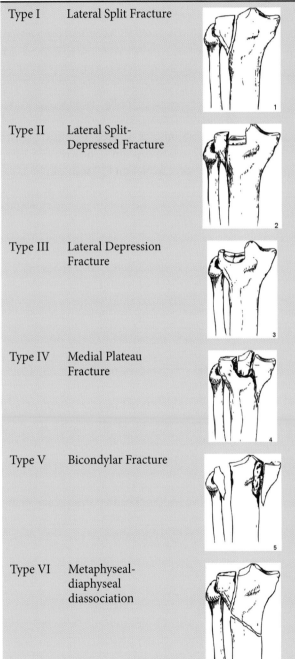

Type I	Lateral Split Fracture
Type II	Lateral Split-Depressed Fracture
Type III	Lateral Depression Fracture
Type IV	Medial Plateau Fracture
Type V	Bicondylar Fracture
Type VI	Metaphyseal-diaphyseal diassociation

9. **B.** The Lachman test is the most sensitive physical exam maneuver to test for ACL laxity. The knee is placed in 20 to 30 degrees of flexion, the femur is stabilized, and an anteriorly directed force is applied to the tibia. The examiner should estimate the distance of translation as well as whether there is an endpoint or not. The pivot shift test and anterior drawer test (options A and C) are other physical examination maneuvers testing the ACL; however, they are not as reliable as the Lachman exam. The McMurray test (option D) and Apley compression test (option E) are a part of physical examinations evaluating the meniscus, not the ACL.

10. **C.** Meniscal tears are the most common associated injury seen with an ACL tear. They occur in 65% to 75% of patients. Lateral meniscal tears are more common in acute ACL injuries. Option B is incorrect because medial meniscus tears are more frequently seen in chronic injuries but less prevalent in acute injuries. Bone bruises or trabecular microfractures (option E) occur in just over half the patient with an ACL injury; however, these are typically located along the lateral femoral condyle and the posterolateral proximal tibia. These so-called pivot-shift contusions are a result of the subluxation and spontaneous reduction of the knee joint that occurs during an injury that leads to knee ligament disruption. Approximately 33% of patients with an ACL tear will have at least one additional ligament injured. Regarding option A, the medial collateral ligament is injured in about 7% of patient with an ACL injury. Medial patellofemoral ligament tears (option D) are associated with acute patellar dislocations, not ACL tears.

11. **C.** The initial treatment for a suspected ACL tear includes pain control, MRI, and physical therapy for mobilization. Pain control with NSAIDS is preferred. Option D is incorrect because prolonged immobilization should be avoided as it may lead to arthrofibrosis. Regarding choice E, the use of an ACL brace continues to be controversial and has become an individualized and optional part of the treatment plan. Patients should be referred to an orthopedic surgeon for counseling of treatment options, but not all patients require surgical repair (option B). The ideal candidate for surgical reconstruction is the patient with an acute ACL deficiency and an active lifestyle as well as one with a chronic injury and functional instability with normal daily activities.

12. A. Stiffness following ACL reconstruction, called arthrofibrosis, is the most common complication after surgical reconstruction. It is likely related to inflammation affecting the synovial lining leading to thickening of the capsule and loss of the normal space within the joint. Proper surgical technique and rehabilitation can help reduced the risk of joint stiffness. Loss of extension is reported to be as high as 59% in some populations and other complications are rare. Graft failure occurs and varies with different populations and different graft types. It ranges from 2% to 5%. The rate of deep venous thrombosis (option C) is approximately 1% to 1.5%, iatrogenic neurovascular injury (option D) incidence is about 1%, and postoperative intra-articular infection (option B) has been reported as low as 0.3% in a large cohort.

13. A. The quadriceps tendon and fascia lata attach to the anterosuperior margin of the patella. The patellar tendon attaches to the inferior margin of the patella. Together, these comprise the knee's extensor mechanism. To test the patient's extensor mechanism, have the patient perform a straight leg raise. They will be unable to do it and an extensor lag will be evident if the extensor mechanism is not intact. In this fracture pattern, the complete transverse fracture with that amount of displacement indicates that the extensor mechanism is not intact, as there is not continuity through the patella. In less displaced fractures where it is not clear from the fracture pattern if the extensor mechanism is intact or not, the patient may be hesitant to perform a straight leg raise secondary to pain. In these cases, the hemarthrosis can be aspirated and local anaesthetic can be injected into the joint in order to provide pain relief and thus encourage better patient participation in the exam.

14. E. Indications for operative fixation of a patella fracture are extensor mechanism failure, open fractures, displaced patella fracture >3 mm, and fracture articular displacement >2 mm. Due to the significant amount of displacement of this fracture, it cannot be treated nonoperatively (options A and B). In cases where there is significant comminution that is not amenable to fixation, parts or the whole of the patella can be excised (a patellectomy) and the tendon can be advanced and repaired back down to preserve the patient's extensor mechanism (options C and D). As a whole, the goal is to preserve the patella whenever possible. In this case, the patient has a fracture pattern that is amendable to open reduction internal fixation (option E).

BIBLIOGRAPHY

Alberty RE, Goodfried G, Boyden AM. Popliteal artery injury with fractural dislocation of the knee. *Am J Surg.* 1981;142:36–40.

Almekinders LC, Logan TC. Results following treatment of traumatic dislocations of the knee joint. *Clin Orthop Relat Res.* 1992;284:203–207.

Andrews JR, Tedder JL, Godbout BP. Bicondylar tibial plateau fracture complicated by compartment syndrome. *Orthop Rev.* 1992;21:317–319.

Anglen JO, Aleto T. Temporary transarticular external fixation of the knee and ankle. *J Orthop Trauma.* 1998;12:431–434.

Azar FM, Brandt JC, Miller RH 3rd, Phillips BB. Ultra-low-velocity knee dislocations. *Am J Sports Med.* 2011;39:2170–2174.

Baer PA, Tenenbaum J, Fam AG, Little H. Coexistent septic and crystal arthritis. Report of four cases and literature review. *J Rheumatol.* 1986;13;604–607.

Bardin T. Gonococcal arthritis. *Best Pract Res Clin Rheumatol.* 2003;17;201–208.

Barei DP, Nork SE, Mills WJ, Henley MB, Benirschke SK. Complications associated with internal fixation of high-energy bicondylar tibial plateau fractures utilizing a two-incision technique. *J Orthop Trauma.* 2004;18;649–657.

Berkson EM, Virkus WW. High-energy tibial plateau fractures. *J Am Acad Orthop Surg.* 2006;14:20–31.

Bonnaig NS, Casstevens C, Archdeacon MT, et al. Fix it or discard it? A retrospective analysis of functional outcomes after surgically treated patella fractures comparing ORIF with partial patellectomy. *J Orthop Trauma.* 2015;29(2):80–84.

Boring TH, O'Donoghue DH. Acute patellar dislocation: results of immediate surgical repair. *Clin Orthop Relat Res.* 1978;136:182–185.

Brogadir SP, Schimmer BM, Myers RA. Spectrum of the gonococcal arthritis-dermatitis syndrome. *Semin Arthritis Rheum.* 1979;8:177–183.

Canadian Orthopaedic Trauma Society. Open reduction and internal fixation compared with circular fixator application for bicondylar tibial plateau fractures. Results of a multicenter, prospective, randomized clinical trial. *J Bone Joint Surg Am.* 2006;88(12):2613–2623.

Cash JD, Hughston JC. Treatment of acute patellar dislocation. *Am J Sports Med.* 1988;16:244–249.

Chan KK, Resnick D, Goodwin D, Seeger LL. Posteromedial tibial plateau injury Including avulsion fracture of the semimembranous tendon insertion site: ancillary sign of anterior cruciate ligament tear at MR imaging. *Radiology.* 1999;211:754–758.

Chang YH, Tu YK, Yeh WL, Hsu RW. Tibial plateau fracture with compartment syndrome: a complication of higher incidence in Taiwan. *Chang Gung Med J.* 2000;23: 149–155.

Cohen AP, King D, Gibbon AJ. Impingement fracture of the anteromedial tibial margin: a radiographic sign of combined posterolateral complex and posterior cruciate ligament disruption. *Skeletal Radiol.* 2001;30:114–116.

Cosgarea AJ, DeHaven KE, Lovelock JE The surgical treatment of arthrofibrosis of the knee. *Am J Sports Med.* 1994;22:184–191.

Cullison TR, Muldoon MP, Gorman JD, Goff WB. The incidence of deep venous thrombosis in anterior cruciate ligament reconstruction. *Arthroscopy.* 1996;12:657–659.

Egol KA, Tejwani NC, Capla EL, Wolinsky PL, Koval KJ. Staged management of high-energy proximal tibia fractures ota types 41: the results of a prospective, standardized protocol. *J Orthop Trauma.* 2005;19:448–455; discussion 56.

Fanelli GC, Stannard JP, Stuart MJ, et al. Management of complex knee ligament injuries. *J Bone Joint Surg Am.* 2010;92:2235–2246.

Freed JF, Nies KM, Boyer RS, Louie JS. Acute monoarticular arthritis. A diagnostic approach. *JAMA.* 1980;243: 2314–2316.

Freedman KB, D'Amato MJ, Nedeff DD, Kaz A, Bach BR Jr Arthroscopic anterior cruciate ligament reconstruction: a metaanalysis comparing patellar tendon and hamstring tendon autografts. *Am J Sports Med.* 2003;31:2–11.

Gable DR, Allen JW, Richardson JD. Blunt popliteal artery injury: is physical examination alone enough for evaluation? *J Trauma.* 1997;43:541–544.

Gardner MJ, Yacoubian S, Geller D, et al. The incidence of soft tissue injury in operative tibial plateau fractures: a magnetic resonance imaging analysis of 103 patients. *J Orthop Trauma.* 2005;19:79–84.

Goldenberg DL, Cohen AS. Acute infectious arthritis. A review of patients with nongonococcal joint infections with emphasis on therapy and prognosis. *Am J Med.* 1976;60:36–77.

Green NE, Allen BL. Vascular injuries associated with dislocation of the knee. *J Bone Joint Surg Am.* 1977;59:236–239.

Greis PE, Bardana DD, Holmstrom MC, Burks RT. Meniscal injury: I. basic science and evaluation. *J Am Acad Orthop Surg.* 2002;10:168–176.

Gupta MN, Sturrock RD, Field M. A prospective 2-year study of 75 patients with adult-onset septic arthritis. *Rheumatology Oxford.* 2001;40:24–30.

Heckman JD, Tornetta P. *Rockwood and Green's fracture in Adults.* Vol. 2. Lippincott Williams & Wilkins; 2010.

Holmes KK, Weisner PJ, Pedersen AH. The gonococcal arthritis-dermatitis syndrome. *Ann Intern Med.* 1971;75: 470–471.

Hoover NW. Injuries of the popliteal artery associated with fractures and dislocations. *Surg Clin North Am.* 1961;41:1099–1112.

Hughes JG, Vetter EA, Patel R, et al. Culture with bactec peds plus/f bottle compared with conventional methods for detection of bacteria in synovial fluid. *J Clin Microbiol.* 2001;39:4468–4471.

Johnson ME, Foster L, DeLee JC. Neurologic and vascular injuries associated with knee ligament injuries. *Am J Sports Med.* 2008;36:2448–2462.

Jones RE, Smith EC, Bone GE. Vascular and orthopedic complications of knee dislocation. *Surg Gynecol Obstet.* 1979;149:554–558.

Koval KJ, Helfet DL. Tibial plateau fractures: evaluation and treatment. *J Am Acad Orthop Surg.* 1995;3:86–94.

LaPrade RF, Wentorf FA, Fritts H, Gundry C, Hightower CD. A prospective magnetic resonance imaging study of the incidence of posterolateral and multiple ligament injuries in acute knee injuries presenting with a hemarthrosis. *Arthroscopy.* 2007;23:1341–1347.

Larson RL, Tailon M. Anterior cruciate ligament insufficiency: principles of treatment. *J Am Acad Orthop Surg.* 1994;2:26–35.

Levy BA, Zlowodzki MP, Graves M, Cole PA. Screening for extermity arterial injury with the arterial pressure index. *Am J Emerg Med.* 2005;23:689–695.

Magnussen RA, Carey JL, Spindler KP. Does operative fixation of an osteochondritis dissecans loose body result in healing and long-term maintenance of knee function? *Am J Sports Med.* 2009;37:754–759.

Manshady BM, Thompson GR, Weiss JJ. Septic arthritis in a general hospital 1966–1977. *J Rheumatol.* 1980;7:523–530.

Margaretten ME, Kohlwes J, Moore D, Bent S. Does this adult patient have septic arthritis? *JAMA.* 2007;297:1478–1488.

Mathews CJ, Kingsley G, Field M, Jones A, Weston VC, Phillips M, et al. Management of septic arthritis: a systematic review. *Postgrad Med J.* 2008;84:265–270.

Mathews CJ, Weston VC, Jones A, Field M, Coakley G. Bacterial septic arthritis in adults. *Lancet.* 2010;375:846–855.

McCutchan JD, Gillham NR. Injury to the popliteal artery associated with dislocation of the knee: palpable distal pulses do not negate the requirement for arteriography. *Injury.* 1989;20:307–310.

McDonough EBJr., Wojtys EM. Multiligamentous injuries of the knee and associated vascular injuries. *Am J Sports Med.* 2009;37:156–159.

Melvin JS, Mehta S. Patellar fractures in adult. *J Am Acad Orthop Surg.* 2011;19(4):198–207.

Miller MD, Thompson SR, Hart JA. *Review of Orthopedics.* Elsevier Saunders; 2012.

Mills WJ, Barei DP, McNair P. The value of the ankle-brachial index for diagnosing arterial injury after knee dislocation: a prospective study. *J Trauma.* 2004;56:1261–1265.

Niall DM, Nutton RW, Keating JF. Palsy of the common peroneal nerve after traumatic dislocation of the knee. *J Bone Joint Surg Br.* 2005;87:664–667.

Nomura E. Inoue M. Cartilage lesions of the patella in recurrent patellar dislocation. *Am J Sports Med.* 2004;32:498–502.

O'Brien JP, Goldenberg DL, Rice PA. Disseminated gonococcal infection: a prospective analysis of 49 patients and a review of pathophysiology and immune mechanisms. *Medicine Baltimore.* 1983;62:395–406.

Petsche TS, Hutchinson MR. Loss of extension after reconstruction of the anterior cruciate ligament. *J Am Acad Orthop Surg.* 1999;7:119–127.

Pierce TP, Kurowicki J, Kelly JJ, et al. Risk factors for requiring a revision anterior cruciate ligament reconstruction: a case-control study. *J Knee Surg.* 2021;34(8):859–863.

Prodromos CC, Fu FH, Howell SM, Johnson DH, Lawhorn K. Controversies in soft-tissue anterior cruciate ligament reconstruction: grafts, bundles, tunnels, fixation, and harvest. *J Am Acad Orthop Surg.* 2008;16:376–384.

Reckling FW, Peltier LF. Acute knee dislocations and their complications. *J Trauma.* 1969;9:181–191.

Rice PA. Gonococcal arthritis disseminated gonococcal infection. *Infect Dis Clin North Am.* 2005;19:853–861.

Rihn JA, Groff YJ, Harner CD, Cha PS. The acutely dislocated knee: evaluation and management. *J Am Acad Orthop Surg.* 2004;12:334–346.

Sallay PI, Poggi J, Speer KP, Garrett WE. Acute dislocation of the patella. A correlative pathoanatomic study. *Am J Sports Med.* 1996;24:52–60.

Shah SN, Karunakar MA. Early wound complications after operative treatment of high energy tibial plateau fractures through two incisions. *Bull NYU Hosp Jt Dis.* 2007;65:115–119.

Sisto DJ, Warren RF. Complete knee dislocation. A follow-up study of operative treatment. *Clin Orthop Relat Res.* 1985;198:94–101.

Swan A, Amer H, Dieppe P. The value of synovial fluid assays in the diagnosis of joint disease: a literature survey. *Ann Rheum Dis.* 2002;61:493–498.

Tjoumakaris FP, Forsythe B, Bradley JP. Patellofemoral instability in athletes: treatment via modified fulkerson osteotomy and lateral release. *Am J Sports Med.* 2010;38:992–999.

Warren RF, Levy IM. Meniscal lesions associated with anterior cruciate ligament injury. *Clin Orthop Relat Res.* 1983;32–37.

Wascher DC. High-velocity knee dislocation with vascular injury. Treatment principles. *Clin Sports Med.* 2000;19:457–477.

Wascher DC, Dvirnak PC, DeCoster TA. Knee dislocation: initial assessment and implications for treatment. *J Orthop Trauma.* 1997;11:525–529.

Welling RE, Kakkasseril J, Cranley JJ. Complete dislocations of the knee with popliteal vascular injury. *J Trauma.* 1981;21:450–453.

Widner M, Dunleavy M, Lynch S. Outcomes following ACL reconstruction based on graft type: are all grafts equivalent? *Curr Rev Musculoskelet Med.* 2019;12(4):460–465.

Williams RJ 3rd, Laurencin CT, Warren RF, Speciale AC, Brause BD, O Brien S. Septic arthritis after arthroscopic anterior cruciate ligament reconstruction. *Diagnosis and management. Am J Sports Med.* 1997;25:261–267.

Yagupsky P, Peled N, Press J. Use of bactec 9240 blood culture system for detection of brucella melitensis in synovial fluid. *J Clin Microbiol.* 2001;39:738–739.

Yagupsky P, Press J. Use of the isolator 1.5 microbial tube for culture of synovial fluid from patients with septic arthritis. *J Clin Microbiol.* 1997;35:2410–2412.

Ziran BH, Becher SJ. Radiographic predictors of compartment syndrome in tibial plateau fractures. *J Orthop Trauma.* 2013;27:612–615.

TRANSPLANT SURGERY

74

Transplant Surgery—Kidney

Joy Sarkar

SCENARIO 1

A 61-year-old female patient with insulin-dependent diabetes mellitus who has recently progressed from Stage IV chronic kidney disease to end-stage renal disease (ESRD) presents for evaluation for kidney transplantation.

1. **Which of the following is true regarding the pre-transplant evaluation process?**

   A. HIV positivity is a contraindication.
   B. Crossmatch testing is used to identify the presence of preformed antibody in the donor's serum that is directed against antigens in the recipient.
   C. Potential recipients with low calculated panel of reactive antibody are anticipated to have a higher risk of graft loss.
   D. A positive complement-dependent cytotoxic (CDC) crossmatch is a contraindication.
   E. Patients become a candidate for kidney transplantation once dialysis therapy begins.

A suitable cadaveric donor is found, and the patient undergoes kidney transplantation; the immediate postoperative course is uncomplicated. Ten days later, the patient presents with an abrupt decrease in urine output, creatinine elevation to 1.5 mg/dL, and has graft tenderness on exam. A fever of 100.9°F is noted.

2. **Which of the following is true about the initial management of this patient's oliguria and elevated serum creatinine?**

   A. Renal biopsy should first be performed.
   B. Doppler ultrasound should be performed.
   C. The dose of cyclosporine should be increased.
   D. Angiography is indicated to evaluate the vascular supply to the graft.
   E. The patient should be promptly taken back to the operating room to salvage the graft.

Cyclosporine levels are drawn on the previous patient and found to be at therapeutic levels. A Doppler ultrasound is obtained and shows arterial and vascular flow with no perinephric fluid collection. Subsequently, a percutaneous biopsy of the graft shows lymphocytes within the renal tubules and vascular endothelium. Immunophenotyping of the biopsy demonstrates T-cell preponderance.

3. **Which of the following is true regarding the postoperative complication experienced by this patient?**

   A. This complication is likely related to a clerical error during the pre-transplant crossmatch.
   B. The treatment involves decreasing immunosuppressive therapy.
   C. Management consists of pulse corticosteroids and changing maintenance therapy from cyclosporine to tacrolimus.
   D. Risk factors for this complication include perioperative hypovolemia, ischemia-reperfusion injury, and the use of an extended-criteria donor.
   E. This viral infection was likely transmitted via leukocytes within the donor.

4. **Which of the following is correct regarding post-renal transplant technical complications?**

A. Renal artery thrombosis in the early postoperative period should be urgently treated with heparin infusion and angioplasty.

B. Renal vein thrombosis may manifest with hematuria in the first week following transplantation.

C. On Doppler ultrasound, identification of a round, sonolucent, septated mass medial to the renal allograft is most consistent with a urine leak.

D. Initial management of a lymphocele involves intra-peritoneal marsupialization

E. Presence of multiple strictures in the transplanted ureter during the early post-operative period is associated with polyoma BK viral infection.

SCENARIO 2

A 68-year-old man who received a living-donor kidney transplant 2 years ago presents for routine follow-up. He has been doing well on maintenance therapy consisting of tacrolimus, prednisone, and mycophenolate, and has no complaints. On exam, he is noted to have a blood pressure of 168/82. Labs are drawn, and are notable for potassium of 5.4 mEq/L, and serum creatinine of 1.65 mg/dL. His blood pressure, potassium level, and serum creatinine were all within normal limits at his last follow-up visit. Tacrolimus trough levels are within the target range. A renal allograft Doppler ultrasound is performed and shows no evidence of ureteral obstruction or renal artery stenosis. A biopsy of the allograft is performed, and demonstrates areas of interstitial fibrosis and obliterative arteriolopathy, without evidence of lymphocytic infiltration or C4d staining.

5. **Based on the workup already done, the next best step in this patient's management is:**

A. Start lisinopril

B. Discontinue mycophenolate and change to azathioprine

C. Pulse high-dose IV glucocorticoids

D. Plasmapheresis followed by intravenous immunoglobulin (IVIG)

E. Reduce tacrolimus dosing by 25%

6. **Regarding the mechanism and use of various immunosuppressive agents, which of the following is correct?**

A. Cyclosporine binds cyclophilin protein and blocks IL-2 production.

B. Azathioprine binds antigens on T cells, causing altered T cell function as well as T cell depletion.

C. Rituximab binds to FK binding protein, and is used in maintenance immunosuppression.

D. Sirolimus inhibits the function of NF-κB, diminishing the response to cytokines.

E. ATGAM binds to CD20, leading to initial cytokine release followed by B-cell depletion.

7. **With regard to complications arising from prolonged immunosuppression, which of the following is correct?**

A. The most common malignancy associated with post-transplantation immunosuppression is lymphoma.

B. Mycophenolate mofetil and azathioprine are associated with diarrhea and leukopenia.

C. Antithymocyte globulin is associated with gingival hyperplasia and hirsutism.

D. Post-transplant activation of cytomegalovirus (CMV) occurs most commonly in patients who tested seropositive for CMV IgG preoperatively.

E. Sirolimus is associated with nephrotoxicity.

ANSWERS

1. **D.** Evaluation of a potential kidney transplant recipient involves a thorough history and physical examination, evaluation of kidney function and comorbidities, and histocompatibility testing. Transplantation is indicated when kidney failure is determined to be irreversible. While chronic dialysis therapy or a GFR ≤ 20 ml/min are criteria for being waitlisted for a cadaveric organ, these are not prerequisites for undergoing kidney transplantation if a suitable living donor is available. In fact, patient and graft survival are improved when transplantation is performed prior to the patient requiring dialysis therapy.

Contraindications to kidney transplantation include active infection, active malignancy, active substance abuse, uncontrolled psychiatric disease, or treatment noncompliance. Controlled HIV is not an absolute contraindication to kidney transplantation, as long as the viral load is undetectable and the CD4 count is ≥200 cells/μL.

The purpose of histocompatibility testing is to identify mismatches between the human leukocyte antigens (HLAs) of potential donors and recipients, which can cause antibody-mediated rejection, such as hyperacute rejection. In general terms, this testing consists of two portions: screening potential recipients for anti-HLA antibodies, and a final crossmatch between a potential donor and recipient pair to identify any donor-specific antibodies (DSA) in the recipient's serum. The calculated panel reactive antibody (cPRA) estimates the percentage of donors who will be crossmatch incompatible with the recipient, and is calculated from the results of the HLA-specific antibodies screening. Patients with a high cPRA wait significantly longer for a compatible organ, and have a higher risk of graft loss once transplanted. A positive complement-dependent cytotoxic (CDC) crossmatch indicates high burden of donor-specific antibodies in the recipient, and is a contraindication to transplantation.

2. **B.** Post-transplant oliguria with elevated creatinine has multiple possible etiologies to include hypovolemia, urinary catheter occlusion, calcineurin inhibitor (tacrolimus, pimecrolimus, or cyclosporine) toxicity, viral infection, delayed graft function, hyperacute or acute rejection, renal artery thrombosis, renal vein thrombosis, urine leak, or ureteral obstruction (e.g., by stricture or lymphocele). The most frequent cause of an elevated creatinine-level post-transplant is calcineurin inhibitor toxicity. After this is ruled out, the next step is to evaluate blood flow and rule out structural problems with Doppler ultrasound. If the ultrasound is normal, it is then appropriate to perform a renal biopsy, which can differentiate rejection, post-transplant lymphoproliferative disorder (PTLD), and acute tubular necrosis (ATN), among other diagnoses. If arterial/venous thrombosis, arterial stenosis, or aneurysm is seen on the ultrasound, angiography is then indicated to confirm the diagnosis. If no blood flow is seen to the transplanted kidney on ultrasound or a nuclear medicine renal scan, then re-exploration is indicated.

3. **C.** T-lymphocytes within the renal tubules and vascular endothelium are characteristic of acute cell-mediated rejection. Each rejection episode decreases the long-term function of the graft, and should be treated with pulse corticosteroids. Also, if the episode of rejection occurred on therapeutic calcineurin inhibitor levels, the maintenance therapy should be changed. In contrast, hyperacute rejection occurs within minutes to hours of reperfusion, manifests with rapid mottling and often graft rupture, and is mediated by preformed anti-HLA antibodies due to ABO incompatibility. Hyperacute rejection is rare due to pre-transplant crossmatching, and is usually due to clerical error. PTLD is associated with EBV, and can be differentiated from acute rejection on biopsy by the preponderance of B lymphocytes; treatment is to decrease immunosuppression. Acute tubular necrosis (ATN) may cause oliguria and elevated creatinine, and risk factors include hypovolemia, reperfusion injury, and use of an extended-criteria donor. Biopsy would show injury of tubular cells and casts within the tubule lumen. CMV infection may be transmitted within donor leukocytes and also can cause oliguria with creatinine elevation; treatment is with ganciclovir. On biopsy, intranuclear or cytoplasmic inclusions are characteristic of viral infections including CMV.

4. **B.** Renal artery thrombosis is a rare complication occurring in 1% of cases, and necessitates return to the operating room for urgent exploration. New onset hematuria may be the first sign of a renal vein thrombosis. Lymphoceles are the result of intraoperative lymphatic disruption and are identifiable on ultrasound as a round, multiseptated mass medial to the graft that may compress the ureter. It is differentiated from urine leak sonographically in that a urine leak would be a nonseptated fluid collection in the pelvis. A lymphocele is initially managed with percutaneous drainage; creation of a peritoneal window can be helpful for drainage if percutaneous drainage does not resolve symptoms. Presence of multiple ureteral strictures in the *late* postoperative period may be due to polyoma BK virus, but early ureteral stenosis is usually due to ischemia or extrinsic compression.

5. **E.** The differential diagnosis of elevated serum creatinine and hypertension occurring in the late post-transplant period includes rejection (both acute and chronic), calcineurin inhibitor (CNI) nephrotoxicity, recurrent primary disease, renal artery stenosis, urinary obstruction, and infections, among other causes. The workup of elevated creatinine is discussed earlier in the answer to question 2, and includes assessment of patient compliance with maintenance therapy, measurement of CNI levels, Doppler ultrasound of the allograft, evaluation for donor-specific antibodies, and, in appropriate cases, biopsy of the allograft. This patient's graft biopsy,

which shows arteriolopathy, fibrosis, and no evidence of lymphocytic infiltration or antibody-mediated process (negative for C4d staining), is suggestive of cyclosporine-mediated nephrotoxicity. CNI nephrotoxicity may occur even in the setting of trough CNI levels in the target range, because local drug levels in the kidney may be higher than in the blood. Appropriate approaches to suspected CNI nephrotoxicity include decreasing the dose or changing to an alternative agent; for example, an mTOR inhibitor such as sirolimus. Administration of a calcium channel blocker may also mediate CNI-induced renal vasoconstriction, and improve renal function and hypertension. In this patient with an elevated serum potassium, an ACE inhibitor such as lisinopril is not the best option, as it may worsen hyperkalemia. Pulse glucocorticoids, plasmapheresis, and IVIG are treatments for acute rejection. The most common reason for discontinuation of mycophenolate mofetil is GI disturbance, such as diarrhea.

6. **A.** Cyclosporine is a calcineurin inhibitor, which functions by binding cyclophilin protein and blocking IL-2 production. Azathioprine functions by converting 6-mercaptopurine to 6-thioinosine-5′-monophosphate, which interferes with DNA and purine synthesis; T-cell antigens are bound and blocked by antilymphocyte globulins such as ATGAM, as well as OKT-3 and several monoclonal antibodies (e.g., basiliximab and dacluzimab). Rituximab binds to CD20 on B cells, causing depletion; tacrolimus and sirolimus (a.k.a. rapamycin) both bind FK binding protein. Corticosteroids bind a nuclear receptor, inhibiting NF-κB and blocking T-cell activation.

7. **B.** Immunosuppression is associated with both drug-specific toxicity as well as susceptibility to infections and malignancy. The most common malignancy associated with post-transplant immunosuppression is skin cancer, specifically squamous cell carcinoma. Post-transplant activation of CMV actually occurs most commonly in patients who tested sero-negative for CMV preoperatively and received a graft from a CMV-seropositive donor. Mycophenolate mofetil and azathioprine are both antiproliferative agents with associated GI toxicity and leukopenia. Antithymocyte globulin is associated with cytokine release syndrome, leukopenia, and serum sickness. Gingival hyperplasia and hirsutism are both associated with cyclosporine. Like cyclosporine, tacrolimus is a calcineurin inhibitor associated with nephrotoxicity, but sirolimus is not, and tacrolimus is more strongly associated with post-transplant diabetes than sirolimus.

BIBLIOGRAPHY

Adams AB, Kirk AD, Larsen CP. Transplantation immunobiology and immunosuppression. In: Townsend CM, Beauchamp D, Evers BM, et al., eds. *Sabiston Textbook of Surgery: The Biological Basis of Modern Surgical Practice*. 19th ed. Elsevier; 2012:617–654.

Becker Y. Kidney and pancreas transplantation. In: Townsend CM, Beauchamp D, Evers BM, et al., eds. *Sabiston Textbook of Surgery: The Biological Basis of Modern Surgical Practice*. 19th ed. Elsevier; 2012:666–681.

Bunnapradist S, Danovitch GM. Evaluation of adult kidney transplant candidates. *Am J Kidney Dis*. 2007;50:890.

Danovitch GM, ed. *Handbook of Kidney Transplantation*. 5th ed. Lippincott Williams & Wilkins; 2009:198–216.

Freise C, Stock P. Renal transplantation. In: Mulholland MW, Lillemoe KD, Doherty GM, et al., eds. *Greenfield's Surgery: Scientific Principles and Practice*. 5th ed. Lippincott Williams & Wilkins; 2011:531–541.

Naesens M, Kuypers DRJ, Sarwal M. Calcineurin inhibitor nephrotoxicity. *CJASN*. 2009;4(2):481–508.

Patel R, Terasaki PI. Significance of the positive crossmatch test in kidney transplantation. *N Engl J Med*. 1969;280(14):735.

Racusen LC, Solez K, Colvin RB, et al. The Banff 97 working classification of renal allograft pathology. *Kidney Int*. 1999; 55:713–723.

Veale JL, Singer JS, Gritsch HA. The transplant operation and its surgical complications. In: Danovitch GM, ed. *Handbook of Kidney Transplantation*. 5th ed. Lippincott Williams & Wilkins; 2009:181–197.

Wilkinson A. The "First Quarter": The first three months after transplantation. In: Danovitch GM, ed. *Handbook of Kidney Transplantation*. 5th ed. Philadelphia, PA: Lippincott Williams & Wilkins; 2009:198–216.

75

Transplant Surgery—Liver

Joy Sarkar

SCENARIO 1

A 52-year-old patient with a long history of hepatitis C (HCV) presents with vague epigastric pain and reports weight loss of 10 pounds over the past 4 months with a serum AFP level of 600 mcg/L. Contrast computerized tomography (CT) scan of the liver shows multiple nodules in the hepatic parenchyma.

1. Which of the following is true regarding the possibility of liver transplantation in a patient with chronic hepatitis C?

A. Preoperative treatment with lamivudine may decrease the rate of HCV recurrence after transplantation.

B. HCV is the second most common indication for liver transplantation worldwide.

C. Up to 30% of patients with active hepatitis C at the time of transplant will experience recurrence of HCV in the transplanted liver.

D. The Model for End-Stage Liver Disease (MELD) score assessment predicts perioperative mortality of transplant recipients.

E. Post-transplantation, progression of HCV infection to cirrhosis is more aggressive than the original infection.

2. Which of the following is a contraindication to liver transplantation in a patient with hepatocellular carcinoma (HCC)?

A. Portal vein thrombosis

B. Hepatorenal syndrome

C. Three tumors within hepatic parenchyma measuring

D. Solitary HCC nodule in peripheral lung measuring 1 cm

E. HIV infection

SCENARIO 2

A previously healthy 24-year-old patient is admitted with a 2-day history of malaise, nausea, vomiting, jaundice, and epigastric pain. Over the next 3 days, she becomes increasingly confused, then obtunded, with associated marked elevation in liver enzymes, bilirubin, and ammonia levels. Her INR rises to 7.1 and Cr to 4.3 mg/dL.

3. Which of the following is true with regard to liver transplantation in this patient?

A. Alcohol-induced hepatitis is the most likely etiology.

B. Without transplantation, the mortality rate approaches 80%.

C. Emergent transplantation is contraindicated due to severe coagulopathy.

D. The MELD score assessment will be used to determine the patient's priority on the transplant waiting list.

E. One-year survival is higher after transplantation for fulminant hepatic failure than for chronic liver failure.

The aforementioned patient undergoes orthotopic liver transplantation. On the first postoperative day, the patient demonstrates no improvement in mental status. Laboratory analysis is notable for acidosis, marked elevation in liver enzymes, elevated INR, and hyperkalemia. Minimal output is noted from the T-tube biliary drainage catheter.

4. **The most likely etiology for this clinical presentation is:**

   A. Acute cell-mediated rejection
   B. Bacterial sepsis
   C. Primary nonfunction of graft
   D. Biliary anastomotic leak
   E. Acute viral hepatitis

5. **The best treatment for the aforementioned condition is:**

   A. Increase in tacrolimus dose
   B. High-dose intravenous corticosteroids
   C. Interferon with ribavirin
   D. Endoscopic retrograde cholangio-oancreatography (ERCP) with biliary stenting
   E. Re-transplantation

SCENARIO 3

A 46-year-old male patient with cirrhosis from prior alcohol abuse undergoes orthotopic liver transplantation, and upon discharge is placed on an immunosuppressive maintenance regimen of tacrolimus and prednisone. Three weeks postoperatively, the patient presents with right upper quadrant abdominal pain and malaise. His temperature is found to be 100.9°F, and laboratory workup is notable for serum bilirubin level of 2.3 mg/dl, ALT 870 units/L, AST 920 units/L. Tests for HBV, HCV, and cytomegalovirus (CMV) are all negative. Ultrasound shows normal flow in the hepatic artery and portal vein, without intrahepatic ductal dilation. A percutaneous biopsy of the graft is performed, showing venous endothelial inflammation, a mixed inflammatory infiltrate of lymphocytes, neutrophils, and eosinophils in the portal triad, and cholangitis with scattered degenerative changes to the ducts.

6. **What is next best step in managing this patient?**

   A. Changing tacrolimus to cyclosporine
   B. Addition of mycophenolate mofetil
   C. Pulse of methylprednisolone
   D. Addition of thymoglobulin
   E. Increasing dose of tacrolimus

7. **Which of the following medications, if taken with the above immunosuppressive regimen of tacrolimus and prednisone, may increase the risk of graft rejection?**

   A. Fluconazole
   B. Phenytoin
   C. Amiodarone
   D. Clarithromycin
   E. Diltiazem

ANSWERS

1. **E.** Worldwide, HCV is the most common indication for liver transplantation. Following liver transplantation, the majority of patients with positive HCV titers will experience recurrence of hepatitis C in the transplanted liver. Preoperative therapy with interferon and ribavirin is helpful in managing symptoms of early HCV infection, but will only achieve viral clearance from serum in a small percentage of patients. Lamivudine is used in post-transplant patients with HBV and has been shown to significantly improve survival rates and overall outcomes. When hepatitis C recurs in the transplanted liver, the progression to cirrhosis is much more aggressive than the original infection, and patients can progress to end-stage liver failure in 6 months. The MELD formula is calculated using logarithms of the serum creatinine, bilirubin, and INR. The MELD score predicts the likelihood of death if the patient does not receive liver transplantation, but does not correlate with non-transplant postoperative survival rates.

2. **D.** The majority of HCC tumors develop in patients with cirrhosis. While liver resection is the treatment of choice for HCC in patients without cirrhosis, orthotopic liver transplantation (OLT) has evolved as the preferred treatment for HCC in the setting of advanced cirrhosis as OLT treats both the tumor and underlying liver dysfunction. The Milan criteria guide patient selection for liver transplantation; patients with a solitary tumor up to 5 cm or three tumors up to 3 cm each are eligible for OLT. Metastatic HCC is an absolute contraindication to transplantation. Portal vein thrombosis is not a contraindication to OLT because the thrombus can be extracted, or a jump graft can be placed to the superior mesenteric vein (SMV). Patients with hepatorenal syndrome may experience recovery of renal function following liver transplantation; even in advanced cases, the patient may be a candidate for combined liver-kidney transplantation. HIV is no

longer considered an absolute contraindication to OLT, provided it is well controlled with antiretroviral therapy, but active sepsis remains a contraindication.

3. **B.** Fulminant hepatic failure is defined as the presence of encephalopathy within 8 weeks of the development of jaundice in the absence of previous liver disease. In the United States and Europe, the most common cause of fulminant hepatic failure is acetaminophen overdose. The King's College criteria are the most widely accepted guideline for transplantation of patients with fulminant hepatic failure. According to the King's College criteria, a patient with fulminant hepatic failure secondary to acetaminophen overdose qualifies for transplantation if either pH <7.3, or all three of the following criteria are met: grade 3–4 encephalopathy, PT >100 s or INR >6.5, or Cr >3.4 mg/dL. In non-acetaminophen overdose, the criteria are either PT >100 s (i.e., INR >6.5) or any three of the following: age <10 or >40 years, non-A/non-B/drug-induced/Wilson disease hepatitis, greater than 7-day transition from jaundice to encephalopathy, PT >50 s (i.e., INR >3.5), or total bilirubin >17.5 mg/dL. Regardless of etiology, the patient in this scenario meets King's College criteria for transplantation based on her severe encephalopathy, INR, and creatinine level.

Without transplantation, the mortality from fulminant hepatic failure approaches 80%. While the MELD score can be additive to the King's College criteria in predicting mortality, and is used to assign priority on the transplant waiting list for patients with chronic liver failure, patients with fulminant hepatic failure are listed as status 1A (highest priority), which supersedes the MELD score assessment. Survival after transplantation for fulminant hepatic failure is lower at 1 year compared to transplantation for chronic liver failure: 73% versus 85%.

4. **C.** Primary nonfunction of the transplanted liver occurs in 2% to 10% of cases and is characterized by absence of bile production, severe acidosis, elevation of liver enzymes, hyperkalemia, hepatic encephalopathy, and eventually multi-organ failure. Possible etiologies are early hepatic arterial thrombosis, prolonged ischemia of the donor liver, poor preservation, advanced donor age, or allograft steatosis. Acute cell-mediated rejection after liver transplantation is a less common cause of graft loss than primary nonfunction or hepatic artery thrombosis.

Rejection may be asymptomatic, or may present with mild symptoms mimicking hepatitis. In fact, recurrent hepatitis C may occur in the early postoperative period due to the immunosuppressive regimen and be difficult to distinguish from acute rejection, although a biopsy can be helpful in this regard. Intraabdominal sepsis may occur, manifesting with fever and peritonitis, and is most often due to biliary anastomotic leak. Biliary leak or stricture is a common postoperative complication occurring in 10% to 30% of cases, and is diagnosed via cholangiography.

5. **E.** Patients with primary nonfunction of the graft are essentially anhepatic, and a majority require retransplantation; patients are relisted as Status 1A. High-dose intravenous corticosteroids are the treatment for acute cell-mediated rejection, except in patients with underlying hepatitis C. These patients should minimize steroids as much as possible to decrease viral replication, and should instead receive an increase in their tacrolimus or mycophenolate mofetil dose. Patients with recurrent hepatitis C may be treated with a combination of interferon and ribavirin. ERCP with biliary stenting is the treatment of choice for a biliary leak or stricture.

6. **E.** Acute cellular rejection after liver transplantation occurs in approximately 15% to 25% of recipients, and is most likely to occur within the first 90 days after transplantation. Patients may present with nonspecific symptoms such as abdominal pain and malaise. Similarly, the laboratory workup will often show a transaminitis and hyperbilirubinemia, but these findings are not specific to rejection. Therefore, the gold standard for diagnosis of acute rejection is biopsy of the graft. The major histologic features of rejection include a mixed infiltrate of predominantly lymphocytes in the portal triad, venous endothelial inflammation, and either destructive or nondestructive cholangitis. Treatment depends on the patient's current immunosuppressive regimen. If the dose of calcineurin inhibitor like tacrolimus is found to be subtherapeutic, rejection may be adequately treated by increasing the dose. Patients on cyclosporine may be changed to tacrolimus, which was found to be superior to cyclosporine in preventing acute rejection and graft loss, and improving overall survival. An antimetabolite, such as mycophenolate mofetil, may be added if the patient is not already taking one. For patients already on triple therapy (tacrolimus,

mycophenolate, and prednisone or other steroid), the first-line therapy is high-dose glucocorticoid, such as methylprednisolone, followed by a taper. Approximately 10% of patients will experience steroid-resistant rejection, and multiple treatment options exist, including thymoglobulin, anti-IL2-receptor antibodies (e.g., basiliximab), mTOR inhibitors (e.g., sirolimus), and anti-CD3 monoclonal antibody (OKT3).

7. **B.** Calcineurin inhibitors such as cyclosporine and tacrolimus are metabolized by enzyme cytochrome P450 3A4 (CYP3A4). Because of this, drugs that inhibit CYP3A4 may lead to increased levels of tacrolimus, causing toxicity, while drugs that induce CYP3A4 may lead to decreased levels, which may potentiate rejection. Well-known inhibitors of CYP3A4 include amiodarone, azole antifungals (e.g., fluconazole), macrolide antibiotics (e.g., clarithromycin, grapefruit juice, some calcium channel blockers such as diltiazem and verapamil, and some medications used to treat HIV such as ritonavir and HIV protease inhibitors. Inducers of CYP3A4 include anti-seizure medications such as carbamazepine, phenytoin, and phenobarbital, rifamycins such as rifampin, and St. John's wort.

BIBLIOGRAPHY

Ascher NL. Liver transplantation. In: Townsend CM, Beauchamp D, Evers BM, et al., eds. *Sabiston Textbook of Surgery: The Biological Basis of Modern Surgical Practice.* 19th ed. Elsevier; 2012:655–665.

Choudhary NS, Saigal S, Bansal RK, Saraf N, Gautam D, Soin AS. Acute and chronic rejection after liver transplantation: what a clinician needs to know. *J Clin Exp Hepatol.* 2017;7(4):358–366.

Locke JE, Cameron AM. Treatment for hepatocellular carcinoma: Resection versus transplantation. In: Cameron JL, Cameron AM, eds. *Current Surgical Therapy.* 11th ed. Elsevier; 2014:334–335.

Lynch T, Price A. The effect of cytochrome P450 metabolism on drug response, interactions, and adverse effects. *Am Fam Physician.* 2007;76(3):391–396.

Moini M, Schilsky ML, Tichy EM. Review on immunosuppression in liver transplantation. *World J Hepatol.* 2015;7(10):1355–1368.

Roberts MS, Angus DC, Bryce CL, Valenta Z, Weissfeld L. Survival after liver transplantation in the United States: a disease-specific analysis of the UNOS database. *Liver Transpl.* 2004;10(7):886–897.

Welling TH, Pelletier SJ. Hepatic transplantation. In: Mulholland MW, Lillemoe KD, Doherty GM, et al., eds. *Greenfield's Surgery: Scientific Principles and Practice.* 5th ed. Lippincott Williams & Wilkins; 2011:542–564.

Trauma and Critical Care

76

Trauma and Critical Care—Roadside Bomb

Rob Conrad

During the annual Memorial Day parade of your hometown, a large explosion occurs along the parade route, with multiple injured persons and fatalities at the scene. Prehospital EMS providers, first responders, and bystanders begin to administer first aid to those injured and start transfer of patients to the local hospital. As an on-call general surgeon, you and your colleagues stand ready in the emergency department while preparing for a potential mass casualty event. Hospital administrators have activated the disaster/mass casualty plan, triage officers are designated, and the incident command plan is in effect.

1. **A prehospital provider encounters an injured female with a below knee traumatic amputation and multiple truncal fragment wounds with labored breathing (Figure 76-1). The first priority in the initial care of this patient should be?**

   A. Airway
   B. Breathing
   C. Circulation/control of life-threatening hemorrhage
   D. Disability
   E. Evacuation

2. **Which of the following pairs of hemorrhage source and preferred management is correct?**

   A. Junctional hemorrhage—Tourniquet placed directly over the injury
   B. Extremity hemorrhage—Hemostatic dressing and direct pressure
   C. Truncal hemorrhage—Permissive hypotension and hemostatic resuscitation

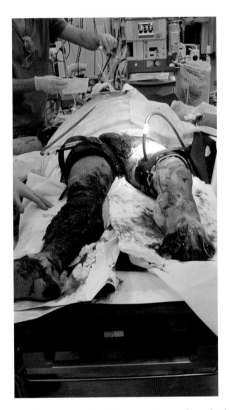

Figure 76-1 Representative injury pattern of roadside bomb or improvised explosive device.

   D. Pelvic hemorrhage—Early use of rFactor VIIa
   E. Intra-cranial hemorrhage—Reversal of hypercoaguable state and neurosurgical intervention

3. **The principles of damage control surgery include which of the following?**

A. Primary focus upon control of hemorrhage only

B. Avoiding the use of temporary abdominal closures

C. Appropriate triage based upon injuries and available resources

D. Colostomy for all colon injuries

E. Definitive repair of all abdominal injuries

4. **The concept of damage control or hemostatic resuscitation includes which of the following?**

A. Limited use of colloid solution resuscitation

B. 3:1:1 PRBC:FFP:Platelet transfusion strategy

C. Empiric transfusion of cryoprecipitate

D. Administration of tranexamic acid (TXA) for treatment of hyperfibrinolysis

5. **Primary blast injuries include which of the following?**

A. Damage to gas filled organs due to extreme pressure changes

B. Truncal injury sustained as victim is thrown through the air by blast

C. Crush injuries from structural collapse due to a blast around the patient

D. Penetrating injury from debris and fragments propelled by the blast force

6. **Unique to mass casualty incidents is the category of the "expectant" patient. Which of the following would triage a patient into the "expectant" category?**

A. Lower extremity amputation

B. Requirement of supplemental oxygen

C. Forty percent total body surface area burns

D. Cardiac arrest on scene

E. Systolic blood pressure of 95

7. **Noncompressible torso hemorrhage is a major cause of mortality in blast injuries. Aortic occlusion can decrease distal bleeding and provide a window of opportunity for definitive hemorrhage control. Options for aortic occlusion include direct clamping through a thoracotomy or laparotomy and resuscitative endovascular balloon occlusion (REBOA). Which of the following is an absolute contraindication to use of resuscitative endovascular balloon occlusion (REBOA)?**

A. Pelvic fracture

B. Penetrating abdominal trauma

C. Penetrating thoracic/neck trauma

D. Pregnancy

E. Peripheral vascular disease

ANSWERS

1. **C.** Traditional teaching of advanced cardiac life support (ACLS) and advanced trauma life support (ATLS) concepts stress the "ABCDE" mantra (airway, breathing, circulation, disability, and exposure), in which airway control is paramount. However, in the setting of combat injuries and civilian catastrophes such as blast injuries, immediate control of life-threatening hemorrhage takes precedence as fatal hemorrhage can rapidly occur while addressing other elements of the primary survey. Hemorrhage remains the leading cause of potentially preventable morbidity and mortality in both military and civilian trauma, reinforcing the importance of prehospital efforts to control bleeding and prevent exsanguination after severe injury. The experiences gained during combat operations in Iraq and Afghanistan have led to a change in the priorities of treatment that are taught to combat medics and first-responders.

As the most likely cause of potentially preventable death in these scenarios is hemorrhage, the standard ATLS approach of focusing first on the airway has been changed to a primary focus on C, or the control of hemorrhage, as the first priority. The next priorities would be on assessing the airway and breathing for life-threatening issues such as airway obstruction, tension pneumothorax, or an open pneumothorax ("sucking chest wound").

2. **C.** Major extremity hemorrhage can be effectively controlled in both the prehospital and hospital setting using an effective proximal tourniquet. Application of tourniquets to control major hemorrhage should be placed as distal as possible yet proximal to the site of injury, to control hemorrhage and limit the extent of tissue ischemia. Hasty tourniquets applied in combat under fire or prior to moving a patient to a safer location may be placed expediently anywhere proximal on the injured extremity and later moved distally. Approximately one-third of bleeding deaths after explosive events are due to extremity hemorrhage, with the remaining two-thirds attributed to junctional bleeding or noncompressible truncal hemorrhage (Figure 76-2). "Junctional" injuries are defined as injuries to the groin, axilla, neck, or perineum. These injuries present major challenges to

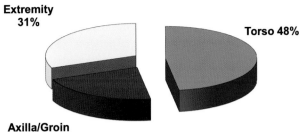

Figure 76-2 Distribution of preventable bleeding deaths from battlefield wounds by the site of hemorrhage.

hemorrhage control as damaged deep vascular structures transition from the extremities to major cavities beyond the effective reach of a proximal tourniquet. Direct pressure and topical hemostatic adjuncts are often the only currently available treatments of potential benefit before proximal surgical control can be achieved. Noncompressible truncal hemorrhage is the most feared and fatal type of bleeding as it is not amenable to prehospital hemorrhage control measures, and requires higher-level interventions such as surgery or angioembolization. Significant pelvic hemorrhage may result from complex bony injuries and damage to the pelvic vasculature. Treatment of pelvic fractures may include pelvic sheeting, commercial or improvised binders, and forms of external fixation that aim to stabilize the pelvic ring. Surgical control of pelvic hemorrhage includes open and catheter-based therapies as well as pre-peritoneal pelvic packing to tamponade hemorrhage. Permissive hypotension is the concept that avoiding normal or elevated blood pressure in a bleeding patient prior to surgical hemorrhage control limits blood loss.

The goal is to maintain an adequate arterial pressure for critical organ perfusion while limiting over-pressurization from vigorous fluid resuscitation that may exacerbate hemorrhage. Although there was initial interest in the use of activated recombinant factor VII (rFactor VIIa) as an adjunctive therapy for bleeding, subsequent studies have found little to no benefit and it also would not be used as a prehospital therapy for pelvic bleeding. The treatment of traumatic intracranial hemorrhage begins with reversal of any identified coagulopathy, not hypercoaguble state, treatment of associated cerebral edema, and possible neurosurgical interventions.

3. **C.** Damage control surgery (DCS) is a concept that includes the principles of limiting further physiologic insult to a severely injured patient through the rapid surgical control of life-threatening hemorrhage and enteric spillage, to minimize further bleeding, restore tissue perfusion, and prevent sepsis. The goal is to avoid prolonged, initial operative procedures that may further exacerbate hypothermia, coagulopathy, or acidosis. Temporary closures of the abdomen and thorax may be employed to shorten the procedure length and allow for urgent or planned reoperation in this population. Once bleeding and gastrointestinal spillage are controlled, there are no further attempts to address other non-life-threatening abdominal injuries at the initial surgery.

The operation is terminated and the patient is returned to the ICU for resuscitation and restoration of normal physiology and coagulation. Following physiologic restoration, these patients are taken back to the operating room for definitive treatments and closure. In mass casualty situations and resource-constrained environments, DCS allows limited surgical personnel to provide critical surgical procedures to severely injured patients rapidly, and then either evacuate them to higher levels of care or clear the operating room for additional patients.

4. **D.** Damage control resuscitation (DCR) or hemostatic resuscitation is the concept of limiting further blood loss before surgical hemorrhage control is obtained, as well as replacing shed-blood volume with a balanced blood product-based resuscitation that restores the capacity to carry and deliver oxygen and addresses derangements of the coagulation system. DCR research has focused upon improved morbidity and mortality with limitation of crystalloid infusion to prevent hemodilution (colloid solutions are, in general, not advocated for trauma resuscitations), acidosis and worsening of coagulopathy, in favor of transfusion ratios approaching 1:1:1 of packed red blood to fresh frozen plasma and platelets. Additional targeted treatment of specific coagulation abnormalities based upon traditional studies (PT/INR, PTT, fibrinogen) and point of care testing such as thromboelastography is recommended, to avoid unnecessary transfusion and appropriate resource utilization.

Permissive hypotension is the concept that avoiding normal or elevated blood pressure in a bleeding patient prior to surgical hemorrhage control limits blood loss. The goal is to maintain an adequate arterial pressure for critical organ perfusion while limiting over-pressurization from vigorous fluid resuscitation that may exacerbate hemorrhage. Previous studies in civilian trauma patients have confirmed a favorable survival advantage by limiting prehospital resuscitation but heterogeneity in clinical trials such as optimal blood pressure target and fluid resuscitation type have yet to yield definitive conclusions.

Current research has identified early derangements of the coagulation system that appear to confer an increased risk of morbidity and mortality after trauma, termed the acute coagulopathy of trauma. Hyperfibrinolysis is a key component of this condition, and targeted pharmacologic intervention with the antifibrinolytic agent, TXA, has been linked to a survival advantage in several studies of bleeding trauma patients. The use of TXA in the setting of major hemorrhage and massive transfusion situations is now recommended in the early treatment (<3 hours from injury) in civilian and combat injuries.

5. **A.** Blast injuries are traditionally classified based upon the discrete mechanism of injury involved. Primary blast injuries involve damage to gas-filled organs such as the intestine, lungs, and middle ear as well as the brain. These injuries result from over-pressurization due to the blast force. Rupture of the tympanic membrane is a frequently encountered primary blast injury, but the absence does not rule out other types of blast injury. Secondary blast injuries result from injury due to flying debris and fragments that are propelled by the blast. These are the most frequently sustained type of blast injuries. Tertiary injuries occur when a person is thrown through the air by the blast, whereas quaternary injuries include other blast effects such as burn injury, inhalation of toxic gases, or injury due to collapse of structures around the person. Lastly, quinary injuries are the result of contamination by chemical, radiological, or biological materials from the blast itself or other injured persons.

In addition to the aforementioned injury classification, the severity of injury sustained after a blast mechanism depends upon the patient's proximity to the blast, the energy of the blast itself, and whether the blast occurred in a closed space. Persons injured by a blast in an enclosed space such as a vehicle or building frequently sustain a higher rate of lethal primary blast injury as well as increased frequency of secondary penetrating injuries.

6. **D.** Unlike conventional trauma care, trauma care during a mass casualty scenario requires a fundamental change in the triage of patients. The ultimate principle of trauma care in the mass casualty setting is to provide the greatest good for the greatest number of patients. By definition, mass casualty incidents are scenarios in which patient care resources are overextended but not overwhelmed. In contrast, mass casualty event are scenarios in which patient care resources are overwhelmed and cannot be expeditiously supplemented. Regardless, demand for patient care resources exceeds supply. Medical triage levels determined by experienced medical providers rapidly categorizes victims based on severity of injuries, likelihood of survival and available resources (personnel, supplies, logistic, and evacuation). Victim are classified into the following categories: Urgent (Red)—immediate lifesaving intervention required; Delayed (Yellow)—no immediate lifesaving intervention needed; Minor (Green)—minimal medical care needed; and Deceased (Black). Lastly, victims can be classified into the "expectant" category although this remain controversial. Victims are classified as "expectant" should they be deemed unlikely to survive due to the nature of their injuries, underlying comorbidities or resource limitations. This category was first developed by the military but is now widely used in large civilian trauma centers. Current criteria for the "expectant" category include cardiac arrest on scene, severe comorbidities, intubation or ventilation on scene, severe head injuries, and > 80% total body surface area burns. Similarly, cardiopulmonary resuscitation (CPR) and massive transfusion protocols (MTP) are often suspended during mass casualty scenarios, given the high burden of personnel and resource utilization.

7. **C.** A major cause of mortality from blast injuries results from noncompressible hemorrhage. Hemorrhage from the chest, abdomen, pelvis, or junctional sites can be difficult to control without operative intervention. Aortic occlusion is an adjunct, which can allow temporary proximal control of hemorrhage allowing time for the patient to be resuscitated and proceed to definitive surgical hemorrhage control. Options for aortic occlusion include direct clamping through a thoracotomy or laparotomy and REBOA. While precise indication for REBOA in trauma remain poorly defined, absolute contraindications include penetrating neck/torso trauma or

suspected supra-diaphragmatic hemorrhage as these can be exacerbated by REBOA placement. Patients who do not meet criteria for resuscitative thoracotomy should also not be considered for REBOA. REBOA has been used for hemorrhage control is both Obstetric and Gynecologic procedures. Occlusion with REBOA can be placed in the aorta from the left subclavian artery to the celiac trunk (Zone I) to control hemorrhage from the abdominal viscera, pelvis, and lower extremities. Similarly, occlusion with REBOA in the infrarenal aorta (Zone III) can control hemorrhage from the pelvis and lower extremities while sparing abdominal ischemia. Further research is needed to determine the ideal patient population for REBOA placement as well as the appropriate timing and duration of occlusion.

BIBLIOGRAPHY

Beekley AC. Damage control resuscitation: a sensible approach to the exsanguinating surgical patient. *Crit Care Med.* 2008;36(7):S267–S274.

Biddinger PD, Glaggish A, Harrington L, et al. Be prepared—the Boston marathon and mass-casualty events. *N E J Med.* 2013;368:1958–1960.

Blackbourne LH. Combat damage control surgery. *Crit Care Med.* 2008;36(7):S304–S310.

Borgman MA, Spinella PC, Perkins JG, et al. The ratio of blood products transfused affects mortality in patients receiving massive transfusions at a combat support hospital. *J Trauma.* 2007;63(4):805–813.

Brenner M, Inaba K, Aiolfi A, et al. Resuscitative endovascular balloon occlusion of the aorta and resuscitative thoracotomy in select patients with hemorrhagic shock: early results from the American Association for the Surgery of Trauma's Aortic Occlusion in Resuscitation for Trauma and Acute Care Surgery Registry. *J Am Coll Surg.* 2018;226:730.

Briggs SM. *Advanced Disaster Medical Response Manual for Providers.* 2nd ed. Cine-Med Publishing, Inc; 2014.

Bulger EM, Snyder D, Schoelles K, et al. An evidence-based guideline for external hemorrhage control: American college of surgeons committee on trauma. *Prehosp Emerg Care.* 2014;18(2):163–173.

Butler FK Jr, Holcomb JB, Giebner SD, et al. Tactical combat casualty care 2007: evolving concepts and battlefield experience. *Mil Med.* 2007;172(11):S1–S19.

Cooper GJ, Maynard RL, Cross NL, et al. Casualties from terrorist bombings. *J Trauma.* 1983;23(11):955–967.

Cothren CC, Osborn PM, Moore EE, et al. Preperitoneal pelvic packing for hemodynamically unstable pelvic fractures: A paradigm shift. *J Trauma.* 2007;62(4):834–839.

Cotton BA, Reddy N, Hatch QM, et al. Damage control resuscitation is associated with a reduction in resuscitation volumes and improvement in survival in 390 damage control laparotomy patients. *Ann Surg.* 2011;254(4):598–605.

CRASH-2 trial collaborators, Shakur H, Roberts I, Bautista R, et al. Effects of tranexamic acid on death, vascular occlusive events, and blood transfusion in trauma patients with significant haemorrhage (CRASH-2): a randomised, placebo-controlled trial. *Lancet.* 2010;376:23–32.

Culley JM, Svendsen E. A review of the literature on the validity of mass casualty triage systems with a focus on chemical exposures. *Am J Disaster Med.* 2014;9(2):137–150.

DePalma RG, Burris DG, Champion HR, et al. Blast injuries. *N Engl J Med.* 2005;352(13):1335–1342.

Eastridge BJ, Mabry RL, Seguin P, Cantrell J, Tops T, Uribe P, et al. Death on the battlefield (2001–2011): Implications for the future of combat casualty care. *J Trauma Acute Care Surg.* 2012;73:S431–S437.

Kauvar DS, Lefering R, Wade CE. Impact of hemorrhage on trauma outcome: An overview of epidemiology, clinical presentations, and therapeutic considerations. *J Trauma.* 2006;60:S3–S11.

Kwan I, Bunn F, Chinnock P, et al. Timing and volume of fluid administration for patients with bleeding. *Cochrane Database Syst Rev.* 2003;(3):CD002245.

Moore LJ, Brenner M, Kozar RA, et al. Implementation of resuscitative endovascular balloon occlusion of the aorta as an alternative to resuscitative thoracotomy for noncompressible truncal hemorrhage. *J Trauma Acute Care Surg.* 2015; 79:523.

Morrison CA, Carrick MM, Norman MA, et al. Hypotensive resuscitation strategy reduces transfusion requirements and severe postoperative coagulopathy in trauma patients with hemorrhagic shock: preliminary results of a randomized controlled trial. *J Trauma.* 2011;70(3):652–663.

Morrisson JJ, Dubose JJ, Rasmussen TE, et al. Military application of tranexamic acid in trauma emergency resuscitation (MATTERs) study. *Arch Surg.* 2012;147:113–119.

Morrison JJ, Rasmussen TE. Noncompressible torso hemorrhage: a review with contemporary definitions and management strategies. *Surg Clin North Am.* 2012;92:843.

Rommens PM, Hofmann A, Hessmann MH. Management of acute hemorrhage in pelvic trauma: an overview. *Eur J Trauma Emerg Surg.* 2010;2:91–99.

Rotondo MF, Schwab CW, McGonigal MD, et al. Damage control: an approach for improved survival in exsanguinating penetrating abdominal injury. *J Trauma.* 1993;35(3): 375–382.

77

Knife Wounds

Rob Conrad

A 35-year-old man is brought to the emergency department after an altercation at a bar. He has a 3-cm stab wound to his right chest, approximately 5 cm lateral to and just superior to his nipple. He is able to tell you that the wound is from a knife. He is oriented and appropriate, although intoxicated, and complains loudly of pain in his right chest. His initial vital signs are as follows: HR 96, BP 110/63, RR 20, 98% saturation on room air.

1. **What is your first step in the management of this patient?**
   A. Perform a tube thoracostomy.
   B. Perform the primary survey and examine for any other wounds.
   C. Perform a FAST (focused assessment with sonography for trauma) scan to identify intra-abdominal injury.
   D. Obtain a chest radiograph to identify presence of pneumothorax or hemothorax.

2. **Despite fluid resuscitation, the patient's blood pressure suddenly becomes 60/palpable. His trachea is midline and his breath sounds are reduced over the right hemithorax, with dullness to percussion. What is the best next step in management?**
   A. Place a 36F chest tube into the right pleural cavity at the second interspace in the midaxillary line.
   B. Place a 36F chest tube into the right pleural cavity at the fifth interspace in the mid- or anterior axillary line.

   C. Place an 18 g angiocath into the second intercostal space at the midclavicular line.
   D. Take the patient immediately to the operating room for thoracotomy.
   E. Initiate a massive transfusion protocol to stabilize the patient for computerized tomography (CT) scan to identify the source of the hypotension.

3. **Which of the following is a correct indicator for operative intervention paired with an appropriate operative approach for this patient?**
   A. Greater than 500 cc blood from the chest tube upon initial placement—right posterolateral thoracotomy in the operating room
   B. Cardiac arrest in the trauma bay—left anterolateral thoracotomy in the emergency room
   C. Persistent transfusion requirements to maintain stable blood pressure—median sternotomy in the emergency room
   D. Second entry wound identified below the costal margin—transverse anterior thoracotomy (clamshell incision) in the operating room
   E. An entry wound medial to the midclavicular line—median sternotomy in the emergency room

4. **If this patient's wound were located in the neck above the cricoid cartilage (but below the angle of the mandible), which of the following diagnostic tests would be indicated?**
   A. None; manage expectantly with admission for serial exams
   B. CT scan of the neck with CT angiography (CTA) of the cervical vessels.

C. CTA or angiography plus bronchoscopy

D. CTA or angiography, bronchoscopy, and esopha-gogastroduodenoscopy (EGD)

5. **The patient has 800 cc initial drainage from the right-sided chest tube, which then slows down over the next few hours. He is admitted to the floor on telemetry for monitoring, and remains stable. A follow-up chest radiograph the next morning demonstrates significant residual basilar fluid. What is the most appropriate next step?**

A. Go to the operating room for a video-assisted thoracoscopic surgery (VATS) to evacuate the retained hemothorax.

B. Go to the operating room for a right anterolateral thoracotomy.

C. Place a pigtail catheter to drain the residual hemothorax.

D. Observation and serial chest X-rays.

6. **A stable patient with a 3-cm stab wound to the right chest undergoes a chest x-ray, which is unremarkable, identifying no pneumothorax or hemothorax. Subsequent CT scan of the chest reveals a small apical pneumothorax. The patient is otherwise stable and asymptomatic. Which of the following correctly pairs this patient's identified injury with an appropriate intervention?**

A. Occult pneumothorax—immediate chest tube

B. Spontaneous pneumothorax—video-assisted thoracoscopic surgery (VATS)

C. Tension pneumothorax—needle decompression

D. Occult pneumothorax—observation

E. Pneumomediastinum—antibiotics and drainage

7. **A patient presents to the Emergency Department with a 2-cm left thoracoabdominal stab wound. The wound is located along the left anterior axillary line, 2 cm below the level of the nipple. The patient is hemodynamically stable and on exam exhibits no peritonitis. The patient undergoes CT scan of the chest, abdomen, and pelvis, which does not identify any intrathoracic or intraabdominal injuries. What is the best next step in management?**

A. Emergent laparotomy

B. Observation alone

C. Observation with delayed laparoscopy

D. Immediate laparoscopy

E. Discharge From Emergency Department

ANSWERS

1. **B.** In any trauma patient, the first priority is to ensure stable ABCs, airway, breathing, and circulation, which may include emergent interventions (e.g., tube thoracostomy). In this patient with stable vital signs, the initial step is to perform a primary and secondary survey—a brief head to toe physical examination. A common mistake in the setting of penetrating trauma is failure to identify multiple injuries. Common locations for missed penetrating injuries can be in the back, axilla, or perineum, so a complete head to toe survey is critical. Most patients can be stabilized enough to undergo a secondary survey, but any problems identified on the primary survey should be immediately addressed. Once all injuries are identified, they can be prioritized for diagnostic imaging or operative repair. Both chest X-ray and FAST scan can be used as adjuncts to the secondary survey, but they do not replace the need for a head-to-toe assessment of the patient. In the initial evaluation of a trauma patient, priorities are: 1. identifying all wounds, 2. determining if urgent lifesaving intervention is indicated, and 3. determining if additional testing is needed.

2. **B.** In the setting of penetrating trauma to the chest, the differential diagnosis for hypotension includes tension pneumothorax, cardiac tamponade, and hemothorax. Classically, a tension pneumothorax will present with deviation of the trachea away from the injury, increased percussion, and decreased breath sounds with distended neck veins. However, these can be late findings and may be difficult to appreciate in a busy and noisy trauma bay. If a tension pneumo-thorax is suspected, the first step would be placing an large bore (14 or 18 gauge) angiocath to needle decompress the thoracic cavity. The diagnosis would be confirmed by a rush of air from the needle, and a chest tube should then be placed.

In this patient, the absence of tracheal deviation along with dullness to percussion makes a hemothorax the more likely diagnosis, and a chest tube the appropriate next step. The preferred method for tube thoracostomy is to enter the "safe triangle" bounded by the anterior border of the latissimus, the lateral border of the pectoralis major, and a horizontal line at the level of the nipple (males) or infra-mammary crease (females). This positioning minimizes the likelihood of entering the abdominal cavity, injuring muscle or breast tissue, or underlying structures such as the internal mammary artery, and avoids the major chest wall musculature that can cause significant pain with chest tube insertion.

3. **B.** Accepted indications for emergency department thoracotomy in the setting of penetrating thoracic trauma are loss of pulses with previously witnessed cardiac activity and unresponsive, persistent, hypotension. In blunt trauma, indications are rapid exsanguination from the chest tube (>1,500 cc on initial placement) with unresponsive hypotension. Survival rates after emergency thoracotomy are up to 30% for penetrating trauma, but closer to 1% for blunt trauma patients. The goals of an emergency department thoracotomy are to control hemorrhage (which may require cross-clamping the descending thoracic aorta), allow access for internal cardiac massage, and treat potential cardiac tamponade. Access to the heart, descending aorta, and mediastinum requires a left thoracotomy incision. Regardless of the side of injury, traumatic arrest warrants a left thoracotomy for access to the mediastinal structures. If necessary, the incision can be extended to the right chest ("clamshell" thoracotomy) for access to the right thoracic cavity.

Stable patients with penetrating trauma may still require exploration in the operating room. Traditionally, anterior abdominal stab wounds warranted mandatory laparotomy to rule out intraabdominal injury, although recent evidence has raised the possibility of expectant management for the stable patient with penetrating injuries. Thoracic injury to "the box," the area defined by nipples, sternal notch, and xiphoid process generally warrants operative exploration as well.

In a stable patient, however, it is reasonable to proceed with additional diagnostic studies. Although some have advocated an extensive workup, including esophagoscopy, bronchoscopy, and a pericardial window, more recent data indicates that a high-quality CT scan provides excellent imaging of the thorax and mediastinum, and additional studies can be performed based on the clinical exam and CT findings. In a patient who undergoes tube thoracostomy, indications to proceed to the operating room are: >1,500 cc on initial placement, >150–200 cc/hr for >3 hours, or hemodynamic instability requiring persistent blood transfusions.

4. **B.** Zone I of the neck extends from the clavicles to the cricoid cartilage, Zone II is from the cricoid cartilage to the angle of the mandible, and Zone III is from the angle of the mandible to the skull base. The majority of penetrating injuries, as with the patient in this case, occur in Zone II. For unstable patients with signs of major vascular or airway injury, management of penetrating neck trauma involves securing an airway and proceeding directly to the operating room for neck exploration. These signs include stridor, massive subcutaneous air, gurgling or bubbling through the wound, hemoptysis/hematemesis, and pulsatile bleeding or rapidly expanding hematoma.

Historically, all Zone II injuries that breached the platysma mandated operative exploration. This is no longer widely practiced, and stable patients with no hard signs of vascular or airway imaging can be managed expectantly with appropriate diagnostic tests. CTA has similar sensitivity to operative exploration for identifying vascular and soft tissue injuries. CT imaging can also provide valuable information about potential injuries to the esophagus or trachea that can guide the selective use of additional studies to evaluate these structures. Esophageal injuries are frequently asymptomatic, and morbidity significantly increases if repair is delayed beyond 24 hours. Contrast esophagography or esophagoscopy is recommended for all Zone II injuries that breach the platysma and have either physical exam or CT scan findings concerning for an esophageal injury. Similarly, flexible bronchoscopy can be used selectively based on any examination or CT imaging findings concerning for airway injury. With the accuracy of CT, bronchoscopy and upper endoscopy are not mandatory, however.

5. **A.** Retained hemothorax is a relatively common problem among patients who present with a moderate or large volume hemothorax with either blunt or penetrating trauma. Although observation only is an option, this carries the risk of developing an infected hematoma (empyema) or fibrothorax. If there is still a significant amount of clotted blood in the thoracic cavity that is not adequately drained by the initial chest tube, then there are several options for management.

These include placement of a second chest tube (or removal and replacement of the initial chest tube) in a better position to evacuate the fluid collection or administration of local lytic therapy

(TPA or urokinase administered through the chest tube) to attempt to break up the clot and allow drainage through the chest tube. Although these can be effective in select cases, they have been associated with relatively high failure rates. Since the retained hemothorax likely consists of clotted blood, a small-bore pigtail catheter is unlikely to achieve adequate drainage. There has been a trend toward the increased use of early VATS to evacuate the hematoma and place a well-positioned chest tube under direct visualization. This approach can also be useful if there is suspicion for an associated diaphragm injury that can be repaired simultaneously. Median sternotomy would not be indicated for evacuation of a retained hemothorax.

6. D. With CT scans being performed more routinely on trauma patients, many previously undetected injuries are now being identified. Occult pneumothorax is defined as a pneumothorax seen on CT scan of the chest but not on plain film x-ray. The stable patient with an occult pneumothorax presents the trauma surgeon with a treatment dilemma. The predicament is trying to determine which occult pneumothorax will progress and which can be safely observed. Retrospective data suggests that placing a chest tube for occult pneumothorax results in longer hospital stays and longer ICU stays. There have been attempts to categorize occult pneumothoraces using scoring systems based on size and location; however, these studies are retrospective and there are no current recommended size cutoffs, which would mandate tube thoracostomy. Another important question has been the factor of positive pressure ventilation and the ability to observe occult pneumothoraces. In a patient with an occult pneumothorax going to the operating room for management of other injuries, will positive pressure ventilation increased the likelihood of progression? While current studies suffer from small sample size, a recent prospective randomized study suggests that the majority of patient with occult pneumothoraces will not have progression regardless of the presence of positive pressure ventilation. Currently, the Eastern Association for the Surgery of Trauma (EAST) has clinical practice guidelines, which provided a Level 3 recommendation, "Occult pneumothorax, those not seen on chest radiograph, may be observed in a stable patient regardless of positive pressure ventilation."

7. C. Historically, penetrating abdominal trauma as defined by abdominal fascial penetration would mandate exploratory laparotomy. However, this dogma resulted in a high negative laparotomy rate and associated complications. A landmark publication from the Kings County Hospital Center in Brooklyn in 1960 changed the general approach to the management of abdominal trauma toward selective nonoperative management. There are now numerous studies supporting the utility of selective nonoperative management of abdominal stab wounds. In summary, adopting the strategy of operating on stab victims based on clinical status decreased unnecessary laparotomy, complications, and hospital length of stay. Current clinical practice guidelines from the EAST recommend that "routine laparotomy is not indicated in hemodynamically stable patients with abdominal stab wounds without signs of peritonitis or diffuse abdominal tenderness." Obviously, patients who are hemodynamically unstable or who have peritonitis should be taken emergently for laparotomy. In patients with penetrating abdominal trauma managed nonoperatively, multiple studies have demonstrated that most serious injuries will declare themselves on clinical assessment. Furthermore, for the vast majority of patients with penetrating abdominal trauma, serial examination over 24 hours was reliable in detecting significant injuries if performed by experienced surgeons. Lastly, for patients undergoing nonoperatively management CT imaging is strongly recommended. Finally, for penetrating trauma to the left thoracoabdominal region, diagnostic laparoscopy should be considered to evaluate for diaphragmatic injuries in those who do not have clear indications for laparotomy. However, diagnostic laparoscopy should not replace laparotomy to identify hollow viscus injuries. A study by Demetriades suggests performing diagnostic laparoscopy greater than 8 hours after admission so that diaphragmatic repair could be performed without concern for missed intraabdominal injury.

BIBLIOGRAPHY

Ball CG. Incidence, risk factors, and outcomes for occult pneumothoraces in victims of major trauma. *J Trauma.* 2005;59:917–924.

Biffl WL, Moore EE. Management guidelines for penetrating abdominal trauma. *Curr Opin Crit Care.* December 2010;16(6):609–617.

Brasel KJ, Stafford RE, Weigelt JA, Tenquist JE, Borgstrom DC. Treatment of occult pneumothoraces from blunt trauma. *J Trauma*. 1999;46:987–990.

Brohi K. Emergency Department Thoracotomy. http://www.trauma.org/index.php/main/article/361/.

Burgess CA, Dale OT, Almeyda R, Corbridge RJ. An evidence based review of the assessment and management of penetrating neck trauma. *Clin Otolaryngol*. February 2012;37(1):44–52.

Collins JC, Levine G, Waxman K. Occult traumatic pneumothorax: immediate tube thoracostomy versus expectant management. *Am Surg*. 1992;58:743–746.

de Moya MA, Seaver C, Spaniolas K, et al. Occult pneumothorax in trauma patients: development of an objective scoring system. *J Trauma*. 2007;63:13–17.

Demetriades D, Rabinowitz B. Indications for operation in abdominal stab wounds: a prospective study of 651 patients. *Ann Surg*. 1987;205:129–132.

Enderson BL, Abdalla R, Frame SB, Casey MT, Gould H, Maull KI. Tube thoracostomy for occult pneumothorax: a prospective randomized study of its use. *J Trauma*. 1993;35:726–729.

Hill SL, Edmisten T, Holtzman G, Wright A. The occult pneumothorax: an increasing diagnostic entity in trauma. *Am Surg*. 1999;65:254–258.

Houshian S, Larsen MS, Holm C. Missed injuries in a level I trauma center. *J Trauma*. April 2002;52(4):715–719.

Ivatury RR, Simon RJ, Stahl WM. A critical evaluation of laparoscopy in penetrating abdominal trauma. *J Trauma*. 1993;34: 822–828.

Laws D, Neville E, Duffy J. BTS guidelines for the insertion of a chest drain. *Thorax*. May 2003;58(Suppl 2): ii53–ii59.

Lowe RJ, Saletta JD, Read DR, et al. Should laparotomy be mandatory or selective in gunshot wounds of the abdomen? *J Trauma*. 1977;17:903–907.

Moore FA, Moore EE. Initial management of life-threatening trauma. In: Souba W, Fink M, Jurkovich G. et al., eds. *ACS Surgery: Principles and Practice*. 6th ed. B.C. Decker Inc; 2007: 1211–1230.

Mowery NT, Gunter OL, Collier BR, et al. Practice management guidelines for management of hemothorax and occult pneumothorax. *J Trauma*. February 2011;70(2): 510–518.

Murray JA, Demetriades D, Asensio JA, et al. Occult injuries to the diaphragm: prospective evaluation of laparoscopy in penetrating injuries to the left lower chest. *J Am Coll Surg*. 1998;187:626–630.

Nance FC, Cohn I Jr. Surgical management in the management of stab wounds of the abdomen: a retrospective and prospective analysis based on a study of 600 stabbed patients. *Ann Surg*. 1969;170:569–580.

Shaftan GW. Indications for operation in abdominal trauma. *Am J Surg*. 1960;99:657–664.

Tisherman SA, Bokhari F, Collier B, et al. Clinical practice guideline: penetrating zone II neck trauma. *J Trauma*. May 2008;64(5):1392–1405.

Wilder JR, Kudchadkar A. Stab wounds of the abdomen: observe or explore? *JAMA*. 1980;243:2503–2505.

78

Penetrating Trauma—Multiple Gunshot Wounds

Erik Criman and Matthew J. Martin

While on trauma call, you receive the following page: 23YOM GSW TO CHEST/ABD/RT THIGH. GCS 15 HR 100 BP 90/P RR30 98%/NRB. ETA 3MIN.

As you reach the trauma bay, your patient arrives in extremis. He is unresponsive with agonal breathing, oxygen saturation in the low 80s despite ventilation with a bag valve mask, and his radial pulse is weakly palpable with a rate of 105 beats per minute. Paramedics have established two large bore peripheral IVs and have begun infusing 2 liters of normal saline. They report that the patient was shot three times at close range with an unknown firearm. The first wound in the right upper chest was characterized as "sucking" on the scene and has been dressed with an occlusive dressing, taped on three sides. They have already performed a needle decompression. The second wound is in the left lower quadrant of the abdomen and is hemostatic. The final wound is located in the right mid-thigh and is presently hemostatic. Paramedics tell you that the bleeding was "pulsatile" prior to the application of a tourniquet.

1. **Your first priority for this patient should be:**
   A. Establishing a definitive airway
   B. Performing a chest X-ray
   C. Removing the tourniquet on the patient's right lower extremity
   D. Placing a left-sided tube thoracostomy
   E. Placing a central venous catheter

2. **Your patient undergoes a rapid sequence intubation, has a left-sided tube thoracostomy placed with prompt return of air and 1,800 mL blood, and has the remainder of the 2 liters of crystalloid infused via Emergency Medical Services. You remove the tourniquet and immediately appreciate pulsatile bleeding. Distal right lower extremity pulses are not palpable prior to the reapplication of this device, which provides hemostasis. The patient's heart rate has increased to 120 beats per minute with a blood pressure of 86/44. With your primary survey completed, which of the following injuries necessitates urgent operative intervention?**
   A. Gunshot wound to the chest only
   B. Gunshot wound to the abdomen only
   C. Right lower extremity injury only
   D. Right lower extremity injury and the chest injury
   E. Right lower extremity injury, abdominal injury, and chest injury

3. **Regarding penetrating chest trauma, which of the following is correct?**
   A. Tamponade physiology requires accumulation of at least 150 cc of blood in the pericardial space.
   B. Eighty-five percent of injuries can be managed with tube thoracostomy alone.
   C. Great vessel injuries are common in penetrating chest trauma.
   D. Lung injury that requires operative intervention is more common following blunt injury.
   E. Prophylactic antibiotic use reduces the incidence of post-traumatic empyema in the setting of retained hemothorax.

4. **Regarding this patient's penetrating abdominal wound, which of the following is correct?**

A. Injuries to the bowel may be primarily repaired if less than 75% of the bowel's circumference being involved.

B. The most common organ injured is the large bowel.

C. FAST (focused assessment with sonography for trauma) examination is poor at detecting hollow viscous injuries.

D. All patients with penetrating abdominal injuries that violate the posterior fascia must undergo an exploration but a laparoscopic one may suffice.

E. The operation of choice in an unstable patient having sustained penetrating abdominal injury is a limited laparotomy with extension only if injuries are suspected.

5. **In this patient with multiple gunshot wounds and physiologic derangement, which of the following would be the most appropriate management of a superficial femoral artery transection?**

A. Temporary intravascular shunt placement
B. Primary end to end arterial anastomosis
C. Ligation
D. Reconstruction using a prosthetic graft
E. Reconstruction using an autogenous reversed greater saphenous vein graft

6. **When compared with other forms of interpersonal injury (OIPI), which of the following is correct regarding patients having sustained gunshot wounds?**

A. Mortality is greater
B. Incidence of ICU admission is lower
C. More likely to have nonoperative management
D. Median hospital charge per admission is lower
E. Have a higher need for surgical intervention

ANSWERS

Gunshot wounds fall under the broad classification of penetrating trauma and comprise up to 10% of all major trauma in the United States. The energy imparted to tissue can be calculated using the kinetic energy equation: $K_e = \frac{1}{2}m(\Delta v)^2$, where m is the mass of the projectile and Δv is the change in velocity before and after contact. Simplistically, it can be inferred that higher caliber firearms and those projecting higher velocities will cause more grievous injury. This assumes, of course, that the entirety of the projectile's kinetic energy is imparted to the tissue. Those bullets that enter and exit do not expend all their kinetic energy on the body. Furthermore, the projectile's behavior in the body is a function of its relative density. Lower-density projectiles (e.g., lead or so-called hollow-point bullets) will tend to expand, creating a progressively enlarging wound tract with a comparatively small entrance wound and a large exit wound. High-density or high-velocity projectiles tend to pass directly through tissue but can cause significant indirect injury via cavitation. Even further, high-density tissue like bone can dramatically alter the initial trajectory, deflecting the projectile in nearly any direction. It is imperative that patients who have sustained gunshot wounds undergo a systematic evaluation with complete anatomic exposure and physical examination.

1. **A.** The primary survey on trauma patients follows an algorithmic approach to prevent overlooking potentially life-threatening pathology. Patients with gunshot wounds are no exception. Evaluation and stabilization of the patient's airway to ensure adequate oxygenation and ventilation represents the first step in resuscitation. Remember the acronym "ABCDE" for the primary survey. This involves assessing the patient's airway and maintaining in-line cervical spine immobilization, ensuring adequacy of the patient's breathing by assessing both oxygenation (via pulse oximetry) and ventilation (evaluating respiratory rate and effort), circulation (pulse examination, addressing life-threatening bleeding), disability (neurologic examination), and exposure (strip patient and perform rapid scan for injuries). It is important to be mindful that with a team approach in a working trauma, much of the aforementioned can be performed simultaneously.

For our patient, his unresponsiveness, agonal breathing, and oxygen desaturation are concerning and a definitive airway is indicated. While a chest X-ray will be performed and the left-sided needle decompression will need to be supplanted by a tube thoracostomy, these are of subsidiary importance to securing the patient's airway. A central venous catheter is not necessary at this time, given the presence of two large bore peripheral IVs. While it will be important to take down the patient's tourniquet to perform a detailed extremity evaluation, the report of pulsatile bleeding in the field is suggestive of vascular injury and given present hemostasis, this can be deferred until the initial resuscitation has been performed.

2. **E.** Knowing the indications for operative intervention is essential to caring for patients having sustained traumatic injuries. For penetrating thoracic trauma, immediate resuscitative thoracotomy (the so-called Emergency Department Thoracotomy) is indicated for witnessed pulseless electrical activity (overall survival 4% to 5% for gunshot wounds vs. 18% to 24% for stab wounds). Urgent thoracotomy (within 1 to 4 hours of admission) is indicated for: initial chest tube output >1,500 mL, evidence of ongoing bleeding at a rate of 200–300 mL/h, massive air leak, or cardiac tamponade.

For abdominal trauma, indications for laparotomy include hemodynamic instability, peritonitis on examination, or evisceration. Strong consideration should also be given to exploration for those patients with an abdomen that cannot be evaluated clinically (e.g., due to altered mental status, distracting injury, and paralytic/sedative administration).

During evaluation of the extremities, hard signs of arterial injury include pulsatile hemorrhage, expanding/pulsatile hematoma, bruit or thrill over wound, absent distal pulses, or evidence to suggest extremity ischemia (pallor, poikilothermia, pain, paralysis). So-called soft signs include non-expanding hematoma, peripheral nerve deficit, history of pulsatile hemorrhage at the time of injury, and unexplained hypotension. Any patient presenting with hard signs of vascular injury should undergo prompt exploration as the positive predictive value of physical examination for arterial injury approaches 100%. In the absence of hard signs, an alternate means of performing a bedside evaluation is with the injured extremity index (analogous to an ankle-brachial index, also known as an arterial pressure index) with a normal value of >0.9 having a reported sensitivity/specificity of 95/97% respectively for major vascular injury. A normal physical examination and injured extremity index virtually exclude major arterial injury.

3. **B.** Most thoracic injuries can be managed with tube thoracostomy; only 10% to 15% of thoracic trauma requires operative intervention. Tamponade physiology classically requires only 50 cc of blood in the pericardial space and is characterized clinically by Beck's Triad (jugular venous distention, muffled heart sounds, hypotension), occasionally with a narrowed pulse pressure, and the presence of an effusion on FAST examination.

Patients with tamponade physiology should receive aggressive volume administration because they will be dependent on their preload to generate cardiac output. Decompressive pericardiocentesis may be performed though in the setting of trauma, but this is often a temporizing measure. Definitive surgical management in this setting of trauma involves the creation of a pericardial window.

The reported incidence of great vessel injury in penetrating chest trauma is only 4%, as most of these patients exsanguinate prior to presentation. Gunshot wounds to the mediastinum should raise suspicion and the diagnosis can be confirmed with CT angiography. If present, urgent exploration is warranted.

Lung injury that requires surgical intervention is more commonly encountered with penetrating trauma. The majority of these injuries can be managed with pulmonary tractotomy (for penetrating non-hilar injuries) or nonanatomic stapled resections. Inadequately evacuated hemothorax can result in secondary infection (post-traumatic empyema) or fibrothorax (entrapped lung). Unfortunately, prophylactic antibiotics do not appear to prevent the secondary development of infection in this setting. Chest tubes are often unsuccessful in removing clotted blood and consideration should be given to operative exploration for patients with retained hemothorax.

4. **C.** While a FAST examination is a useful bedside adjunct to detect the presence of free intra-abdominal or pericardial fluid, it is operator dependent and has a poor sensitivity with respect to hollow viscous, retroperitoneal, and diaphragmatic injuries. A negative FAST examination does not rule out intra-peritoneal injury. There is evidence to suggest that hemodynamically stable patients with abdominal gunshot wounds and no evidence of peritonitis on exam may undergo evaluation via computerized tomography of the abdomen to determine whether further operative intervention is required. Even if the posterior fascia is violated, elective nonoperative management with observation and serial examinations is a safe alternative to reflex operative exploration in a major trauma center with in-hospital surgical support.

In general, primary repairs can be done on both small and large bowel if 50% or less of the circumference is damaged. The most injured abdominal organ with penetrating trauma is the small bowel. For unstable patients with penetrating abdominal injuries, a full laparotomy incision should be made so that all injuries can be identified quickly.

5. **A.** Temporary intravascular shunts have served as a valuable adjunct in vascular trauma for decades. With increasing evidence to support a damage control approach to trauma, shunts offer the ability to temporize an injury that would otherwise require ligation (and associated morbidity) or a lengthy operative reconstruction. With increased use in both civilian and military trauma, shunts have been found to improve chances for limb salvage with minimal added operative time and no additional morbidity. In this scenario, ligation would place the patient at significant risk for critical limb ischemia and dramatically increase the chance of eventual amputation. The other modalities discussed would likely add operative time and potentially worsen the patient's existing physiologic derangement. In general, the surgeon should use the largest possible shunt and not routinely anticoagulate these patients.

6. **E.** While many societies have endeavoured to mitigate the individual impact of gunshot wounds, the cost to health care systems and society at large remains high. A recent study out of Los Angeles, California, demonstrated that patients sustaining gunshot wounds were more than five times more likely to die, two times more likely to require surgical intervention, and had a greater chance of ICU admission, longer overall length of stay, and on average, had more than twice the median hospital charge per admission when compared with patients sustaining other forms of interpersonal injury.

BIBLIOGRAPHY

American College of Surgeons Committee on Trauma. *Advanced Trauma Life Support (ATLS) Student Course Manual.* 9th ed. American College of Surgeons; 2012.

Boulanger BR, Kearney PA, Tsuei B, Ochoa JB. The routine use of sonography in penetrating torso injury is beneficial. *J Trauma.* 2001;51(2):320.

Champion HR, Copes WS, Sacco WJ, et al. The major trauma outcome study: establishing national norms for trauma care. *J Trauma.* 1990;30(11):1356.

Cohn SM. Pulmonary contusion: review of the clinical entity. *J Trauma.* 1997;42(5):973–979.

Como JJ, Bokhari F, Chiu WC, et al. Practice management guidelines for selective nonoperative management of penetrating abdominal trauma. *J Trauma.* 2010;68(3):721.

Demetriades D. Penetrating injuries to the thoracic great vessels. *J Card Surg.* 1997;12(2):173–179.

Demetriades D, Hadjizacharia P, Constantinou C, et al. Selective nonoperative management of penetrating abdominal solid organ injuries. *Ann Surg.* 2006;244(4):620–628.

Demetriades D, Velmahos GC. Penetrating injuries of the chest: indications for operation. *Scand J Surg.* 2002;91(1):41–45.

Eger M, Goleman L, Goldstein A, Hirsch M. The use of a temporary shunt in the management of arterial vascular injuries. *Surg Gynecol Obstet.* 1971;132:67–70.

Foran CP, Clark DJ, Henry R, et al. Current burden of gunshot wound injuries at two Los Angeles county level I trauma centers. *J Am Col Surg.* 2019;229(2):141–149.

Fox N, Rajani RR, Bokhari F, et al. Penetrating lower extremity arterial trauma, evaluation and management of. *J Trauma.* 2012;73(5):S315–S320.

Frykberg ER, Dennis JW, Bishop K, Laneve L, Alexander RH. The reliability of physical examination in the evaluation of penetrating extremity trauma for vascular injury: results at one year. *J Trauma.* 1991;31(4):502.

Hines MH, Meredith JW. Special problems of thoracic trauma. In: Ritchie WP, Steele G Jr., Dean RH, et al. eds. *General Surgery.* JB Lippincott; 1995:859–872.

Hoth JJ, Burch PT, Bullock TK, et al. Pathogenesis of posttraumatic empyema: the impact of pneumonia on pleural space infections. *Surg Infect (Larchmt).* 2003;4(1):29–35.

Isenhour JL, Marx J. Advances in abdominal trauma. *Emergency Clinics of North America.* 2007;25:713.

Johansen K, Lynch K, Paun M, Copass M. Non-invasive vascular tests reliably exclude occult arterial trauma in injured extremities. *J Trauma.* 1991;1(4):515–519.

Karmy-Jones R, Jurkovich GJ. Blunt chest trauma. *Curr Probl Surg.* 2004;41:211–380.

Karmy-Jones R, Jurkovich GJ, Shatz DV, et al. Management of traumatic lung injury: A western trauma association multicenter review. *J Trauma.* 2001;51(6):1049–1053.

Maxwell RA, Campbell DJ, Fabian TC, et al. Use of presumptive antibiotics following tube thoracostomy for traumatic hemopneumothorax in the prevention of empyema and pneumonia: a multi-center trial. *J Trauma.* 2004;57(4):742–748.

Meredith JW, Hoth JJ. Thoracic trauma: when and how to intervene. *Surg Clin North Am.* 2007;87(1):95–118.

Natarajan B, Gupta PT, Cemaj S, Sorensen M, Hatzoudis GI, Forse RA. FAST scan: is it worth doing in hemodynamically stable blunt trauma patients? *Surgery.* 2010;148(4):695.

Pryor JP, Reilly PM, Dabrowski GP, Grossman MD, Schwab CW. Nonoperative management of abdominal gunshot wounds. *Ann Emerg Med.* 2004;43(3):344.

Subramanian A, Vercruysse G, Dente C, et al. A decade's experience with temporary intravascular shunts at a civilian Level I trauma center. *J Trauma.* 2008;65:316–326.

Taller J, Kamdar JP, Greene JA, et al. Temporary vascular shunts as initial treatment of proximal extremity vascular injuries during combat operations: the new standard of care at Echelon II facilities? *J Trauma.* 2008;65:595–603.

Velmahos GC, Constantinou C, Tillou A, Brown CV, Salim A, Demetriades D. Abdominal computed tomographic scan for patients with gunshot wounds to the abdomen selected for non-operative management. *J Trauma.* 2005;59(5):1155.

Velmanos GC, Demetriades D, Toutouzas KG, et al. Selective nonoperative management in 1856 patients with abdominal gunshot wounds: should routine laparotomy still be the standard of care? *Ann Surg.* 2001;234(3):395.

Wall MJ Jr, Hirschberg A, Mattox KL. Pulmonary tractotomy with selective vascular ligation for penetrating injuries to the lung. *Am J Surg.* 1994;168(6):665–669.

79

Cervical Spine Clearance

Matthew R. Fusco, Ajith J. Thomas, Christopher S. Ogilvy, and Rob Conrad

A 60-year-old male restrained driver is involved in a high-speed head-on motor vehicle collision. He is heavily intoxicated and uncooperative, therefore he is intubated at the scene and brought to the nearest Level I trauma center. Upon arrival, he is able to shrug his shoulders to questions. Initial vital signs indicate a pulse of 48 bpm and a blood pressure of 78/39 mmHg. His respiratory status appears stable on the current ventilator settings and initial primary trauma evaluation fails to reveal any major external signs of injury.

Subsequent secondary trauma survey reveals the patient is able to shrug his shoulders but demonstrates no motor or sensory function below his deltoids. Questionable rectal tone is present. A cervical collar is in place, but the patient demonstrates tenderness to palpation in the midline of the cervical spine.

1. **What is the most likely cause of this patient's hypotension?**

   A. Splenic rupture
   B. Cardiac tamponade
   C. Flail chest
   D. Spinal shock
   E. Beta-blockade

2. **Which of the following is not a component evaluated by the NEXUS criteria for clearing a patient's cervical spine from injury such that the cervical collar can be removed? Which of the following would allow a patient's cervical spine to be cleared without radiologic assistance?**

   A. No pain with passive motion of the patient's neck
   B. Limited use of medications like ambien and Benadryl
   C. Fractures limited to small bones of the hands and feet
   D. History of intact mental status at the scene of the accident
   E. Low velocity mechanism of injury

3. **Which of the following therapeutic measures is considered a current standard treatment for this patient's shock?**

   A. Limited boluses of normal saline or LR
   B. Bed rest
   C. Selective vasopressor treatment to keep MAPs >85
   D. Administration of methylprednisolone bolus at 30 mg/kg followed by continuous infusion at 5.4 mg/kg/hr for 23 hours

4. **Imaging reveals a fracture dislocation of the mid cervical spine with a resultant spinal cord injury. Computed tomographic angiography (CTA) reveals a traumatic vertebral artery dissection. Which of the following is associated with a markedly increased chance of cervical vascular injury and thus requires an evaluation with CTA?**

   A. Neurological examination out of proportion with CT scan head findings
   B. Seat belt sign
   C. C5 spinous process fracture
   D. Glascow coma scale <10
   E. Le Fort I fracture

5. **For an obtunded patient, which of the following is the best option for clearing his cervical spine of injury?**

   A. Clearance of the cervical spine after negative Flexion/Extension (F/E) radiography of the cervical spine

   B. Clearance of the cervical spine after negative magnetic resonance imaging (MRI) of the cervical spine and a negative clinical examination

   C. A Reliable Clinical Exam Must Be Done

   D. A negative CT scan of the cervical spine

6. **During the primary survey of a trauma patient in the emergency room, which of the following patient requires cervical spine immobilization?**

   A. A 85-year-old female who is neurologically intact after a ground-level fall while on apixaban

   B. A 21-year-old male restrained driver s/p a motor vehicle collision (MVC) at 25 mph

   C. Gunshot wound (GSW) to the head

   D. A 36-year-old male pedestrian involved in an auto versus pedestrian (AVP) accident

ANSWERS

1. **D.** Spinal cord injury following a traumatic cervical spine injury typically results from blunt compression injury to the cord itself. Typically the central gray matter is affected first while the peripherally located white matter fiber tracts may be relatively spared. If the spinal cord injury is severe enough, neurogenic or spinal shock may occur. The most basic definition of this is inadequate tissue perfusion due to paralysis of vasomotor input, most commonly due to loss of sympathetic tone and significant disruption of the vasodilator and vasoconstrictor balance. It is commonly characterized by bradycardia, hypotension, decreased peripheral vascular resistance, and decreased cardiac output. Common physical examination findings demonstrate flaccid paralysis of the extremities with no sensory function, lack of rectal tone, lack of foley catheter sensation, and priapism in males. If the spinal cord injury occurs at C5 or above, then respiratory depression may occur. As this patient demonstrates some deltoid function, this indicates a lower cervical cord injury. Presence of a shoulder shrug should not fool the examiner. This motor function is provided by the 11th cranial nerve. The most common classification of spinal cord injuries occurs via the ASIA system:

A = Complete	No motor or sensory function is preserved in the sacral segments S4–S5
B = Incomplete	Sensory but no motor function is preserved below the neurological level and includes the sacral segments S4–S5
C = Incomplete	Motor function is preserved below the neurological level, and more than half of key muscles below the neurological level have a muscle grade less than 3
D = Incomplete	Motor function is preserved below the neurological level, and at least half of key muscles below the neurological level have a muscle grade of 3 or more
E = Normal	Motor and sensory function are normal

2. **E.** Any patient suspected of a cervical spine injury and therefore a potentially unstable cervical spine should be placed in cervical immobilization with a rigid collar. Maintenance of in-line cervical alignment during intubation as well as log-roll precautions must be upheld during transfers. Per the NEXUS criteria, a patient can be cleared with a 99.8% negative predictive value for cervical spine injury if the following criteria are met:

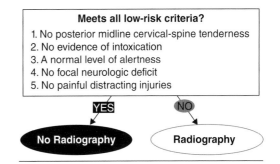

3. **C.** Current treatment protocols for spinal shock involve the mainstays of aggressive fluid resuscitation and vasopressors. Vasopressor choice is left to the discretion of the treating physician based on the patient's co-morbid factors. A goal MAP of >85 sustained for 7 days has demonstrated some promise for improving a patient's outcome. Usage of high-dose steroids in acute spinal cord injury is a controversial topic and has been for quite some time. Various large trials (NASCIS I, II, III) have demonstrated mild benefits with the administration of methylprednisolone bolus of 30 mg/kg followed by 23 hours of continuous infusion at 5.4 mg/kg/hour. However, these studies have also demonstrated significant deleterious side effects with high-dose steroids leading to the Congress of Neurosurgeons to declare that high-dose steroids' risks outweigh their benefits, and are thus not recommended.

4. **A.** Blunt carotid or vertebral artery injuries can be a potentially lethal injury if missed upon initial trauma evaluation. Level II evidence exists for neck CTA screening in trauma patients with an exam out of proportion to their cranial imaging (i.e., a comatose patient with minimal traumatic intracranial damage). Level III evidence exists for such screening in trauma patients with GCS 8 or below, petrous bone fractures, diffuse axonal injury, C1–3 fractures, any cervical spine fracture with subluxation, cervical spine fracture through the foramen transervsarium, or Le Fort II/III injuries. Surprisingly, despite its widely believed association with cervical vascular injuries, presence of an isolated "seat belt sign" with no other aforementioned listed injuries is only associated with a 1% yield for blunt cervical vascular injuries. Treatment of such blunt injuries attempts to prevent intracranial ischemic injuries. Previously aggressive treatment with open surgical or endovascular repair, often in the form of stenting or coiling, provided the mainstay of treatment. However, current emerging evidence suggests these lesions, if diagnosed prior to evidence of ischemia, can be quite benign if treated with antithrombotic medications. Currently, either anticoagulation via heparin/Coumadin or anti-platelet medications via aspirin 325 mg daily are widely used.

5. **B.** Cervical spine clearance in the obtunded trauma patient is a difficult clinical situation for any surgeon. The possibility of a missed cervical spine injury can be devastating. However, prolonged cervical spine immobilization also has significant risks. Obviously, cervical collars should be removed as soon as safe and feasible after trauma. For the awake patient without neurologic deficits, neck pain/tenderness, altered mental status or distracting injury, cervical spine imaging is not mandatory and cervical spine clearance can be performed by clinical examination alone. For the obtunded patient with a negative cervical spine CT scan, there are a number of options for cervical spine clearance. Options include, leaving a cervical collar in place until a clinical examination can be performed, to remove the cervical collar on the basis of negative cervical spine CT alone or to obtain MRI. If the cervical spine MRI is negative, the cervical spine can be safely cleared and it does not require a clinical exam. In the setting of a negative cervical spine CT, the risk of missed injury is also quite low. The incidence of missed ligamentous injury after negative cervical spine CT is <5%, with the incidence of clinically significant injuries as defined by those requiring surgical interventions approaching zero. The largest study to date found that cervical spine CT had negative predictive values of 98.9% for ligamentous injury and 100% for unstable cervical spine injury. With a negative MRI or CT scan of the cervical spine, a clinical exam is not required.

Recent studies have addressed F/E radiography of the cervical spine, and the overwhelming majority recommends that it is almost always inadequate and may even be dangerous. In the obtunded trauma patient, F/E radiography of the cervical spine was found to reliably diagnosis injuries in only 4% of patients.

6. **C.** Indications for cervical spine immobilization include dangerous mechanisms of injury. High-risk mechanisms as defined by the Canadian C-spine Rules (CCR) include fall from greater than 3 feet, high-speed MVC (high speed is >35 mph), MVC rollover/ejection, bicycle collisions, and AVP or recreational vehicle accidents. Given the high rate of cervical spine injuries associated with the aforementioned mechanisms, cervical spine immobilization should be implemented until advanced imaging and a thorough neurologic exam can be obtained. However, in patients with penetrating trauma to the brain, cervical spine immobilization is not necessary unless the trajectory suggests direct injury to the spine. Many patients with penetrating head injuries will require emergency airway management, which may be complicated or delayed by cervical spine immobilization. Numerous studies have shown patients with gunshot wounds limited to the head have an exceedingly low incidence of cervical spine injuries. In a study by Kaups and Davis, with over 200 patients sustaining a gunshot wound to the head, none sustained indirect blast-or fall-related spinal injuries.

BIBLIOGRAPHY

Aarabi B, Hadley MN, Dhall SS, et al. Management of acute traumatic central cord syndrome (ATCCS). *Neurosurgery.* 2013;72(2):195–204.

Bachulis BL, Long WB, Hynes JD, Johnson MC. Clinical indications for cervical spine radiographs in the traumatized patient. *Am J Surg.* 1987;153:473–478.

Bolinger B, Shartz M, Marion D. Bedside fluoroscopic flexion and extension cervical spine radiographs for clearance of the cervical spine in comatose trauma patients. *J Trauma.* 2004;56:132–136.

Chong CL, Ware DN, Harris JH Jr. Is cervical spine imaging indicated in gunshot wounds to the cranium? *J Trauma.* 1998;44:501–502.

Dumont RJ, Okonkwo DO, Verma S, et al. Acute spinal cord injury, part I: patho-physiologic mechanisms. *Clin. Neuropharmacol.* 2001;24:254–264.

Harrigan MR, Hadley MN, Dhall SS, et al. Management of vertebral artery injuries following non-penetrating cervical trauma. *Neurosurgery.* 2013;72(2):234–243.

Hogan GJ, Mirvis SE, Shanmuganathan K, Scalea TM. Exclusion of unstable cervical spine injury in obtunded patients with blunt trauma: is MR imaging needed when multi-detector row CT findings are normal? *Radiology.* 2005;237:106–113.

Hurlbert RJ, Hadley MN, Walters BC, et al. Pharmacological therapy for acute spinal cord injury. *Neurosurgery.* 2013;72(2):93–105.

Kaups KL, Davis JW. Patients with gunshot wounds to the head do not require cervical spine immobilization and evaluation. *J Trauma.* 1998;44:865–867.

Michaleff ZA, Maher CG, Verhagen AP, Rebbeck T, Lin C-WC. Accuracy of the Canadian C-spine rule and NEXUS to screen for clinically important cervical spine injury in patients following blunt trauma: a systematic review. *CMAJ Can. Med. Assoc. J. J. Assoc. Medicale Can.* 2012;184: E867–E876.

Stiell IG, Clement CM, McKnight RD, et al. The Canadian C-spine rule versus the NEXUS low-risk criteria in patients with trauma. *N Engl J Med.* 2003;349:2510–2518.

80

Management of Elevated Intracranial Pressure

Matthew R. Fusco, Ajith J. Thomas, Christopher S. Ogilvy, and Kristopher G. Hooten

A 32-year-old male, unrestrained driver is involved in a high-speed motor vehicle collision. After a prolonged extraction, the patient is found to be somnolent and is intubated on the scene. After arrival in the trauma center, a complete evaluation, including a whole-body trauma CT reveals a non-displaced linear skull fracture and multiple areas of intracranial contusions with diffuse edema but no large mass lesions. No other systemic injuries are discovered. His neurologic exam demonstrates small but reactive pupils; presence of corneal, gag, and cough reflexes; lack of eye opening to voice or painful stimulation; and brisk withdrawal of both legs and his right arm to painful stimulation as well as localization of his left arm to painful stimulation.

1. **What is the patient's Glasgow Coma Scale (GCS)?**

   A. 5
   B. 6
   C. 7
   D. 8
   E. 9

2. **Which of the following is an indication for the use of intracranial pressure monitoring in traumatic brain injury?**

   A. Intracranial injury demonstrated on computerized tomography (CT) scan and GCS of 8 or below
   B. Lack of intracranial injury on CT scan, but age <40, and motor posturing on exam
   C. Lack of neurologic examination due to intoxication
   D. Patients undergoing nonoperative management of other injuries

3. **Which of the following should be implemented in this patient following intracranial pressure monitor placement and admission to the ICU?**

   A. Elevation of the head of bed to up to 10 degrees
   B. Maintaining hemoglobin levels >10 g/dL
   C. Maintenance of a cerebral perfusion pressure of 60 or above
   D. Permissive hypercapnia
   E. Administration of high levels of positive end-expiratory pressure (PEEP) to aid in oxygenation

4. **On post-admission day 2, the patient's intracranial pressures rise to the low 30s. Which of the following maneuvers can be used to reduce his intracranial pressure?**

   A. Decrease sedation
   B. Administration of hypertonic saline
   C. Permissive hypotension
   D. Transient periods of hypoventilation
   E. Administration of methylprednisolone

5. **Despite the previous treatment, the patient's intracranial pressure continues to rise. Which of the following maneuvers can be used to reduce his intracranial pressure?**

   A. Lumbar puncture
   B. Electroencephalography (EEG)
   C. Carbonic anhydrase inhibitor administration
   D. Vasoactive administration
   E. Placement of an external ventricular drain for cerebrospinal fluid (CSF) diversion

ANSWERS

1. **C.** GCS is the most basic method of quickly communicating a patient's neurologic examination. It comprises three components.

   Thus, a nonresponsive comatose patient has a GCS of 3, whereas an awake, oriented patient would

Eye Opening (E)	Verbal Response (V)	Motor Response (M)
4 = opens spontaneously	5 = normal conversation	6 = normal
3 = opens to voice	4 = disoriented conversation	5 = localizes pain
2 = opens to pain	3 = words, incoherent	4 = withdraws from pain
1 = none	2 = incomprehensible sounds	3 = decorticate posturing
	1 = none	2 = decerebrate posturing
		1 = none

demonstrate a GCS of 15. Intubated patients automatically receive just 1 point for verbal response. If a patient's motor exam is asymmetric, the best response is used for grading. Thus, this patient's exam is E1, V1, M5 for a total "GCS of 7." For intubated patients, many providers use the convention of adding a "T" following the GCS score, so this patient would be described as a "GCS 7T."

2. **A.** The Brain Trauma Foundation Guidelines Level II recommendation for ICP monitor placement is a patient with a traumatic intracranial injury on imaging and a GCS of 8 or less. These patients will have an elevated ICP 60% of the time. Also, ICP monitor placement is recommended for a patient with a normal head CT OVER 40 years of age who demonstrates posturing on examination and hypotension. Patients meeting these criteria have demonstrated elevated ICP 13% of the time. Insertion of an intracranial pressure monitor can be used to evaluate and treat elevated ICP in patients with an abnormal head CT or as a surrogate for a neurologic examination in those who require sedation or chemical paralysis for other injuries (e.g., a trauma patient with an open abdomen on paralytics), but it is not required.

3. **C.** The Monro-Kellie doctrine states that the skull is a fixed compartment with three basic components: brain (80%), cerebrospinal fluid (10%), and blood (10%). An increase in any one of these components requires an equal decrease in one or both of the other two to prevent an increase in intracranial pressure. Typical cerebral blood flow compromises 15% to 20% of the cardiac output; a decrease in this may result in unmet cerebral metabolic demands. The primary goal of treatment of severe brain injury is to prevent

secondary injury by maintaining adequate cerebral blood flow and oxygen delivery. Cerebral blood flow can be roughly estimated by cerebral perfusion pressure ($CPP = MAP - ICP$), and is commonly used to guide therapy.

In uninjured patients, the brain will maintain cerebral perfusion via autoregulation over estimated CPP ranges of 50 to 150. Patients with severe brain injury, however, will commonly exhibit loss of autoregulation, which means that their cerebral blood flow will be directly dependent on an adequate mean arterial pressure (MAP) and a normal intracranial pressure (ICP). This is why there is so much attention paid to maintaining a normal to slightly elevated blood pressure and aggressive measures to avoid ICP elevations in patients with severe brain injury.

All attempts at treating elevated intracranial pressure keep this Monro-Kellie hypothesis and its relationship with cerebral perfusion pressure in mind. The first steps toward the treatment of a patient with elevated intracranial pressure begin with many simple bedside maneuvers. Initial steps should include endotracheal intubation and mechanical ventilation, elevation of the head of bed 30–45° to aid cerebral venous outflow, seizure prophylaxis for 1 week only (in the absence of an indication to continue), maintenance of hemoglobin of at least 7 g/dL or above, hyponatremia avoidance, fever avoidance, adequate pulmonary support, and avoidance of elevated intra-abdominal pressure. Pulmonary support should focus of avoidance of hypoxia, hypercapnia, and excessive PEEP. Elevated levels of $PaCO_2$ lead to intracranial vasodilation and cerebral blood volume, thus elevated ICP. Excessive PEEP may lead to increased intra-thoracic pressure and thus impaired cerebral venous outflow.

4. B. Treating ICP > 22 mmHg is recommended as values above this level are associated with increased mortality. If elevated ICP occurs, more aggressive methods of treatment include hypertonic saline, sedation (via propofol or barbituates to decreased cerebral metabolic demands), paralytics, and mannitol for both rheologic and osmotic effects. Cautions with treatments include hypotension with mannitol, sodium fluctuations with hypertonic saline, porofol infusion syndrome with prolonged used, and decreased cardiac output with barbiturates. "Steroids should be avoided in intracranial trauma. Despite the usage of dexamethasone with other causes of cerebral edema, steroids are associated with elevated mortality in trauma patients with severe brain injury due to the myriad of side effects." Hypotension should be avoided to help maintain the CPP. Hyperventilation can be used as a temporizing measure but prolonged use can cause cerebral ischemia.

5. E. Treating ICP > 22 mmHg is recommended as values above this level are associated with increased mortality. External ventricular drains (EVDs) may be placed in conjunction with intracranial pressure monitors. These devices offer CSF diversion, which can lower ICP by removing CSF from the intracranial space and can be used in combination with medical therapy to lower ICP. Lumbar puncture would be contraindicated in the setting of cerebral edema. EEGs while may be used in the setting of TBI are not therapeutic. Vasoactive drug may be needed to maintain CPP and avoid hypotension, but may elevate ICPs with the loss of cerebral autoregulation. Carbonic anhydrase inhibitors may lower ICP but are not used in the acute setting.

BIBLIOGRAPHY

Brain Trauma Foundation, American Association of Neurological Surgeons, Congress of Neurological Surgeons, et al. Guidelines for the management of severe traumatic brain injury, fourth edition. 3. Hyperosmolar therapy. *Neurosurgery.* 2017;80(1):6–15. https://braintrauma.org/uploads/03/12/Guidelines_for_Management_of_Severe_TBI_4th_Edition.pdf

Brain Trauma Foundation, American Association of Neurological Surgeons, Congress of Neurological Surgeons, et al. Guidelines for the management of severe traumatic brain injury, fourth edition. 4. Cerebrospinal fluid drainage. *Neurosurgery.* 2017;80(1):6–15. https://braintrauma.org/uploads/03/12/Guidelines_for_Management_of_Severe_TBI_4th_Edition.pdf

Brain Trauma Foundation, American Association of Neurological Surgeons, Congress of Neurological Surgeons, et al. Guidelines for the management of severe traumatic brain injury, fourth edition. 5. Ventilation therapies. *Neurosurgery.* 2017;80(1):6–15. https://braintrauma.org/uploads/03/12/Guidelines_for_Management_of_Severe_TBI_4th_Edition.pdf

Brain Trauma Foundation, American Association of Neurological Surgeons, Congress of Neurological Surgeons, et al. Guidelines for the management of severe traumatic brain injury, fourth edition. 6. Anesthetics, analgesics, and sedatives. *Neurosurgery.* 2017;80(1):6–15. https://braintrauma.org/uploads/03/12/Guidelines_for_Management_of_Severe_TBI_4th_Edition.pdf

Brain Trauma Foundation, American Association of Neurological Surgeons, Congress of Neurological Surgeons, et al. Guidelines for the management of severe traumatic brain injury, fourth edition. 7. Steroids. *Neurosurgery.* 2017;80(1):6–15. https://braintrauma.org/uploads/03/12/Guidelines_for_Management_of_Severe_TBI_4th_Edition.pdf

Brain Trauma Foundation, American Association of Neurological Surgeons, Congress of Neurological Surgeons, et al. Guidelines for the management of severe traumatic brain injury, fourth edition. 11. Seizure prophylaxis. *Neurosurgery.* 2017;80(1):6–15. https://braintrauma.org/uploads/03/12/Guidelines_for_Management_of_Severe_TBI_4th_Edition.pdf)

Brain Trauma Foundation, American Association of Neurological Surgeons, Congress of Neurological Surgeons, et al. Guidelines for the management of severe traumatic brain injury, fourth edition. 12. Intracranial pressure monitoring. *Neurosurgery.* 2017;80(1):6–15. https://braintrauma.org/uploads/03/12/Guidelines_for_Management_of_Severe_TBI_4th_Edition.pdf

Brain Trauma Foundation, American Association of Neurological Surgeons, Congress of Neurological Surgeons, et al. Guidelines for the management of severe traumatic brain injury, fourth edition. 15. Blood pressure thresholds. *Neurosurgery.* 2017;80(1):6–15. https://braintrauma.org/uploads/03/12/Guidelines_for_Management_of_Severe_TBI_4th_Edition.pdf

Brain Trauma Foundation, American Association of Neurological Surgeons, Congress of Neurological Surgeons, et al. Guidelines for the management of severe traumatic brain injury, fourth edition. 16. Intracranial pressure thresholds. *Neurosurgery.* 2017;80(1):6–15. https://braintrauma.org/uploads/03/12/Guidelines_for_Management_of_Severe_TBI_4th_Edition.pdf

Brain Trauma Foundation, American Association of Neurological Surgeons, Congress of Neurological Surgeons, et al. Guidelines for the management of severe traumatic brain injury, fourth edition. 17. Cerebral perfusion pressure thresholds. *Neurosurgery.* 2017;80(1):6–15. https://braintrauma.org/uploads/03/12/Guidelines_for_Management_of_Severe_TBI_4th_Edition.pdf

Edwards P, Arango M, Balica L, et al. Final results of MRC CRASH, a randomised placebo-controlled trial of intravenous corticosteroid in adults with head injury-outcomes at 6 months. *Lancet.* 2005;365: 1957–1959.

Hawryluk GWJ, Aguilera S, Buki A, et al. A management algorithm for patients with intracranial pressure monitoring: the Seattle International Severe Traumatic Brain Injury Consensus Conference (SIBICC). *Intensive Care Med.* 2019;45(12):1783–1794.

81

Ortho-Trauma—Pelvic Fracture

William J. Jordan and John S. Mayo

A 27-year-old female presents to the emergency department after a motorcycle crash. She was hemodynamically unstable on arrival and is currently receiving 2 L of crystalloid via large bore peripheral IVs. Glasgow Coma Scale (GCS) is 12. She is breathing spontaneously and has no obvious extremity trauma. Initial radiographs demonstrate normal cervical alignment without fracture, right-sided fractures of ribs 4 to 8, a small right-sided pulmonary contusion, no free air under the diaphragm, and a pelvis film that shows widening of the pubic symphysis by 4 cm along with diastasis of the left sacroiliac joint. Abdominal ultrasound is negative for free fluid. The patient is currently on her menses.

1. **With regard to the pelvic injury, the patient's hemodynamic instability is most likely related to:**

    A. Disruption of the anastomosis of the external iliac/deep epigastric and obturator vessels (the Corona Mortis)

    B. Arterial injury of the superior gluteal artery and vein at the level of the greater sciatic notch

    C. Post-traumatic closed soft tissue degloving injury in which the skin and subcutaneous tissue separate from the fascia superficial to the underlying musculature (Morel-Lavallee lesion)

    D. Disruption of the anterior sacral venous plexus

    E. Rupture of the pelvic floor structures (sacrospinous and sacrotuberrous ligaments) with vaginal laceration by the anterior pubic symphysis fragments

2. **What percentage of vascular injuries from high-energy pelvic trauma are arterial in nature?**

    A. <5%

    B. 10% to 15%

    C. 50%

    D. 60% to 75%

    E. >85%

3. **Regarding the hemodynamic instability of pelvic fractures, what is the fracture pattern associated with the highest severity of hemorrhage?**

    A. Anteroposterior compression (APC III) fracture patterns

    B. Lateral compression (LC III) fracture patterns

    C. Vertical sheer (VS) fracture patterns

    D. Combined APC/VS patterns

    E. Open pelvic fractures

4. **Regarding the mortality of displaced pelvic fractures, the highest mortality rates are seen in:**

    A. Anteroposterior compression (APC III) fracture patterns

    B. Lateral compression (LC III) fracture patterns

    C. Vertical sheer (VS) fracture patterns

    D. Combined APC/VS patterns

    E. Open pelvic fractures

5. **A speculum examination of the vaginal mucosa demonstrates a 2-cm laceration on the left wall of the vagina and proctoscopy shows a rectal laceration. Which of the following should occur early in the treatment of this injury?**

    A. Urgent primary closure of vaginal laceration

    B. Repair of the rectal laceration and diverting colostomy

    C. Repair of the rectal laceration and drainage

D. Repair of likely associated bladder and urethral injuries

E. Urine diversion

6. **With which pelvic radiograph finding would a pelvic binder worsen pain and fracture displacement?**

   A. Unilateral superior displacement of the ilium relative to the sacrum

   B. Anterior sacroiliac joint disruption

   C. Internal rotation fracture with overriding pubic symphysis

   D. Pubic symphysis widened to 4 cm without associated sacroiliac injury

   E. Bilateral superior displacement of the ilium

ANSWERS

1. **D.** Hemodynamic instability after blunt trauma is due to ongoing hemorrhage until proven otherwise, with the common locations being the chest, abdomen, pelvis, or extremity/external bleeding. The normal chest X-ray and abdominal ultrasound in conjunction with the abnormal pelvis X-ray make the pelvis the most likely source of bleeding in this patient. Although arterial injuries in association with major pelvic trauma can occur, the majority of bleeding occurs at the venous plexus located on the anterior aspect of the sacrum and sacroiliac joints. This historically has responded best to pelvic packing or fracture reduction, rather than immediate angiography. Injuries to the superior gluteal arteries posteriorly and the Corona Mortis anteriorly have been reported and can be devastating, but they are far outnumbered by the venous lacerations of the presacral venous plexus. Morel-Lavallee lesions are common after blunt force trauma but do not typically lead to hemodynamic instability seen from the deep pelvic venous lacerations.

2. **B.** The current management of pelvic fracture patients who are hemodynamically unstable consists of aggressive resuscitation, mechanical stabilization, and angioembolization. Despite this multidisciplinary approach, mortality rates of these high-risk patients can exceed 40%. Initial maneuvers to reduce the pelvic fracture and decrease the pelvic volume include placement of a pelvic binder, wrapping the pelvis with a sheet, or application of an external fixation device. Binders also help with fracture reduction and stabilization, which works to improve pain.

However, it is important to note the correct placement of pelvic binders, which should be centered over the greater trochanters. If binders are incorrectly placed, they can worsen fracture dislocation and pain. Preperitoneal pelvic packing (PPP) via laparotomy can directly address the venous bleeding that compromises 85% of pelvic fracture hemorrhage and does not respond to the initial maneuvers listed earlier. The remaining 15% of vascular injuries are arterial and may best be addressed via angiography in the event of continued hemodynamic instability following pelvic packing.

3. **A.** In an antero-posterior compression fracture (APC), the fracture propagates from anterior to posterior. This widens the symphysis pubis and depending on the level of force can widen the anterior sacroiliac joint or disrupt it entirely. In an APC III injury, the pelvic floor ligaments (sacrospinous and sacrotuberous) are disrupted and can lead to instability and increased volume in the pelvic cavity. Disruption and displacement of the sacroiliac joint has the potential to lead to massive hemorrhage from the anterior sacral venous plexus that is closely approximated to the joint. Major hemorrhage in patients with pelvic fractures can reliably be predicted based on a pulse greater than 130, a hematocrit of 30 or less, and wide diastasis of the pubic symphysis.

4. **E.** Open pelvic fractures are potentially lethal injuries with a reported mortality rate of 30% to 50%. Open fractures of the pelvis by definition communicate with the rectum, the vagina, or the outside environment by disruption of the skin. They are often associated with the disruption of the pelvic floor, leading to loss of tamponade and persistent bleeding. An additional concern is pelvic infection and sepsis due to the open communication with the rectum, vagina, or skin. Clinical suspicion of an open fracture and any rectal or vaginal bleeding mandates a thorough examination of the pelvis, perineum, rectum/anal complex, and vagina in females.

   In addition to visual inspection and digital examination, full evaluation should include rigid proctoscopy or flexible sigmoidoscopy, and speculum examination in females. Management of major open pelvic fractures includes administration of intravenous antibiotics, washout and debridement of open wounds, and consideration for a possible diverting colostomy to prevent fecal contamination of the open fracture.

5. **B.** Early diagnosis of an open pelvic fracture is essential and a thorough examination must be done so that no such injuries are missed. While it is not difficult to diagnose an open fracture when massive wounds of the skin and perineum are present, a small vaginal or rectal tear that communicates with and contaminates the fracture may be missed unless it is sought specifically. Rectal injuries must be sought, particularly in patients with a sacral fracture, because the fragments of bone frequently traverse the rectal wall.

Classically, an open pelvic fracture prompts recommendations for colostomy to prevent soft-tissue sepsis in an expanded perineum. It has recently been suggested that fecal diversion in an open pelvic fracture can be applied selectively, according to the actual location, nature, and size of the cutaneous wound. For open fractures with an associated rectal injury, immediate diverting colostomy and repair of the rectal laceration (if possible) are indicated. Anterior wounds of the groin, anterior thigh, iliac crest, or pubis do not require diversion. Injuries to the vagina must also be repaired, but it is not as essential with regard to reducing sepsis. Urinary tract injuries can also occur, should be expected with hematuria or blood at the urethral openings, and should also be repaired but delaying repair does not necessarily increase the risk of sepsis.

6. **E.** Although pelvic binders are now routinely applied for suspected or proven pelvic fractures, they may have no benefit or may even cause additional harm in select types of fractures. The AP pelvic radiograph will identify injuries that may benefit from provisional stabilization with external compression with a sheet or pelvic binder. In general, lateral compression (LC) injuries with internal rotation or iliac wing fractures will not respond to binder placement, whereas APC and VS injuries will. APC and VS injuries can be suspected from the mechanism but also have distinct characteristics on plain films.

APC injuries are hallmarked by a widened pubic symphysis. Anterior disruption without associated posterior injury will only allow the symphysis to widen to about 2.5 cm. To widen further, there must be associated injuries to the sacrospinous, sacrotuberous, and anterior sacroiliac ligaments to widen further. In VS injuries, the sacrum is displaced relative to the iliac wing resulting in superior displacement of the ilium and pubis. This can happen on one side or bilaterally.

LC fractures are the most common pelvic fractures and are hallmarked by horizontal fracturing of the pubic rami, internal rotation of the injured side of the pelvic including the hip, and posterior fracturing of the ilium. More severe fractures can extend the disruption to the other side of the pelvis. Compression of an LC injury is potentially damaging as it may induce additional lateral compression and fracture dislocation or bleeding.

BIBLIOGRAPHY

Alton TB, Gee AO. Classifications in brief; Young and Burgess classification of pelvic ring injuries. *Clin Orthop Relat Res.* Aug 2014;472(8):2338–2342.

Blackmore CC, Cummings P, Jurkovich GJ, Linnau KF, Hoffer EK, Rivara FP. Predicting major hemorrhage in patients with pelvic fracture. *J Trauma.* August 2006;61(2):346–352.

Cothren CC, Osborn PM, Moore EE, Morgan SJ, Johnson JL, Smith WR. Perperitoneal pelvic packing for hemodynamically unstable pelvic fractures: a paradigm shift. *J Trauma.* 2007;62(4):834–842.

Cullinane DC, Schiller HJ, Zielinski MD, et al. Eastern Association for the Surgery of Trauma practice management guidelines for hemorrhage in pelvic fracture—update and systematic review. *J Trauma.* 2011;71(6):1850–1868.

Fallinger MS, McGanity PL. Unstable fractures of the pelvic ring. *J Bone Joint Surg Am.* June 1992;74(5):781–791.

Langford JR, Burgess AR, Liporace FA, Haldukewych GJ. Pelvic fractures: part 1: evaluation, classification, and resuscitation. *J Am Acad Orthop Surg.* August 2013;21(8):448–457.

Mohanty K, Musso D, Powell JN, Kortbeek JB, Kirkpatrick AW. Emergent management of pelvic ring injuries: an update. *Can J Surg.* February 2005;48(1):49–56.

Tai DK, Li W-H, Lee K-Y, et al. Retroperitoneal pelvic packing in the management of hemodynamically unstable pelvis fractures: level 1 trauma center experience. *J Trauma.* October 2011;71(4):E79–E86.

82

Intracranial Hematomas

Ahmed B. Bayoumi, Fares Nigim, Ekkehard M. Kasper, and Kristopher G. Hooten

CASE 1

A 44-year-old female patient presented to the emergency department after a fall while hiking. She reports hitting her head directly on a large rock with a history of profuse bleeding from her scalp. She denied any loss of consciousness or seizures. The bleeding was controlled by a gauze dressing and compression bandage at the site of the injury. She was hemodynamically stable and had a Glasgow Coma Scale (GCS) of 15/15. On neurological examination, she had no motor deficits except for right-sided lower motor neuron (LMN) facial palsy. A large, parietal lacerated scalp wound was visible 3 cm away from the midline on the left, measuring about 2 cm in length. A computerized tomography (CT) of her head and key image is demonstrated in Figure 82-1.

1. **Which of the following is an indication for surgical intervention in open depressed skull fractures?**

   A. Depression that exceeds 5 mm
   B. Such fractures associated with a >1-cm intracranial hematoma
   C. Such fractures overlying a dural venous sinus
   D. Dural injury with persistent cerebrospinal fluid (CSF) leak

2. **Regarding the management of open depressed skull fracture, which of the following is true?**

   A. Early surgical intervention may decrease the risk of primary traumatic brain injury.
   B. In the presence of suspected wound contamination, primary bone replacement (cranioplasty) is recommended.

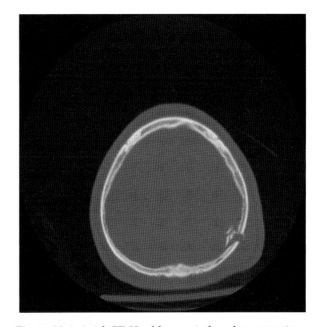

Figure 82-1 Axial CT Head bone window demonstrating a depressed skull fracture.

   C. Early surgical intervention may decrease the risk of infection.
   D. Severe cosmetic deformity requires urgent surgery.

CASE 2

A 34-year-old male patient presented to the emergency department after a fall while. Witness reports fall of 20 to 30 feet over a cliff while attempting a selfie. Patient was found unconscious with profuse bleeding from his scalp. By the time of arrival to emergency department,

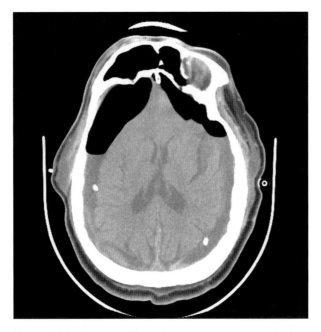

Figure 82-2 Axial CT Head demonstrating a frontal sinus fracture, pneumocephalus and a subdural hematoma

patient was confused but otherwise neurologically intact. He was hemodynamically stable and had a GCS of 14/15. On examination, patient was noted to have a deep left forehead laceration and no other focal deficits.

His head CT is demonstrated in Figure 82-2.

1. **Regarding initial management in this patient with an open skull fracture, Which of the following would be a contraindication to bedside debridement and closure of scalp laceration?**

   A. Depression that is measured at 7 mm
   B. Associated intracranial hematoma with significant mass effect
   C. Involvement of the frontal sinus
   D. Absence of pneumocephalus
   E. Disruption of the galea

2. **On hospital day 2, patient noted a salty taste in his mouth and dripping of clear fluid from nares when leaning forward. Which of the following is true?**

   A. Urgent surgical intervention is recommended.
   B. Magnetic resonance imaging (MRI) is the most sensitive procedure to localize the injury.
   C. Meningococci are the most common pathogen that may cause meningitis.
   D. This injury is less likely to persist compared to spontaneous ones.
   E. This fluid would have a lower concentration of glucose than mucus.

CASE 3

A 3-year-old male with no significant past medical history presents to the emergency department with altered level of consciousness following direct trauma to the head by a heavy object about 3 hours prior to arrival. He was brought in by his parents, who said that he had loss of consciousness for a minute after which he woke up complaining of headache and blurry vision. He vomited once before becoming somnolent and again about 30 minutes later.

On general examination, his vital signs were as follows: BP = 170/85 mmHg, RR = 18 cycle/min, Pulse = 48 beat/min, and GCS = 9/15. Bruises and swelling were seen over the left scalp. On neurological examination, the patient opened his eyes and moaned to stimulation with round, equal, and reactive pupils. The patient localized to painful stimuli on the left and was not moving his extremities on the right.

No other injuries were noted on trauma evaluation. Cranial imaging via CT is demonstrated in Figure 82-3.

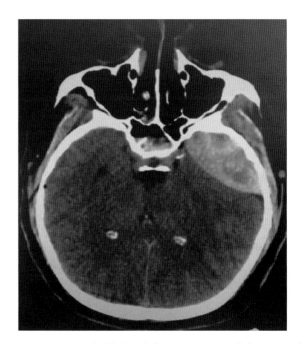

Figure 82-3 Axial CT Head demonstrating a left temporal traumatic hemorrhage

1. **What is the cause of the patient neurologic decline?**

   A. Subdural hematoma (SDH)
   B. Infection
   C. Hydrocephalus
   D. Tension pneumocephalus
   E. Epidural hematoma (EDH)

2. **Regarding the management of this patient, which of the following is correct?**

   A. Lumbar puncture is recommended to alleviate elevated ICP symptoms.

   B. Lesions of this type exceeding 30 cm^3 should be surgically evacuated regardless the conscious level of the patient.

   C. These lesions can never be managed conservatively.

   D. These lesions are usually evacuated in the operating room by two widely spaced burr holes rather than a craniotomy.

   E. Palliative care is recommended as these lesions carry a worse prognosis than other types of intracranial hemorrhage.

3. **Regarding the clinical findings for this patient, which of the following is concerning?**

   A. Respiration rate of 18

   B. Systolic blood pressure of 170

   C. Age of the patient

   D. The gender of this patient

   E. The lucid interval

4. **Regarding the underlying etiology for these lesions, which of the following is true?**

   A. A rare source of bleeding in these lesions is the middle meningeal artery.

   B. These lesions cannot be caused by injury of dural venous sinuses.

   C. These lesions are commonly associated with a skull fracture.

   D. The bridging cortical veins are usually torn with associated extensive brain lacerations.

   E. These lesions are most commonly seen in elderly patients due to age-related brain atrophy.

CASE 4

A 21-year-old male Caucasian patient was brought into the emergency room by his girlfriend after a motorbike accident. She reports an episode of a left face and arm twitching an hour after the accident. The patient had a transient loss of consciousness. Upon regaining consciousness, he complained only of a headache before he developed the seizure. On general examination, vital signs were found to be within normal limits. On neurological examination, he was found to still be in postictal status but without any motor deficit. Intravenous fosphenytoin was administered and a non-contrast head CT scan was performed and can been seen in Figure 82-4.

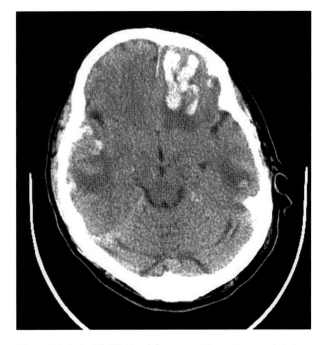

Figure 82-4 Axial CT Head demonstrating a traumatic intracranial hemorrhage.

1. **What type of intracranial hemorrhage is present?**

   A. Epidural hemorrhage

   B. Subdural hemorrhage

   C. Subarachnoid hemorrhage (SAH)

   D. Hemorrhagic brain contusions

   E. Intraventricular hemorrhage

2. **Regarding this type of traumatic intracranial hemorrhage, which of the following is correct?**

   A. It occurs most commonly in the occipital and parietal poles of the brain.

   B. Lesion progression after initial imaging is rare.

   C. Surgical evacuation is only indicated in case of progressive neurological deterioration.

   D. Temporal involvement has a lower threshold for surgery than the other sites.

   E. IV Dexamethasone is part of the medical management for this type of head injury.

3. **Regarding outcomes of patients with this type of traumatic brain injury, which of the following is a poor predictor of outcome in this patient?**

   A. History of seizure

   B. Waxing and waning of the patient's GCS

   C. Amount of fractured skull

   D. Speed at which he was traveling

   E. Effacement of basal cisterns

4. **Which of the following is considered for initial management in this patient?**

   A. Elevation of the head of bed to up to 10°
   B. Admission to the ICU
   C. Maintenance of a cerebral perfusion pressure (CPP) of 40 or below
   D. Permissive hypercapnia
   E. Noninvasive ventilation

CASE 5

A 26-year-old Hispanic male was brought to the emergency room after being involved in a motor vehicle accident 2 hours prior. He appeared confused and complaining of an intense headache and nausea. He was a known cocaine addict. The patient had unremarkable vital signs and a GCS of 13/15. On neurological examination, he was agitated and confused with post-traumatic amnesia. He had no apparent motor or sensory deficit except for right-sided pupillary dilation and ptosis since the accident. A thorough examination was done to exclude associated injuries and a non-contrast CT study of the head was done, which revealed the image seen (Figure 82-5).

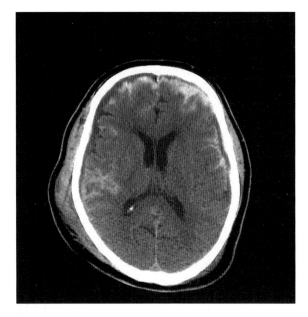

Figure 82-5 Axial CT Head demonstrating a bilateral intracranial hemorrhage pattern.

1. **What type of intracranial hemorrhage is present?**

   A. Epidural hemorrhage
   B. Subdural hemorrhage
   C. SAH
   D. Hemorrhagic brain contusions
   E. Intraventricular hemorrhage

2. **What is the most common cause of this type of intracranial hemorrhage?**

   A. Trauma
   B. Aneurysmal rupture
   C. Ruptured arteriovenous malformation (AVM)
   D. Coagulopathy
   E. Cocaine abuse

3. **Regarding the clinical presentation of this type of intracranial hemorrhage, which of the following is correct?**

   A. The patient usually presents with high ICP symptoms secondary to hemorrhagic mass effect
   B. Seizures are not a part of the course of the disease.
   C. Sudden onset of unilateral ptosis with pupillary dilation may indicate a cerebral aneurysm.
   D. Patients do not present with focal neurological deficits.

4. **If this patient had no obvious history of head trauma, what would be the gold standard study to identify the underlying cause of hemorrhage?**

   A. Magnetic resonance angiography (MRA)
   B. MRI diffusion study (DWI)
   C. Catheter cerebral angiography
   D. CT perfusion study
   E. Transcranial doppler study

5. **If the patient's conscious level deteriorates, what is the most likely cause of this deterioration?**

   A. Hydrocephalus
   B. Cerebral vasodilation
   C. Hypernatremia
   D. Undiagnosed carotid injury
   E. Seizures prophylaxis

CASE 6

A 75-year-old female on clopidogrel for a remote stroke was brought to the emergency room by her daughter. The patient has been complaining of confusion, forgetfulness, and headaches over the last month and her symptoms got worse over the last week. She denies vomiting, nausea, speech difficulties, or visual changes. She fell 2 months prior to admission and had a minor head trauma, which was cared for without medical attention. During history taking, the patient reported that she had a stroke 2 years ago, which left her with slight weakness in the left upper and lower extremities. She also has a history of congestive heart failure (CHF) with an ejection fraction of 28% noted on echocardiogram done 4 months ago.

On physical examination, her vital signs show BP 135/90 mmHg; temperature of 98°F (36.7°C); RR of 16/minute; HR 76/minute and regular. Head, eye, ear, nose, and throat (HEENT) exam is normocephalic but showing a large bruise on her left temple. PERRLA shows no fundoscopic abnormalities. Her neck is supple, with no carotid bruits and her heart rate and rhythm is normal S1/S2, with no murmurs, rubs, or gallops.

The neurological examination shows mental status is alert and oriented × 3. Her GCS is 13/15 and the cranial nerves are 2–12 grossly intact. Her strength is 5/5 in all muscle groups except 3/5 in the left arm throughout. Her DTRs are asymmetric 3+ in left upper and lower extremities and 1+ on the right. There was no Babinski sign bilaterally. The cerebellar exam was negative, as was Romberg's test. Her gait is normal and her sensation is intact to pinprick and light touch.

A thorough physical examination was done to exclude skull bone fractures and spine injuries. Head CT-scan imaging showed the images provided in Figure 82-6.

1. **What type of intracranial hemorrhage is present?**
   A. Epidural hemorrhage
   B. Subdural hemorrhage
   C. SAH
   D. Hemorrhagic brain contusions
   E. Intraventricular hemorrhage

2. **Which of the following is considered to be the highest risk factor for development of these lesions after head trauma?**
   A. Seizure history
   B. Anticoagulation/antiplatelet therapy
   C. Gender
   D. Alcohol abuse
   E. Age >65

3. **Which of the following statements is correct with regard the options for management of these lesions?**
   A. Conservative treatment is suitable in lesions with less than 10-mm thickness even with the presence of focal neurologic signs.
   B. Burr-hole drainage with the placement of subdural drain is not as effective as a craniotomy.

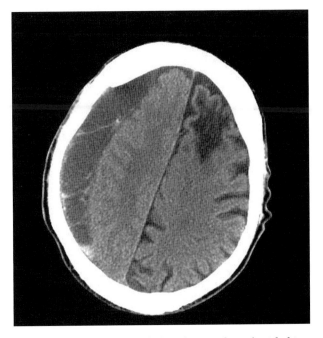

Figure 82-6 Axial CT head demonstrating left frontal encephalomalacia and a right sided intracranial hemorrhage

C. Percutaneous twist-drill bedside drainage is indicated.

D. Burr-hole drainage requires intubation or heavy sedation.

4. **Which of the following risk factors is associated with higher recurrence rate of chronic subdural hematoma (CSDH)?**

A. Significant brain atrophy
B. Etiology
C. Time interval to surgery
D. Gender
E. Age

ANSWERS

Answers to Case 1

1. **D.** Figure 82-1 is an axial cut of CT head (bone window) showing a left parietal compound depressed bone fracture. A depressed skull fracture greater than the thickness of the calvarium (>1 cm), an intracranial hematoma with mass effect are considered recommendations for surgical intervention. Treatment is recommended to reduce secondary injury and prevent CNS infection. It is recommended to manage patients with skull fractures overlying a dural venous sinuses conservatively only if there is no neurological deficit or CSF leak. The high probability of vessel wall laceration with subsequent profuse bleeding during surgery is the main cause of perioperative mortality. Meier and his colleagues reported 100% mortality rate of cases with skull fractures lacerating the posterior third of the superior sagittal sinus and a 50% mortality rate in cases in which the middle third was afflicted. Patients with open depressed cranial fractures may be treated nonoperatively if there is no clinical or radiographic evidence of dural penetration (pneumocephalus), significant intracranial hematoma, frontal sinus involvement, gross cosmetic deformity, wound infection, or gross contamination.

2. **C.** Early surgery has been recommended to reduce the risk of infection but it does not affect the extent of primary traumatic brain injury. It may reduce the risk of secondary injury, however. There is no evidence that bone elevation following open skull fractures necessarily decreases the incidence of post-traumatic seizures, which probably occur as a direct result of the initial brain injury. Antibiotics are part of the

management strategies of compound depressed fractures and are currently recommended. Same session cranioplasty or repair of autologous bone is accepted only if there is no evidence of infection. Marked cosmetic deformity may warrant elective but not urgent surgical skull reconstruction.

Answers to Case 2

1. **B.** Figure 82-2 is an axial cut of CT head (bone), which shows a case of minimally displaced frontal sinus fracture. In addition, there is a small overlying EDH. As noted previously, nonoperative management can be considered if there is no evidence of dural penetration, significant mass effect from an associated hematoma or bone fragment. The presence of a hematoma with mass effect should be addressed emergently with surgical intervention. The absence of pneumocephalus suggests intact dura. Pneumocephalus is defined as the presence of air within the intracranial cavity. Frontal sinus involvement, while historically considered an indication for surgery, is not an absolute indication, and conservative management can be considered in the absence of significant mass effect, without significant displacement of the fracture, and in the absence of a persistent CSF leak.

2. **D.** This is a CSF leak. Initial treatment of traumatic CSF leaks is typically conservative as most post-traumatic CSF leaks subside within 72 hours to 1 week without surgical intervention. Spontaneous CSF fistula cases are more likely to persist. Detection of β_2-transferrin in rhinorrhea-fluid corroborates the presence of a CSF fistula. Tahir and colleagues reported that CT-cisternography has the highest sensitivity and specificity when compared to MRI in detecting the site of a CSF leak. Pneumococci are the most common causative organisms in cases of meningitis following a CSF fistula. Glucose urine strips could help in identifying CSF due to its high glucose concentration ($\geq$40 mg/dl) when compared to low glucose levels (<5 mg/dl) found in mucus secretions.

Answers to Case 3

1. **E.** CT demonstrates a left frontal EDH with significant mass effect correlating with history of lucid interval and clinical findings. The classic appearance of EDH is a homogeneous hyperdense extra-axial lenticular mass with convex borders. EDH is usually localized to a limited part of the calvarium since it is

confined by the skull sutures (not the falx). On the other hand, a SDH is characterized on head CT as a crescentic mass with biconcave shape, diffusely spanning a large area of the brain convexity and is not limited by the sutures. This difference is illustrated in Figure 82-7.

2. B. An EDH measuring more than 30 cm³ in volume should be surgically evacuated regardless the GCS. A midline shift of more than 5 mm is also a critical radiological sign of brain compression, which usually indicates the need for surgical intervention. A patient with a GCS of more than 8 and a hematoma less than 30 cm³, less than 15 mm in thickness, with less than 0.5 cm midline shift, and without focal deficit can be managed by close observation. Acute intracranial hematomas are evacuated by cranitomies or craniectomies as the fresh blood is almost always clotted. On the other hand, chronic SDH are usually liquefied and can be surgically drained by one or two burr holes. Dural tenting/tack-up/hitching stitches (that holds the dura to bone) are recommended to close the epidural space in order to prevent EDH re-accumulation. However, hemostasis is still the most relevant aspect to prevent rebleeding and there is no compelling evidence to support the role of dural tenting for all intracranial operations.

Lumbar puncture may lead to life-threatening central or tonsillar herniation and is therefore not used in cases in which there is high ICP and a pressure gradient between the intracranial and intraspinal compartments.

3. B The systolic blood pressure of 170, especially in a young healthy patient, can be concerning for a Cushing reflex and pending brain herniation. Increasing systolic and pulse pressure with bradycardia and respiratory irregularity are signs of increased intracranial pressure, leading to cerebral herniation and fatal brainstem compression. EDH are more common in males and in the young adult and pediatric populations. Age is typically considered a good prognostic factor in traumatic brain injury. Preoperative GCS is a predictive factor for outcome with the higher GCS correlating with an improved clinical outcome in the treatment of EDH. The classic lucid interval is seen in only 21% of traumatic EDH cases and can be seen in other expanding intracranial lesion. In regard to clinical exam findings of hemiparesis as noted in this scenario, it is important to note that weakness can be a false localizing sign with cerebral herniation. While suspected to be contralateral weakness, ipsilateral weakness occurs when the contralateral cerebral

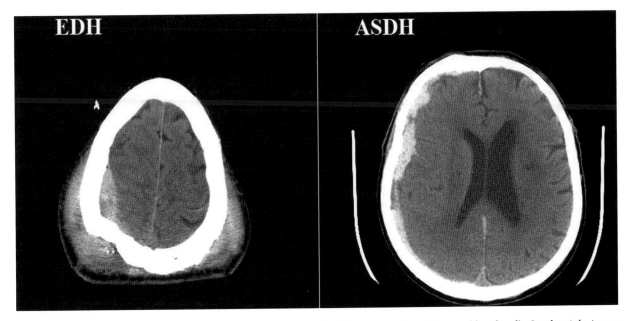

Figure 82-7 Axial cuts of CT head. On the left image: Acute epidural hematoma (lenticular and localized). On the right image: Acute subdural hematoma (crescentic and diffuse).

peduncle is compressed against the edge of tentorial incisura during uncal herniation. Uncal herniation usually occurs in middle cranial fossa masses where the uncus herniates medially compressing the occulomotor nerve, cerebral peduncles of the mid-brain, and posterior cerebral arteries, which may cause unilateral ptosis with mydriasis, hemiparesis, and hemianopia, respectively.

4. C. Associated cranial fractures have been reported in retrospective series ranging from 50% to 95% of cases. When an EDH is identified, the CT scan should be examined to evaluate the calvarium for fractures. EDH can result from injury to the middle meningeal artery, middle meningeal vein, diploic veins, or the venous sinuses. Historically, the most common cause is the middle meningeal artery; however, this varies depending on the location, cause, and age of the patient. Tearing or avulsion of the bridging cortical veins is one of the causes of SDH. Hemorrhagic brain contusions or lacerations might be another source of SDH. EDH are rarely in seen elderly patients > 65 years old likely due to adherence of the dura to the inner table of the skull, thus sealing firmly the epidural space.

Answers to Case 4

1. D. Figure 82-4 is an axial cut of CT head showing multiple hemorrhagic brain contusions (left frontal and bitemporal). It is also known as post-traumatic intracerebral hemorrhage/hematoma and usually appears on CT scanning as an intra-axial hyperdensity indicating fresh blood within the brain parenchyma. Sometimes injured brain tissues or part of a contusive lesion can appear normal (isodense) or as a hypodensity. Because of continued bleeding of microvessels fractured at the time of primary injury, reports demonstrate 30% to 50% of lesions will have some growth on imaging within the first 24–72 hours post injury.

2. D. The degree of temporal involvement often plays a critical role due to its proximity to the brain stem, whereas mass effect is better tolerated in affected supratentorial brain areas. Therefore, the development of temporal hematomas carries a lower threshold for surgical intervention. The indications for surgery in cases of traumatic brain contusions include hematoma causing progressive neurological deterioration; signs of significant mass effect on CT; medically refractory intracranial hypertension;

patients with GCS scores of 6 to 8 with a frontal or temporal contusion greater than 20 cm³ in volume and with a midline shift of at least 5 mm or cisternal compression on CT scan, and patients with any lesion greater than 50 cm³ in volume. Patients with such features should be treated operatively with decompression and possible resection of the affected area.

Cerebral contusions most frequently develop after a mechanical impact of distinct skull areas onto the rather soft brain substance during trauma. Frontal and temporal lobe tips are most commonly affected by such focal hemorrhagic contusions following translational acceleration. Glucocorticoids are not recommended to improve the outcome or lower the ICP in patients with severe traumatic brain injury.

3. E. Traumatic intracranial hematomas / contusions are a heterogeneous group of traumatic lesions that can evolve resulting in secondary brain injury and mass effect. Similar to other traumatic brain injuries, increased age and decreased GCS are predictors of poor outcomes. Clinical deterioration in the first hours after injury is associated with contusion enlargement. Radiographic predictors include significant mass effect (same size criteria 30 cm³ and >5 mm of shift?) with midline shift and effacement of basal cisterns. Patients with Glasgow Coma Scale (GCS) scores of 6 to 8 with frontal or temporal contusions greater than 20 cm³ in volume with midline shift of at least 5 mm and/or cisternal compression on CT scan, and patients with any lesion greater than 50 cm³ in volume should be treated operatively.

4. B. Because of the risk for hematoma expansion and clinical decline, patients with traumatic intracranial hematomas should be observed closely for neurologic decline. Routine serial imaging is controversial and has not been proven to alter management. Initial steps should include admission to unit capable of close neurologic monitoring, elevation of the head of bed 30°–45° to aid cerebral venous outflow, seizure prophylaxis for 1 week only (in the absence of an indication to continue), maintenance of hemoglobin of at least 7 g/dL or above, hyponatremia avoidance, fever avoidance, adequate pulmonary support, and avoidance of elevated intra-abdominal pressure. Endotracheal intubation and mechanical ventilation in intubated for GCS < 9. Pulmonary support should focus of avoidance of hypoxia, hypercapnia, and excessive PEEP. Elevated levels of PaCO₂ lead to intracranial vasodilation and cerebral blood volume and thus elevated ICP. Excessive PEEP may lead to increased intra-thoracic pressure and thus impaired cerebral venous outflow. It is also not recommended to use hyperventilation vigorously to lower $PaCO_2$ to less than 25 mmHg as a $PaCO_2$ of less than 30 mmHg may lower the CBF or distort cerebral autoregulation without consistently lowering ICP. The goal is to keep $PaCO_2$ at the lower end of eucapnia (35 mmHg). The recommended CPP is between 60 and 80 mmHg. CPP is the MAP–ICP, so MAP elevation is as important as lowering the ICP in order to maintain perfusion to the brain.

Answers to Case 5

1. C. Figure 82-5 is an axial cut of CT head and shows diffuse post-traumatic SAH. This is a case of SAH shown in the CT in the form of a hyperdense blood film in the subarachnoid cisterns. Underlying causes and subarachnoid blood distribution pattern should be considered when evaluating these patients.

2. A. Trauma is the most common cause of SAH. Aneurysmal rupture is the most common cause of spontaneous SAH. Ruptured AVM usually presents in the form of intracerebral hemorrhage or intraventricular hemorrhage. SAH occurs in about 5% of AVM cases. Other causes may include pituitary apoplexy, coagulopathy, and cocaine abuse.

3. C. Unilateral ptosis with pupillary dilation indicates a cranial nerve III (oculomotor nerve) injury. While this may be from underlying uncal herniation in the setting of trauma, occulomotor nerve compression secondary to a posterior communicating artery (P-comm) aneurysm should also be considered in a patient with SAH or those without a history of trauma. Nine percent of P-comm aneurysms present with unilateral occulomotor nerve palsy, which may indicate impending rupture and prompt intervention by a specialized neurovascular team. Patients with SAH may present with increased ICP symptoms, seizures, or neurological deficit. Elevated ICP is unlikely from a SAH, but more likely from other traumatic intracranial hemorrhages.

4. C. The four-vessel cerebral angiogram or catheter cerebral angiography is the gold standard study for the evaluation of cerebral aneurysms. CT angiography (CTA) with three-dimensional reconstruction imaging may be used instead of catheter angiography in some centers as the sole imaging diagnostic study before major surgical intervention. CTA is a noninvasive tool that may provide prompt, accurate, and versatile diagnostic and anatomical information on which clipping can be based.

MRA can also detect cerebral aneurysms, but it has lower sensitivity and specificity compared to the catheter cerebral angiogram especially for aneurysms less than 3 mm diameter. MRA is also useful in screening high-risk patients. MRI Diffusion (DWI) is the best imaging study for detection of acute brain ischemia within the first hours especially when it involves the brain stem or cerebellum. CT perfusion identifies the area surrounding the infarction called potentially salvageable penumbra that allows for better outcomes if interventional treatment modalities are available. Transcranial doppler (TCD) is a noninvasive semiquantitative technique of ultrasound derived blood velocity measurements within major cerebral vessels (e.g., MCA) through thin regions of skull bones providing a window. TCD is usually used in SAH to detect cerebral vasospasm early prior to the clinical delayed ischemic neurological deficit.

5. A. SAH has numerous possible complications that may cause neurological deterioration. It is believed that proteinaceous blood products may occlude the arachnoid granulations causing secondary communicating hydrocephalus in 20% of SAH survivors. Angiographic cerebral vasospasm is a contributing factor of delayed neurological deficit in patients with SAH. Broderick and his colleagues reported on the causes of morbidity and mortality following aneurysmal SAH. In their study, rebleeding was the most important preventable cause of death.

It is also well-known that seizures may occur early following SAH mostly due to the presence of blood in the cisterns, which may irritate the cerebral cortex, but the explanation of late-onset seizures remains unclear. Medications to prevent seizures are not known to decrease the GCS. The prevalence rate of hyponatremia following SAH is about 30% to 55%. Hyponatremia may lead to seizures, vasospasm, altered mental status, or death. It may occur due to syndrome of inappropriate ADH (SIADH) secretion or glucocorticoid deficiency. However, correction of hyponatremia should always be gradual and monitored, as rapid corrections may cause central pontine myelinolysis (osmotic demyelinating syndrome). An associated carotid injury would be a rare cause of a complication to an SAH.

Answers to Case 6

1. B. Figure 82-6 is an axial cut of CT head and shows right frontoparietal acute on SCDH. Lesion is convex in shape and spanning sutures.

2. B. Patients with chronic anticoagulation/antiplatelet therapies are considered to be at high risk for SCDH from mild head trauma. Those patients are prone to develop subdural bleeding within days or weeks after small head trauma. The mechanism is not yet very well understood, although alteration in the blood-hematoma components was found in most anticoagulation treated patients.

Although patients with uncontrolled seizure episodes are more prone to frequent head traumas from potential recurrent seizure episodes, those patients don't have higher incidence of SDH after trivial trauma compared to patients with chronic anticoagulation therapy. There is higher incidence of CSDH in male compared to female, but gender does not seem to influence the development of CSDH after slight head trauma. History of alcohol abuse does not show a strict correlation with CSDH after trauma as coagulation therapies do. Patients with an age >65 years have a higher incidence of CSDH, but use of anticoagulation or antiplatelet is a greater risk factor.

3. C. The decision for nonoperative versus surgical management should be influenced by the clinical exam (GCS), CT parameters, and salvageability of the patient. Indications for surgery for an acute subdural hematoma (ASDH) include a thickness greater than 10 mm or midline shift greater than 5 mm. For ASDH, craniotomy is recommended over burr-hole drainage. For CSDH, surgical treatment is also recommended with mass effect greater than 5-mm midline shift or thickness greater than 10 mm, but conservative treatment can be considered in patients without focal neurologic deficit or mental status changes. Burr-hole drainage can be a safe and effective treatment with the placement of subdural drain. Percutaneous twist-drill bedside drainage is the least invasive technique of the aforementioned techniques. It requires a 0.5-cm incision in the scalp and has been shown to be a safe technique. CSDH is more frequent among the elderly, the treatments diverge regarding the perioperative risks related to general anesthesia; burr-hole and twist drill drainage can be performed without the need for general anesthesia so patients comorbidities have to be taken in consideration.

4. A. Brain atrophy, hydrocephalus, midline shift, and hematoma density on CT (e.g., high, iso, or low) all influence the outcome of CSDHs. Traumatic causes, sex, hematoma location, and age have not been shown to correlate with CSDHs outcome. For ASDH, similar to severe TBI, increase in poor outcomes is seen in patients over 60 years of age and poor neurologic exam (low GCS) on presentation. Timing of surgery should be based on clinical and radiographic findings. Length of time from clinical deterioration to operative treatment is related to outcome.

BIBLIOGRAPHY

Agid R, Andersson T, Almqvist H, et al. Negative CT angiography findings in patients with spontaneous subarachnoid hemorrhage: when is digital subtraction angiography still needed? *AJNR Am J Neuroradiol.* 2010;31:696–705.

Ajlan A, Marcoux J. Intracranial pressure management. In: Nader R, Sabbagh AJ, eds. *Neurosurgery Case Review.* Thieme; 2010:174–177.

Alahmadi H, Vachhrajani S, Cusimano MD. The natural history of brain contusion: an analysis of radiological and clinical progression. *J Neurosug.* 2010 May;112(5):1139–1145.

Araujo JL, Aguiar Udo P, Todeschini AB, Saade N, Veiga JC. Epidemiological analysis of 210 cases of surgically treated traumatic extradural hematoma. *Revista do Colegio Brasileiro de Cirurgioes.* 2012;39(4):268–271.

Baechli H, Nordmann A, Bucher HC, Gratzl O. Demographics and prevalent risk factors of chronic subdural haematoma: results of a large single-center cohort study. *Neurosurg Rev.* 2004;27:263–266.

Bricolo AP, Pasut LM. Extradural hematoma: toward zero mortality. A prospective study. *Neurosurgery.* 1984;14(1):8–12.

Broderick JP, Brott TG, Duldner JE, Tomsick T, Leach A. Initial and recurrent bleeding are the major causes of death following subarachnoid hemorrhage. *Stroke.* 1994;25:1342–1347.

Brown CV, Weng J, Oh D, et al. Does routine serial computed tomography of the head influence management of traumatic braininjury? A prospective evaluation. *J Trauma.* 2004 Nov;57(5):939–943.

Bullock MR, Chesnut R, Ghajar J, et al. Surgical management of depressed cranial fractures. *Neurosurgery.* 2006;58: S56–S60; discussion Si–iv.

Bullock MR, Chesnut R, Ghajar J, et al. Surgical management of epdidural hemtaoms. *Neurosurgery.* 2006;58:S7–S15; discussion Si–iv.

Bullock MR, Chesnut R, Ghajar J, et al. Surgical management of traumatic parenchymal lesions. *Neurosurgery.* 2006;58:S25–S46; discussion Si–iv.

Bullock MR, Chesnut R, Ghajar J, et al. Surgical management of acute subdural hematomas. *Neurosurgery.* 2006;58: S16–S24; discussion Si–Siv.

Chen PR, Amin-Hanjani S, Albuquerque FC, McDougall C, Zabramski JM, Spetzler RF. Outcome of oculomotor nerve palsy from posterior communicating artery aneurysms: Comparison of clipping and coiling. *Neurosurgery.* 2006;58:1040–1046; discussion 1040–1046.

da Rocha AJ, da Silva CJ, Gama HP, et al. Comparison of magnetic resonance imaging sequences with computed tomography to detect low-grade subarachnoid hemorrhage: Role of fluid-attenuated inversion recovery sequence. *J Comput Assist Tomogr.* 2006;30:295–303.

Daele JJ, Goffart Y, Machiels S. Traumatic, iatrogenic, and spontaneous cerebrospinal fluid (CSF) leak: Endoscopic repair. *B-ENT 7.* 2011;17:47–60.

Dorai Z, Hynan LS, Kopitnik TA, Samson D. Factors related to hydrocephalus after aneurysmal subarachnoid hemorrhage. *Neurosurgery.* 2003;52:763–769; discussion 769–771.

Dunn LT. Raised intracranial pressure. *J Neurol Neurosurg Psychiatry.* 2002;73(1):i23–i27.

Edlow JA, Caplan LR. Avoiding pitfalls in the diagnosis of subarachnoid hemorrhage. *N Engl J Med.* 2000;342:29–36.

Fodstad H, Kelly PH, Buchfelder M. History of the cushing reflex. *Neurosurgery.* 2006 Nov;59(5):1132–1137; discussion 1137.

Gade GF, Becker DP, Miller JD, Dwan PS. Pathology and pathophysiology of head injury. In: Youmans JR, ed. *Youmans Neurological Surgery.* 6th ed. Elsevier Saunders; 1990:1965–2016.

Germanwala AV, Huang J, Tamargo RJ. Hydrocephalus after aneurysmal subarachnoid hemorrhage. *Neurosurg Clin N Am.* 2010;21:263–270.

Gharaibeh KA, Craig MJ, Koch CA, Lerant AA, Fulop T, Csongradi E. Desmopression is an effective adjunct treatment for reversing excessive hyponatremia overcorrection. *World J Clin Cases.* 2013;1:155–158.

Glaser N, Bundros A, Anderson S, Tancredi D, Lo W, Orgain M, et al. Brain cell swelling during hypocapnia increases with hyperglycemia or ketosis. *Pediatr Diabetes.* 2014;15(7):484–493.

Greenberg MS. *Handbook of Neurosurgery.* Thieme Publishers; 2010.

Gurdjian ES. Cerebral contusions: re-evaluation of the mechanism of their development. *J Trauma.* 1976;16:35–51.

Hackney DB, Lesnick JE, Zimmerman RA, Grossman RI, Goldberg HI, Bilaniuk LT. MR identification of bleeding site in subarachnoid hemorrhage with multiple intracranial aneurysms. *J Comput Assist Tomogr.* 1986;10:878–880.

Hamilton MG, Rashidi A, Rezaii J, et al. The role of postoperative patient posture in the recurrence of traumatic chronic subdural hematoma after burr-hole surgery. *Neurosurgery.* 2007;61(4):794–797; discussion 797.

Hannon MJ, Behan LA, O'Brien MM, et al. Hyponatremia following mild/moderate subarachnoid hemorrhage is due to SIAD and glucocorticoid deficiency and not cerebral salt wasting. *J Clin Endocrinol Metab.* 2014;99:291–298.

Hasan D, Schonck RS, Avezaat CJ, Tanghe HL, van Gijn J, van der Lugt PJ. Epileptic seizures after subarachnoid hemorrhage. *Ann Neurol.* 1993;3:286–291.

Heula A-L, Ohlmeier S, Sajanti J, Majamaa K. Characterization of chronic subdural hematoma fluid proteome. *Neurosurgery.* August 2013;73(2):317–331.

Hoen B, Viel JF, Gerard A, Dureux JB, Canton P. Mortality in pneumococcal meningitis: a multivariate analysis of prognostic factors. *Eur J Med.* 1993;2:28–32.

Iaccarino C, Schiavi P, Picetti E, Goldoni M, Cerasti D, Caspani M, et al. Patients with brain contusions: predictors of outcome and relationship between radiological and clinical evaluation. *J Neurosurg.* 2014 Apr;120(4):908–918.

Jamieson KG, Yelland JD. Surgically treated traumatic subdural hematomas. *J Neurosurg.* 1972;37(2):137–149.

Jennette B. *Epilepsy After Non-missile Head Injuries.* London: Heinemann Medical; 1975:179.

Kentaro M, Minoru M. Surgical treatment of chronic subdural hematoma in 500 consecutive cases: clinical characteristics, surgical outcome, complications, and recurrence rate. *Neurol Med Chir.* August 2001;41(8):371–381.

Kim HS, Hur JW, Lee JW, Lee HK. Extraordinarily long-term post-traumatic cerebrospinal fluid fistula. *J Korean Neurosurg.* 2007;42:403–405.

Kolias AG, Sinha R, Park H, et al. Surgical management of chronic subdural hematomas: In need of better evidence. *Acta Neurochir.* 2013;155:183–184.

Lackner P, Vahmjanin A, Hu Q, Krafft PR, Rolland W, Zhang JH. Chronic hydrocephalus after experimental subarachnoid hemorrhage. *PLoS One.* 2013;8:e69571.

Laviv Y, Rappaport ZH. Risk factors for development of significant chronic subdural hematoma following conservative treatment of acute subdural hemorrhage. *Br J Neurosurg.* May 2014;19:733–738.

Lee KS. The pathogenesis and clinical significance of traumatic subdural hygroma. *Brain Inj.* 1998;12:595–603.

Lee KS, Bae WK, Doh JW, Bae HG, Yun IG. Origin of chronic subdural haematoma and relation to traumatic subdural lesions. *Brain Inj.* 1998;12:901–910.

LeFeuvre D, Taylor A, Peter JC. Compound depressed skull fractures involving a venous sinus. *Surg Neurol.* 2004;62:121–125; discussion 125–126.

Leggate JR, Lopez-Ramos N, Genitori L, Lena G, Choux M. Extradural haematoma in infants. *Br J Neurosurg.* 1989;3(5):533–539.

Lind CR, Lind CJ, Mee EW. Reduction in the number of repeated operations for the treatment of subacute and chronic subdural hematomas by placement of subdural drains. *J Neurosurgery.* 2003;99:44–46.

Lindegaard KF, Nornes H, Bakke SJ, Sorteberg W, Nakstad P. Cerebral vasospasm after subarachnoid haemorrhage investigated by means of transcranial Doppler ultrasound. *Acta Neurochir Suppl.* 1988;42:81–84.

Lindvall Peter, Koskinen Lars-Owe D. Anticoagulants and antiplatelet agents and the risk of development and recurrence of chronic subdural haematomas. *J Clin Neurosc.* 2009;16:1287–1290.

Macdonald RL. Delayed neurological deterioration after subarachnoid haemorrhage. *Nat Rev Neurol.* 2014;10:44–58.

Malik NK, Makhdoomi R, Indira B, Shankar S, Sastry K. Posterior fossa extradural hematoma: Our experience and review of the literature. *Surg Neurol.* 2007;68(2):155–158; discussion 158.

Meier U, Gartner F, Knopf W, Klotzer R, Wolf O. The traumatic dural sinus injury: a clinical study. *Acta Neurochir.* 1992;119:91–93.

Morgan M, Sekhon L, Rahman Z, Dandie G. Morbidity of intracranial hemorrhage in patients with cerebral arteriovenous malformation. *Stroke.* 1998;29:2001–2002.

Morgenstern LB, Luna-Gonzales H, Huber JC Jr., et al. Worst headache and subarachnoid hemorrhage: prospective, modern computed tomography and spinal fluid analysis. *Ann Emerg Med.* 1998;32:297–304.

Nabavi DG, Cenic A, Craen RA, et al. CT assessment of cerebral perfusion: experimental validation and initial clinical experience. *Radiology.* 1999;213:141–149.

Obrist WD, Langfitt TW, Jaggi JL, Cruz J, Gennarelli TA. Cerebral blood flow and metabolism in comatose patients with acute head injury. Relationship to intracranial hypertension. *J Neurosurg.* 1984;61:241–253.

Ozer FD, Yurt A, Sucu HK, Tektas S. Depressed fractures over cranial venous sinus. *J Emerg Med.* 2005;29:137–139.

Perry JJ, Stiell IG, Sivilotti ML, et al. Clinical decision rules to rule out subarachnoid hemorrhage for acute headache. *JAMA.* 2013;310:1248–1255.

Phonprasert C, Suwanwela C, Hongsaprabhas C, Prichayudh P, O'Charoen S. Extradural hematoma: analysis of 138 cases. *J Trauma.* 1980;20(8):679–683.

Rahman M, Friedman WA. Hyponatremia in neurosurgical patients: clinical guidelines development. *Neurosurgery.* 2009;65(5):925–935; discussion 935–936.

Riesgo P, Piquer J, Botella C, Orozco M, Navarro J, Cabanes J. Delayed extradural hematoma after mild head injury: report of three cases. *Surg Neurol.* 1997;48(3):226–231.

Rivas JJ, Lobato RD, Sarabia R, Cordobes F, Cabrera A, Gomez P. Extradural hematoma: Analysis of factors influencing the courses of 161 patients. *Neurosurgery.* 1988;23(1):44–51.

Ross JS, Masaryk TJ, Modic MT, Ruggieri PM, Haacke EM, Selman WR. Intracranial aneurysms: evaluation by MR angiography. *Am J Neuroradiol.* 1990;11:449–455.

Ryall RG, Peacock MK, Simpson DA. Usefulness of beta 2-transferrin assay in the detection of cerebrospinal fluid leaks following head injury. *J Neurosurg.* 1992;77:737–739.

Saramma P, Menon RG, Srivastava A, Sarma PS. Hyponatremia after aneurysmal subarachnoid hemorrhage: Implications and outcomes. *J Neurosci Rural Pract.* 2013;4:24–28.

Sawiris N, Venizelos A, Ouyang B, Lopes D, Chen M. Current utility of diagnostic catheter cerebral angiography. *J Stroke Cerebrovasc Dis.* 2014;23(3):e145–e150.

Shapiro SA, Scully T. Closed continuous drainage of cerebrospinal fluid via a lumbar subarachnoid catheter for treatment or prevention of cranial/spinal cerebrospinal fluid fistula. *Neurosurg.* 1992;30:241–245.

Stanisic M, Lyngstadaas SP, Pripp AH, et al. Chemokines as markers of local inflammation and angiogenesis in patients with chronic subdural hematoma: A prospective study. *Acta Neurochir.* 2012;154:113–120.

Strong EB. Frontal sinus fractures: current concepts. *Craniomaxillofac Trauma Reconstr.* 2009 Oct;2(3):161–175.

Tahir MZ, Khan MB, Bashir MU, Akhtar S, Bari E. Cerebrospinal fluid rhinorrhea: an institutional perspective from Pakistan. *Surg Neurol Int.* 2011;2:174.

Tsai FY, Teal JS, Hieshima GB. *Neuroradiology of Head Trauma.* University Park Press; 1984.

van Gijn J, Kerr RS, Rinkel GJ. Subarachnoid haemorrhage. *Lancet.* 2007;369:306–318.

Wilberger JE Jr., Harris M, Diamond DL. Acute subdural hematoma: morbidity, mortality, and mortality, and operative timing. *J Neurosurg.* 1991;74(2):212–218.

Winston KR. Efficacy of dural tenting sutures. *J Neurosurg.* 1999;91(2):180–184.

83

Neurosurgery—Hyponatremia/Hypernatremia

Albert Jesse Schuette and Kristopher G. Hooten

CASE 1

A 38-year-old male presents to the trauma bay with a Glasgow coma scale (GCS) of 15 following a motor vehicle crash. The patient underwent a computed tomography (CT) scan of the head demonstrating a traumatic subarachnoid hemorrhage and a right frontal lobe contusion. He was admitted to the ICU for evaluation, and trauma evaluation did not reveal additional injuries. The patient remained stable for the first 24 hours and was downgraded to the floor. Hospital day 3, the patient becomes slightly more agitated and confused. Current GCS is 13. A follow-up CT scan showed no change in his intracranial injuries. Further workup with a chemistry panel shows a sodium level of 129 mmol/L.

1. **Regarding the results of his chemistry panel, which of the following is most correct?**

   A. Electrolyte imbalance is rare in the setting of traumatic brain injury (TBI).
   B. Further workup is indicated for all patients with sodium levels less than
   C. 135 mmol/L.
   D. Hyponatremia is defined as sodium levels less than 140 mmol/L.
   E. Chronic hyponatremia is clinically more dangerous than acute hyponatremia.
   F. In TBI patients, the majority of cases result from syndrome of inappropriate antidiuretic hormone secretion (SIADH).

2. **Which of the following statements is true regarding the neurological signs and symptoms associated with severe hyponatremia?**

   A. Symptoms are not apparent until Na^+ drops below 115 mmol/L.
   B. If the hyponatremia is chronic, the patient is more likely to be symptomatic.
   C. Hyponatremia is not a cause of seizures.
   D. Mild symptoms may include headache, confusion, and poor concentration.
   E. Hyponatremia is not lethal.

3. **After determining that the effective serum osmolality was within the normal range and urine osmolality was greater than 100 mOsm/kg, what is the next best step in determining the cause of the hyponatremia in this patient?**

   A. Assess the patient's volume status.
   B. Determine the liver function and cardiac output.
   C. Check pituitary function assays for cortisol derangements.
   D. Obtain the hormone levels of antidiuretic hormone (ADH) and natriuretic peptides.
   E. Measure the serum lithium level.

4. **You determine the patient to be minimally/asymptomatic from his hyponatremia. Based on your diagnosis, what treatment would you begin to correct the low serum sodium level?**

   A. Fluid bolus
   B. Hypertonic saline
   C. Fluid restriction
   D. Vaptan therapy
   E. IV steroid

CASE 2

A 36-year-old male presents to the trauma bay with a GCS of 4 following a non-helmeted motorcycle crash. The patient underwent a CT scan of the demonstrating a severe traumatic brain injury with diffuse cerebral edema, traumatic subarachnoid hemorrhage, basilar skull fractures, and evidence of diffuse axonal injury. An intracranial pressure (ICP) monitor and external ventricular drain was placed for management of his elevated ICP. After initial resuscitation, he was admitted to the ICU for treatment. Over the first 12 hours, the patient's urine output has noted acutely increase to over 300 mL/hr. Serum sodium has increased to over 150 mmol/L.

5. **What is the likely cause of abnormal serum sodium?**

   A. Nephrogenic diabetes insipidus
   B. Neurogenic diabetes insipidus
   C. SIADH
   D. Cerebral salt wasting (CSW)
   E. Cannot determine without further laboratory evaluation

6. **Which of the following is the next best treatment option for this patient?**

   A. Monitor fluid intake and output hourly and draw the serum sodium every 24 hours.
   B. Place on a basal fluid rate with hypotonic solution with replacement for urine output above the basal rate.
   C. Administer DDAVP first and assess impact on urine output.
   D. Allow the patient's thirst mechanism to control the Na level.
   E. Restrict the fluid.

ANSWERS

1. **E.** Hyponatremia is a common electrolyte disorder encountered in the ICU patients with neurotrauma or recent neurosurgical procedures. Acute hyponatremia is clinically more dangerous than chronic hyponatremia with a risk of higher morbidity and mortality. Hyponatremia clinically presents with impaired consciousness, seizures, elevated ICP, cerebral herniation; patients, however, may also be asymptomatic initially. The cause of hyponatremia is frequently multifactorial, but most commonly related to SIADH. Hyponatremia is defined as sodium levels less than 135 mmol/L, but recommendations for hyponatremia treatment and further investigation is when the serum sodium level is less than 131 mmol/L. Treatment should be directed by the proper diagnosis.

2. **D.** This question relates to the symptoms and general treatment options of hyponatremia. The neurologic symptoms of mild hyponatremia or chronic hyponatremia involve headaches, confusion, poor concentration, anorexia, and muscle weakness. The more acute and severe hyponatremia cases can lead to cerebral edema, nausea, seizures, respiratory arrest, coma, and death from transtentorial herniation. Symptoms generally commonly seen below Na^+ 125 mmol/L. Symptoms are more apparent with acute onset (<48 hours in duration) as there is less time for mechanisms of the brain to compensate. For that reason, chronic hyponatremia (>48 hours) can be relatively asymptomatic even at low Na levels.

3. **A.** The diagnosis for the cause of hyponatremia is generally reached in an algorithmic fashion. Evaluation of hyponatremia should include a combination of clinical exam, basic laboratory studies, and invasive monitoring when available. After a lab measurement shows serum sodium less than 131 mmol/L, one must determine the effective serum osmolality. This rules out hyperglycemia, hypertriglyceridemia, and hyperproteinemia (so-called pseudohyponatremia) as the cause of the abnormal laboratory value.

   The patient's volume status must be ascertained. This is extremely important in a neurologic patient as it will help differentiate the most common neurologic causes of hyponatremia: SIADH and CSW. While unlikely in an inpatient setting, polydipsia (water intoxication) can be ruled out by evaluating urine osmolality and urine sodium levels to ensure that the patient is not suffering from water intoxication. If urine is dilute (Uosm < 100 mOsm/kg), then the cause is water intoxication. If urine osmolality is > 200 mOsm/kg and urine sodium is > 25 mmol/L, then fluid balance is needed to differentiate CSW and SIADH. Figure 83-1 provides a brief overview of this algorithm. One must also consider, other systemic causes of hypotraemia, including extra-renal sodium losses including blood loss, N/V, diarrhea as well as hypervolemia causes such as cirrhosis or congestive heart failure.

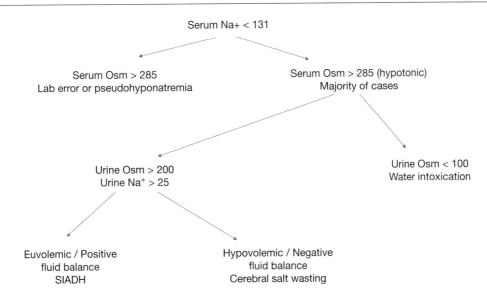

Figure 83-1

4. **C.** As with the diagnosis, the treatment for SIADH also runs as an algorithm. Again, the patient must be confirmed to be euvolemic as the treatment for CSW involves fluid resuscitation and for SIADH often involves fluid restriction. In the case of a patient with mild hyponatremia (125–135 mmol/L) with no or minimal symptoms, treatment should involve fluid restriction. If the patient is symptomatic in the acute setting, they should receive hypertonic saline with close monitoring of the sodium levels. In the chronic setting, oral salt replacement is an option for correction as well. Newer medications such as the vaptan class, which act as a vasopressin antagonist, can be used in severe cases typically in consultation with nephrology. The rate of correction even in symptomatic and acute cases should not exceed 1 to 2 mmol/L/hr and 8–10 mmol/L in 24 hours to avoid central pontine myelinolysis. CSW is treated with fluid and sodium replacement with oral sodium tablets or hypertonic IV saline. In severe or refractory cases, fludrocortisone may be used.

5. **B.** Hypernatremia is defined as a serum sodium >150 mEq/L. In patients with neurologic injuries, this is commonly due to diabetes insipidus (DI). DI is due to low levels of ADH or renal insensitivity to ADH. Diabetes insipidus is defined by high urine output or inappropriately dilute urine. The diagnosis can be reached with elevated serum sodium (hypernatremia) in the setting of consistent high output of urine with high _____. The two major etiologies are neurogenic DI and nephrogenic DI. The primary causes of nephrogenic DI are medications, renal disease, hypokalemia, and hypercalcemia. Neurogenic DI can be idiopathic, posttraumatic, tumors, infections, vascular, and autoimmune. In a post-traumatic patient who has worsening mental status, the cause is most likely due to herniation from pituitary stalk injury or hypothalamic injury from impending brain death.

6. **B.** After arriving at the diagnosis of neurogenic diabetes insipidus, it is essential to begin treatment of the patient. In a conscious and ambulatory patient, often their thirst mechanisms will compensate for the hypernatremia. In a comatose patient such as this one in the acute setting, the volume status should be corrected and free water deficit can be replaced commonly with IV hypotonic saline or free water. The definitive treatment is replacing ADH with pharmacologic analogues. These include vasopressin and longer acting, DDAVP. However, the patient in this scenario is unable to drink or compensate with his thirst mechanism. If the patient is not able to drink, he or she should be monitored for intake and output should be monitored hourly with serial sodium monitoring. To deal with the fluid loss, the patient should be placed on a basal fluid rate of hyptonic NS

with replacement for urine output above the base rate. If the fluid replacement continues to fall behind and the hypernatremia worsens, ADH therapy can be initiated. With the exception of fluid restriction (which is not a treatment of diabetes insipidus), the other choices are possible answers in the treatment of DI; however, the best option is to start with hypotonic solution.

BIBLIOGRAPHY

Adrogue HJ, Madias NE. Hyponatremia. *N Engl J Med.* May 25 2000;342(21):1581–1589.

Chanson P, Salenave S. Treatment of neurogenic diabetes insipidus. *Annales d'endocrinologie.* December 2011;72(6): 496–499.

Cole CD, Gottfried ON, Liu JK, Caouldwell WT. Hyponatremia in the neurosurgical patient: diagnosis and management. *Neurosurg Focus.* 2004;16(4)1–9.

Greenberg MS. *Handbook of Neurosurgery.* Thieme Publishing Company; 2010.

Hannon MJ, Thompson CJ. Neurosurgical hyponatremia. *J Clin Med.* 2014;3(4):1084–1104.

Maghnie M. Diabetes insipidus. *Hormone research.* 2003; 59(1):42–54.

Peri A, Giuliani C. Management of euvolemic hyponatremia attributed to SIADH in the hospital setting. *Minerva Endocrinologica.* March 2014;39(1):33–41.

Petersen RC. Acute confusional state. Don't mistake it for dementia. *Postgrad Med.* 1992;92(8):141–148.

Powers CJ, Friedman AH. Diagnosis and management of hyponatremia in neurosurgical patients. 2007;29(20)1–5.

Rahman M, Friedman WA. Hyponatremia in neurosurgical patients: clinical guidelines development. *Neurosurgery.* 2009;65(5):925–935; discussion 935–936.

Upadhyay UM, Gormley WB. Etiology and management of hyponatremia in neurosurgical patients. *J Intensive Care Med.* 2012;27(3):139–144.

84

Ophthalmology Trauma

Morohunranti O. Oguntoye and Robert A. Mazzoli

There is an ammonium nitrate explosion at a local fertilizer plant, with multiple injured persons and fatalities at the scene. Prehospital EMS providers, first responders, and bystanders begin to administer first aid to the injured and start transfer of patients to the local hospital. As the on-call emergency medicine physician, you and your colleagues stand ready in the emergency department while preparing for a potential mass casualty event. As part of the report for incoming injuries, you are notified that there are multiple face and eye injuries. The on-call ophthalmologist is on his way, but he is being delayed by the traffic that was caused by the explosion. You have been designated to manage ophthalmic injuries until he arrives.

1. **A 35-year-old male involved in the explosion was splashed in the face with ammonia. His face was irrigated with water at the scene, but he complains of persistent eye pain and decreased vision. What should the first priority in the initial care of the patient be?**

    A. Obtaining visual acuity
    B. Neutralization of pH with an acidic solution
    C. Copious irrigation with non-caustic solution
    D. Obtaining eye pressure
    E. Pain control

2. **You examine a 45-year-old female worker who fell during the explosion, striking her eye on the side of a work bench. On gently retracting the lids, the globe appears soft and irregular with diffuse subconjunctival hemorrhage and swelling. She can only count fingers with that eye. You suspect a ruptured globe and begin management**

until the ophthalmologist arrives. Which of the following would be contra-indicated in the initial management of this patient?

    A. Ultrasound
    B. Fox shield/rigid eye shield
    C. Antibiotics
    D. X-ray/CT
    E. Tetanus shot

3. **A worker is hit in the left eye/orbit with a large piece of flying debris. The patient is in severe pain, and is unable to open his eye. Gentle palpation of the left eye reveals a markedly swollen orbit that is difficult to retropulse. The eyelids are tense but you are able to gently open the lids with a retractor. Vision is light perception only. You note the pupil dilates when you shine light in it, but the contralateral pupil then constricts as you swing the light to it. Extraocular motility is severely limited. What is your diagnosis and plan for management?**

    A. Open globe—lateral canthotomy and cantholysis
    B. Orbital blowout fracture—orbital decompression
    C. Retrobulbar hemorrhage—pressure patch in anticipation of surgical intervention
    D. Retrobulbar hemorrhage—lateral canthotomy and cantholysis
    E. Periorbital ecchymosis—ice packs and pain control

4. There is an elementary school next to the fertilizer plant. A 7-year-old child was struck in the right face and orbit with flying debris, resulting in a brief loss

of consciousness. He has minimal bruising on his face and he has no complaints other than mild discomfort around that eye. As you conduct your exam, you note that he avoids looking at you, preferring to keep his eyes shut. His vision, intraocular pressure (IOP), and pupil exam appear normal, but when you instruct him to look up as part of the exam, he immediately vomits. You continue your exam and note that his heart rate drops dramatically whenever you ask him to move his eyes, prompting you to discontinue the exam. You suspect an orbital fracture but the eye and lid are otherwise unremarkable. What is your concern and urgency?

A. Intracranial hemorrhage: emergent
B. Orbital floor ("blowout") fracture: emergent
C. Orbital floor ("blowout"): nonurgent
D. Retrobulbar hemorrhage: emergent
E. Carotid dissection: nonurgent

5. The on-call ophthalmologist has called to get an update on the patients you have seen. Which of the following physical exam or imaging techniques would be indicated for the given pathology?

A. Best corrected visual acuity in a retrobulbar hemorrhage
B. Relative afferent pupillary defect (RAPD) with an open globe injury
C. IOP exam in a chemical burn
D. Ultrasound when computerized tomography (CT) scan is not available in a suspected globe rupture
E. CT scan of orbit and brain with intraorbital foreign body

6. One of the survivors, a 42-year-old male, suffered significant inhalational injuries and was intubated upon arrival in the ED. Two weeks later, he remains hospitalized for his injuries. Because of fevers and high white blood cell count blood cultures were obtained and he was found to have a *Candida albicans* bloodstream infection. He was placed on systemic fluconazole. On review of systems, the patient has no visual complaints. What additional measures should be taken?

A. Ophthalmology consult if patient develops visual complaints
B. Observation if patient has no visual complaints
C. Topical antifungal ophthalmic drops and consultation if patient has visual complaints

D. Ophthalmology consult despite no visual complaints
E. Ophthalmology consult upon discharge from the hospital

7. Another blast survivor is taken to the OR emergently for isolated orthopedic injuries. Upon awakening from surgery, the 65-year-old female complains of eye pain and decreased vision. She normally wears glasses, but neither the pain nor the decreased vision improve with glasses. You suspect a corneal abrasion. How would you confirm your suspicion?

A. Fluorescein and Wood's lamp
B. Atropine and Wood's lamp
C. Irrigation with normal saline and recheck vision
D. Fluoride and Wood's lamp
E. Erythromycin ointment

ANSWERS

1. **C.** A chemical injury is a true ophthalmic emergency. While visual acuity and IOP are the "vital signs" of ophthalmology, in the case of a chemical injury, diluting and removing the chemical agent takes priority. Copious but gentle irrigation with any non-caustic fluid should begin in the prehospital setting and continue at the hospital until the pH of the ocular surface has normalized to between 7.0 and 7.2. In an emergency department setting, Lactated Ringer's or normal saline are the preferred fluids for irrigation, but tap water can be used, if necessary. Irrigation should last for at least 30 minutes and may require several liters of irrigant.

If there is any suspicion for an open globe, irrigation should be gentle but thorough and tap water should be avoided because of potential intraocular damage. Never use acidic solutions to neutralize alkalis or vice versa, as these can generate harmful substrates. Topical anesthetic can be used to facilitate the irrigation process and provide the patient some comfort, but it should not delay care. A lid speculum may be necessary to keep eyes open for irrigation. Upper and lower eyelid fornices should be everted and irrigated. Particulate matter should be flushed out or manually removed. The conjunctival fornices should be swept with moistened cotton-tipped applicators to remove any particles or caustic materials. Check the pH in the fornices 5 to 10 minutes after irrigation and resume irrigation if the pH is not within the normal range. Retained material should be suspected if the pH remains abnormal.

The pH should be rechecked 15 to 30 minutes after stabilization. It is also important to identify the chemical agent and the time of the injury. Alkali materials (e.g., sodium hydroxide/lye, ammonia, calcium hydroxide/lime, and industrial/chemical detergents) cause more damage to the eye than acidic materials due to deeper penetration. Once the pH has been neutralized, a full eye exam should be conducted. Worrisome findings for extensive damage include significantly decreased visual acuity (irrigation itself may cause a temporary keratitis and mild decrease in vision), increased IOP, partial and full-thickness burns to the surrounding skin, conjunctival swelling, conjunctival blanching, full thickness penetration/open globe, and an opaque cornea. A shield should be applied and the patient transferred to an ophthalmologist immediately for further care.

2. **A.** A history suspicious for open globe will often include a blunt or penetrating trauma to the eye, a feeling of loss of fluid from the eye, pain, and decreased vision. Determining whether there is an open globe is one of the most important aspects of the ocular trauma evaluation, as this requires meticulous initial care to prevent additional injury and an emergent evaluation by an ophthalmologist. Signs that are concerning for open globe include a soft or irregular-appearing globe, an irregular or peaked pupil, hemorrhagic swelling of the conjunctiva (especially if 360 degrees), positive Seidel's sign on the cornea (leakage of fluid seen upon staining with fluorescein), hyphema (blood in the anterior chamber), a shallow or deep anterior chamber (compared to the uninjured eye), decreased extraocular motility, foreign body tract, and severe vision loss.

Figure 84-1 shows a patient who presented to the emergency department after being hit in the eye with a branch. He complained of fluid leakage from his eye, mild to moderate eye pain, and decreased vision. Note the irregular, cloudy pupil, flat anterior chamber, and the leakage of intraocular fluids (vitreous) at the 5 o'clock position of the eye. Also note the examiner's finger positioning, with the fingers at the brow and maxilla used to hold open the eye. This allows for a proper examination without applying pressure

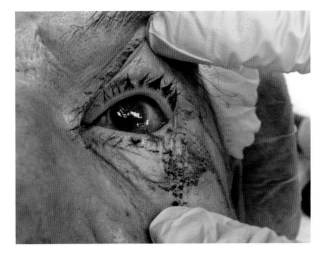

Figure 84-1 Signs of an open globe injury after blunt trauma to the eye: irregular pupil, flat anterior chamber, and leakage of intraocular fluids from the eye. Note the examiner's finger positioning, minimizing pressure on the globe. Source: Dr. Morohunranti O. Oguntoye.

to the globe, which could lead to further extrusion of intraocular contents.

Once the diagnosis of an open globe is made, further examination should be deferred to the ophthalmologist, who can address the injury at the time of surgical repair. A visual acuity may be obtained (light perception, hand motion, count fingers are appropriate measures if the patient cannot see letters on a near card) but measurement of IOP should not be attempted. No pressure should be applied to an eye with a suspected open globe, to include an ultrasound probe, especially when other clinical findings strongly point to the diagnosis and disposition. Ask the patient not to strain or squeeze their eyelids. Do not remove any penetrating objects. A rigid eye shield should be applied over the patient's eye to prevent further injury. If a rigid eye shield is not available, alternatives include the bottom of a paper cup, moldable splints (e.g., SAM splints), or sunglasses/eye protection. Do not apply patches or gauze pads to an open globe. Do not use topical anesthetics or ointments. Anti-nausea medications should be given with any pain medications to prevent valsalva or vomiting. Imaging (preferably an axial face and orbit CT scan with coronal reconstructions) should be obtained to rule out concomitant injuries or unidentified retained foreign bodies.

Antibiotics should be given within 6 hours of the injury (4th-generation fluoroquinolones IV have excellent vitreous penetration and are preferred in adults; Cefazolin 25 to 50 mg/kg/day IV in 3 divided doses and Gentamicin 2 mg/kg IV q8h for children). A tetanus shot should be given if necessary. Remembering how to deal with an open globe can be facilitated by using the acronym FACT: Fox shield, Antibiotics/Anti-emetics/Analgesia, CT scan, and tetanus shot. The eye should be shielded and the patient should be transferred immediately to the nearest ophthalmologist for further care.

3. **D.** In a patient who has had recent blunt trauma or surgery to the eye/orbit, findings of intense pain, decreased vision, an RAPD (the affected pupil paradoxically dilates to light, while the normal pupil constricts to it), inability to open eyelids due to swelling, and loss of color vision should raise a strong suspicion for retrobulbar hemorrhage, which is a true ocular emergency. In contrast to the open globe, the exam will reveal a tense, proptotic globe that is resistant to retropulsion on gentle palpation. In the case of an orbital blowout fracture, the globe is usually enophthalmic (sunken in) and there is pain on eye movement, but the visual acuity is usually normal or only slightly decreased. A patient with periorbital ecchymosis ("black eye") may have some periorbital tenderness and swelling but should not have globe proptosis, significantly elevated eye pressure, or visual acuity changes.

Retrobulbar hemorrhage is an orbital compartment syndrome that can rapidly and permanently damage the optic nerve and retina leading to permanent vision loss if not identified and treated immediately. The retina's ischemic tolerance time is roughly 90 minutes. Retrobulbar hemorrhage is a clinical diagnosis and does not require any additional imaging. The key to effective management of a retrobulbar hemorrhage is timely and aggressive decompression with a lateral canthotomy and cantholysis *by the first provider that is able to perform the decompression* (see Figure 84-2). The goal is to disinsert the lower eyelid sling from its periosteal attachments at the lateral canthus. The only two instruments needed are tissue forceps, and blunt scissors. If available, local anesthetic and a hemostat can facilitate a smoother procedure.

A detailed description of lateral canthotomy and cantholysis is found within the article by Ballard et al.

Following a successful lateral canthotomy and cantholysis, additional measures to reduce the orbital pressure should be instituted, including applying ice packs to the orbit, elevation of the head, and administration of systemic analgesia and anti-emetics.

4. **B.** This is what is known as a "white-eyed blow out fracture" or trapdoor fracture with oculocardiac reflex, and represents an ocular emergency.

Children's bones are flexible, and their orbital bones can break and bend, allowing the rectus muscle to pass below the broken but non-displaced bone. This can result in a fracture in which the rectus muscle is trapped below what appears to be an intact orbital floor. The external signs can be minimal: there may be no periorbital edema but the patient will exhibit significant extraocular muscle restriction. A child will often not complain of double vision, rather he may simply close one or both eyes.

The oculocardiac reflex can occur when extraocular muscles are pulled. Immediate signs and symptoms can include nausea, vomiting, and bradycardia with eye movement. Bradycardia can be so profound as to cause syncope or asystole. The manifestation of this reflex is an ocular emergency and an ophthalmologist should be consulted immediately for definitive management.

Adults with orbital floor fractures will complain of pain on attempted eye movement, binocular vertical diplopia, and hypoesthesia in the distribution of the infraorbital nerve V_2 (ipsilateral cheek and upper lip). Signs may include enophthalmos, crepitus, subcutaneous emphysema, restricted eye movement, nosebleeds, bony point tenderness, and step-off deformities of the orbital rim. If the patient had an intracranial hemorrhage, dilated pupils and rapidly declining mental status should be expected. A retrobulbar hemorrhage or carotid dissection would cause an RAPD. Periorbital ecchymosis should not cause vomiting or bradycardia. While orbital blowout fractures in children can be an ocular emergency, in adults without an RAPD or oculocardiac reflex, ophthalmic referral can be delayed up to 24 to 48 hours. An RAPD, flashes, floaters, photophobia, or decreased vision should prompt an immediate ophthalmic consult.

5. **E.** Ultrasound is contraindicated in an open globe because pressure on the globe may lead to extrusion of intraocular contents. The initial visual acuity in

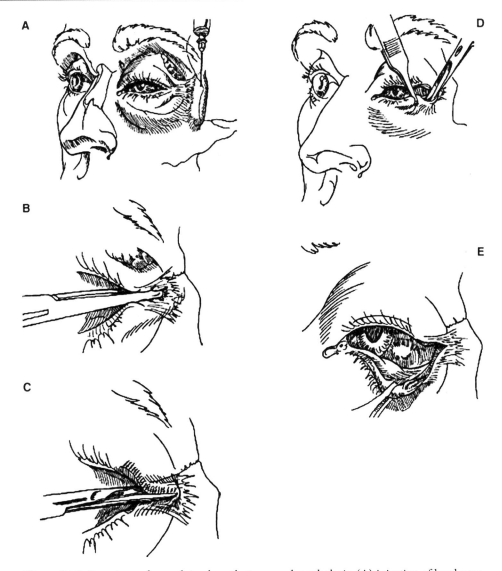

Figure 84-2 Steps to perform a lateral canthotomy and cantholysis. (**A**) injection of local anesthesic, (**B**) crush the lateral canthus with straight hemostat, (**C**) divide the lateral canthon tendon, (**D**) pull the lower eyelid away from face and divide the inferior crus of the canthal tendon, (**E**) divide any remaining attachments so lower eyelid pulls away freely from face (Reproduced from Department of Defense. Ocular injuries. In: *Emergency War Surgery Manual*. 4th ed. San Antonio, Texas: Borden Institute; 2013:14.8).

an open globe correlates with trauma severity and is highly predictive of final visual outcome. The RAPD in a patient with a retrobulbar hemorrhage indicates ocular compartment syndrome, requiring emergent decompression. Fluorescein exam in a chemical burn indicates the extent of the corneal damage. In the case of penetrating ocular or orbital injury, a CT scan should always be obtained to determine the location of intraorbital foreign bodies and to

rule out optic nerve or central nervous system involvement.

An eye exam can be broken down into a "primary survey" (identifying sight-threatening injuries) and a "secondary survey" (the complete ophthalmic exam). The primary survey is performed using a muscle light/penlight, fluorescein with Wood's lamp, a visual acuity card, an IOP instrument, and an ophthalmoscope. The secondary survey is performed using a slit lamp and an ophthalmoscope.

Key findings on the primary survey include:

- Best corrected visual acuity: Count fingers (CF), hand motion (HM), and no light perception (NLP) from best to worst if the patient is unable to visualize the far or near charts.
- IOP: not elevated (>21) or decreased (<10) (Note: do not perform if suspecting open globe).
- Globe: well-formed, no leakage of fluid, free extraocular motility, no proptosis, not tense to retropulsion, no foreign bodies, enophthalmos/exophthalmos, no oculocardiac reflex.
- Cornea: fluorescein exam without evidence of uptake or leakage, no corneal clouding, no foreign bodies (Note: contact lenses should be removed).
- Conjunctiva: no swelling, no blanching, no subconjunctival hemorrhage.
- Anterior chamber: well formed, no inflammation, no blood (hyphema).
- Pupil: reactive to light and accommodation, not peaked/irregular/torn.
- Posterior segment: no optic nerve swelling, no vitreous hemorrhage.
- Key findings on the secondary survey:
- Orbit/Globe: crepitus, step-offs/deformities, numbness on cheek, teeth, or forehead.
- Lids: laceration, medial canthus rounding, canalicular lacerations, epiphora, tense lids, ecchymosis, fornix evaluation, singed lashes.
- Conjunctiva: laceration.
- Cornea: corneal edema.
- Iris: iris tears, photophobia.
- Anterior segment: lens dislocation.
- Posterior segment: retinal detachment.

6. **D.** This patient has a fungal bloodstream infection and is at risk for ocular involvement of the fungemia. The only way to determine if there is ocular involvement is with an immediate ophthalmology consultation. Ocular involvement of fungemia can cause chorioretinits and endophthalmitis. Patients with history of indwelling catheters, long-term antibiotic treatment, immunosuppressive therapy, history of hyperalimentation, recent abdominal surgery, or diabetes mellitus are at risk for endogenous yeast endophthalmitis. In patients who develop fungal endophthalmitis, up to two-thirds lose useful vision. In patients with ocular manifestations of fungemia, in addition to systemic antifungals to treat the underlying cause, intraocular (not topical) antifungal medications and eye surgery (vitrectomy) may be needed. Topical antifungal eye drops play no role in the treatment of intraocular involvement of the fungemia.

The presence of visual complaints should play no part in whether the consultation is placed. In one retrospective study, the majority of patients with ocular fungal involvement (54.5%) were either asymptomatic or unable to communicate. Of those who were able to communicate, 71.4% had visual complaints. The most common symptoms are fairly mild, including blurred vision and floaters. Fungal ocular involvement also confers a poorer systemic prognosis and should extend the duration of the systemic antifungal treatment to 4 to 6 weeks after evidence of resolution of the intraocular infection.

7. **A.** Fluorescein dye is used to stain the cornea and, with the aid of a Wood's lamp, will highlight an abrasion on the cornea. Fluorescein drops (rather than fluorescein strips) have the added benefit of having an anesthetic solution in the drops, so the patient will usually get some temporary relief with the use of the fluorescein drops. This temporary pain relief with the use of liquid fluorescein would also support the diagnosis of a corneal abrasion. The blurred vision is usually due to the corneal defect and should resolve once the defect has healed.

To treat the corneal abrasion, an antibiotic ophthalmic ointment such as erythromycin or a fluoroquinolone is necessary. PO analgesia may also be needed, as any topical anesthetic tends to wear off within 15 minutes. The eye should be reexamined within 24 hours to look for improvement in symptoms and shrinkage in the size of the abrasion. The patient should be seen by an optometrist or ophthalmologist.

Atropine has no role in diagnosis of eye injuries.

If a foreign body is seen or suspected, irrigation with normal saline may be used to dislodge the foreign body. Fluorescein with Wood's lamp should then be used to look for abrasions. If an abrasion is found, it should be treated with a fluoroquinolone antibiotic to cover for pseudomonas.

Fluoride has no role in the diagnosis of eye injuries.

BIBLIOGRAPHY

Bagheri N, Wajda, BN. *The Wills Eye Manual: Office and Emergency Room Diagnosis and Treatment of Eye Disease.* 7th ed. Wolters Kluwer; 2017.

Ballard S, Enzenauer R, O'Donnell T, Fleming JC, Risk G, Waite AN. Emergency lateral canthotomy and cantholysis: a simple procedure to preserve vision from sight threatening orbital hemorrhage. *J Spec Oper Med.* 2009;9:26–32.

Gerstenblith AT, Rabinowitz MP. *The Wills Eye Manual: Office and Emergency Room Diagnosis and Treatment of Eye Disease.* Lippincott Williams & Wilkins; 2012.

Hemmati HD, Colby KA. Ophthalmic pearls: cornea. treating acute chemical injuries of the cornea. American Academy of Ophthalmology *EyeNet Magazine*; October 2012.

Joint Theater Trauma System Clinical Practice Guideline. Initial care of ocular and adnexal injuries by non-ophthalmologists at Role 1, Role 2, and non-ophthalmic Role 3 Facilities. *CENTCOM*; November 2014.

Lima V, Burt B, Leibovitch L, Prabhakaran V, Goldberg RA, Selva D. Orbital compartment syndrome: the ophthalmic surgical emergency. *Surv. Ophthalmol.* July–August 2009;54(4):441–9.

McCannel Colin A. *American Academy of Ophthalmology Basic and Clinical Science Course Section 12: Retina and Vitreous.* American Academy of Ophthalmology; 2016. Chapter 21.

Murtaza, AK, Vahedi S, Nichols MM, et al. Inpatient ophthalmology consultation for fungemia: prevalence of ocular involvement and necessity of funduscopic screening. *Am. J. Ophthalmol.* November 2015;160:1078–1083.e2.

85

Cardiothoracic Trauma

Mia DeBarros

1. A 22-year-old male who sustained a gunshot wound to the chest arrives in the emergency room at your facility. He is hemodynamically stable and has an entry wound just below his right nipple and probable exit wound just below the tip of the left scapula. Supine chest film shows no retained bullet fragments, contusion of the lung, and moderate left apical pneumothorax. A FAST exam shows no effusion or other abnormality. The initial diagnostic workup and management of this injury should include:

   A. Computerized tomography angiogram (CTA) of the chest and placement of left chest thoracostomy tube
   B. Placement of left thoracostomy tube and observation on the ward
   C. Trans-esophageal echocardiogram, non-contrast CT scan of the chest, and left chest thoracostomy tube
   D. Bronchoscopy, CT chest with oral contrast, CT angiography to evaluate the great vessels, and left chest thoracostomy tube
   E. Immediate surgical exploration via a median sternotomy

2. A 50-year-old male is brought to a local emergency room after a motor vehicle collision. He is complaining of mild mid-sternal chest pain and has some bruising over the sternum. He is a healthy male with no cardiac history. CT scan of the chest, abdomen, and pelvis are unremarkable other than a sternal body fracture. Electrocardiogram shows sinus tachycardia rhythm with a heart rate of 110 bpm. His pain is well controlled and there appear to be no other reasons for his tachycardia. What is the most appropriate management of this patient?

   A. Admit to the intensive care unit with continuous telemetry.
   B. Admit for observation with continuous telemetry and obtain echocardiogram to evaluate cardiac wall motion.
   C. Discharge home with instructions to return to the hospital if the symptoms worsen.
   D. Admit and consult with cardiologist for suspected acute coronary syndrome.
   E. Repeat CT scan of the chest in 12 hours and then discharge home if no new findings.

3. A 20-year-old male is brought in by EMS with a stab wound to the left chest just lateral to the mid-sternum. He is tachycardiac to 120 BPM and tachypneic with hypotension but responds with 1L bolus of lactated ringers. His physical exam is notable for JVD. A FAST exam is performed and significant for pericardial effusion. What is the next step in management?

   A. Obtain CT angiography to evaluate for thoracic injuries.
   B. Transfer to operating room and perform median sternotomy with cardiac surgery on backup.
   C. Perform pericardiocentesis to relieve the pericardial effusion.
   D. Perform anterior lateral thoracotomy in the trauma bay.
   E. Place a left-sided chest tube and admit to ICU for continued resuscitation.

4. A 21-year-old helmeted male on a motorcycle struck a tree traveling at 60 mph. His injuries include fractures of ribs 2 through 6 on the right, right clavicle fracture and right large pneumothorax and moderate pulmonary contusion with overlying subcutaneous emphysema. A right-sided chest tube is placed for large pneumothorax. Repeat chest film shows a persistent pneumothorax so a second chest tube was placed. A third set of chest films show that the lung has re-expanded slightly but a moderate apical pneumothorax remains. He is awake with a Glasgow Coma Scale (GCS) = 14, tachypneic on 6L with oxygen saturation of 92%. The two chest tubes have a persistent large air leak present. The next step in this patient's management should be:

A. Oxygenate with 100% oxygen for 24 hours to allow pneumothorax to resolve spontaneously and nonoperative treatment for rib fractures if they are non-displaced.

B. Obtain chest CT now and consider video-assisted thoracic surgery (VATS) for repair/resection of parenchymal lung laceration.

C. Have urgent bronchoscopy and fiber-optic intubation.

D. Admit to ICU with continued observation with 100% oxygenation, aggressive pain control, and pulmonary toilet.

E. Right thoracotomy for repair of probable large parenchymal lung laceration.

5. A 25-year-old male presents the emergency department after being stabbed multiple times in the left flank and left upper abdomen with a box cutter during a bar fight. He is hemodynamically stable. A CXR demonstrates pneumothorax and chest tube is placed. A FAST exam is negative. CT chest and abdomen demonstrate a small to moderate diaphragm defect, but no other obvious signs of injury. What is the next step in management of this patient?

A. Admit for continued resuscitation and observation and laparotomy if he becomes unstable.

B. Admit and repeat chest x-ray in 12 hours. If pneumothorax and hemothorax are resolved, remove the chest tube and discharge with return precautions.

C. Refer to the OR for laparoscopic exploration and repair of the diaphragmatic defect.

D. Observe in the emergency department, washout the stab wounds in the emergency department, repeat CXR in 4 to 6 hours, and remove the chest tube and discharge home.

E. Refer to the OR for thorascopic exploration and possible repair of the diaphragmatic defect.

6. A 33-year-old female was admitted after being involved in a motor vehicle collision. She had a left chest tube placed upon admission for a hemothorax that was seen on CXR. She underwent a CT chest as part of her initial evaluation, which demonstrated improvement but not resolution of her hemothorax. She was admitted to the ICU for continued resuscitation and observation. Initially, 150 cc of blood was evacuated at chest tube placement but after 24 hours only additional 100 cc has drained. A repeat CT scan of the chest on hospital day 3 still shows retained hemothorax. The most appropriate management of this patient at this time would be:

A. VATS to evacuate the hemothorax.

B. VATS if hemothorax does not resolve in 3 more weeks of observation.

C. Instill thrombolytic agent into the chest cavity via the chest tube to break up the clot.

D. Thoracotomy for decortication and evacuation of hemothorax.

E. CT-scan guided aspiration of retained hemothorax.

7. A 65-year-old male sustained multiple bilateral rib fractures and a moderate pulmonary contusion after a motorcycle crash. He was intubated after developing respiratory failure due to aspiration and poor respiratory mechanics. He is hemodynamically stable and oxygenating well but is unable to wean from the ventilator after 24 hours due to tachypnea. A CT chest shows several mildly displaced ribs. Trauma evaluation did not reveal any other injuries. The appropriate management of this patient should be:

A. Continue current management with daily spontaneous breathing trials, and aggressive pain control with opioids and antibiotics for aspiration.

B. Extubate to noninvasive positive pressure, increase opioids, add ketorolac and ketamine.

C. Consult anesthesia for thoracic epidural and add ketorolac to his opioids.

D. Operative fixation of rib fractures.

E. Perform early tracheostomy.

ANSWERS

1. A. Transmediastinal penetrating trauma represents a difficult problem for the trauma surgeon. All patients should be treated according to ATLS protocol regardless of the type of injury they present with. Unstable patients should proceed to the operating room for exploration. The difficulty in the unstable patient with a transmediastinal penetrating trauma is determining what approach to start with and relies on clinical judgment. Patients who are hemodynamically stable should proceed with a primary and organized secondary survey to elicit all possible injuries. In the past, this subset of patients required extensive workup to evaluate all components of the mediastinum: echocardiogram, bronchoscopy, esophagoscopy, esophagram, and angiography. With significant advancements in diagnostic imaging, workup can proceed quickly and less invasively. A FAST exam is the first line diagnostic tool to rule out pericardial effusion or tamponade, followed by CXR or FAST to rule out pneumothorax. If these are negative, a CTA is obtained. The current CT scanners have high sensitivity for great vessel injuries, pneumothorax, hemothorax, pneumomediastinum, pneumopericardium, pericardial and cardiac injuries, cardiac luxation, wound trajectories, and foreign bodies. The findings on CT can assist in further workup if needed such as bronchoscopy and esophagram or esophagoscopy for aerodigestive injuries. If the CT is negative, then no further workup is required. The patient in this question has a left pneumothorax and a negative FAST exam. Following placement of a tube thoracostomy, the next step in initial management is obtaining CTA of the chest.

2. A. The true incidence of blunt cardiac injury is unknown, but ranges from 8% to 71% in the literature. The most common injury is myocardial contusion. The location or distribution of injury is related to the position of the heart within the bony thorax. The right side of the heart is more anterior and sustains injury more frequently. The most common mechanism of injury is motor vehicle crashes and pedestrian vs. car and less commonly falls from great heights, crush injuries, assault, and direct blows to the chest. Blunt cardiac injury is rarely seen in isolation and typically associated with other injuries such as rib and sternal fractures, pneumothorax, hemothorax, and pulmonary contusions. If these injuries are present, blunt cardiac injury should be suspected and ruled out. EAST guidelines recommend an EKG as first line diagnostic technique. Patients with abnormal EKG findings should be admitted for 24 to 48 hours of observation with continuous EKG telemetry. Patients who are unstable with suspected blunt cardiac injury should undergo TTE (level II evidence). FAST exam may also be utilized to evaluate for wall motion abnormalities, but there is no level I evidence to support its use in the diagnosis of blunt cardiac injury=BCI. Troponin may be used to enhance the negative predictive value of EKG but is not recommended in all patients with blunt cardiac trauma.

3. B. Penetrating cardiac trauma is life-threatening injury. The mortality is 40% with outcomes dependent on massive transfusion protocols and the immediate availability of surgical staff. The most common mechanisms are stabbings and gunshot wounds. The most commonly injured location is the right ventricle due to its anterior location. Fortunately, this type of injury also has the best outcome with the literature reporting 60% of all patients surviving to discharge. Multi-chamber injury is considered an independent predictor of mortality. Diagnosis begins with physical exam and evaluating entry and exit wounds. A high index of suspicion should be present if the wounds fall within the "cardiac box," which traditionally was the clavicles to the xiphoid and laterally to the nipples. Newer studies have developed a "3D cardiac box" incorporating the lateral and posterior thorax as well (patients can be stabbed and shot in the side and back). Hypotension, jugular venous distension, and muffled heart sounds should also raise concern that there is a cardiac injury. Diagnosis is aided by use of FAST, which can reliably detect pericardial effusion. CXR can be utilized to determine the trajectory of the missile. CT is only if patients are hemodynamically stable and can help to define anatomy and evaluate for other thoracic injuries. EAST guidelines recommend ED or anterior lateral thoracotomy if patient has penetrating injury with loss of signs of life prior to arrival or in the emergency department. The specific recommendation of within 15 minutes of arrival is no longer recommended and requires clinical judgment. The purpose is to relieve life-threatening tamponade and obtain temporary hemostasis either by repairing a cardiac laceration or cross-clamping the descending aorta until transportation to the operating room for definitive exploration and hemostatic control. If the patient is stable to transport to the emergency department and the cardiac injury appears to be isolated, a median sternotomy in the operating room provides better exposure to all four chambers of the heart and the possibility of going on cardio-pulmonary bypass if more complex injuries are encountered. Simple lacerations can be temporarily controlled with digital occlusion. Foley catheters should not be used as they can make the injury bigger and interfere with cardiac function. Skin staples have been used for damage control but should be used with caution. The laceration should be repaired with simple interrupted monofilament sutures with pledgets to prevent tearing of the suture through the myocardium. Lacerations near the coronary arteries should be closed with horizontal mattress sutures taking care not to include the artery in the suture. Pericardium may also be harvested to use as a pledget. Expert consultation from cardiac surgery should be obtained if the injury involves multiple chambers, the great vessels or the valves.

4. **C.** Tracheobronchial injuries are rare in thoracic trauma but maybe life-threatening if not recognized and treated rapidly. Mechanisms for trauma include penetrating or blunt. The exact mechanism for blunt trauma is unknown but believed to be the result of rapid deceleration resulting in airway laceration near a fixed point. The majority of penetrating injuries occur in the cervical trachea (75%–80%). Blunt injuries occur in the thoracic trachea or main stem bronchi usually within 2 cm of the carina (a fixed point). On physical exam, patients have respiratory distress, subcutaneous emphysema, or dyspnea. Imaging findings suspicious for tracheobronchial injury include subcutaneous emphysema, pneumomediastinum, and pneumothorax. Tracheal defects may be apparent on CT chest. A chest tube placed for pneumothorax that does not resolve or has a persistent and continuous air leak is highly suspicious for a tracheobronchial injury. Definitive diagnosis is made by flexible bronchoscopy. Treatment is focused on securing the airway first and then management of the injury. Patients should undergo fiberoptic intubation with the use of bronchoscopy and not direct laryngoscopy. The bronchoscope is used to safely direct the endotracheal tube past the injury under direct vision to prevent further injury. If the injury is located in the carina or main stem bronchus, the bronchoscope can guide the endotracheal tube into the contra-lateral and uninjured main stem or guide a bronchial blocker into place to prevent continued ventilation to injured airways. Surgical repair for all injuries regardless of location is mandatory, but more severe life-threatening injuries should be repaired first once the airway is secured. Most injuries are able to be repaired primarily with a tissue flap as a buttress. Cervical injuries are repaired through a collar incision while the thoracic trachea, carina, right main stem, and proximal left main stem are repaired through a right thoracotomy and the distal left main stem is repaired via a left thoracotomy.

5. **C.** Diaphragmatic injury is rare, occurring in 0.5% of all traumas. The most common mechanism is penetrating from stab wounds or gun shot wounds. Blunt injury accounts for 1.5% of all traumatic diaphragmatic injuries and is typically a marker of severe poly-trauma. Diagnosis is difficult particularly in small defects; however, the natural history of small defects is enlargement of the defect over time and eventual herniation of abdominal contents into the thoracic cavity resulting in obstruction and possible strangulation. This may occur decades after the traumatic event. All diaphragm defects should be repaired when they are discovered assuming no other contraindications to surgery are present at time of diagnosis. In this patient who has been stabbed in the abdomen and flank, laparoscopy would be more helpful to evaluate for intra-peritoneal injuries and allow the diaphragm to be directly visualized and repaired. The diaphragm can also be repaired via the thoracic approach (VATS or thoracotomy); however, this does not allow evaluation of the abdominal cavity to look for missed injuries.

6. **A.** Hemothorax is a common occurrence in thoracic trauma particularly when rib fractures are present. The first-line treatment for hemothorax is placement of tube thoracostomy, which is therapeutic and diagnostic. The traditional teaching recommends thoracic exploration for >1,500 mL or 200 mL per hour for 4 hours. The drainage of a hemothorax prevents the development of pneumonia, empyema, or fibrothorax. Retained hemothorax is typically defined as hemothorax present greater than 72 hours after tube thoracostomy. If tube thoracostomy is not successful in complete evacuation of the hemothorax,

VATS is recommended. EAST guidelines (level I evidence) currently recommend the use of early VATS to prevent retained hemothorax and the associated sequalae. Since the MIST 2 trial utilizing tPA and DNAse to treat parapneumonic effusions nonoperatively was published, there has been interest in utilizing tPA to treat retained hemothorax nonoperatively. A recent meta-analysis of 10 studies with 225 patients found that use of lytic therapy avoided surgery in 87% of cases; however, the study authors could not conclude that lytic therapy was superior to surgery for management of retained hemothorax. Another meta-analysis evaluated the timing of VATS and noted that VATS performed within 3 days of admission was more successful than VATS after 7 days of admission with less tube thoracostomy duration and length of stay and less incidence of conversion to thoracotomy. Furthermore, the use of prophylactic antibiotics to prevent pneumonia and empyema from hemothorax while tube thoracostomy is in place is no longer recommended. The aforementioned patient has failed a trial of conservative management with tube thoracostomy. She should undergo VATS to evacuate her hemothorax if there are no contraindications to VATS.

7. **D.** In patients with multiple rib fractures, flail chest and pulmonary contusions are at high risk for further pulmonary complications and mortality. This is particularly acute in the geriatric population. Current EAST guidelines support the operative fixation of flail chest in patients in order to decrease duration of mechanical ventilation, ICU length of stay, pneumonia, and need for tracheostomy. The guidelines are a meta-analysis of 22 studies, many of which excluded severely injured patients with multi-organ injury and head trauma. The patients appeared to benefit the most when operative fixation occurred within 72 hours of presentation. It is important to evaluate the patient and treat life-threatening injuries first. If a patient is not able to have operative fixation of his or her ribs within 72 hours due to hemodynamic instability, this does not preclude operative fixation at a later time once he or she has recovered sufficiently. It is important that this procedure is undertaken by a team that is familiar with thoracic anatomy and operative fixation techniques to obtain the best outcome. The EAST guidelines could not make a recommendation on non-flail chest rib fixation due to lack of studies, but recent studies have indicated that there may be a benefit to surgery in patients with multiple rib fractures that are non-flail chest.

BIBLIOGRAPHY

Bellister SA, Dennis BM, Guillamodegui OD. Blunt and Penetrating Cardiac Trauma. *Surg Clin N Am*. 2017;97(5):1065–1076.

Clancy K, Velopulos C, Bilanuik JW, et al. EAST screening for blunt cardiac injury *J Trauma*. 2012;73(5):S301–S306.

Cook A, Hu C, Ward G, et al. AAST antibiotics in tube thoracostomy study group presumptive antibiotics in tube thoracostomy for traumatic hemothorax: a prospective multi-center American Association for Surgery of Trauma Study. *Trauma Surg Acute Care Open*. 2019;4(1):e000356.

Dennis BM, Bellister SA, Guillamondegui OD. Thoracic trauma. *Surg Clin N Am*. 2017;97(5):1047–1064.

Durso AM, Caban K, Munera F. Penetrating thoracic injury *Radiol Clin North Am*. 2015;53(4):675–693.

Furák J, Athanassiadi K. Diaphragm and transdiaphragmatic injuries. *J Thorac Dis*. 2019;11(Suppl 2):S152–S157.

Hendrickson Kuroki MT, Armen SB. Lytic therapy for retained hemothorax systemic review and meta-analysis. *Chest*. 2019;155(4):805–815.

Huis in't Veld MA, Craft CA, Hood RE. Blunt Cardiac trauma. *Card Clin*. 2018;36(1):183–191.

Kasotakis G, Hasenboehler EA, Streib EW. Operative fixation of rib fractures after blunt trauma: A practice management guideline from the Eastern Association for the Surgery of Trauma. *J Trauma Acute Care Surg*. 2017;82(3):618–626.

Mowery NT, Gunter OL, Collier BR. Practice management guidelines for management of hemothorax and occult pneumothorax. *J Trauma*. 2011;70(2):510–518.

Ziapour B, Mostafidi E, Sadeghi-Bazargani H, Kabir A, Okereke I. Timing to perform VATS for traumatic-retained hemothorax (a systematic review and meta-analysis). *Eur J Trauma Emerg Surg*. 2020;46(2):337–346.

86

Sepsis and Multi-Organ Failure

Robert Shawhan, Matthew Eckert, Matthew J. Martin, and Christopher B. Horn

A 68-year-old female is brought into the emergency department by her son for evaluation of altered mental status. The son reports that his mother rarely goes to the doctor, is an alcoholic, and has been a smoker as long as he can remember. She has occasionally had intermittent bouts of diverticulitis that have been treated with oral antibiotics. Her most recent bout was 2 weeks ago for which she recently finished a course of antibiotics. For the past 2 days she has had frequent stools and increasing abdominal pain over the past 48 hours. Today she was noted to be somnolent and difficult to arouse by her son.

On exam, her vitals show a temperature of 101.8°F, with a heart rate of 121 per minute. Her blood pressure is 83/54 and respiratory rate of 24, O2: 83% on RA. She is lethargic, lungs are coarse bilaterally; her abdomen is distended, and she grimaces with palpation of her lower abdomen. Her skin is pale and cool, and she has flat neck veins. Labs are significant for a white blood cell count (WBC) of 24, creatinine of 3.2, and lactate of 5.8. An arterial blood gas is obtained that pH of 7.30, pCO_2 of 80, and pO_2 of 67 with a base deficit of 10. Her central venous oxygen saturation ($ScvO_2$) is 55%.

1. **The patient is intubated and transfer to the intensive care unit (ICU) is being arranged. Which of the following is the best answer regarding the initiation of goal-directed therapy?**

   A. Antibiotic therapy should be delayed until a causative organism is identified.
   B. Lactate is a poor guide for resuscitation.
   C. The patient should receive an initial fluid bolus of 30 cc/kg of crystalloid solution.
   D. In intubated patients, a higher CVP (12 to 15 mmHg) should be considered pathologic.
   E. Early initiation of targeted goal-directed therapy in sepsis does not survival.

2. **Despite receiving 3 liters of crystalloid, the patient remains hypotensive with a systolic blood pressure of 75 and a $ScvO_2$ of 60. Her hematocrit is 41%. Which of the following is the appropriate next step?**

   A. Switching to using a hydroxyethyl starch solution
   B. High-dose phenylephrine infusion and titration to a MAP of 65 mmHg
   C. Levophed (norepinephrine) infusion
   D. Intravenous hydrocortisone
   E. Obtain an echocardiogram

3. **Initial cultures were sent on admission. Because of a recent history of antibiotic use and diarrhea, a polymerase chain reaction (PCR)–based *Clostridium difficile* toxin test was sent as well. Despite initiating broad spectrum antibiotics, the patient remains in shock. Twelve hours after admission, the lab reports the patient positive for *Clostridium difficile* (*C. difficile*) toxin. Which of the following statements is true regarding the management of this patient?**

   A. Repeat the test for *C. difficile* because PCR-based tests have a high false positive rate.
   B. Anti-fungal agents should be started.
   C. Pro brain natriuretic peptide (BNP) can help the decision to start antibiotics.

D. Surgical intervention for this pathology would include a total abdominal colectomy and end ileostomy.

E. Once a source of infection is identified, source control should be initiated after antibiotics have taken effect and the patient is no longer septic.

4. **Upon arrival to the ICU, a chest x-ray is obtained and is shows bilateral infiltrates. The ventilator is set to assist control mode with a peep of 5, tidal volume of 8 cc/kg, and FiO$_2$ of 60%. On these settings, her most recent PaO$_2$ is 55. You suspect acute respiratory distress syndrome (ARDS). Which of the following is true regarding ARDS?**

A. ARDS requires the presence of a focal and uni-lateral infiltrate on radiologic examination.

B. Corticosteroid use has been shown to reduce the overall mortality rates.

C. Use of high tidal volumes and low positive end-expiratory pressure (PEEP) is the main ventilator strategy used to ventilate patients.

D. Treatment options for refractory ARDS include high-frequency ventilation.

E. Airway pressure release ventilation has been shown to improve mortality.

5. **In patients treated for septic shock, there are consequences of a prolonged ICU stay and can include progressive dysfunction and even failure of multiple organ systems. Regarding outcomes of multi-organ dysfunction syndrome (MODS), which of the following is true?**

A. For such patients that develop delirium, the use of benzodiazepines is preferred.

B. Acute kidney injury is an independent risk factor for death.

C. Parental nutrition has been shown to be benefi-cial when initiated early.

D. Stress ulcer prophylaxis with proton-pump inhibitors is not associated with any adverse events or complications.

E. Critical illness polyneuropathy typically affects cranial nerves.

6. **Despite completing appropriate treatment for *C. difficile*, the patient continues to have loose stools. Repeat PCR is positive for recurrent *C. difficile*. Which of the following is the best option for treating recurrent *C. difficile* infections?**

A. Probiotics along with intravenous antibiotics.

B. Fidaxomicin

C. Metronidazole

D. Fecal microbiota transplants

E. Bezlotoxumab

7. **Despite adequate resuscitation and the addition of both norepinephrine and vasopressin, the patient remains hypotensive and tachycardic. Which of the following is most accurate regarding the use of steroids in patients in septic shock?**

A. The addition of vitamin C and thiamine to hydro-cortisone significantly decreases mortality versus steroids alone.

B. The addition of vitamin C and thiamine to hydrocortisone significantly decreases vasopressor use.

C. Corticosteroid use significantly decreases ICU and hospital length of stay but has minimal or no effect on long-term survival.

D. Corticosteroid use requires a positive cortisol stimulation test.

E. Corticosteroid use significantly decreases ICU length of stay, hospital length of stay, and long-term survival.

ANSWERS

1. **C.** The main principles of sepsis therapy are early recognition/diagnosis and to begin both treatment and resuscitation immediately upon identification of sepsis or suspected sepsis. The current criterion for diagnosis of sepsis is infection plus evidence of end-organ hypoperfusion and injury, which is defined as a change of 2 points or greater on the sequential organ failure assessment (SOFA) scoring system. Treatment consists of early initiation of empiric broad spectrum antibiotics and initial broad spectrum antibiotic administration, and does not require identification of the exact causative organism. When sepsis is suspected, early initiation of resuscitation with the goal of reversing tissue induced hypoperfusion has been previously shown to improve patient survival in patients presenting with septic shock. The current Surviving Sepsis Campaign Guidelines recommends an initial fluid bolus of 30 cc/kg of isotonic crystalloid solution for initial resuscitation. The goals of resuscitation should be to achieve a CVP 8–12 mmHg, MAP ≥65 mmHg, urine output ≥0.5 mL/kg/hr, and improved markers

of end-organ perfusion (e.g., lactate) within 6 hours. In mechanically ventilated patients, venous return can be impeded and as a result a higher target for CVP (12 to 15 mmHg) is recommended. Note that there is no arbitrary systolic blood pressure as a primary goal of resuscitation.

Lactate is also a marker of metabolic acidosis and tissue hypoperfusion and is seen in a majority of patients presenting in septic shock. When a patient presents with hypotension and an elevated lactate (≥4), he or she has an increased mortality over elevated lactate or hypotension alone. If a patient presents with an elevated lactate, it can be monitored until it reaches normal levels and can be used along with other markers, to guide resuscitation. Base deficit is another measure of metabolic acidosis that may be used to gauge the severity of illness and to guide resuscitation. It is often used as a surrogate for lactate, but there are many other factors that can impact the base deficit (renal failure, alcohol, bicarbonate losses), making it a less specific measure of tissue hypoperfusion and lactic acidosis.

In addition to restoring tissue hypoperfusion, a source of the patient's sepsis should be sought, and appropriate antibiotics should be administered. Each hour antibiotics administration is delayed results in a measurable increase in patient mortality. Ideally, cultures should be obtained prior to giving antibiotics with the goal of administering antibiotics within 1 hour of presenting with sepsis. However, if obtaining appropriate cultures would delay the administration of antibiotics beyond 1 hour, then antibiotics should be given prior to obtaining cultures.

2. **C.** Many studies have been conducted comparing synthetic starches to isotonic crystalloid based solutions. The results of these studied have varied. Some studies have shown no mortality difference, others have shown increased mortality or increased rates of renal replacement therapy. None have shown a benefit, and recent data suggest increased renal failure and mortality with administration of hydroxyethyl starch solutions. There is also a concern for the potential impact of these solutions on platelet function and coagulation. As a result, starch-based solutions are not recommended for resuscitation.

Vasopressor therapy is recommended for use in hypotensive septic patients after adequate volume resuscitation to maintain perfusion pressures. Norepinephrine (Levophed) is currently the initial vasopressor of choice for septic shock, as it provides a balanced pressure and cardiac inotrope effect. Dopamine is associated with increased short-term mortality and serious adverse events compared to norepinephrine. Pure vasopressors such as phenylephrine should be avoided as the unopposed vasoconstriction can often further worsen the ongoing tissue hypoperfusion and lead to severe extremity or bowel ischemia. If the patient remains hypotensive after starting norepinephrine, then starting a low dose infusion of vasopressin at 0.03 U/min can be used to decrease the dose of norepinephrine and enhance organ perfusion. If the patient remains in septic shock despite fluids and appropriate vasopressor therapy, then corticosteroid administration can be considered.

Based on the presentation, there is a high suspicion of septic shock and no clinical or physical exam signs of cardiogenic shock. While an echocardiogram may be useful in certain situations, the treatment for septic shock should not be delayed. Delaying treatment of septic shock and can result in increased patient mortality.

3. **D.** This patient has a *C. difficile* infection and likely toxic megacolon secondary to the infection. PCR-based *C. difficile* toxin as well as most current tests for C. difficile are extremely sensitive and specific for the diagnosis of an active *C. difficile* infection and repeat testing is not necessary. The severity of *C. difficile* infections can range from mild to severe. In very severe cases, patients can present with shock and sepsis known as fulminant *C. difficile* colitis or toxic megacolon. Over the past two decades, this diagnosis has become more common, and more patients are requiring surgical intervention.

While we do not know from the description if there is perforation or peritoneal signs, this patient is clearly in shock. Antibiotic therapy should be targeted at the suspected diagnosis and the patient should be immediately evaluated for surgical intervention. Surgical intervention for toxic megacolon from any cause typically mandates resection of the entire colon (total abdominal colectomy) and placement of an end ileostomy. A less invasive option is a diverting loop ileostomy and then colonic lavage with vancomycin via the ileostomy, but there is controversy over the appropriateness of this option. Antifungal agents should not be routinely started in septic patients or for *C. difficile* colitis. They should be used only in patients that are at risk of or suspected of having a fungal infection. Patients that are immunocompromised, neutropenic, or live in at-risk areas should be considered for the implementation of antifungal agents. However, there is nothing in this patient's history that would lead us to suspect she is at an increased for a fungal infection.

Once a source of infection is identified, then antimicrobial therapy should be targeted at the suspected source. If there a specific anatomical source of infection such as an abscess and cholangitis, that is driving a patient's sepsis, then emergent-targeted therapy should be initiated within 12 hours; not after antibiotics have taken effect. However, if no source of infection is identified and the patient improved with empiric antibiotic therapy, then procalcitonin levels (not pro BNP levels) can be used to help a clinician determine when to stop antimicrobial therapy.

4. D. In 2012, an updated clinical definition of ARDS (known as the Berlin Definition) was published. The presence of bilateral chest opacities is needed to make the diagnosis of ARDS, and either a chest radiograph or a CT scan is an acceptable way to evaluate for this. A focal unilateral infiltrate or consolidation on chest x-ray would be more consistent with lobar pneumonia than ARDS. According to the most recent ARDS definition outlined by the ARDS task force, the diagnosis of ARDS must be made within one week of a known clinical insult, and typically the diagnosis is made within 72 hours. After the diagnosis is made, the use of low tidal volumes (4 to 6 mL/kg) should be initiated as this is the only mode of ventilation shown to improve mortality in randomized controlled trials of patients with ARDS. As part of this strategy, high PEEP is often utilized to increase alveolar recruitment and improve oxygenation but has not been shown to improve overall mortality. Additional factors that have been found to improve mortality in randomized studies include prone positioning and the use of neuromuscular blockade. These options should be considered in patients who are not responding to standard ARDS ventilation and management protocols.

Many other strategies are utilized to try and improve outcomes in patients with refractory ARDS. One treatment that has been studied is the use of corticosteroids. The ARDSNet trial showed that while corticosteroids reduced then mean number of days on a ventilator and increased the number of shock-free days, they had no effect on overall survival and were harmful when given more than two weeks after the diagnosis of ARDS was made. Meduri et al. used low dose corticosteroids, and while ICU mortality was significantly reduced overall, mortality was not. For the patient in ARDS who is refractory to standard mechanical ventilation, salvage or rescue options include switching to APRV, high frequency or "jet" ventilation, and even ECMO. Other rescue therapies include prone positioning, neuromuscular blockade, and inhaled nitric oxide. While these treatments are used as rescue therapies in severe ARDS and have been shown to produce improved oxygenation, they have not been shown to improve mortality in controlled trials.

5. B. There are many challenges that are encountered when managing a critically ill patient, and delirium is a commonly encountered complication in the ICU setting. Severely ill and older patients are at particularly high risk for developing delirium, and this has been shown to adversely impact morbidity and mortality. While benzodiazapenes are effective for delirium acutely, their use has been shown to increase ICU length of stay and as a result they should be avoided whenever possible. Rather the primary treatment for agitation and delirium is non-pharmacologic and includes reorientation and maintenance of sleep-wake cycles. If this is ineffective then anti-psychotics such as haloperidol or the newer atypical antipsychotics are preferred to benzodiazepines.

Another area that can challenge the management of septic patients is predicting which patients are likely to have a worse outcome. There are many scoring systems that are utilized to predict outcomes in these patients, including the well-described APACHE score. One such system that is specific for multi-organ failure is the SOFA score. This system independently grades the severity of organ dysfunction for six different organ systems: respiratory, coagulation, liver, cardiovascular, central nervous system, and renal. The individual scores are then added to give a total score.

Higher overall SOFA scores directly correlate with a worse outcome (Figure 86-1). Mortality has been shown to directly increase with the number of organ systems that are failing and approaches 100% when four or more organ systems have failed. Among individual organ systems, one of the strongest predictors

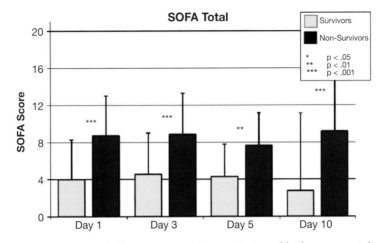

Figure 86-1 Graph demonstrating the association of higher sequential organ failure assessment (SOFA) scores with mortality at all time points during ICU admission. (Reprinted with permission from Fueglistaler P, Amsler F, Schuepp M, et al.)

of ICU morbidity and risk of mortality is the development of acute kidney injury or renal failure.

Many critically ill patients are at increased risk of upper gastrointestinal bleeding, and stress ulcer prophylaxis is indicated for patients with prolonged mechanical ventilation (>48 hours) or other risk factors. The risk of bleeding from stress ulceration or gastritis in this patient population must be weighed against the risk of treatment with either proton pump inhibitors (PPI) or histamine receptor blockers (H_2 blockers). Multiple studies have shown that patients that receive stress ulcer prophylaxis are at increased risk of adverse events and complications such as *C. difficile* infections, ventilator associated pneumonia, and thrombocytopenia (H_2 blockers).

Although hypermetabolism and a prolonged catabolic state are characteristic of sepsis and MODS, there has been no demonstrated survival benefit of administration of parenteral nutrition. Multiple series have demonstrated that overall infectious complications are lower among patients given enteral nutrition versus total parenteral nutrition, and the gut should be the preferred route for nutritional support whenever possible. Another important problem that is seen in patients with septic shock is critical illness polyneuropathy. The highly morbid condition is more common in patients with prolonged ICU stays and among patients who received steroids or neuromuscular blocking agents. It can present with muscle atrophy, limb weakness, peripheral sensory deficits,

and difficulty weaning patients from mechanical ventilation. However, cranial nerve function is usually spared.

6. **E.** Bezlotoxumab is a monoclonal antibody against *C. difficile* toxin B. This and actoxumab, a monoclonal antibody targeting *C. difficile* toxin A, were evaluated in the MODIFY I and MODIFY II studies. In MODIFY I, bezlotoxumab, actoxumab, and a combination of both were compared to placebo in adults receiving standard of care treatment for *C. difficile*. Both bezotoxumab and the combination regimen had a significantly lower recurrence rate than the placebo group. There was no difference between recurrence rates in the placebo group and the actoxumab group. MODIFY II evaluated bezlotoxumab and a combination of bezlotoxumab and actoxumab to placebo. There was no added benefit to the addition of actoxumab.

Current IDSA guidelines recommend Fidaxomicin or oral vancomycin for first-line therapy of non-severe or severe *C. difficile* infection. Fidaxomicin is also recommended for first and subsequent recurrences. Either it or a tapered and pulsed vancomycin regimen may be used for a recurrent *C. difficile* infection. Metronidazole is not recommended for recurrent *C. difficile* infections. Fecal transplants are only recommended for those patients who have multiple recurrences and have failed antibiotic therapy. While probiotic use in the prevention of *C. difficile* infections is currently an area of active investigation, the IDSA notes insufficient evidence to make a recommendation for or against use of prophylactic probiotics.

7. C. A recent Cochrane review analyzed the use of corticosteroids in sepsis. They found a small decrease in 28 days and hospital mortality. They further found decreases in ICU and hospital length of stay. Despite this, long-term mortality was not affected by corticosteroid use. There has been significant interest in the use of vitamin C, hydrocortisone, and thiamine after the publication of a single, retrospective before-and-after study suggested lower SOFA score, lower pressor use and lower mortality after early infusion of the so-called HAT (hydrocortisone, ascorbic acid, and thiamine) protocol. The recently published VITAMINS trial of the therapy, a prospective, controlled, randomized trial, did not show any differences in short- or long-term mortality or ventilator use of HAT therapy over corticosteroids alone. Steroids should be considered for patients with persistent hypotension despite adequate initial fluid resuscitation and vasopressor administration. Although previous recommendations included performing testing of the adrenocortical axis (e.g., a "cortisol stim test"), current guidelines recommend empiric initiation and continuation or discontinuation based on clinical response.

BIBLIOGRAPHY

The Acute Respiratory Distress Syndrome Network. Ventilation with lower tidal volumes as compared with traditional tidal volumes for acute lung injury and the acute respiratory distress syndrome. *N Engl J Med.* 2000;342(18):1301–1308.

Adhikari NKJ, Dellinger RP, Lundin S, et al. Inhaled nitric oxide does not reduce mortality in patients with acute respiratory distress syndrome regardless of severity: systematic review and meta-analysis. *Crit Care Med.* 2014;42(2):404–412.

Annane D, Bellissant E, Bollaert PE, et al. Corticosteroids for treating sepsis in children and adults. Cochrane *Database Syst Rev.* 2019;12(12):CD002243.

Brower RG, Lanken PN, MacIntyre N, et al. Higher versus lower positive end-expiratory pressures in patients with the acute respiratory distress syndrome. *N Engl J Med.* 2004;351(4):327–336.

Cohen SH, Gerding DN, Johnson S, et al. Clinical practice guidelines for Clostridium difficile infection in adults: 2010 update by the Society for Healthcare Epidemiology of America (SHEA) and the Infectious Diseases Society of America (IDSA). *Infect Control Hosp Epidemiol.* 2010;31(5):431–455.

De Backer D, Aldecoa C, Njimi H, Vincent JL. Dopamine versus norepinephrine in the treatment of septic shock: a meta-analysis. *Crit Care Med.* 2012;40(3):725–730.

De Backer D, Biston P, Devriendt J, et al. Comparison of dopamine and norepinephrine in the treatment of shock. *N Engl J Med.* 2010;362(9):779–789.

Delaloye J, Calandra T. Invasive candidiasis as a cause of sepsis in the critically ill patient. *Virulence.* 2014;5(1):161–169.

Dellinger RP, Levy MM, Rhodes A, et al. Surviving Sepsis Campaign: international guidelines for management of severe sepsis and septic shock, 2012. *Intensive Care Med.* 2013;39(2):165–228.

Ferreira FL, Bota DP, Bross A, Mélot C, Vincent JL. Serial evaluation of the SOFA score to predict outcome in critically ill patients. *JAMA.* 2001;286(14):1754–1758.

Friedrich O. Critical illness myopathy: sepsis-mediated failure of the peripheral nervous system. *Eur J Anaesthesiol Suppl.* 2008;42:73–82.

Fueglistaler P, Amsler F, Schuepp M, et al. Prognostic value of sequential organ failure assessment and simplified acute physiology II score compared with trauma scores in the outcomes of multiple-trauma patients. *Am J Surg.* 2010;200:204–214.

Fujii T, Luethi N, Young PJ, et al. Effect of vitamin C, hydrocortisone, and thiamine vs hydrocortisone alone on time alive and free of vasopressor support among patients with septic shock. The VITAMINS randomized clinical trial. *JAMA.* 2020;323(5):423–431.

Girard TD, Bernard GR. Mechanical ventilation in ARDS: a state-of-the-art review. *Chest.* 2007;131(3):921–929.

Guidet B, Martinet O, Boulain T, et al. Assessment of hemodynamic efficacy and safety of 6% hydroxyethylstarch 130/0.4 versus 0.9% NaCl fluid replacement in patients with severe sepsis: the CRYSTMAS study. *Crit Care.* 2012;16(3):R94.

Heyland DK, Johnson AP, Reynolds SC, Muscedere J. Procalcitonin for reduced antibiotic exposure in the critical care setting: a systematic review and an economic evaluation. *Crit Care Med.* 2011;39(7):1792–1799.

Marik PE, Khangoora V, Rivera R, et al. Hydrocortisone, vitamin C, and thiamine for the treatment of severe sepsis and septic shock. *Chest.* 2017;151(6):1229–1238.

Marik PE, Vasu T, Hirani A, Pachinburavan M. Stress ulcer prophylaxis in the new millennium: a systematic review and meta-analysis. *Crit Care Med.* 2010;38(11):2222–2228.

Maung AA, Kaplan LJ. Airway pressure release ventilation in acute respiratory distress syndrome. *Crit Care Clin.* 2011;27(3):501–509.

McDonald LC, Gerding DN, Stuart Johnson S, et al. Clinical practice guidelines for Clostridium difficile infection in adults and children: 2017 update by the Infectious Diseases Society of America (IDSA) and Society for Healthcare Epidemiology of America (SHEA). *Clin Infect Dis.* 2018 Mar 19;66(7):e1–e48.

Meduri GU, Golden E, Freire AX, et al. Methylprednisolone infusion in early severe ARDS results of a randomized controlled trial, 2007. *Chest.* 2009;136(5 Suppl):e30.

McConnell KW, Coopersmith CM. Organ failure avoidance and mitigation strategies in surgery. *Surg Clin North Am.* 2012;92(2):307–319, ix.

Myburgh JA, Finfer S, Bellomo R, et al. Hydroxyethyl starch or saline for fluid resuscitation in intensive care. *N Engl J Med*. 2012;367(20):1901–1911.

Perner A, Haase N, Guttormsen AB, et al. Hydroxyethyl starch 130/0.42 versus Ringer's acetate in severe sepsis. *N Engl J Med*. 2012;367(2):124–134.

Ranieri VM, Rubenfeld GD, Thompson BT, et al. Acute respiratory distress syndrome: the Berlin Definition. *JAMA*. 2012;307(23):2526–2533.

Rivers E, Nguyen B, Havstad S, et al. Early goal-directed therapy in the treatment of severe sepsis and septic shock. *N Engl J Med*. 2001;345(19):1368–1377.

Russell JA. Bench-to-bedside review: vasopressin in the management of septic shock. *Crit Care*. 2011;15(4): 226.

Sartelli M, Di Bella S, McFarland LV, et al. 2019 update of the WSES guidelines for management of *Clostridioides* (*Clostridium*) *difficile* infection in surgical patients. *World J Emerg Surg*. 2019;14:8

Sprung CL, Annane D, Keh D, et al. Hydrocortisone therapy for patients with septic shock. *N Engl J Med*. 2008;358(2): 111–124.

Stanley JD, Bartlett JG, Dart BW, Ashcraft JH. Clostridium difficile infection. *Curr Probl Surg*. 2013;50(7):302–337.

Steinberg KP, Hudson LD, Goodman RB, et al. Efficacy and safety of corticosteroids for persistent acute respiratory distress syndrome. *N Engl J Med*. 2006;354(16):1671–1684.

Vincent JL, de Mendonça A, Cantraine F, et al. Use of the SOFA score to assess the incidence of organ dysfunction/ failure in intensive care units: Results of a multicenter, prospective study. Working group on "sepsis-related problems" of the European Society of Intensive Care Medicine. *Crit Care Med*. 1998;26(11):1793–1800.

Wilcox M, Gerding D, Poxton I, et al. Bezlotoxumab alone and with Actoxumab for prevention of recurrent Clostridium difficile infection in patients on standard of care antibiotics: integrated results of 2 phase 3 studies (MODIFY I and MODIFY II). *Open Forum Infect Dis*. 2015;2(suppl 1):67.

87

Major Burns and Smoke Inhalation

Tovy Haber Kamine, Stephen R. Odom, Felicia N. Williams, Rabia Nizamani, and Booker T. King

A 20-year-old man arrives in the emergency department after being pulled from a burning vehicle after motor vehicle collision. On initial evaluation in the emergency room, he is noted to be agitated, with singed hair around his mouth and coughing up black sputum. Bilateral lower extremities were circumferentially burned with thick leathery skin, from his bilateral lower extremities and trunk, both circumferentially. His vital signs are a temperature of 95.3°F with a heart rate of 140/min. Blood pressure is 80/50 mmHg with a respiratory rate of 30, and Sat 89% on 15 L/min by nasal cannula. The patient is subsequently intubated and placed on mechanical ventilation. Two large bore intravenous lines were placed in his antecubital fossae without difficulty. A secondary survey is performed, which reveals a patent airway, equal breath sounds, and no additional injuries. The patient's weight is 60 kg.

1. **The patient is started on 1,080 cc/hr of lactated ringers (LR) and transferred to the intensive care unit (ICU). A Foley catheter is placed and after 2 hours, he is noted to have 0 cc of urine output for 2 hours. Select the next most appropriate step in management.**

   A. Continue LR at 1,080 cc/hr for 8 hours total, then decrease to 540 cc/hr for the following 16 hours.

   B. Increase LR to 1,440 cc/hr, then monitor urine output over the next hour.

   C. Bolus LR and titrate to a urine output of 30 to 50 cc/hr.

   D. Bolus LR and titrate to a urine output of 100 to 200 cc/hr.

2. **The patient is placed on 100% FiO_2. An arterial blood gas is performed with the following results: pH: 7.04; pCO_2: 70 mmHg; pO_2: 460 mmHg; HCO_3: 12 mEq/L; Base Excess: −12 mEq/L; Lactate: 12 mmol/L. Which of the following is the most appropriate next step in management?**

   A. Sodium bicarbonate

   B. Hyperbaric oxygen

   C. Activated charcoal

   D. Chest escharotomy

   E. Decrease FiO_2

3. **After 4 hours in ICU, the patient's physical exam was as follows: bilateral lower extremities were noted to be cold, without palpable pulses, and he had dark amber urine. His vitals at this point are: temperature: 97.5; HR: 140/min; BP: 90/40 (mean arterial pressure [MAP]: 57) mmHg; Sat: 100% on assist control/volume control (AC/VC) mechanical ventilation: FiO_2: 60%; RR: 20/min; tidal volume (TV): 400 cc; positive end-expiratory pressure (PEEP): 8 mmHg. Which is the next most appropriate step in management?**

   A. Bedside escharotomies of bilateral lower extremities, possible fasciotomies.

   B. Urgent transfer to the operating room for fasciotomies of the right lower extremity.

   C. Initiation of vasopressor therapy to target a MAP of 65 mmHg.

   D. Excision of bilateral lower extremity burns with split thickness skin graft from any available donor sites.

4. Your patient is a 40-year-old male with type II DM who sustained a 53% total body surface area burn and inhalation injury in a structural fire 2 days ago. On admission his burn wounds were placed in mafenide acetate and his fluid resuscitation was successfully completed at 24 hours. An arterial blood gas was obtained for a respiratory rate of 35 breaths per minute: $pH = 7.20$, $pCO_2 = 21$ meq/L, $O_2 = 108$ mmHg, $HCO_3^- = 10$ meq/L, base excess $= -15$ meg/L and a lactate of 1.5 mmol/L. The anion gap is 12 mEq/L and $K^+ = 4.1$ mEq/l. What is the cause of the acidosis?

   A. Severe septic shock due to invasive burn wound infection
   B. Diabetic ketoacidosis due to poorly controlled diabetes mellitus
   C. Use of topical agent on the burn wounds
   D. Acute kidney injury caused by severe hypovolemia
   E. Latrogenically caused by resuscitation with normal saline

5. You admit a 23-year-old 80-kg male who sustained chemical burns after an accident at a hydraulic fracking site. The patient was not wearing the proper personal protective equipment. He is transported to your burn center by ground and arrives 2 hours after the injury and has received little resuscitation. After addressing the burn wounds, you determine the patient has deep partial and full-thickness burns involving the face, both upper extremities circumferentially and both lower extremities anteriorly. You decide to use the Parkland formula for resuscitation and initiate fluid resuscitation at a rate of:

   A. 400 ml/hr LR
   B. 200 ml/hr 5% albumin
   C. 800 ml/hr LR
   D. 600 ml/hr normal saline
   E. 1,080 ml/hr LR

6. The patient above has completed his third hour of burn resuscitation and is noted to have a urine output ranging from 33 to 45 ml/hr. What should you do next?

   A. The urine output is marginal so give 500 ml bolus of LR.
   B. Start a 5% albumin infusion at 30 ml/hr.
   C. Increase the LR infusion to 1,300 ml/hr.

   D. Keep LR infusion at current rate and continue to monitor the urine output.
   E. Start high dose vitamin C infusion anticipating a complex resuscitation.

ANSWERS

1. **B.** The rule of nine's or the Lund Browder Chart is used to calculate the percentage body surface area (BSA) burned in adults. Only second- and third-degree burns are included in the calculation of total BSA burned; first-degree burns are not included in the calculation.

   The most commonly used formula for calculating crystalloid resuscitation needs in the first 24 hours is the Parkland formula:

   $$\text{First 24 resuscitation} = 4 \text{ cc} \times \text{total body surface area burned (\%)} \times \text{body weight (kg)}$$

   Half of this fluid is given in the first 8 hours after injury, and half in the next 16 hours.

   In this case, resuscitation $= 4$ cc $\times 72\%$ (18% [right lower extremity] $\times$ 18% [left lower extremity] $\times$ 18% [anterior trunk] $\times$ 18% [posterior trunk]) $\times$ 60 kg $= 17,280$ cc.

   8,640 cc given in first 8 hours $= 1,080$ cc/hr $\times$ 8 hrs then 8,640 given over next 16 hours $= 540$ cc/hr $\times$ 16 hrs.

   It is important to note that the Parkland formula is only a guideline and intravenous fluid needs should be titrated to urine output of 30 to 50 cc/hr in most adults. If this urine output range is not achieved, the IV fluid rate should be adjusted $-/+$ 33% each hour until the desired urine output is reached. Fluid boluses should be avoided unless the patient is hypotensive as it could lead to over-resuscitation. Factors such as inhalation injury, and concomitant injuries will increase fluid requirements.

2. **D.** Full-thickness or deep-partial-thickness burns that are circumferential around an extremity or chest will prevent normal elastic movement of the skin. Edema after fluid resuscitation can cause tissue pressure to rise underneath this leathery skin and impair circulation. For this patient with poor ventilation ($pCO_2 = 70$ mmHg), the treatment is escharotomy, which involves a full-thickness incision through the burned skin (epidermis and dermis down to subcutaneous fat). The incision is made along the medial or

lateral aspect of the limb, or, in the chest, in the mid-axillary line, to decompress underlying structures. The incisions should only be through the eschar, as they should not involve the deeper fascia. Although escharotomy is often confused with fasciotomy, the majority of circumferential extremity burns resulting in signs of elevated compartment pressures require only an escharotomy, and not a fasciotomy.

3. **A.** Full-thickness or deep-partial-thickness burns that are circumferential around an extremity or chest will prevent normal elastic movement of the skin. Edema after fluid resuscitation can cause tissue pressure to rise underneath this leathery skin and impair circulation. This has resulted in compromise to the patient's arterial supply to his lower extremities. The treatment, therefore, is escharotomy, which involves a full-thickness incision through the burned skin (epidermis and dermis down to subcutaneous fat). The incision is made along the medial or lateral aspect of the limb, or, in the chest, in the mid-axillary line, to decompress underlying structures. The incisions should only be through the eschar, as they should not involve the deeper fascia. Although escharotomy is often confused with fasciotomy, the majority of circumferential extremity burns resulting in signs of elevated compartment pressures require only an escharotomy, and not a fasciotomy. Factors that may suggest the need for a fasciotomy are indicators of rhabdomyolysis, or significant muscle breakdown that may lead to renal failure. If there is evidence of deeper injury, indicated by ischemic or necrotic muscle encountered during an escharotomy, a fasciotomy may be indicated.

4. **C.** The most likely cause of metabolic acidosis is the mafenide acetate cream used on the burn wounds. Mafenide acetate can cause metabolic acidosis if applied to a large surface area because it inhibits carbonic anhydrase thereby preventing the conversion of CO_2 gas to HCO_3^- in the tissues.

$$CO_2 + H_2O \rightarrow HCO_3^- + H^+$$

Severe septic shock from invasive burn wound infection is rare at this early stage and would likely result in elevated lactate levels. Diabetic ketoacidosis is also not likely given the normal anion gap. Acute kidney injury, although possible, would not usually follow a "successful" fluid resuscitation. Resuscitation with a large volume of normal saline can cause a metabolic acidosis due to the excessive amount of chloride ion that enters the cells and displaces H^+. These patients, however, would have a concomitant hypokalemia.

5. **E.** The areas of burn—face (4.5%), bilateral upper extremities (18%), and anterior legs bilaterally (18%)—result in a 40.5% total body surface area of burn wound. Burn resuscitation with the Parkland formula:

$$4 \text{ ml} \times 80 \text{ kg} \times 40.5\% = 12,960 \text{ ml}$$

Half of this volume is given in first 8 hours (6,480 ml) and the remainder given in the subsequent 16 hours. Since the resuscitation was delayed by 2 hours, you now have 6 hours to complete the first half of the resuscitation yielding a fluid infusion rate of 1,080 ml/hr. LR is the most widely used crystalloid for burn resuscitation as it is isotonic and has similar electrolyte distribution as plasma. Normal saline is not the preferred burn resuscitation fluid as it can cause hypernatremia and metabolic acidosis if infused at high volumes. There is no indication to initiate an albumin infusion at this time.

6. **D.** The goal urine output in the adult patient is 0.5/ml/kg/hr or 30 to 50 ml in most adults. The patient's urine output is within that range therefore no adjustment to the intravenous fluid rate is needed. The practice of giving intravenous bolus during burn resuscitation should be discouraged except in the face of hemodynamic instability. The excess fluid leaves the intravascular space through "leaky" capillaries and enters the interstium increasing the risk of compartment syndromes. An albumin infusion is not necessary at this time. High-dose vitamin C can be considered if the patient is having a difficult resuscitation and urine output goals are not being achieved despite high-fluid resuscitation volumes. It is not indicated in this situation.

BIBLIOGRAPHY

Asch MJ, White MG, Pruitt BA Jr. Acid base changes associated with topical Sulfamylon therapy: retrospective study of 100 burn patients. *Ann Surg.* 1970 Dec;172(6):946–950.

Matsuda T, Tanaka H, Williams S, Hanumadass M, Abcarian H, Reyes H. Reduced fluid volume requirement for resuscitation of third-degree burns with high-dose vitamin C. *J. Burn Care Rehabil.* 1991;12(6):525–532.

Orgill DP, Piccolo N. Escharotomy and decompressive therapies in burns. *J. Burn Care Res.* 2009;30(5):759–768.

Pham TN, Cancio LC, Gibran NS. American Burn Association practice guidelines burn shock resuscitation. *J. Burn Care Res.* 2008;29(1):257–266.

Pruitt BA, Dowling JA, Moncrief JA. Escharotomy in early burn care. *Arch Surg.* 1968;96(4):502–507.

Saffle JR. The phenomenon of "fluid creep" in acute burn resuscitation. *J. Burn Care Res.* 2007;28(3):382–395.

88

Surgical Nutrition

Julia B. Greer and John S. Mayo

A 49-year-old woman who has medically refractory Crohn's disease and high ileostomy output (2,200 mL/day) is referred to your clinic. She has undergone several abdominal surgeries for complications of her Crohn's and she currently has a diverting ileostomy and approximately 120 cm of her small bowel. She has been unable to tolerate any inflammatory bowel disease medications aside from corticosteroids.

The patient was admitted to an outside hospital twice in the last 3 months for rehydration and repletion of sodium, potassium, and magnesium. She now comes to your institution complaining of increased ostomy output, lightheadedness, fatigue, and nausea. She reports a recent weight loss of approximately 20 pounds (approximately 15% of total body weight). A Hickman catheter is placed in her right subclavian vein and she receives 3 days of parenteral nutrition without complications. She is discharged home on parenteral nutrition. You would like to perform an ileostomy takedown but would like to improve her nutritional status first.

1. **Compared to enteral nutrition, parenteral nutrition (PN):**
   A. Is less expensive
   B. Does not suffer from product shortages
   C. Preserves immunologic function of gut
   D. Is not associated with metabolic bone dysfunction
   E. Is less likely to cause diarrhea

2. **Basic parenteral nutrition formulations include:**
   A. Sucrose
   B. Amino acids
   C. 30% IV fat emulsion
   D. Omega-3 fatty acids
   E. Insulin

3. **After 8 weeks at home receiving parenteral nutrition, your patient develops hair loss, a pustular rash around her mouth, and darkening of her skin creases. The most likely cause is:**
   A. Copper deficiency
   B. Hyperkalemia
   C. Hyperglycemia
   D. Magnesium deficiency
   E. Zinc deficiency

4. **All individuals who receive total parenteral nutrition for >13 weeks will develop:**
   A. Venous thrombosis
   B. Steatohepatitis
   C. Gallbladder sludge
   D. Cholelithiasis
   E. Refeeding syndrome

5. **If this patient on parenteral nutrition suddenly spikes a fever, the most important entity to rule out is:**
   A. A Crohn's disease flare
   B. A catheter line infection
   C. An infection at the ostomy site
   D. *Clostridium difficile* colitis
   E. A urinary tract infection

6. **A 1-L bag of your patient's TPN contains 10% dextrose, 10% protein, and 10% fat emulsion. How many calories does this represent?**

A. 2,000 cal
B. 1,800 cal
C. 1,600 cal
D. 1,400 cal
E. 1,200 cal

7. **The patient in this stem has developed a critical illness and requires ICU admission. You decide to calculate a modified Nutrition Risk in Critically Ill (mNUTRIC) Score to help predict 28-day mortality and duration of mechanical ventilation. Which of the following indicates a higher risk mNUTRIC score?**

A. Age >40
B. APACHE II of 15-19
C. SOFA >10
D. 3 or more comorbidities
E. >5 ICU days

ANSWERS

1. **E.** Compared to enteral nutrition, parenteral nutrition (PN) is less likely to cause diarrhea. Enteral nutrition is delivered directly to the GI tract and its hyperosmolarity may result in diarrhea, especially in patients with an underlying condition that causes malabsorption. Diarrhea has been shown to occur in as many as 95% of patients who receive enteral feeds. PN is considerably more expensive than enteral nutrition. Shortages of many forms of product, especially vitamin and trace mineral components, has been causing delays in initiation of PN as well as inconsistent "mixing and matching" of different brands of product, which may result in certain micronutrient deficiencies if the provider does not have expertise with PN. Because it completely bypasses the GI tract, PN does not preserve the immunologic function of the gut. PN has been associated with metabolic bone dysfunction and abnormal bone metabolism and some patients have been shown to develop osteoporosis and osteomalacia.

2. **B.** Standard components of PN formulas include amino acids, dextrose, a 10% or 20% IV fat emulsion to provide essential fatty acids, electrolytes (sodium phosphate, sodium chloride, sodium acetate, potassium phosphate, potassium chloride, potassium acetate, magnesium sulfate, and calcium gluconate), multicomponent vitamins, and multicomponent trace minerals. Some potential additives include cysteine, regular insulin, and additional trace vitamins or elements as required. Although omega-3 fatty acid–enriched PN formulations have been studied as a potential means of decreasing inflammation and increasing immune function in certain subsets of patients, standard PN formulations do not contain them at this time.

3. **E.** A pathognomonic sign of zinc deficiency is hair loss. Skin lesions, including acne, a perioral pustular and darkening of skin folds, are frequently observed. Loss of appetite, decreased motor skills, and decreased immunity may characteristic of low dietary zinc. PN must be formulated to address deficiencies at initiation as well as those that may occur over the course of hyperalimentation. While electrolyte levels are routinely monitored, one should be aware of the potential for vitamin and trace mineral deficits. Individual with high output fistula or ostomy can develop metabolic disturbances. This patient may have had a zinc deficiency prior to receiving PN, which should have been addressed and monitored.

Because copper works with iron to form red blood cells, an early sign of copper deficiency is anemia. Low body temperature, osteoporosis, low white blood cell count, irregular heartbeat, loss of skin pigmentation, and thyroid problems may also occur due to a deficiency of copper. Hyperkalemia is associated with a slow or irregular heartbeat and weakness. Signs of hyperglycemia include weakness, nausea, excessive thirst/urination/appetite, headache, irritability, and abdominal pain. Severe hyperglycemia can lead to unconsciousness. A magnesium deficiency often manifests as cardiac and muscle irregularities, including arrhythmia, weakness, muscle cramps or spasms, restless leg syndrome, and general agitation; additional signs and symptoms of low magnesium include nausea, vomiting, insomnia, and confusion.

4. **C.** Catheter-related venous thrombosis is a fairly rare complication of PN, occurring in 1% to 3% of individuals per catheter-year. Deleterious effects of PN on the liver and gallbladder are well known to clinicians. Hepatic steatosis, which may manifest as fatty liver infiltration, may occur in PN patients within 1 to 2 weeks of initiating PN. It is reversible and can be managed by limiting the fat content. Liver function tests (LFTs) should be checked weekly for individuals on PN and if they are elevated, lipids should be minimized to <1 g/kd/day and total or

peripheral PN should be cycled over 12 hours to rest the liver.

If total bilirubin is >5–10 mg/dL due to hepatic dysfunction, trace elements should be discontinued due to the potential for toxicity of manganese and copper. Cholestasis is inevitable during PN because there are no intestinal nutrients to stimulate hepatic bile flow. Cholestasis typically occurs 2 to 6 weeks after starting PN and is indicated by progressive increases in total bilirubin and elevated serum alkaline phosphatase. While cholelithiasis is not uncommon during PN, it is certainly not ubiquitous. Re-feeding syndrome is a complication that begins rapidly after starting PN in a severely malnourished individual, typically a person who has been in a starvation state for >7–10 days. This syndrome is characterized by a severe shift in fluid and serum electrolyte levels, especially hypophosphatemia, resulting from intracellular electrolyte movement. Severe systemic complications, and even death, can result from re-feeding syndrome. Correcting electrolyte abnormalities prior to initiating PN is preventative for re-feeding syndrome. Although the previous complications may occur for some individuals on PN, *all* PN patients will develop gallbladder sludge after receiving PN for 13 weeks.

5. **B.** Any of the entities listed in question 5 may cause this patient to become febrile but catheter-related bloodstream infections (CR-BSI) are the most common and most serious complication of PN. Adequate nutrition is a cornerstone for strength preservation and immune system function in patients with serious gastrointestinal illnesses and proper training of family members and ancillary health personnel for home PN is essential. Sterile technique when manipulating the catheter is imperative. Not all patients with a CR-BSI will present with pyrexia but a sudden increase in body temperature and an elevated C-reactive protein provide a high index of suspicion. High white blood cell count, low albumin, or elevated total bilirubin may be present. Catheter maintenance for home parenteral nutrition patients and repeated removal/reinsertions can result in loss of venous access. Whenever possible, salvage of an infected tunneled catheter, such as the Hickman catheter used in this patient, should be attempted. The most effective way to prove the existence of a CR-BSI is to simultaneously draw blood cultures from the central

Points	0	1	2	3
Age	<50	50–74	≥ 75	
APACHE II	<15	15–19	20–27	≥ 28
SOFA	<6	6–9	≥ 10	
Number of Co-morbidities	0–1	≥ 2		
Days in ICU	0	≥ 1		

catheter and from a peripheral source. Other sources of fever should be investigated.

6. **D.** Ten percent dextrose of 1,000 mL is 100 g of dextrose, which at 3.4 cal/g is 340 cal. Ten percent protein then is 100 g of protein and at 4 cal/g is 400 cal. Ten percent fat likewise is 100 g of fat and at 9 cal/g is 900 b. Adding up the components, 100 cal dextrose + 400 cal protein + 900 cal fat = 1,400 total cal.

7. **C.** All of the listed points are components of the modified NUTRIC score, or mNUTRIC—the original NUTRIC score included IL-6 testing). The mNUTRIC has been validated as a tool for prediction of 28-day mortality and ventilator duration for critically ill patients. The components are:

APACHE II scores >28 have the most influence and age >75, SOFA scores >10, and APACHE II scores from 20 to 27 have significant influence also. In this question, a SOFA score of >10 is therefore the correct answer.

Scores >5 for the mNUTRIC are associated with worse outcomes and indicate the need for more aggressive nutritional therapy. These patients should be given nutrition by 24 to 48 hours and advanced toward at least 80% of calculated requirements within 48 to 72 hours. During this time, they should also be monitored closely for re-feeding syndrome. With lower scores <5 exclusive parenteral nutrition can be withheld for up to 7 days.

BIBLIOGRAPHY

Ayers P, Adams S, Boullata J, et al. A.S.P.E.N. Parenteral nutrition safety consensus recommendations: translation into practice. *Nutr Clin Practice.* June 2014;29(3):277–282.

Buchman AL, Howard LJ, Guenter P, et al. Micronutrients in parenteral nutrition: Too little or too much? The past, present, and recommendations for the future. [Erratum appears in Gastroenterology. April 2010;138(4):1633. Note: Dosage error in article text.]. *Gastroenterology.* November 2009;137(5 Suppl):S1–S6.

Chang A, Enns R, Saqui O, et al. Line sepsis in home parenteral nutrition patients: are there socioeconomic risk factors? A Canadian study. *JPEN*. November–December 2005;29(6):408–412.

Chang SJ, Huang HH. Diarrhea in enterally fed patients: Blame the diet? *Curr Opin Clin Nutr Metab Care*. September 2013;16(5):588–594.

Clare A, Teubner A, Shaffer JL, et al. What information should lead to a suspicion of catheter sepsis in HPN? *Clin Nutr*. August 2008;27(4):552–556.

Dibb M, Teubner A, Theis V, et al. Review article: the management of long-term parenteral nutrition. *Aliment Pharm & Ther*. March 2013;37(6):587–603.

Dimick JB, Swoboda S, Talamini MA, et al. Risk of colonization of central venous catheters: Catheters for total parenteral nutrition versus other catheters. *Amer J Crit Care*. July 2003;12(4):328–335.

Gastmeier P, Weist K, Ruden H. Catheter-associated primary bloodstream infections: Epidemiology and preventive methods. *Infection*. 1999;27(Suppl 1):S1–S6.

Guenter P, Holcombe B, Mirtallo JM, et al. Parenteral nutrition utilization: response to drug shortages. *JPEN*. January 2014;38(1):11–12.

Hamilton C, Seidner DL. Metabolic bone disease and parenteral nutrition. *Curr Gastroenterol Rep*. August 2004;6(4):335–341.

Lee JW. Fluid and electrolyte disturbances in critically ill patients. *E & BP*. December 2010;8(2):72–81.

Maroulis J, Kalfarentzos F. Complications of parenteral nutrition at the end of the century. *Clin Nutr*. October 2000;19(5):295–304.

McWhirter D. Parenteral nutrition line sepsis: the difficulty in diagnosis. *Proc Nutr Soc*. November 2010;69(4):508–510.

Messing B. Gallbladder sludge and lithiasis: complication of bowel rest. *Nutrition*. March–April 1990;6(2):190–191.

Messing B, Bories C, Kunstlinger F, Bernier JJ. Does total parenteral nutrition induce gallbladder sludge formation and lithiasis? *Gastroenterology*. May 1983;84(5 Pt 1):1012–1019.

McClave SA, Taylor BE, Martindale RG, et al. Guidelines for the provision and assessment of nutrition support therapy in the adult critically ill patient: Society of Critical Care Medicine (SCCM) and American Society of Parenteral and Enteral Nutrition (A.S.P.E.N). *JPEN J Parenter Enteral Nutr*. 2016;40(2):159–211.

Mirtallo JM. Consensus of parenteral nutrition safety issues and recommendations. *JPEN*. March 2012;36(2 Suppl):62S.

Radrizzani D, Bertolini G, Facchini R, et al. Early enteral immunonutrition versus parenteral nutrition in critically ill patients without severe sepsis: A randomized clinical trial. *Intensive Care Med*. August 2006;32(8):1191–1198.

Sabiston D Jr, Lyerly HK. Metabolism in surgical patient. In: Sabiston D Jr, Lyerly HK, eds. *Textbook of Surgery: The Biological Basis of Modern Surgical Practice*. 15th ed. Elsevier Saunders; 1997:137–175.

Seres DS, Valcarcel M, Guillaume A. Advantages of enteral nutrition over parenteral nutrition. *Ther Adv Gastroenterol*. March 2013;6(2):157–167.

Whelan K, Schneider SM. Mechanisms, prevention, and management of diarrhea in enteral nutrition. *Cur Opin Gastroenterol*. March 2011;27(2):152–159.

89

Blood Products and Transfusion

Stephen R. Odom, Christopher B. Horn, and Matthew J. Martin

SCENARIO 1

A 28-year-old male is involved in a high-speed motorcycle collision. He is ejected from his vehicle and sustains an open left femoral fracture. Bystanders report that he was lying in a "puddle of blood." En route, EMS reports ongoing bleeding from the wound. On arrival, he is maintaining his airway and has normal respirations and breath sounds. He is tachycardic in the 130 s and hypotensive with SBP in the 90 s. On exam, he is diaphoretic and has a Glasgow coma score of 13. After 1 liter of normal saline is transfused, a hemoglobin is 9.2 g/dL; however, the patient remains tachycardic, hypotensive and has altered mental status. Resuscitation with whole blood is begun.

1. **Which of the following interventions has been shown to decrease transfusion requirements?**

    A. Prehospital administration of plasma
    B. Prehospital tourniquet use
    C. Aggressive use of crystalloids prior to blood transfusion.
    D. Use of tranexamic acid
    E. Resuscitation with colloids rather than crystalloids.

2. **Which of the following is most accurate regarding the use of whole blood as compared to component therapy?**

    A. In combat, it does not show a difference in 24-hour or 30-day mortality.
    B. It is equivalent to 1:1:1 component therapy in terms of hematocrit, coagulation activity, and platelet count.

    C. It requires significant resources and is not feasible in civilian trauma settings outside of clinical trials.
    D. It decreases transfusion requirements outside of patients with head injuries.
    E. Due to the risk of donor antibodies, it must be crossmatched prior to use.

SCENARIO 2

A 33-year-old female (G3P2), 31 weeks pregnant, with severe vaginal bleeding, is taken emergently to the operating room for cesarean section. Intraoperatively, a percreta is identified with involvement of the bladder and pelvic wall. After delivery of the baby, an emergent hysterectomy is performed for massive bleeding. Blood loss was estimated at 15 liters. The patient was given 7,000 mL of crystalloid, along with 40 units of packed red blood cells, 10 units of fresh frozen plasma, and 20 units of platelets.

3. **Which of the following is an indication for blood transfusion?**

    A. Serum hemoglobin <10 g/dL
    B. Central venous oxygen concentration <55%
    C. Trauma score >14
    D. Loss of 20% of total body blood volume
    E. Systolic blood pressure <90 mmHg

4. **Which of the following is true of transfusion-related acute lung injury (TRALI)?**

    A. Improvement when well-resuscitated takes >2 weeks.
    B. It is caused by anti-HLA-antibodies in blood products that activate recipient leukocytes.

C. Acute respiratory illness arises within 2 days of transfusion of blood products.

D. Is easy to differentiate from acute respiratory distress syndrome (ARDS).

E. It is not associated with the number of transfusions or the age of blood.

5. **Which of the following non-transfusion strategies is of proven benefit in reducing blood product transfusion in stable trauma patients?**

A. Avoidance of hypothermia

B. Pelvic binders

C. Blood substitutes

D. Recombinant Factor V concentrate

E. Tranexamic acid

6. **Which of the following statements regarding heparin-induced thrombocytopenia (HIT) is true?**

A. HIT is an IgA antibody-mediated response to heparin-platelet factor IV complexes.

B. Procine unfractionated heparin (UFH) is more likely to cause HIT than bovine UFH.

C. The combined sensitivity and specificity of ELISA and serotonin functional assay is about 70%.

D. Treatment of confirmed HIT involves stopping heparin and initiation of warfarin therapy.

E. Patients with remote history of HIT can be safely treated with heparin.

7. **Which of the following statements regarding complications of blood transfusion is true?**

A. Risk of hepatitis C infection per unit of packed red blood cells is one in one million.

B. Hyperkalemia is a rare but frequently fatal disorder seen in massive blood transfusion.

C. Citrate can lower serum calcium and magnesium.

D. Massive transfusion frequently causes acidosis.

E. ABO incompatible blood transfusion is a rare cause of hemolytic reaction.

ANSWERS

1. **B.** While tourniquet use has been considered contraindicated in traumatically injured patients, recent military data has led to increased use in the civilian population. No prospective data exists regarding the impact on blood transfusions; however, in a retrospective, case-matched study, patients who received prehospital tourniquets for penetrating vascular injury had significantly fewer units of packed red blood cells and fresh frozen plasma than those who did not receive prehospital tourniquet placement.

Few other hemorrhage control interventions have been as effective. A recent Cochrane review evaluated the use of colloids versus crystalloids. Starches were found to increase transfusion requirements when compared to crystalloids. There was no difference in transfusion requirements between albumin, gelatins or dextrans, and crystalloids. Large-volume resuscitation of hemorrhage with crystalloid solutions should be avoided when possible and would likely result in an increased transfusion requirement. Crystalloid lacks both clotting factors and platelets. Use of crystalloid can cause further bleeding and increased transfusion requirements.

The CRASH-2 Trial demonstrated a mortality benefit in the use of tranexamic acid in trauma patients. In subgroup analysis, this effect was most pronounced when given within 3 hours of injury. However, TXA was not shown to decrease transfusion requirements when compared to patients who received placebo and this finding has led to additional research attempting to identify the mechanism of the TXA benefit in survival. Two recent studies of TXA administration for trauma patients with severe traumatic brain injury have also found a benefit in terms of outcomes, but not a reduced transfusion requirement.

Two trials have evaluated the prehospital use of plasma in traumatically injured patients. The COMBAT trial randomized injured patients undergoing ground transportation by EMS to either saline placebo or prehospital plasma. It resulted in a statistically insignificant difference in mortality between the treatment and study groups. Similarly, the PAMPER study randomized injured patients undergoing aeromedical transportation to placebo or prehospital plasma. In contrast, to COMBAT, PAMPER demonstrated a significant survival benefit to prehospital plasma administration. Neither study demonstrated a statistically significant reduction in transfusion requirements.

2. **D.** In the initial study of whole blood in civilian settings, the UT Houston group demonstrated no difference in transfusion requirement between the whole blood group and the standard of care group. Sensitivity analysis demonstrated that if patients with head injuries were excluded, patients receiving

whole blood received significantly fewer blood transfusions. Recent experience has further shown that whole blood can be used without crossmatching and that cold-stored whole blood is feasible in civilian trauma centers.

While 1:1:1 component therapy is meant to replicate whole blood, there are significant differences in the end composition. One unit of packed blood has a hematocrit >40% and $>150 \times 10^9$ platelets/L. When a unit of blood is split into components, preservative is added. If the resulting components are each given, the mean hematocrit is under 30%, coagulation factors are diluted to about 60% and platelets are diluted to 80×10^9/L.

Interest in whole blood springs from lessons learned in treating combat wounded. A retrospective study compared whole blood therapy with supplemental BCs and plasma to patients who received traditional 1:1:1 component therapy. Patients who received whole blood had similar units of PRBCs and similar PRBC to FFP ratios. Patients who received whole blood used less platelets than the component therapy group. Patients who received fresh whole blood had significantly increased 24-hour and 30-day survival. In multivariate regression, each unit of WFWB was associated with a significant increase in 30-day survival.

3. E. Specific triggers for blood transfusions have been the subject of a large amount of research, and the decision to transfuse is not always clear. Data indicate that in a patient without cardiac or lung disease and hemodynamic stability, a hemoglobin ≥7 g/dL is satisfactory to minimize blood transfusion without adversely affecting mortality. What is clear from these studies is that a liberal transfusion strategy is not helpful for oxygen delivery but has a negative effect on the immune system. In addition, class of hemorrhage by itself is not an indication for transfusion unless systemic hypotension, refractory tachycardia, oliguria, and lactic acidosis are present with evidence of ongoing bleeding.

Systemic venous oxygen saturation (SvO_2) is an attractive measure of oxygen consumption but cannot be associated with parameters of blood loss or severity of injury and so, by itself, cannot represent a reason to transfuse a patient.

The trauma score is a physiologic score that represents the sum of scores for respiratory rate and effort, capillary refill, systolic blood pressure, and Glasgow coma score. In this scoring system, a higher number is a less severe injury. Recent data suggest that over 90% of patients with a trauma score >14 did not need a blood transfusion. Both the revised trauma score and the ISS have been shown, interestingly, to predict the need for transfusion is severe pelvic trauma.

The only reliable criteria for the need to transfuse include clinical criteria, like ongoing bleeding, refractory tachycardia, decreased systolic blood pressure, oliguria, lactic acidosis, and elevated base deficit. A single criterion has been elusive.

4. B. Transfusion-related acute lung injury (TRALI) is an acute respiratory complication of blood transfusion that occurs within 4 to 6 hours of transfusion of product and cannot be traced to another acute lung injury risk factor. The syndrome is very similar to ARDS of other etiologies, and often cannot be differentiated. Overlapping syndromes include transfusion associated circulatory overload (TACO). TRALI is an anti-HLA-antibody mediated reaction from recipient leukocytes. Once complement is activated, acute lung injury ensues. Other theories, including the roles of nonpolar lipids and activated platelets, are less well supported in the literature. Resolution in a well-resuscitated patient normally occurs within 48 hours. Mortality is around 6% (as compared to much higher mortalities seen with ARDS from other causes). Risk factors for the development of TRALI include increased number of transfusions (particularly plasma products), possibly age of blood transfused, female plasma donor, and anti-HLA-antibody complement. Patient risk factors include higher IL-8 level, shock, liver surgery, cirrhosis, positive fluid balance, elevated peak airway pressures, and current smoking.

5. A. There are multiple non-transfusions options in surgical patients, many of which have proven beneficial in decreasing number of transfusions required. Initially, careful surgical technique (minimize blood loss, avoid hypothermia and coagulopathy, damage control, etc.) and careful treatment of preoperative anemia are clearly associated with decreased need for transfusion. While pelvic binders are recommended by the American College of Surgeons, there are no clinically relevant data to support their use. Blood substitutes, including human products, bovine products, and genetically engineered hemoglobin are available. Of these products, the genetically engineered hemoglobin is promising, in that the crossmatch is avoided (timely administration), osmotic pressure is increased (resuscitative fluid), and blood pressure is increased (vasopressor activity), but it remains to be determined that these products are beneficial in reducing blood transfusions in traumatically injured or critically ill patients.

Recombinant factor VII concentrate, not factor V, enhances thrombin generation and platelet activation and has been shown to decrease the need for massive transfusion of the severely injured trauma patients. A multicenter Phase III trial demonstrated a decrease in blood product usage, but did not demonstrate a mortality difference from placebo. It seems reasonable to avoid its use in elderly patients (>75 years old) as they have increased risk of arterial thrombosis. Tranexamic acid is an antifibrinolytic agent that blocks binding of plasmin to fibrin. In the CRASH-2 trial, over 20,000 major trauma patients were evaluated. Early use of tranexamic acid decreased death rate without demonstrated major side effects. Use after 3 hours is not beneficial. Tranexamic acid has also been shown to decrease the size of intracranial bleeding lesions in trauma patients (CRASH-2 collaborators).

6. **E.** HIT is an IgG-mediated disease directed at heparin-platelet factor IV (PF-4) complexes. Bovine UFH increases risk of HIT compared to porcine derived UFH. Orthopedic surgery/injury, cardiac surgery, especially heart transplant, the use of UFH as compared to low molecular weight heparin all increase the risk of HIT. Obstetric patients are at very low risk of developing HIT.

The ELISA test for HIT detects antibodies that react with the heparin-P-F-4 epitope while functional platelet assays (like the serotonin assay) use radiolabeled platelets mixed with patient's serum and heparin. The supernatant is then evaluated for radiolabeled material. Specificity and sensitivity of the ELISA test is 50% to70% and 90%, respectively. Specificity and sensitivity of functional assays are 95% and 90%, respectively. Used in conjunction, the sensitivity and specificity for HIT approach 100%. The results must be put into clinical context because between 20% and 60% of patients will form the heparin-PF-4 complexes that can be seen on the EISA test without the clinical syndrome. Once the diagnosis has been made, all heparin must be stopped.

Even after stopping heparin, patients are at increased risk for thrombotic complications for up to 100 days while the complexes persist, and require treatment with a direct thrombin inhibitor (only argatroban and lepirudin are FDA approved). Factor Xa inhibitors (dancparoid) are options, but not available in the United States.

Ancrod (pit viper venom), a glycoprotein IIb/IIIa inhibitor, has been evaluated in HIT, and was found to be without efficacy and may increase thrombotic risk. Vitamin K antagonists are contraindicated in the acute phase of HIT, but have a role in the long-term management of thrombotic complications. After about 100 days free from heparin, the heparin-PF-4 complexes have cleared and patients with previous episodes of HIT can be safely treated with heparin provided ELISA testing is negative. The IgG response is not amnestic and previous HIT does not increase risk for future HIT.

7. **C.** Transmission of infectious diseases by transfusion in the United States is rare. Bacterial infection is clinically apparent in 1:80,000 cases. Storage of platelets at room temperature may increase risk of bacterial infection after infusion of platelets. Current rates of viral transmission are as follows (per unit transfused): Hepatitis A (1:1 million), Hepatitis B (1:250,000), Hepatitis C (1:150,000), and HIV (1:2 million). Cytomegalovirus (CMV) is present in 50% of the population, and is transmitted in 5% in the infected units. The rate of transmission of prion disease is not known, but is presumably very, very low. Hyperkalemia after massive transfusion can be seen in up to 38.5% in trauma patients but is rarely associated with clinical sequelae. After transfusion, new red blood cell counts can take up potassium resulting in post-transfusion hypokalemia, so electrolytes should be closely monitored before, during, and after transfusion. Citrate (3 g/unit) is used in stored blood, and can bind calcium in the blood, resulting in hypocalcemia after massive transfusion.

Clinical signs of hypocalcemia include widened QT interval, decreased ventricular contractility, hypotension (related to a decrease in peripheral vascular resistance), muscle tremors, and even PEA arrest. Hypomagnesemia can also be responsible for prolonged QT seen after transfusion. The pH of stored blood often decreases to 6.6 to 6.8 because of increasing CO_2. However, the most frequent acid–base problem seen after massive transfusion is alkalosis because of the large amount of citrate in stored blood. Acidosis seen after massive transfusion should be concerning for ongoing tissue hypoperfusion rather than a result of the transfusion itself. ABO incompatible transfusion and the resultant hemolytic reaction is the most common preventable potentially fatal complication of blood transfusion. The most common cause is error along the chain of identification of the unit, the patient, or both.

BIBLIOGRAPHY

Aboudara MC, Hurst FP, Abbott KC, Perkins RM. Hyperkalemia after packed red blood cell transfusion in trauma patients. *J Trauma*. February 2008;64(2 Suppl): S86–S91.

Armand R, Hess JR. Treating coagulopathy in trauma patients. *Transfus Med Rev*. 2003;17(3):223–231.

Bannon MP, O'Neill CM, Martin M, Ilstrup DM, Fish NM, Barrett J. Central venous oxygen saturation, arterial base deficit, and lactate concentration in trauma patients. *Am Surg*. August 1995;61(8):738–745.

Baron JF. Blood substitutes. Haemoglobin therapeutics in clinical practice. *Crit Care*. 1999;3(5):R99–R102.

Boffard KD, Riou B, Warren B, et al. Recombinant factor VIIa as adjunctive therapy for bleeding control in severely injured trauma patients: two parallel randomized, placebo-controlled, double-blind clinical trials. *J Trauma*. July 2005;59(1):8–15.

Cotton BA, Podbielski J, Camp E, et al. A randomized controlled pilot trial of modified whole blood versus component therapy in severely injured patients requiring large volume transfusions. *Ann. Surg*. 2013;258(4)527–533.

CRASH-2 Collaborators, Intracranial Bleeding Study. Effect of tranexamic acid in traumatic brain injury: a nested randomised, placebo controlled trial (CRASH-2 Intracranial Bleeding Study). *BMJ*. July 1, 2011;343:d3795.

CRASH-2 Trial Collaborators, Shakur H, Roberts I, et al. Effects of tranexamic acid on death, vascular occlusive events, and blood transfusion in trauma patients with significant haemorrhage (CRASH-2): a randomised, placebo-controlled trial. July 3, 2010;376(9734):23–32.

Davenport RD. Pathophysiology of hemolytic transfusion reactions. *Semin Hematol*. July 2005;42(3):165–168.

Francis JL, Palmer GJ 3rd, Moroose R, Drexler A. Comparison of bovine and porcine heparin in heparin antibody formation after cardiac surgery. *Ann Thorac Surg*. January 2003;75(1):17–22.

Hauser CJ, Boffard K, Dutton R, et al. Results of the CONTROL trial: Efficacy and safety of recombinant activated Factor VII in the management of refractory traumatic hemorrhage. *J Trauma*. September 2010;69(3):489–500.

Hébert PC, Wells G, Blajchman MA, et al. A multicenter, randomized, controlled clinical trial of transfusion requirements in critical care. Transfusion requirements in critical care investigators, Canadian Critical Care Trials Group. *N Engl J Med*. 1999;340(6):409–417.

Hirsh J, Raschke R. Heparin and low-molecular-weight heparin: the seventh ACCP conference on antithrombotic and thrombolytic therapy. *Chest*. September 2004;126(3 Suppl): 188S–203S.

Lanzarotti S, Weigelt JA. Heparin-induced thrombocytopenia. *Surg Clin North Am*. December 2012;92(6):1559–1572.

Levi M, Levy JH, Andersen HF, Truloff D. Safety of recombinant activated factor VII in randomized clinical trials. *N Engl J Med*. November 4, 2010;363(19):1791–1800.

Lewis SR, Pritchard MW, Evans DJW, et al. Colloids versus crystalloids for fluid resuscitation in critically ill people. *Cochrane Database of Syst Rev*. 2018;3CD000567.

Looney MR, Gilliss BM, Matthay MA. Pathophysiology of transfusion-related acute lung injury. *Curr Opin Hematol*. September 2010;17(5):418–423.

Moore HB, Moore EE, Chapman MP. Plasma-first resuscitation to treat haemorrhagic shock during emergency ground transportation in an urban area: a randomised trial. *Lancet*. 2018 July 28;392(10144):283–291.

Perkins RM, Aboudara MC, Abbott KC, Holcomb JB. Resuscitative hyperkalemia in noncrush trauma: a prospective, observational study. *Clin J Am Soc Nephrol*. March 2007; 2(2):313–319.

Popovsky MA, Moore SB. Diagnostic and pathogenetic considerations in transfusion-related acute lung injury. *Transfusion*. 1985;25(6):573–577.

Roberts I, Shakur H, Afolabi A, et al. The importance of early treatment with tranexamic acid in bleeding trauma patients: an exploratory analysis of the CRASH-2 randomised controlled trial. *Lancet*. 2011;377(9771):1096–1101, 1101.e1–2.

Sayah DM, Looney MR, Toy P. Transfusion reactions: newer concepts on the pathophysiology, incidence, treatment, and prevention of transfusion-related acute lung injury. *Crit Care Clin*. July 2012;28(3):363–372.

Sihler KC, Napolitano LM. Complications of massive transfusion. *Chest*. January 2010;137(1):209–220.

Sperry JL, Guyette, FX, Brown, JB, et al. Prehospital plasma during air medical transport in trauma patients at risk for hemorrhagic shock. *N Engl J Med*. 2018;379:315–326.

Spinella PC, Perkins JG, Grathwohl KW, et al. Warm fresh whole blood is independently associated with improved survival for patients with combat-related traumatic injuries. *J Trauma*. 2009;66(4 Suppl):S69–S76.

Starr AJ, Griffin DR, Reinert CM, et al. Pelvic ring disruptions: Prediction of associated injuries, transfusion requirement, pelvic arteriography, complications, and mortality. *J Orthop Trauma*. September 2002;16(8):553–561.

Teixeira PGR, Brown CVR, Emigh B, et al. Civilian prehospital tourniquet use is associated with improved survival in patients with peripheral vascular injury. *J Am Coll Surg*. 2018;226(5):769–776.

Toy P, Gajic O, Bacchetti P, et al. Transfusion-related acute lung injury: incidence and risk factors. *Blood*. 2012;119(7): 1757–1767.

Vincent JL, Baron JF, Reinhart K, et al. Anemia and blood transfusion in critically ill patients. *JAMA*. 2002;288(12): 1499–1507.

West HC, Jurkovich G, Donnell C, Luterman A. Immediate prediction of blood requirements in trauma victims. *South Med J.* 1989;82(2):186–189.

Yazer M, Jackson B, Sperry J, et al. Initial safety and feasibility of cold-stored uncrossmatched whole blood transfusion in civilian trauma patients. *J. Trauma Acute Care Surg.* 2016;81(1):21–26.

Zentai C, Grottke O, Spahn DR, Rossaint R. Nonsurgical techniques to control massive bleeding. *Anesthesiol Clin.* March 2013;31(1):41–53.

90

Necrotizing Fasciitis

Allyson L. Berglund, John M. Giurini, and Michael Charles

SCENARIO 1

A 33-year-old female with a 19-year history of type 2 insulin dependent diabetes complicated by peripheral neuropathy, peripheral vascular disease, and chronic kidney disease presents to the emergency room complaining of worsening right foot pain and swelling over the last 3 days. She has a history of charcot deformity to her right foot with a chronic right foot ulceration that has been treated with weekly debridements and wound care. She endorses subjective fevers and chills.

On examination, she has a 1 cm × 1 cm × 3 cm deep plantar midfoot ulceration with probing and tracking noted dorsally to the midfoot. There is a strong malodor and her entire foot is significantly edematous and erythematous with significant pain on palpation of the midfoot and lower leg. She has biphasic Dopplerable pulses.

1. **Regarding clinical presentation, which of the following is true?**

   A. Necrotizing fasciitis has the same incidence in both adult and pediatric populations.

   B. Initial signs of necrotizing fasciitis include skin necrosis with a blue or purple discoloration, crepitus, and bullae.

   C. The most constant clinical feature is pain, out of proportion, to physical findings.

   D. When the borders of infection appear ill-defined, a diagnosis of erysipelas is more likely than necrotizing fasciitis.

2. **With regard to the diagnostic tools that are available, which of the following is true?**

   A. Plain radiographs demonstrating subcutaneous gas is present in about 25% of cases.

   B. A computerized tomography (CT) scan has a sensitivity of about 50%.

   C. A LRINEC score of 4 indicates an over 50% chance of necrotizing fasciitis.

   D. A good physical exam will differentiate among cellulitis, an abscess, and necrotizing fasciitis.

3. **When necrotizing fasciitis is suspected, immediate operative debridement is indicated. Which of the following is true regarding surgical exploration?**

   A. Surgical exploration should be delayed until vascular status can be evaluated and optimized.

   B. In dubious cases, surgical exploration should be avoided until the diagnosis is confirmed to limit unnecessary large incisions and tissue debridement.

   C. Repeated surgical debridements are not necessary if the patient is on appropriate intravenous antibiotics.

   D. Macroscopic findings include gray necrotic tissue, "dishwater" pus, and a positive "finger test."

4. **Which of the following is true regarding isolated organisms and antibiotic therapy?**

   A. Broad spectrum intravenous antibiotics are enough to stop the spread of infection.

   B. The most commonly isolated organism is *Clostridium*, and antibiotic therapy should always include coverage for this organism.

   C. Long-term intravenous antibiotics for >4 weeks is standard practice when necrotizing fasciitis has been diagnosed and the patient is free from systemic symptoms.

D. Clindamycin may be useful in controlling exotoxin production especially in cases complicated by streptococcal toxic shock syndrome.

5. **In regard to prognosis, which of the following is true?**

A. Patients infected with *Clostridia* have lower mortality and limb loss rates compared to those with a polymicrobial or other monocrobial infection.

B. The single most important factor that negatively influences prognosis is delayed surgical debridement.

C. Hyperbaric oxygen therapy (HBO) has been shown to dramatically decrease limb loss.

D. Diabetes, even in those presenting in diabetic ketoacidosis, does not have higher mortality or longer hospital stays.

SCENARIO 2

A 67-year-old man was admitted into the VA hospital system 3 days ago with exacerbation of COPD and blood glucose 300 mg/di. He has a 45 "pack year" history of tobacco use and was recently told that he has a "lung mass that needs to be looked into." Since hospitalization, he has required intermittent bladder straight catheter placement for drainage. On rounds early this AM, you find the patient confused, febrile with a heart rate of 118 bpm and systolic blood pressure 90 mmHg. On exam, you noticed tense, red, edematous lower abdominal wall skin that extends into his perineum, gluteal muscles, and scrotum. The scrotum itself is firm and tense to a point that you cannot differentiate specific scrotal contents.

6. **Which of the following is true regarding this clinical scenario?**

A. It is difficult to differentiate from testicular trauma such a torsion, post-vasectomy pain, or an inguinal hernia.

B. Immediate trans-scrotal exploration is required to restore the vascular supply to the testis.

C. This usually involves only gram negative organisms

D. Imaging studies should not delay surgical exploration

7. **Which of the following patient characteristics have been shown to correlate with increased mortality in patients with necrotizing fasciitis?**

A. Obesity

B. Diabetes mellitus

C. Age

D. Renal impairment

8. **Regarding surgical treatment for necrotizing fasciitis. Which of the following is true?**

A. Blood cultures must be drawn before empiric antibiotics are started.

B. As long as the surgical debridement has commenced within the first 24 hours, the overall mortality of NF is significantly reduced.

C. Initial aggressive surgical debridement and fasciotomy is usually enough to remove the nonviable tissue.

D. In NF of the limbs, amputation as a surgical option is associated with less blood loss than necrosectomy.

ANSWERS

1. **C.** Pain, out of proportion to physical findings, has been well documented as a constant recurring feature of necrotizing fasciitis. When present, necrotizing fasciitis should always be considered in the differential diagnosis. Keys that lead to diagnosis include pain out of proportion to the degree of dermal involvement as well as severe pain that appears to extend beyond the apparent borders of infection.

   Necrotizing fasciitis is more common in the adult population, with a reported incidence of 0.40 cases per 100,000 as compared to 0.08 per 100,000 pediatric cases per year. While skin necrosis with a blue or purple discoloration, crepitus, and bullae are perhaps the more well recognized signs and symptoms of necrotizing fasciitis, these are late features of the disease, not initial presenting symptoms. Initial presenting signs are often less specific and include erythema, warmth, myalgia, edema, and pain out of portion. As such, this often can lead to delayed diagnosis and delayed surgical debridement. Erysipelas is different from necrotizing fasciitis in that erysipelas involves infection of the superficial layers of the skin and cutaneous lymphatics, leading to a well-demarcated and often raised border.

2. **A.** Subcutaneous gas seen on plain radiographs is a specific, but not sensitive finding. It has been documented that subcutaneous gas on radiographs is found in as low as 25% of cases, and its absence

should not exclude the diagnosis of necrotizing fasciitis.

The diagnosis of necrotizing fasciitis can often be delayed and mistaken for cellulitis or abscess. Given many of the initial signs and symptoms are nonspecific, both clinical findings and laboratory values in addition to advanced imaging if needed should be used in conjunction to help assist in early diagnosis. In 2004, Wong et al. developed a scoring system LRINEC, which classifies patients into risk categories that determine necrotizing fasciitis probability, as seen in Table 90-1. LRINEC scores ≥6 have a positive predictive value (PPV) of 92% and a negative predictive value (NPV) of 96% for necrotizing fasciitis.

Magnetic resonance imaging (MRI) has been documented to be the most useful imaging technique when differentiating necrotizing from non-necrotizing infections. Specific findings on an MRI include thickening of the soft tissue and a hyperintense signal on T-2 weighted images at the level of the deep fascia and muscle. CT imaging has been reported to be more sensitive than plain radiographs,

Table 90-1 LABORATORY RISK INDICATORS FOR NECROTIZING FASCIITIS (LRINEC) SCORE

Variable, Units	Score
C-Reactive Protein, mg/L	
<150	0
≥150	4
Total white cell count, per mm^2	
<15	0
15–25	1
>25	2
Hemoglobin, g/dL	
>13.5	0
11–13.5	1
<11	2
Sodium, mmol/L	
≥135	0
>141	2
Creatinine, μmol/L	
</= 1.6	0
>1.6	2
Glucose, mmol/L	
</= 180	0
>180	1

with the ability to identify abscesses and other inflammatory changes, with up to 80% sensitivity.

3. **D.** Gross intraoperative findings include thin, watery gray necrotic fluid often described as "dishwater pus," a foul smelling odor, and necrotic muscle, which fails to respond to electrocautery. A positive "finger test" is also characteristic, in which there is ease of dissecting the subcutaneous layer off of the deep fascia with the surgeon's fingers.

Surgical debridement should never be delayed for optimization of vascular perfusion, nor until there is a definitive diagnosis as delay in surgical management has been shown to be both limb and life threatening. A delay in surgical debridement of more than 24 hours has been shown to be an independent risk factor for mortality. Furthermore, repeated surgical debridement may be necessary in order to remove all necrotic tissue, lessen the bacterial load, and expose the tissues to oxygen to aid in reduction of anaerobic bacteria, all helping to facilitate a more rapid recovery.

4. **D.** Clindamycin is a protein synthesis inhibitor that inhibits M protein and exotoxin production. As such, administration of clindamycin has been shown to be especially useful in cases with severe inflammatory responses, which include cases complicated by streptococcal toxic shock syndrome. Initial management of suspected necrotizing fasciitis cases include broad spectrum IV antibiotics. Duration of IV antibiotics after the source has been controlled and the patient is free of systemic signs of inflammation and infection is typically 14 days.

It should be noted that IV antibiotics alone are not enough to control infection. Using only IV antibiotics, mortality approaches 100% because the antibiotics may not reach the affected area due to the thrombosis of vessels. As a result of improved sanitation, *Clostridium* species are now a rare cause of necrotizing fasciitis. Rather, *Streptococcus* is the number one isolated organism, followed by the staphylococcus species.

5. **B.** HBO therapy has been considered as an adjunct therapy in the treatment of necrotizing fasciitis. This is based on the theory that necrotizing infections are associated with decreased oxygen tension and ischemia. As such, it is believed that HBO treatment can reverse these effects by increasing oxygen tension and helping to deliver antibiotic therapy

across the bacterial cell wall. However, various studies have failed to show any benefits, including mortality or hospital stay, with the addition of HBO treatment.

As previously mentioned, a delay in surgical debridement is the single most important factor with regard to a negative prognosis; a delay of over 24 hours is an independent predictor of mortality. It is well known that diabetes in itself is a risk factor for necrotizing fasciitis. Those with a history of type 2 diabetes and who present in diabetic ketoacidosis have been shown to have longer rates of hospital stays and higher rates of mortality. This is likely due to poor glycemic control, which contributes to the pathogenesis and has been correlated to the extent of disease and poor outcomes. Similarly, in a large retrospective cohort study, patients with isolated *Clostridium* infections have been shown to have increased mortality rates, up to four times that when compared to other monocrobial or polymicrobial infections.

6. D. Imaging studies should not delay surgical exploration when there is clinical evidence of progressive soft tissue infection. Clinical presentation as described in this scenario represents necrotizing fasciitis of the perineum, also known as Fournier's gangrene, and it should always be at the top of one's differential diagnosis. Fournier's gangrene requires an accurate diagnosis and emergent surgical debridement of nonviable tissue. CT scans are useful to differentiate deep organ pathology when determining necrotic from viable tissue.

Magnetic resonance imaging has been reported to be >80% sensitive in determining healthy from necrotizing tissue infections but often will delay surgical management.

It is true that testicular torsion is a urologic emergency, which is more common in neonates and postpubertal boys than adults. The onset of testicular pain from torsion is usually acute onset and may range from mild to severe. On physical examination, the classic finding is an asymmetrically high-riding testis and a color Doppler ultrasound is useful in making the diagnosis.

Fournier's gangrene most often involves mixed aerobic/anaerobic organisms. Clinical presentation often includes edematous skin, blisters/bullae, crepitus, and subcutaneous gas, extending into the perineum and involves the scrotum. It is characterized by severe pain that generally starts on the anterior abdominal wall and migrates into the gluteal muscles, scrotum, and penis.

7. C. In a multicenter study published in Feb. 2017 that reviewed patient characteristics of patients with necrotizing fasciitis regarding their correlation with mortality, several interesting facts became clear. Univariate analysis of comorbidities such as diabetes mellitus, hypertension, obesity, and liver cirrhosis showed no statistically significant correlation with mortality. Their results did indicate an association between renal impairment and chronic heart failure and mortality, but this did not reach statistical significance (P = 0.08). The univariate analysis did demonstrate that advanced age (>65) as well as female gender were both statistically significant when correlated with mortality. Interestingly, numerous studies have shown that there is a preference of NF for men, possibly from the increased incidence of Fournier's gangrene in men, but this does not result in an increase in mortality in the male gender. While patients with necrotizing soft tissue infections often suffer from diabetes mellitus (40.3% of all patients in this study), the correlation with overall mortality is not statistically significant (P = 0.1). The correlation between gender and mortality in patients with NF is unclear. Two small studies this author reviewed did show a female proprondence, but in larger studies, female sex did not seem to affect mortality in patients with NF.

8. D. In NF of the limbs, there is always a difficult decision between amputation of the affected limb v. wide, aggressive surgical debridement, which often involves extensive soft tissue and wide fasciotomy. This wide debridement will potentially leave the extremity nonfunctional.

Amputation is associated with less blood loss than a radical debridement and can be a life-saving procedure in the face of septic shock.

Blood cultures, while an important adjunct in guiding antibiotic therapy, should never delay life- or limb-saving surgical debridement, early fluid resuscitation, or early administration of empiric antibiotics based on suspected microbiology associated with NF.

Emergency surgical debridement of all nonviable tissue should be performed in all patients within 12–15 hours after admission. The mortality rate of patients having a delay of >24 hours for surgical debridement has been reported to be *nine times higher* than when the surgery is performed within the first 12–15 hours.

Early, aggressive surgical debridement combined with wide fasciotomy are the gold standard for the treatment of necrotizing soft tissue infections. Commonly, a repeat surgical debridement is needed within 24 hours with often serial operations required to debride "new, now nonviable" tissue that perhaps looked healthy at the termination of the last operative experience. NF that requires a single surgical debridement is the exception, not the norm.

BIBLIOGRAPHY

Anaya DA, McMahon K, Nathens AB, et al. Predictors of mortality and limb loss in necrotizing soft tissue infections. *Arch Surg.* 2005;140:151–157.

Andreasen TJ, Green SD, Childers BJ. Massive infectious soft-tissue injury: diagnosis and management of necrotizing fasciitis and purpura fulminans. *Plast Recontstr Surg.* 2001;107:1025–1035.

Bisno AL, Stevens DL. Streptococcal infections of skin and soft tissues. *N Engl J Med.* 1996;334(4):240–246.

Brown DR, Davis NL, Lepawsky M, Cunningham J, Kortbeek J. A multicenter review of the treatment of major truncal necrotizing infections with and without hyperbaric oxygen therapy. *Am J Surg.* 1994;167(5):485–489.

Childers BJ, Potyondy LD, Nachreiner R, et al. Necrotizing fasciitis: a fourteen-year retrospective study of 163 consecutive patients. *Am Surg.* 2002;68:109–116.

Edlich RF, Cross CL, Dahlstrom JJ, Long WB III. Modern concepts of the diagnosis and treatment of necrotizing fasciitis. *J Emerg Med.* 2010;89:7–36.

Fustes-Morales A, Gutierrez-Castrellon P, Duran-McKinster C, et al. Necrotizing fasciitis: report of 390 pediatric cases. *Arch Dermatol.* 2002;138:893–899.

Hassan Z, Mullins RF, Friedman BC, et al. Treating necrotizing fasciitis with or without hyperbaric oxygen therapy. *Undersea Hyperb Med.* 2010;37:115–123.

Kaafarani HM, King DR. Necrotizing skin and soft tissue infections. *Surg Clln North Am.* 2014;94:155–163.

Lancerotto L, Tocco I, Salmaso R, Vindigni V, Bassetto F. Necrotizing fasciitis: classification, diagnosis and management. *J Trauma.* 2011;72(3):560–566.

Levine EG, Manders SM. Life-threatening necrotizing fasciitis. *Clin Dermatol.* 2005;23:144–147.

Lim YJ, Yong FC, Wong CH, Tan ABH. Necrotising fasciitis and traditional medical therapy—a dangerous liaison. *Ann Acad Med Singap.* 2006;35(4):270–273.

Misiakos EP, Bagias G, Papadoulos I, et al. Early diagnosis and surgical treatment for necrotizing fasciitis: a multicenter study. *Frontiers in Surg.* 2017;4:5.

Oncul O, Erenoglu C, Top C, et al. Necrotizing fasciitis: a life threatening clinical disorder in uncontrolled type 2 diabetic patients. *Diabetes Res Clin Pract.* 2008;80(2):218–223.

Ozalay M, Ozkoc G, Akpinar S, Hersekli MA, Tandogan RN. Necrotizing soft-tissue infection of a limb: clinical presentation and factors related to mortality. *Foot Ank Int.* 2006;27(8):598–605.

Shupak AO, Shoshani I, Goldenber A, et al. Necrotizing fasciitis: an indication for hyperbaric oxygen therapy? *Surgery.* 1995;118(5):873–878.

Stevens DL, Bisno AL, Chambers HF, et al. Practice guidelines for the diagnosis and management of skin and soft tissue infections: 2014 update by the Infectious Diseases Society of America. *Clin Infect Dis.* 2014;59:147.

Stevens DL, Bryant AE. Necrotizing soft-tissue infections. *N Engl J Med.* 2017;377:2253.

Urschel JD, Takita H, Antkowiak JG. Necrotizing soft tissue infections of the chest wall. *Ann Thorac Surg.* 1997;64:276–279.

van Sambeek CHL, van Stigt SF, Brouwers L, Bemelman M. Necrotising fasciitis: a ticking time bomb. *BMJ Case Rep.* 2017;2017:bcr2017221770.

Vijayakumar A, Pullagura R, Thimmappa D. Necrotizing fasciitis: diagnostic challenges and current practices. *ISRN Infectious Diseases.* 2014; Article ID 208072.

Wang YS, Wong CH, Tay YK. Staging of necrotizing fasciitis based on the evolving cutaneous features. *Int J Dermatol.* 2007;46:1036–1041.

Wong CH, Chang HC, Pasupathy S, et al. Necrotizing fasciitis: clinical presentation, microbiology, and determinates of mortality. *J Bone Joint Surg Am.* 2003;85:1454–1460.

Wong CH, Khin LW, Heng KS, Tan KC, Low CO. The LRINEC (laboratory risk indicator for necrotizing fasciitis) score: a tool for distinguishing necrotizing from other soft tissue infections. *Crit Care Med.* 2004;32:1535–1541.

Wysoki MG, Santora TA, Shah RM, Friedman AC. Necrotizing fasciitis: CT characteristics. *Radiology.* 1997; 203:859–863.

91

Genitourinary Trauma

Victoria Maxon

A 35-year-old man presents to the emergency department as a trauma alert, after a motorcycle accident. On primary survey, he has no life-threatening injuries. His vital signs are stable, with a heart rate of 85, blood pressure of 126/84, and a room air oxygen saturation of 99%. On secondary survey, he is noted to have blood at the urethral meatus, perineal bruising, and bruising over the left flank. He has pain over the pubic symphysis and he is in a pelvic binder. His abdomen is mildly distended and bladder is palpable. His rectal examination reveals no blood, normal rectal tone, and a high riding prostate. He has not voided since the incident.

1. **What is the next step in diagnosis and management of blood at the urethral meatus?**

   A. Passage of a coude-tipped Foley catheter
   B. Passage of a three-way Foley catheter
   C. Placement of a suprapubic catheter
   D. Retrograde urethrography
   E. Voiding cystourethrogram

2. **The patient has a severe posterior urethral injury and pelvic fracture. What is the acute management of his distended bladder?**

   A. Passage of Foley catheter
   B. Exploration and primary repair of urethral injury
   C. Placement of suprapubic catheter
   D. Bilateral percutaneous nephrostomy tube placement
   E. Endoscopic realignment of urethral injury

3. **The patient's urine appears grossly bloody. Which imaging test is most appropriate in evaluating his other possible genitourinary injuries?**

   A. Fluoroscopic cystogram
   B. FAST (focused assessment with sonography for trauma) scan
   C. Computerized tomography (CT) scan of the abdomen and pelvis with IV contrast and CT cystogram
   D. CT cystogram
   E. CT scan of the abdomen with and without IV contrast

4. **A CT cystogram demonstrates loops of bowel outlined by contrast. What is the next step in management of this injury?**

   A. Suprapubic tube placement for 14 days
   B. Large bore Foley catheter placement for 14 days
   C. Open exploration and cystorraphy
   D. Laparoscopic exploration and cystorraphy
   E. Bilateral percutaneous nephrostomy tube placement

5. **What is the appropriate management of a simple extraperitoneal bladder rupture?**

   A. Suprapubic tube placement for 7 days
   B. Large bore Foley catheter placement for 14 days
   C. Open exploration and cystorraphy
   D. Laparoscopic exploration and cystorraphy
   E. Observation

6. **CT scan of the abdomen and pelvis with IV contrast is indicated to rule out a renal injury in which clinical scenario(s)?**

   A. Blunt trauma with gross hematuria
   B. Blunt trauma with microscopic hematuria and normal blood pressure

C. Blunt trauma with microscopic hematuria and shock (SBP <90)

D. High-energy mechanism of injury

E. A, C, and D

7. **This patient has a grade 3 left renal injury and is hemodynamically stable. What is the appropriate initial management of that injury?**

A. Open renal exploration

B. Renal angiography

C. Serial examination, serial vital signs, and serial CBC monitoring

D. Ureteral stent placement

E. Nephrectomy

ANSWERS

1. D. Retrograde urethrography is essential in any case of blood at the urethral meatus, as blood at the meatus may be a sign of a urethral disruption or laceration. Inability to urinate, palpable bladder, perineal bruising representing a butterfly hematoma and high-riding prostate can all be signs of possible urethral injury. Passage of a Foley catheter blindly in the setting of a urethral injury may exacerbate a laceration or lead to placement of the catheter outside of the bladder. If the retrograde urethrogram shows the urethra is intact, then Foley placement can be attempted.

2. C. In the setting of a patient with a posterior urethral injury and pelvic fracture, acute decompression of the bladder is essential. Suprapubic tube placement is the first step. Primary realignment of the urethral injury may be attempted after SP tube placement in a hemodynamically stable patient with pelvic fracture if no other life-threatening injuries are identified.

3. C. This patient is at risk for both bladder and renal injury, so imaging will be required to assess those organs. The bladder is best imaged with either a retrograde gravity cystogram or a CT cystogram. The kidneys are best imaged with a contrast-enhanced CT scan of the abdomen and pelvis, as well as with delayed images of the ureters to assess for ureteral injury. A gravity cystogram can also be done with a C-arm in the operating room if the patient needs operative intervention. It is critical that gravity cystography involve oblique views as well as a post drainage film, to assess for leakage posterior to the

bladder. Also, the patient should be filled via gravity to a volume of at least 300 to 400 mL, to adequately distend the bladder. Awake patients should be filled to a sense of bladder fullness. Roughly 90% of all patients with a bladder injury in a blunt trauma setting will have both gross hematuria and a pelvic fracture. Additionally, nearly 30% of patients with gross hematuria and a pelvic fracture will have a bladder injury, so imaging the bladder is essential in those patients. A minority of patients with a bladder injury will have only hematuria or only an isolated pelvic fracture, so the decision to image the bladder in those situations is based on clinical judgment. Certainly any signs or symptoms of bladder perforation, such as low urine output, abdominal distension, or acute kidney injury would warrant cystography.

The indications for renal imaging in blunt trauma patients include gross hematuria, microscopic hematuria (3 to 5 RBCs per high powered field on urinalysis) with systolic BP <90 mmHg, and a mechanism with high energy that could lead to renal injury. A contrast-enhanced CT scan with delayed images of the ureters is the best imaging test in a trauma setting. In the event of urgent exploration, a one-shot intravenous pyelogram (IVP) can be performed with 2 cc/kg of IV contrast and a single plain abdominal film 10 minutes later, to assess for the presence of two kidneys and to provide a pyelogram of each renal unit.

4. C. Bowel loops outlined by contrast represent an intraperitoneal bladder rupture. This requires immediate exploration and repair. Intraperitoneal urine leak can cause peritonitis and may lead to abscess formation. Operative repair of bladder trauma is associated with a significant reduction in mortality.

5. B. A simple extraperitoneal bladder injury can be readily managed with a Foley catheter drainage alone. The catheter must be large enough to allow the egress of clots and be unlikely to occlude. Most clinicians would allow 2 weeks of drainage for healing to occur and would perform a cystogram prior to catheter removal. Operative management is only needed if the patient is otherwise being explored or if there are mitigating factors that will preclude healing, such as fragments of the bone in the bladder injury. In addition, if there are lacerations to the rectum, vagina, or the bladder injury involves the bladder neck, operative repair is best performed to prevent a fistula and allow appropriate healing.

6. E. The guidelines for renal imaging in blunt trauma are very well established. In the absence of gross hematuria, with an insignificant mechanism of injury, and without a systolic blood pressure <90 mmHg and microscopic hematuria (>3–5 RBCs per HPF), there is a 99.7% chance the patient does not have a significant renal injury. A contrast-enhanced CT with delayed images is the optimal imaging test in this setting.

7. C. Most renal injuries can be managed with non-operative intervention. Operative intervention, including open exploration with repair of a renal injury or nephrectomy, ureteral stent or percutaneous nephrostomy placement for urinary extravasation, or angiography, is required for patients with hemodynamic instability or for urinary leaks that do not heal or are complicated by issues such as infection. The majority of renal injuries, especially grade 1 to 3 injuries can be managed without surgical intervention.

BIBLIOGRAPHY

Brandes SB, Eswara JR. Upper urinary tract trauma. In: Morey AF, Zhao LC, eds. *Campbell-Walsh-Wein Urology.* 12th ed. Elsevier Saunders; 2021:90, 1982–2004.

Broghammer JA, Fisher MB, Santucci RA. Conservative management of renal trauma: a review. *Urology.* 2007;70(4):623–629.

Deibert CM, Spencer BA. The association between operative repair of bladder injury and improved survival: results from the National Trauma Data Bank. *J Urol.* 2011;186:151–155.

Morey AF, Brandes S, Dugi DD III, et al. Urotrauma: AUA guideline. *J Urol.* 2017;192(2):1–27.

Morey AF, Simhan J. Genital and lower urinary tract trauma. In: Morey AF, Zhao LC, eds. *Campbell-Walsh-Wein Urology.* 12th ed. Elsevier Saunders; 2021:133, 3048–3061.

92

Foley Trauma

Victoria Maxon

A 64-year-old male with a history of spinal cord injury, hypertension, DM2, and tobacco abuse is scheduled to undergo a video-assisted thoracoscopic surgery (VATS) for resection of a suspicious lung mass. He voids using clean intermittent catheterization (CIC) and has been doing so for the past 8 years. Prior to the start of the case, the nurse attempts to insert a Foley catheter. She meets resistance while advancing the catheter and does not get return of urine.

1. **The next best step for the nurse would be to:**
   A. Slowly force the catheter past the resistance.
   B. Dilate a possible stricture by slowly inflating the catheter balloon.
   C. Assume the positioning is correct and inflate the catheter balloon.
   D. Remove the catheter.
   E. Attempt to pass a larger size catheter.

2. **The nurse repeatedly tries to force the catheter without success before removing the catheter. The urology team is called for consultation. Which of the following is the next best step?**
   A. Attempt to blindly dilate the urethra
   B. Perform cystoscopy
   C. Attempt to pass a larger size catheter
   D. Perform a retrograde urethrogram
   E. Placement of suprapubic tube

3. **What is the most likely cause of difficult Foley catheter placement in this patient?**
   A. Obesity
   B. Benign prostatic hyperplasia
   C. Poor technique during Foley catheter placement
   D. Bladder neck contracture
   E. Urethral stricture

4. **The patient has a prolonged hospital stay and now has the same Foley catheter for 4 weeks. The nurse is advised to remove the catheter and resume CIC. The nurse is unable to deflate the balloon. What is the next step?**
   A. Pass a wire through the balloon port
   B. Cut the balloon port
   C. Bladder ultrasound
   D. Suprapubic puncture of the balloon port with a 22G spinal needle
   E. Cut the main drainage port and balloon port

5. **Which of the following patients is most appropriate for the placement of an 18Fr Coude catheter?**
   A. 21-year-old male with history of posterior urethral injury
   B. 70-year-old male with history of bladder neck contracture
   C. 75-year-old male with history of BPH
   D. 35-year-old female with history of neurogenic bladder
   E. 30-year-old male with history of morbid obesity

ANSWERS

1. **D.** The most appropriate course of action would be to remove the catheter. Confirmation of appropriate catheter placement requires flow of urine and the balloon should not be inflated until this time. In a

male, the catheter balloon may not be inflated until the catheter is completely hubbed at the penis and there is flow of urine. Inflating the balloon at the first flow of urine may result in inflating the balloon in the prostatic urethra. Continuing to advance the catheter after meeting resistance could result in creation of a false passage. You should never inflate the balloon intentionally within the urethra. If a stricture is identified, it may require dilation by a urologist with urethral sounds or dilators.

2. **B.** The safest option would be to examine the urethral anatomy using cystoscopy. This facilitates placement of a guidewire beyond any identified stricture over which a catheter can be placed or dilation of a stricture under direct vision. Attempting to pass a larger catheter in a patient who is suspected to have a stricture would likely result in further trauma. Placement of a smaller bore catheter would also be an appropriate choice. Retro-grade urethrogram is a contrasted X-ray study to evaluate the urethra that is often ordered when urethral trauma is suspected. Although this study could show evidence of urethral stricture, it would not be the best choice while in the operating room. This study may be obtained to further assess the anatomy of the urethra particularly if surgical intervention is planned to treat urethral stricture.

3. **E.** It is important to do a thorough history and physical to identify patients at risk for difficult catheter placement. Urologic procedural history should be reviewed along with any documentation of prior difficult catheter placement. In men, voiding symptoms such as decreased or intermittent urinary stream, valsava to initiate urination, and nocturia may indicate obstructive pathology such as benign prostatic hypertrophy. History of repeated urethral manipulation with CIC or indwelling catheter such as the patient in our scenario should prompt suspicion for prior urethral trauma and possible difficult Foley placement. The incidence of urethral injury and chronic complications increases with prolonged duration of CIC. Considering the patient's known history of prolonged CIC, urethral stricture would be high on the differential for the etiology of the encountered resistance during the nurse's attempt at Foley placement. Studies comparing long-term CIC use versus indwelling catheter for urinary drainage reveals an increased risk for development of urethral stricture in patients with an indwelling catheter, but interestingly no significant difference in the risk for false passage between the two groups.

4. **B.** Cutting the balloon port is the recommended first step in troubleshooting a catheter that will not come out. This should allow a release of fluid from the balloon. If this is unsuccessful, a wire can be placed down the balloon port in an attempt to puncture the balloon or free the channel from sediment. The balloon can also be punctured through a suprapubic approach using a 22G spinal needle in men. This can be performed with or without ultrasound guidance. If these methods fail, imaging of the bladder should be obtained. The patient may have significant encrustation or stone formation that will require surgical intervention.

5. **C.** Alternate catheter types can provide advantages over straight-tipped catheters such as Foley catheters. A Coudé catheter, which has a curved tip, assists in traversing the prostatic urethra in gentlemen with benign prostatic hyperplasia.

BIBLIOGRAPHY

Daneshmand S, Youssefzadeh D, Skinner EC. Review of techniques to remove a Foley catheter when the balloon does not deflate. *Urology*. 2002;59:127–129.

Jacob JM, Sundaram CP. Lower urinary tract catheterization. In: Morey AF, Zhao LC, eds. *Campbell-Walsh-Wein Urology*. 12th ed. Elsevier Saunders; 2021;11:152–159.

Perrouin-Verbe B, Labat J, Richard I, et al. Clean intermittent catheterization from the acute period in spinal cord injury patients. Long-term evaluation of urethral and genital tolerance. *Paraplegia*. 1995;33:619–624.

Singh R., Rohilla RK, Sangwan K, et al. Bladder management methods and urological complications in spinal cord injury patients. *Indian J Orthop*. 2011;45:141–47.

Villanueva C, Hemstreet GP III Difficult male urethral catheterization: a review of different approaches. *Int Braz J Urol*. 2008;34:401–412.

UROLOGY

93

Nephrolithiasis

Peter L. Steinberg, David W. Barham, and Joseph R. Sterbis

A 30-year-old pregnant woman in the second trimester presents to the obstetrics clinic with acute flank pain and nausea. Her urinalysis is negative for nitrites and demonstrates 20 red blood cell per high-power field (RBC/hpf) and 0 white blood cell per hpf (WBC/hpf). Ultrasound demonstrates a 5 mm proximal ureteral stone.

1. **What is the preferred management option of ureteral stones in pregnancy?**

    A. Observation
    B. Medical expulsive therapy
    C. Ureteroscopy
    D. Ureteral stent placement
    E. Percutaneous nephrostomy

2. **A 33-year-old female presents to the ER with right flank pain. She has a past surgical history of a Roux-en-Y gastric bypass. She is found to have a 4-mm distal right ureteral stone with moderate hydronephrosis on CT. Her temperature is 101°F, heart rate 120 bpm, and blood pressure 100/64 mmHg. Urinalysis shows 70 RBC/hpf and 80 WBC/hpf. What is the best treatment option?**

    A. Urgent cystoscopy and right ureteral stent placement
    B. Medical expulsive therapy
    C. Ureteroscopy with laser lithotripsy
    D. Shock wave lithotripsy
    E. 7 day course of oral ciprofloxacin

3. **What is the preferred analgesia for the acute management of renal colic?**

    A. Acetaminophen
    B. NSAIDS
    C. IV opiates
    D. Oral opiates
    E. NSAIDS and IV opiates

4. **Patients who undergo Roux-en-Y gastric bypass are predisposed to which type of nephrolithiasis?**

    A. Xanthine
    B. Calcium oxalate
    C. Calcium phosphate
    D. Cystine
    E. Struvite

5. **During ureteroscopy with laser lithotripsy for a 7-mm distal ureteral stone, you notice a ureteral perforation. This is confirmed on retrograde pyelogram, with obvious extravasation of contrast. A safety wire is in place. Which of the following is the preferred management option?**

    A. Laparoscopic ureteroureterostomy with JP drain placement
    B. Open ureteroureterostomy with JP drain placement
    C. Ureteral stent placement
    D. Percutaneous nephrostomy placement
    E. Observation

6. **After stent placement in the aforementioned patient, she complains of left-sided abdominal pain attributable to the ureteral stent. Which of the following medications is best for ureteral stent pain?**

A. IV morphine
B. oxycodone
C. Gabapentin
D. nifedipine
E. tamsulosin

ANSWERS

1. **A.** The evaluation and management of stone disease in pregnant women is complex and a multidisciplinary approach is recommended. These patients should be managed in conjunction with obstetrics. Observation is the recommended initial therapy provided the patient is not infected. Medical expulsive therapy and surgical options incur risks to the mother and fetus.

2. **A.** This patient has findings consistent with obstructive pyelonephritis. Although microscopic hematuria is a common finding in patients with ureteral stones, pyuria should raise concern for concomitant urinary tract infection. This patient's fever and tachycardia are concerning for pyelonephritis and sepsis. In the setting of obstruction, urgent drainage of the collecting system is required because these patients can decompensate quickly. This can be accomplished with retrograde ureteral stent placement or nephrostomy tube placement. Antibiotics alone is not sufficient. Ureteroscopy, shock wave lithotripsy, and medical expulsive therapy are contraindicated in the setting of infection.

3. **E.** Patients with acute renal colic presenting to the emergency room generally require parenteral analgesia. In that setting, combination therapy with NSAIDs and IV opiates is more efficacious than either agent used on its own.

4. **B.** Gastric bypass increases the risk of calcium oxalate stones through a triad of low urine volume, hypocitraturia, and hyperoxaluria. Malabsorbed fat saponifies enteric calcium. With less luminal calcium available to bind oxalate, there is increased enteric absorption of oxalate, yielding hyperoxaluria. Hypocitraturia is due to metabolic acidosis.

5. **C.** When possible, ureteral stent placement is the preferred management method of a ureteral injury sustained during endoscopic surgery. In most instances, the ureter will heal over the stent without need for further intervention.

6. **E.** Alpha blockers such as tamsulosin and anticholinergics are the most effective medications for stent-related pain. NSAIDs may also be of benefit. Narcotic pain medications are less effective. They may be required as adjuncts to anticholinergics, alpha blockers, and NSAIDs but should rarely be used as mono-therapy.

BIBLIOGRAPHY

Assimos D, Krambeck A, Miller NL, et al. Surgical management of stones: American Urological Association/Endourological Society Guideline, part II. *J Urol.* 2016;196:1161–1169.

Canales BK, Gonzalez RD. Kidney stone risk following Roux-en-Y gastric bypass surgery. *Transl Androl Urol.* 2014;3(3):242–249.

Fischer KM, Louie M, Mucksavage P. Ureteral stent discomfort and its management. *Curr Urol Rep.* 2018;11:64.

Fulgham PF, Assimos DG, Pearle MS, Preminger GM. Clinical effectiveness protocols for imaging in the management of ureteral calculous disease: AUA technology assessment. *J Urol.* April 2013;189(4):1203–1213.

Pearle MS, Goldfarb DS, Assimos DG, et al. Medical management of kidney stones: AUA guideline. *J Urol.* 2014;192(2):316–324.

Safdar B, Degutis LC, Landry K, et al. Intravenous morphine plus ketorolac is superior to either drug alone for treatment of acute renal colic. *Ann Emerg Med.* August 2006;48(2):173–181, 181.e1.

Steinberg PL, Nangia AK, Curtis K. A standardized pain management protocol improves timeliness of analgesia among emergency department patients with renal colic. *Qual Manag Health Care.* January–March 2011;20(1):30–36.

94

Bladder Cancer

Joseph R. Sterbis, Timiyin M. E-Nunu, and John E. Musser

A 64-year-old Caucasian male coal miner with a prior 20 pack per year smoking history, diabetes mellitus, hypertension, and hyperlipidemia presents for evaluation of urinary frequency. A urinalysis demonstrates 2 white blood cells per high-power field (WBC/hpf), 10 red blood cells per hpf (RBC/hpf), and is negative for all other components. No red blood cell casts or dysmorphic red blood cells are present on urine microscopy.

1. **Microscopic hematuria is defined as which of the following?**

    A. Positive urine dipstick test
    B. 1 cell/hpf
    C. 3 cells/hpf
    D. 5 cells/hpf

2. **Which of the following is the best initial workup of microscopic hematuria?**

    A. Cystoscopy, urine cytology
    B. Renal ultrasound and bladder barbotage
    C. Computerized tomography (CT) intravenous pyelogram
    D. Cystoscopy, CT intravenous pyelogram
    E. Urine cytology, urine culture

3. **Which of the following is a risk factor for urinary malignancies?**

    A. Alcohol consumption
    B. Family history of tuberous sclerosis
    C. Smoking
    D. Anagelsic abuse
    E. Artificial sweetener consumption

4. **Cystoscopy revealed a large bladder tumor. A transurethral biopsy of his tumor reveals muscle invasive, high-grade bladder cancer. The patient then undergoes a radical cystectomy and ileal conduit. Which of the following electrolyte abnormalities is expected after urinary diversion with ileum?**

    A. Hypokalemic, hyperchloremic metabolic acidosis
    B. Hypokalemic, hypochloremic metabolic alkalosis
    C. Hyperkalemic, hypochloremic, hyponatremic metabolic acidosis
    D. Hypokalemic, hypernatremic metabolic alkalosis

5. **The most common cause of serious bowel complication is:**

    A. Lack of mechanical bowel prep
    B. Lack of antibiotic bowel prep
    C. Having a resident involved in the case
    D. Long operative duration
    E. Use of irradiated bowel

6. **The patient returns to clinic 18 months after surgery with recurrent gross asymptomatic hematuria. Which of the following sites is the likely location for cancer recurrence?**

    A. Ileal conduit
    B. Kidney
    C. Psoas muscle
    D. Left renal pelvis

ANSWERS

1. C. Asymptomatic microscopic hematuria (AMH) is defined as three or greater RBC/hpf on a clean catch midstream urinary specimen in the absence of any other benign cause. A positive dipstick does not define AMH and microscopic examination of the urinary specimen is mandatory for diagnosis. The likelihood of a urologic malignancy in the presence of microscopic hematuria is approximately 10%.

2. D. The complete workup for hematuria includes cystoscopy and CT intravenous pyelogram. With this evaluation strategy, the cause for hematuria is identified in 80% of cases. Patients with persistent hematuria after a negative initial evaluation warrant repeat evaluation at 48 to 72 months. If the patient cannot obtain a CT intravenous pyelogram, then alternative acceptable imaging studies include intravenous pyelogram, retrograde pyelography, or magnetic resonance urography.

3. C. A risk factors for developing bladder cancer is smoking. Intensity and duration of smoking is linearly related to the risk of developing bladder cancer. Chronic irritation, exposure to aromatic amines, and radiation have been associated with the development of bladder cancer. Tuberous sclerosis is associated with kidney cancer. There is no convincing evidence that alcohol consumption, ingestion of artificial sweetners, or analgesic are associated with development of bladder cancer.

4. A. Hypokalemic, hyperchloremic metabolic acidosis is the electrolyte abnormality present when ileum as a urinary conduit. When urine comes into contact with the bowel wall, ammonia, chloride, and hydrogen are reabsorbed. Depending on which bowel wall, this results in different metabolic and electrolyte abnormalities. In the stomach, sodium and bicarbonate are secreted in exchanged for the resorbed hydrogen and chloride. This results in hypochloremic, hypokalemic metabolic acidosis. In the jejunem, sodium and chloride are secreted with increased absorption of hydrogen and potassium. This results in hyponatremic, hypochloremic, hypekalemic metabolic acidosis. In the ileum and colon, ammonium is broken down to ammonia and hydrogen. Hydrogen is absorbed in exchange for sodium. The ammonia prevents the absorption of potassium and increases the absorption of chloride resulting in a hypokalemic, hyperchloremic metabolic acidosis.

5. E. The use of previously irradiated bowel is associated with serious bowel complications. Among urological operations, radical cystectomy is a major operation that is accompanied with high postoperative complication. The high rates of morbidity are mainly associated with the characteristics of the patients, particularly being of advanced age and having underlying comorbidities. Despite accounting for the comorbidities, use of irradiated bowel leads to dire complications.

6. D. The patient has developed an upper urinary tract tumor. According to SEER data, the relative risk for upper urinary tract tumors for white men and women was listed as 64.2% and 75.4% at or before 2 years; 44.3% and 40.5% at 2 to 5 years; 50.8% and 42.1% at 5 to 10 years; and 43.2% and 22.2% at more than 10 years, respectively. Upper-tract surveillance after a bladder tumor is necessary and is more likely to occur with high-grade bladder cancer. It can be performed with CT urography.

BIBLIOGRAPHY

Castro JE, Ram MD. Electrolyte imbalance following ileal urinary diversion. *Br J Urol.* 1970;42:29–32.

Douglas MD, McDougal WS. Use of intestinal segments in urinary diversion. In: Wein AJ, Kavoussi LR, Novick AC, Partin AW, Peters CA, eds. *Campbell-Walsh Urology.* 10th ed. Saunders; 2007;2411–2449.

Fontaine E, Barthelemy Y, Houlgatte A, et al. Twenty-year experience with jejunal conduits. *Urology.* 1997;50:207–213.

Golimbu M, Morales P. Jejunal conduits: technique and complications. *J Urol.* 1975;113:787–795.

Grossfeld GD, Litwin MS, Wolf JS Jr, et al. Evaluation of asymptomatic microscopic hematuria in adults: the American urological association best practice policy—part I. Definition, prevalence and etiology. *Urology.* 2001;57:599.

Grossfeld GD, Litwin MS, Wolf JS Jr, et al. Evaluation of asymptomatic microscopic hematuria in adults: the American urological association best practice policy—part II. Patient evaluation, cytology, voided markers, imaging, cystoscopy, nephrology evaluation and follow-up. *Urology.* 2001;57:604.

Grossfeld GD, Wolf JS, Litwin MS, et al. Asymptomatic microscopic hematuria in adults: summary of the AUA best practice policy recommendations. *Am Fam Physician.* 2001;63(6). http://www.aafp.org/afp/2001/0315/p1145.html

Kurzrock EA, Baskin LS, Kogan BA. Gatrocystoplasty: long-term follow-up. *J Urol.* 1998;160:2182–2186.

Navai N, Dinney CP. Transurethral and open surgery for bladder cancer. In: McDougal WS, Wein AJ, Kavoussi LR, Partin AW, Peters CA, eds. *Campbell-Walsh Urology*. 11th ed. Elsevier; 2015:2242–2253 Review E-Book.

Rabbani F, Perrotti M, Russo P, Herr HW. Upper-tract tumors after an initial diagnosis of bladder cancer: argument for long-term surveillance. *J Clin Oncol*. 2001;19:94–100.

Wright JL, Hotaling J, Porter MP. Predictors of upper tract urothelial cell carcinoma after primary bladder cancer: a population based analysis. *J Urol*. 2009;181:1035–1039.

Yun EJ, Meng MV, Carroll PR. Evaluation of the patient with hematuria. *Med Clin North Am*. March 2004;88(2):329–343.

95

Renal Tumors

Joseph R. Sterbis

A 39-year-old Caucasian male with a history of poorly controlled hypertension, asthma, and hyperlipidemia obtains a CT of his abdomen and pelvis to evaluate for vague right-sided abdominal pain and is found to have a right renal mass, measuring 8 × 6 × 7 cm in size. A complete workup reveals renal cell carcinoma (RCC) with a single lung metastasis. His glomerular filtration rate (GFR) was calculated to be 30 mL/min.

1. **With regards to renal cancer, this patient's GFR:**

   A. will positively affect outcomes
   B. has a decreased cardiovascular risk
   C. will improve after surgery
   D. has an increased risk of death

2. **Which of the following patients would most likely benefit from a cytoreductive nephrectomy?**

   A. Those with metastases limited to the lungs
   B. Those with poor performance status
   C. Those with poor prognostic features
   D. Those with multiple hepatic metastases

3. **The patient's family history is significant for von Hippel-Lindau disease (VHL). He is tested and is found to have VHL type 2B. He also reports having intermittent headaches, occasional palpitations, and diaphoresis, which he attributed to his poorly controlled hypertension. What is the likely source of his symptoms?**

   A. Retinal hemangioblastoma
   B. Cerebellar hemangioma
   C. Pancreatic cysts
   D. Pheochromocytoma

4. **Which of the following is the most reliable method to distinguish RCC from an upper tract urothelial tumor?**

   A. Retrograde urography
   B. CT urography
   C. Non-contrast renal CT
   D. Urine cytology

ANSWERS

1. **D.** An independent, graded association has been documented between a reduced estimated GFR and the risk of death, cardiovascular events, and hospitalization. This patient's GFR of 30 mL/min, which is significantly less that normal (60 mL/min) which puts him at risk for these events. At the same time, the decreased GFR may be due to the renal cancer itself and as such, may improve after kidney resection. Alternative, one-third of patients develop chronic kidney disease after renal resection. Thus the outcome of kidney function after removal is hard to predict.

2. **a.** Cytoreductive nephrectomy preceding systemic therapy is performed in the setting of advanced metastatic disease. In the cytokine era, retrospective evidence suggests that good performance status, good prognostic features, and metastases limited to the lungs are more likely to benefit from cytoreductive nephrectomy.

3. **D.** Pheochromocytoma occurs in 10% to 17% of patients with VHL. VHL type 2 differs from type 1 in that affected family members are at high risk to

develop pheochromocytomas. VHL type 2 is further divided into types 2A, 2B, and 2C. Individuals in families with VHL type 2A develop pheochromocytomas but have a low risk for RCC. Those with VHL type 2B develop pheochromocytomas and have a high risk for RCC.

4. B. Upper tract urothelial carcinoma (UT-UC) is a relatively uncommon form of cancer arising from the urothelial lining of the renal pelvis and calyces. UT-UC of the renal pelvis is an aggressive tumor, which may invade the renal parenchyma and mimic primary RCC. Advanced RCC can also invade the pelvicalyceal system. Distinguishing these primary lesions from each other can be difficult, and correct diagnosis is needed to determine appropriate surgery and medical treatment.

CT urography is easier to perform than intravenous pyelography and has a higher degree of accuracy in detecting renal parenchymal lesions. The sensitivity for detecting upper tract malignant disease has been reported to approach 100% with CT urography. CT urography also has a specificity of 60% and a negative predictive value of 100%. Retrograde urography has an accuracy of 75% in diagnosis of an upper tract malignant neoplasm. Ureteroscopy is reserved for situations when the diagnosis is unclear after conventional radiographic studies and for patients in whom the treatment plan may be changed on the basis of the ureteroscopic findings, for example, those who may be amenable to endoscopic resection. Accuracy estimates of the sensitivity of cytology range from about 20% for grade 1 tumors to 45% and 75% for grade 2 and grade 3 tumors, respectively. Non-contrast CT does not allow for distinction between parenchymal and urothelial lesions.

BIBLIOGRAPHY

Bloom HJ. Proceedings: hormone-induced and spontaneous regression of metastatic renal cancer. *Cancer.* 1973;32:1066–1071.

Caoili EM, Cohan RH, Korobkin M, et al. Urinary tract abnormalities: initial experience with multi-detector row CT urography. *Radiology.* 2002;222:353.

Culp SH, Tannir NM, Abel EJ, et al. Can we better select patients with metastatic renal cell carcinoma for cytoreductive nephrectomy? *Cancer.* 2010:116:3378–3388.

Flanigan RC, Salmon SE, Blumenstein BA, et al. Nephrectomy followed by interferon alfa-2b compared with interferon alfa-2b alone for metastatic renal-cell cancer. *N Engl J Med.* 2001;345:1655–1659.

Friedel G, Hurtgen M, Penzenstadler M, et al. Resection of pulmonary metastases from renal cell carcinoma. *Anticancer Res.* 1999;19:1593–1596.

Go AS, Chertow GM, Fan D, McCulloch CE, Hsu CY. Chronic kidney disease and the risks of death, cardiovascular events, and hospitalization. *N Engl J Med.* September 23, 2004;351(13):1296–1305. Erratum in: *N Engl J Med.* 2008;18(4):4.

Horton WA, Wong V, Eldridge R. Von Hippel-Lindau disease: clinical and pathological manifestations in nine families with 50 affected members. *Arch Intern Med.* 1976;136:769.

Levine E, Collins DL, Horton WA, et al. CT screening of the abdomen in von Hippel-Lindau disease. *AJR Am J Roentgenol.* 1982;139:505.

Marcus SG, Choyke PL, Reiter R, et al. Regression of metastatic renal cell carcinoma after cytoreductive nephrectomy. *J Urol.* 1993;150:463–466.

Middleton AW Jr. Indications for and results of nephrectomy for metastatic renal cell carcinoma. *Urol Clin North Am.* 1980;7:711–717.

Middleton RG. Surgery for metastatic renal cell carcinoma. *J Urol.* 1967;97:973–977.

Milestone B, Freidman AC, Seidmon EJ, et al. Staging of ureteral transitional cell carcinoma by CT and MRI. *Urology.* 1990;36:346.

Murthy SC, Kim K, Rice TW, et al. Can we predict long-term survival after pulmonary metastasectomy for renal cell carcinoma? *Ann Thorac Surg.* 2005;79:996–1003.

Motzer RJ, et al. Kidney Cancer, Version 3.2022, NCCN clinical practice guidelines in oncology. J Natl Compr Canc Netw. 2022 Jan;20(1):71–90.

Russo P, Synder M, Vickers A, et al. Cytoreductive nephrectomy and nephrectomy/complete metastasectomy for metastatic renal cancer. *Sci World J.* 2007;7:768–778.

Sella A, Swanson DA, Ro JY, et al. Surgery following response to interferon-alpha-based therapy for residual renal cell carcinoma. *J Urol.* 1993;149:19–21; discussion 21–22.

Snow RM, Schellhammer PF. Spontaneous regression of metastatic renal cell carcinoma. *Urology.* 1982;20:177–181.

Walther MM, Yang JC, Pass HI, et al. Cytoreductive surgery before high dose interleukin-2 based therapy in patients with metastatic renal cell carcinoma. *J Urol.* 1997;158:1675–1678.

Wein AJ, Kavoussi LR, Novick AC, Partin AW, Peters CA. Chapter 49: Malignant renal tumors. In: Steven CC, Brian RL, eds. *Campbell-Walsh Urology.* 2012 ed. Elsevier Saunders; 2007;1413–1474.

Zbar B, Kishida T, Chen F, et al. Germline mutations in the von Hippel-Lindau disease (VHL) gene in families from North America, Europe and Japan. *Hum Mutat.* 1996;8(4):348–357.

96

Testicular Lump

Joseph R. Sterbis

A 22-year-old Caucasian male presents to general surgery clinic for evaluation and treatment of a left inguinal hernia. During the physical examination, the hernia is identified, but a 3-cm left testicular mass is also noted. It is painless and firm. The patient has not noted it previously.

1. The initial radiographic assessment should consist of what test?

A. Scrotal magnetic resonance imaging (MRI)
B. Pelvic and scrotal computerized tomography (CT)
C. Testicular ultrasound
D. PET scan

2. Imaging has confirmed a testicular mass concerning for malignancy. Pending urologic evaluation, a serum β-hCG, alpha-fetoprotein (AFP), and lactate dehydrogenase (LDH) tests are ordered, all of which are significantly elevated above normal limits. Radical orchiectomy will be performed via which incision and will demonstrate which most likely pathology?

A. Scrotal incision; seminoma
B. Scrotal incision; non-seminoma
C. Inguinal incision; seminoma
D. Inguinal incision; non-seminoma

3. What is the primary landing zone for retro-peritoneal metastases in a left-sided testicular germ cell tumor?

A. Paracaval lymph nodes
B. Interaortocaval lymph nodes
C. Para-aortic lymph nodes
D. Inguinal nodes

4. Following the orchiectomy and staging imaging which demonstrated a retroperitoneal mass, the patient was treated with three cycles of BEP (bleomycin, etopside, and cisplatin). This history should prompt which concern for subsequent operative procedures?

A. Pulmonary fibrosis
B. Cardiomyopathy
C. Nephrotoxicity
D. SIADH

5. Following his course of chemotherapy, the patient has a residual retroperitoneal mass, prompting his urologist to perform a retroperitoneal lymph node dissection. The patient should be counseled regarding what potentially permanent outcome as a result of this particular procedure?

A. Urinary retention
B. Detrusor overactivity
C. Reduced penile sensation
D. Erectile dysfunction
E. Retrograde ejaculation

6. A 22-year-old male patient is referred to you for a large retroperitoneal mass. Your initial evaluation should include:

A. Needle biopsy of the mass. Why would one not ask for this test as part of the initial management especially if a sarcoma is still a concern.
B. Testicular exam
C. Serum AFP, HCG, and LDH
D. All of the above

E.   A and B

F.   B and C

ANSWERS

1. C. The imaging study of choice in testicular cancer is a scrotal ultrasound. Classically, testicular cancer will present as a painless testis mass, confirmed with a corresponding hypoechoic lesion on ultrasound. The patient should have an accompanying posterior-anterior (PA) and lateral chest radiograph. Once a malignant diagnosis is confirmed, a CT of the abdomen and pelvis with IV and oral contrast will complete the radiographic staging by assessing for retroperitoneal metastases.

2. D. Testicular cancer is managed with a radical orchiectomy, which consists of a high ligation of the spermatic cord at the level of the internal inguinal ring performed via an inguinal incision. A long permanent suture is placed on the proximal end of the spermatic cord before it is tucked into the internal ring so that it may be later identified during a retroperitoneal lymph node dissection. The inguinal incision allows for complete excision of the cord, along with potential microscopic metastases, as well as avoiding contamination of the scrotal lymphatics, reducing rates of local recurrence. One meta-analysis demonstrated a local recurrence rate of 2.9% for those with scrotal violation vs. 0.4% with inguinal incisions. Care should also be taken to avoid violation of the tunica vaginalis in order to reduce the risk of local tumor recurrence.

The presence of an elevated AFP indicates that the patient will be treated as though he has a non-seminomatous germ cell tumor as pure seminoma will never produce AFP. Seminoma will express hCG in approximately 15% of patients. Choriocarcinoma and embryonal carcinoma, non-seminomatous subtypes, can also produce hCG. Serum LDH is nonspecific, but it can correlate with disease volume.

3. C. Left-sided tumors predominantly metastasize to the para-aortic lymph nodes, whereas right-sided tumors will generally metastasize to the para-caval and interaortocaval lymph nodes. In either case, metastasis can occur to the opposite side, but such crossing metastases are more common with right-sided tumors. Generally, testis cancer metastasizes in an organized, progressive manner, beginning with the retroperitoneal lymph nodes. One exception is choriocarcinoma, which can spread in a hematogenous manner.

4. A. SIADH, the syndrome of inappropriate anti-diuretic hormone can occur after the use of vincristine and cyclophosphamides Cardiomyopathy occurs commonly after the use of anthracycline chemotherapeutic agents like doxorubicin and mitozantrone.

Cisplatin causes nephrotoxicity in up to 33% of patients and may cause renal failure in post nephrectomy patients. However, hydration is usually enough to treat this toxicity and it does not typically affect the patient long-term or for subsequent operations.

5. E. Retrograde ejaculation is a well-known side effect from retroperitoneal lymph node dissection (RPLND). The post-ganglionic sympathetic nerves responsible for ejaculation (T12-L3) are disrupted during a RPLND. This side effect may be avoided by performing a template RPLND in low-stage disease or by performing a bilateral nerve-sparing RPLND. In the former, the predictable metastatic pattern of testicular germ cell tumors allow either the right or left sympathetic nerves to be spared, thus preserving ejaculation. Alternatively, a bilateral nodal dissection can be performed, with care taken to preserve the individual nerves along with the hypogastric plexus anterior to the aorta, just below the origin of the inferior mesenteric artery. With appropriate nerve sparing, ejaculation can be preserved in nearly all patients.

An additional complication of RPLND is that of chylous ascites, due to lymphatic leakage. This can be prevented by meticulous attention to lymphostasis.

6. F. Patients with retroperitoneal masses are not uncommonly referred to general surgeons with presumed sarcoma. In young men in particular, the patients should be considered for a germ cell tumor origin.

BIBLIOGRAPHY

Capelouto CC, et al. A review of scrotal violation in testicular cancer: is adjuvant local therapy necessary? *J Urol.* March 1995;153(3 Pt 2):981–985.

Donat SM, et al. Bleomycin associated pulmonary toxicity: is perioperative oxygen restriction necessary. *J Urol.* October 1998;160:1347–1352.

Eggener SE, et al. Incidence of disease outside modified retroperitoneal lymph node dissection templates in clinical stage I or IIA nonseminomatous germ cell testicular cancer. *J Urol.* March 2007;177(3):937–942.

Jules-Elysee K, et al. Bleomycin-induced pulmonary toxicity. *Clin Chest Med.* 1990;11:1.

Klein EA. Open technique for nerve-sparing retroperitoneal lymphadenectomy. *Urology.* January 2000;55(1):132–135.

Gilligan T, et al. Testicular Cancer, version 2.2020, NCCN clinical practice guidelines in oncology. J Natl Compr Canc Netw. 2019 Dec;17(12): 1529–54.

97

Traumatic Ureteral Injury—During Colectomy

David W. Barham, Raffaella DeRosa, and Joseph R. Sterbis

A 30-year-old male is brought to the emergency room following a gunshot wound to the left lower quadrant. Initially he is stable and a computerized tomography (CT) scan of his abdomen suggests a left colonic and left retroperitoneal injury. He undergoes an exploratory laparotomy at which time a colonic injury is identified, requiring resection of the injured segment and a diverting colostomy. During further assessment, a left ureteral transection is noted in the mid-ureter.

1. **During the case, the patient becomes acidotic and hypothermic. He starts to require pressor support. He has no other apparent injuries. The treatment of choice in this setting is which of the following?**

   A. Transureteroureterostomy
   B. Ureteroureterostomy
   C. Boari flap
   D. Ligation of the ureteral stumps with permanent suture
   E. Psoas hitch with ureteral reimplant

2. **His preoperative CT scan demonstrated a 5-mm left lower pole renal calculus. Which of the following treatment options is contraindicated?**

   A. Transureteroureterostomy
   B. Ureteroureterostomy
   C. Boari flap
   D. Ligation of the ureteral stumps
   E. Psoas hitch with ureteral reimplant

3. **Which of the following considerations is true when performing an ureteroureterostomy?**

   A. A tension-free anastomosis is not required.

   B. Spatulating opposing ends of the ureteral segments can be done selectively.
   C. Fine, permanent suture is required.
   D. Placement of a double-J ureteral stent across the anastomosis is recommended.
   E. In the setting of a gunshot wound, a ureteroureterostomy cannot be done.

4. **Which of the following is true regarding ureteroneocystostomy?**

   A. The reimplant should be placed on the base of the bladder.
   B. A refluxing reimplant has a higher risk of stricture.
   C. This is the treatment of choice for distal ureteral injuries.
   D. Stay sutures should be placed in the ureter to avoid tissue handling.
   E. If a psoas hitch is required, the ipsilateral bladder pedicle may need to be ligated to achieve sufficient mobilization of the bladder.

5. **Which of the following is true about ureteral injury due to external trauma from gunshot wounds?**

   A. Ureteral injuries associated with external trauma will always present with hematuria.
   B. The diagnosis is usually made by a CT cystogram.
   C. High-velocity gunshot wounds (>350 m/second) can create a surrounding energy wave 30 to 40 times the missile diameter.
   D. Injury from missiles and bullets can be located only along the path of tissue penetration.
   E. Blast injuries to the urinary drainage system will usually present as an increase in output

from surgically placed drains immediately (<24 hours) after the surgery.

6. **In a stable patient with gross hematuria and a suspected urologic injury, the ideal imaging modality is:**

    A. One-shot plain film intravenous pyelogram

    B. Renal bladder ultrasound

    C. IV contrast enhanced CT abdomen/pelvis with delayed images

    D. Magnetic resonance (MR) urogram

7. **Fourteen days after his ureteral repair and diverting ostomy placement, the patient develops abdominal pain, ileus, leukocytosis, and fever. His hemoglobin and hematocrit are stable, images reveal extravasation in the left mid-ureter suggestive of ureteral injury. The best treatment choice is:**

    A. Cystoscopy and left ureteral stent placement

    B. Abdominal exploration with ureteroureterostomy

    C. Auto-transplant

    D. Foley catheter drainage only

    E. Abdominal exploration with psoas hitch

ANSWERS

1. **D.** If recognized at the time of surgery, surgical division of the ureter or partial ureteral excision should be managed based on the location and length of injury. Options for repair include ipsilateral ureteroureterostomy, ureteral reimplantation with or without a psoas hitch, and trans ureteroureterostomy. In occasions when the patient is unstable, the ureter can be ligated with sutures, a nephrostomy tube is placed, and reconstruction can occur within the next 48 to 72 hours. If the patient is hemodynamically unstable, then damage control is recommended and delayed ureteral repair can be performed. In this patient, he has the lethal triad in trauma and he should be resuscitated before any definitive repairs are done.

2. **A.** Transureteroureterostomy places the contralateral renal unit at risk and is contraindicated in patients with a prior history of urinary stone disease. Both upper tracts are at risk if there is any problem distal to the transureteroureterostomy anastomotic site. The other reconstructive surgeries can be implemented in the setting of known stone disease.

3. **D.** The use of permanent sutures within the urinary tract is a nidus for stone formation. The proximal and distal ends of the ureters should be spatulated and sewn together in a tension-free fashion with absorbable monofilament suture. A stent should be placed across the water-tight anastomosis. Contusions or damaged areas of the ureter need to be debrided until the edges bleed prior to performing ureteral anastomoses.

4. **D.** Short defects involving the distal ureter should be repaired with ureteroneocystostomy. Non-refluxing ureteral implants have a higher risk of stricture than refluxing ureteral implants; but refluxing anastomoses show no increase in complications related to urine reflux. The principles of repair include spatulation, lack of tension, stenting, postoperative drainage, and a water-tight anastomosis with fine nonreactive absorbable suture. The contralateral bladder pedicle can be ligated when performing a psoas hitch to provide enough mobilization to perform a ureteroneocystostomy. Stay suture can improve tissue handling and preserve the blood supply to the ureter. Re-implanted ureters are usually placed at the dome of the bladder.

5. **C.** The missile or bullet can tumble during penetration and cause damage to the surrounding tissues at a significant distance from its path. High-velocity bullets or missiles can create an energy wave that penetrates and injures distant tissues. Hematuria is not always present after ureteral injury. Triphasic CT can be used to evaluate tissue trauma and for ureteral injury. CT cystogram will usually identify a bladder injury. Damage to the ureters can present 3 to 5 days after injury as increased drainage from the surgically placed drains. This fluid can be sent to pathology for a creatinine level.

6. **C.** Stable trauma patients with gross hematuria should be suspected of having a urologic injury. The American Urological Association Urotrauma Guidelines recommend IV contrast enhanced CT abdomen/pelvis with immediate and delayed imaging. Delayed films are important to evaluate for an injury to the collecting system, renal pelvis, or ureter. One-shot IVP may be used intraoperatively during retroperitoneal exploration when considering nephrectomy to demonstrate the presence of a normal contralateral kidney. Renal bladder ultrasound and MR urogram play no role in the workup

of traumatic urologic injuries. CT non-contrast is suboptimal in identifying injuries to the collecting system or ureters.

7. **A.** When ureteral injury is identified in a delayed fashion, cystoscopy with retrograde placement of ureteral stent should be attempted. If unable to place ureteral stent retrograde, then nephrostomy tube placement can be performed. Open repair is discouraged in the delayed setting. Foley catheter placement alone will not help the ureteral injury.

BIBLIOGRAPHY

Al-Ali M, Haddad L. The late treatment of 63 overlooked or complicated ureteral missile injuries: the promise of nephrostomy and role of autotransplantation. *J Urol.* 1996;156:1918–1921.

Carver B, Bozeman C, Venable D. Ureteral injury due to penetrating trauma. *South Med J.* 2004;97:462–464.

Elliot S, McAninch JW. Ureteral injuries: external and iatrogenic. *Urol Clin North Am.* 2006;33:55–66.

Fugita OE, Kavoussi L. Laparoscopic ureteral reimplantation for ureteral lesion secondary to transvaginal ultrasonography for oocyte retrieval. *Urology.* 2001;58:281.

Ghali A, El Malik E, Ibrahim A, et al. Ureteric injuries: diagnosis, management, and outcome. *J Trauma.* 1999;46:150–158.

Iwaszko MR, Krambeck AE, Chow GK, Gettman MT. Transureteroureterostomy revisited: long-term surgical outcomes. *J Urol.* March 2010;183(3):1055–1059.

Kristjánsson A, Mânsson W. Refluxing or nonrefluxing ureteric anastomosis. *BJU Int.* 1999;84(8):905–910.

Kunkle D, Kansas B, Pathak A, et al. Delayed diagnosis of traumatic ureteral injuries. *J Urol.* 2006;176:2503–2507.

Medina D, Lavery R, Ross S, Livingston D. Ureteral trauma: preoperative studies neither predict injury nor prevent missed injuries. *J Am Coll Surg.* 1998;186:641–644.

Minervini A, Boni G, Salinitri G, et al. Evaluation of renal function and upper urinary tract morphology in the ileal orthotopic neobladder with no antireflux mechanism. *J Urol.* 2005;173(1):144–147.

Modi P, Goel R, Dodiya S. Laparoscopic ureteroneocystostomy for distal ureteral injuries. *Urology.* 2005;66:751.

Morey AF, Brandes S, Dugi DD, et al. Urotrauma: AUA Guideline. *J Urol.* 2014;192:327–335.

Noble IG, Lee KT, Mundy AR. Transuretero-ureterostomy: a review of 253 cases. *Br J Urol.* January 1997;79(1):20–23.

Palmer JK, Benson GS, Corriere JN Jr. Diagnosis and initial management of urological injuries associated with 200 consecutive pelvic fractures. *J Urol.* 1983;130:712–714.

Partin AW, Dmochowski RR, Kavoussi LR, Peters CA. Chapter 90, Upper urinary tract trauma. *Campbell-Walsh-Wein Urology.* 2021 ed. Elsevier; 2020;1982–2004.

Perez-Brayfield M, Keane T, Krishnan A, et al. Gunshot wounds to the ureter: a 40-year experience at Grady Memorial Hospital. *J Urol.* 2001;166:119–121.

Reddy PK, Evans RM. Laparoscopic ureteroneocystostomy. *J Urol.* 1994;152:2057.

Schimpf MO, Wagner JR. Robot-assisted laparoscopic boari flap ureteral reimplantation. *J Endourol.* 2008;22:2691.

Velmahos G, Degiannis E. The management of urinary tract injuries after gunshot wounds of the anterior and posterior abdomen. *Injury.* 1997;28:535–538.

Wessells H, Deirmenjian J, McAninch J. Preservation of renal function after reconstruction for trauma: quantitative assessment with radionuclide scintigraphy. *J Urol.* 1997;157:1583–1586.

Wiesner C, Thuroff JW. Techniques for uretero-intestinal reimplantation. *Curr Opin Urol.* 2004;14(6):351–355.

98

Prostate Cancer

Joseph R. Sterbis, Lauren P.K. Muramoto, and John E. Musser

A 58-year-old male is diagnosed in urology clinic with clinical T2a Gleason $3 + 2 = 5$ prostate cancer. His serum prostate specific antigen is 4.2. He has a history of hypertension and no prior surgical history. He has no prior history of radiation or chemotherapy administration.

1. **Which treatment option is most recommended?**
   A. Radical prostatectomy with bilateral pelvic lymph node dissection
   B. External beam radiation therapy
   C. Brachytherapy seed implants
   D. Active surveillance

2. **The patient elects for a radical prostatectomy with bilateral pelvic lymph node dissection. During the pelvic lymph node dissection, the left obturator nerve is accidentally divided during sharp dissection. It is recognized immediately. How do you address this complication?**
   A. Because the division was done sharply, leave the two ends.
   B. Reapproximate the two ends with fine, permanent suture.
   C. Perform a nerve graft, approximating the two ends.
   D. Approximate both ends to a nearby surrounding nerve.

3. **During the apical prostatic dissection, a small 1-cm full-thickness rectal injury is incurred. Which of the following is the best course of action at this time?**
   A. Omental flap coverage following primary repair
   B. Resection of the injured rectum, followed by primary anastomosis
   C. Resection of the injured rectum, primary anastomosis, and diverting ileostomy
   D. Diverting colostomy after resection even in a patient without prior radiation therapy
   E. Double layer, air-tight closure of the rectal injury

4. **Four months later, the patient is scheduled for a laparoscopic cholecystectomy. The operating room nurse has difficulty placing a foley catheter. What is the most likely source for this difficulty?**
   A. Anastomotic contracture at the bladder neck
   B. Prostate cancer recurrence at the bladder neck
   C. Urethral stricture
   D. Rectourethral fistula

5. **At his 6-month follow-up, the patient states he has been doing well but still reports difficulty achieving and maintaining erections. Which of the following would not lower his risk of post prostatectomy erectile dysfunction?**
   A. Avoid use of thermal energy during dissection of the neurovascular bundle
   B. Careful dissection of vascular pedicles
   C. Pretreatment with PDE-5 inhibitor
   D. Use a robotic platform

6. **The patient experiences a disease recurrence and is initiated on androgen deprivation therapy (ADT). Which of the following is true regarding this treatment?**
   A. The patient is at reduced risk for cardiac morbidity.

B. The patient is at increased risk for loss of lean muscle.

C. The patient is at reduced risk for osteoporosis.

D. The patient is at increased risk for loss of body fat.

7. Besides ADT, what should be offered to the patient at this time?

A. Continued surveillance only

B. Pelvic exploration with bilateral pelvic lymph node dissection

C. Salvage XRT

D. Platinum-based chemotherapy

A year after his radical prostatectomy, he presents with abdominal pain and dysuria. His vital signs are as follows: BP 145/70, HR 104, RR 22, SpO2 95% on RA, and temperature 101.4°F. On his labs, he has an elevated leukocytosis, urine is positive for nitrites and leukocyte esterase. His PMHx is significant for open prostatectomy 4 months ago. He is admitted and treated for urosepsis. A voiding cystourethrogram is obtained and shows contrast within the sigmoid colon.

8. The next step is:

A. Diverting colostomy

B. Rectal tube and low residue diet

C. Primary repair with omental pedicle flap

D. Transanal repair with rectal advancement flap

ANSWERS

1. D. Active surveillance is appropriate for men with low-risk prostate cancer, defined as having organ-confined pathology, <0.2 mL, a Gleason sum less than or equal to 6, and a Gleason grade < 4 or 5 in the biopsy specimen.

2. B. If the obturator nerve is accidentally divided, it should be reanastamosed with fine, non-absorbable sutures. The patient can make a full functional recovery.

3. A. Rectal injury is a serious intraoperative complication. If a rectal injury occurs, the prostatectomy should be completed. Small injuries that are less than 50% of the circumference of the rectum can be treated without resection. The rectum can be closed primarily, and a piece of omentum should be placed between the rectal closure and the vesicourethral anastomosis to reduce the incidence of rectourethral fistula. The rectal defect should be closed in two layers and the wound copiously irrigated with antibiotic solution. If the patient has had radiation therapy prior to surgery, a diverting colostomy should be performed.

4. A. Two to five percent of patients develop a bladder neck contracture approximately 6 to 12 weeks after an open prostatectomy. The initial management includes dilation with urethral sounds or a direct vision incision of the bladder neck.

5. D. Post-prostatectomy erectile dysfunction continues to be a challenging side-effect to manage and can have significant impact on quality of life. Though in the literature it has been reported that erectile function can take up to 5 years to recover, a significant portion of patients will fail to recover potency. Success of recovery is thought to depend on several factors to include age, prior baseline erectile function, surgeon experience, and use of nerve sparing technique. The most common location where the nerves involved in erectile function can be damaged is at the apical dissection of the prostatic capsule from the neurovascular bundle. Avoidance of excessive surgical monopolary energy is also key during a nerve sparing procedure. Lastly, penile rehabilitation with a low-dose PDE-5 inhibitor starting nightly 2 weeks before surgery and continued in the postoperative period have been used to preserve erectile tissue.

6. B. General complications of androgen ablation include osteoporosis, hot flashes, and decline in cognitive function, increased cardiovascular morbidity and mortality, and changes in body habitus. Bone mineral density can decrease, and the longer the patient remains on ADT, the greater the risk of fracture. ADT has been linked to cognitive decline in men with prostate cancer. Men treated with ADT have demonstrated a loss of muscle mass and increase in percentage of body fat. ADT can adversely affect body habitus, glucose metabolism, lipid profiles, and increase cardiovascular morbidity and mortality.

7. C. Based on the 2020 NCCN guidelines, patients who experience biochemical recurrence evidenced by rise in post-prostatectomy PSA levels should undergo risk stratification and imaging to rule out any metastatic disease or local recurrence. Salvage radiation should be offered to all patients with non-metastatic prostate cancer who experience a rise in post-prostatectomy PSA levels and has been shown to improve disease specific survival significantly compared to observation alone. There is no role for surgical exploration or platinum-based chemotherapy in this situation.

8. A. The VCUG demonstrates a colovesical fistula which represents an uncommon complication of prostatectomy. The patient is likely uroseptic from fecal contamination due to this colovesical fistula. Definitive repair will be required as this fistula will likely not close on its own. In this setting of active infection, repair at this time would likely be unsuccessful therefore a period of fecal diversion is necessary to allow for wound healing. Afterwards, one can attempt repair through a variety of techniques described.

BIBLIOGRAPHY

Borland RN, Walsh PC. The management of rectal injury during radical retropubic prostatectomy. *J Urol.* 1992;147:905–907.

Daniell HW, Dunn SR, Ferguson DW, et al. Progressive osteoporosis during androgen deprivation therapy for prostate cancer. *J Urol.* 2000;163:181–186.

De Ridder DJMK, Greenwell T. Urinary tract fistulae. *Campbell-Walsh Urology.* 2021;129:2924–2963.e10.

Epstein JI, Walsh PC, Carmichael M, et al. Pathologic and clinical findings to predict tumor extent of nonpalpable (stage T1c) prostate cancer. *JAMA.* 1994;271:368–374.

Jenkins LC, Mulhall JP. Impact of prostate cancer treatments on sexual health. Mydlo JH, Godec CJ, eds. *Prostate Cancer Science and Clinical Practice.* 2nd ed. Academic Press; 2016.

Krupski TL, Smith MR, Lee WC, et al. Natural history of bone complications in men with prostate carcinoma initiating androgen deprivation therapy. *Cancer.* 2004;101: 541–549.

Nelson CJ, Lee JS, Gamboa MC, Roth AJ. Cognitive effects of hormone therapy in men with prostate cancer. *Cancer.* 2008;113:1097–1106.

Saigal CS, Gore JL, Krupski TL, et al. Androgen deprivation therapy increases cardiovascular morbidity in men with prostate cancer. *Cancer.* 2007;110:1493–1500.

Spaliviero M, Steinberg AP, et al. Laparoscopic injury and repair of obturator nerve during radical prostatectomy. *Urology.* November 2004;64(5):1030.

Trock BJ, Han M, Freedland SJ, et al. Prostate cancer-specific survival following salvage radiotherapy vs observation in men with biochemical recurrence after radical prostatectomy. *JAMA.* 2008;299:2760–2769.

Tubaro A, Hind A, Vicentini C, Miano L. A prospective study of the safety and efficacy of suprapubic transvesical prostatectomy in patients with benign prostatic hyperplasia. *J Urol.* 2001;166(1):172–176.

Van Londen G, Levy ME, Perera S, et al. Body composition changes during androgen deprivation therapy for prostate cancer: a 2-year prospective study. *Crit Rev Oncol/Hematol.* 2008;68:172–177.

Varkarakis I, Kyriakakis Z, Delis A, Protogerou V, Deliveliotis C. Long-term results of open transvesical prostatectomy from a contemporary series of patients. *Urology.* 2004;64(2):306–310.

Vasilev SE. Obturator nerve injury: a review of management options. *Gynecol Oncol.* 1994 May;53(2):152–155.

Wedmid A, Mendoza P, Sharma S, et al. Rectal injury during robot-assisted radical prostatectomy: incidence and management. *J. Urol.* 2011;186:1928–1933.

VASCULAR

99

Carotid Artery Disease

Vernon Horst and Kelly Kempe

A 72-year-old female is referred to your office for evaluation and recommendations after incidental findings on a neck computerized tomography angiogram (CTA) performed as part of a workup for a neck mass. She has a history of diabetes mellitus and essential hypertension, both well controlled with medical therapy. Her CTA shows an occluded left internal carotid artery (ICA), and 60% stenosis of the right internal carotid artery. Further questioning reveals history of right-sided weakness lasting only for 2 hours, which occurred 2 years ago. The neck mass was determined benign and she is undergoing imaging surveillance for this.

1. **The best treatment option for this patient is:**
    A. Right internal carotid endarterectomy
    B. Right internal carotid stent
    C. Left carotid endarterectomy
    D. Left common to external carotid endarterectomy, patch angioplasty, and ICA lumen obliteration
    E. Addition of anti-platelet therapy and high-dose statin to her current medical regimen

2. **The aforementioned patient did not want surgery and chose medical optimization. She presents to the emergency department 2 months after the initial visit. She has had three episodes of right arm paralysis since her office visit, the last one occurring 8 hours prior to presentation. She currently has no neurologic deficits. Head CT scan shows no evidence of intracranial infarction, and her neck CTA is unchanged. The best treatment plan at this time is:**

    A. Right internal carotid endarterectomy
    B. Right internal carotid stent
    C. Left carotid endarterectomy
    D. Left common to external carotid endarterectomy, patch angioplasty, and ICA exclusion
    E. Staged right internal and left external carotid endarterectomy

3. **Three years later, this same patient develops worsening right asymptomatic ICA stenosis (right ICA peak systolic velocity 370 cm/sec, ICA/CCA ratio 5:6; contralateral side <50% ICA stenosis). You perform a right carotid endarterectomy under general anesthesia. Completion angiogram demonstrates no abnormality. Postoperatively, the patient awakens in the operating room but fails to move her left side on neurologic examination. Your next step is:**

    A. Transfer to radiology for STAT neck and head CTA
    B. Immediate administration of protamine
    C. Immediate carotid exposure with Doppler imaging
    D. Transfemoral cerebral angiogram
    E. Transfer to neurovascular intensive care unit for serial neurovascular checks

4. **You evaluate a 78-year-old patient in the neurovascular intensive care unit 24 hours after she presented to the emergency department with a right hemispheric cerebrovascular accident (CVA). Her neck CTA demonstrates 60% stenosis of the right ICA and 85% stenosis of the left ICA**

per NASCET criteria. Duplex imaging confirms these findings. She is neurologically stable at this time, with interval improvement of her symptoms compared to her admission exam. The best treatment plan for this patient, along with initiation of high-dose statin and dual antiplatelet therapy, is

A. Immediate right carotid endarterectomy, followed by elective left carotid endarterectomy
B. Right carotid endarterectomy within 2 weeks of presentation but after neurologic symptoms plateau, followed by elective left carotid endarterectomy
C. Left carotid endarterectomy to this admission, followed by right carotid endarterectomy 6 weeks after presentation
D. Elective left carotid endarterectomy only
E. Right carotid endarterectomy within 2 weeks of presentation but only if neurologic symptoms worsen

5. A 60-year-old patient with diabetes and hypertension is found to have 90% right ICA stenosis on CTA after presenting to the emergency department for a TIA. He has no further neurologic symptoms. His hospitalist ordered a cardiac workup. A positive stress test leads to a cardiac catheterization. The patient was found to have a 95% left main coronary ostial lesion with left anterior descending artery (LAD) 90% stenosis, and right circumflex artery 70% stenosis. The best operative plan for this patient is:

A. Coronary stenting followed by elective carotid endarterectomy (CEA) later this admission
B. Coronary artery bypass graft (CABG) followed by elective CEA
C. Awake CEA under regional anesthesia, followed by CABG later this admission
D. Carotid artery stenting (CAS)
E. CEA and CABG under the same anesthesia during this admission.

ANSWERS

1. **E.** Optimal medical therapy should be part of the treatment of all patients with carotid artery disease, regardless of plans for surgical intervention. This includes optimal treatment of diabetes, hypertension, hypercholesterolemia, and smoking cessation to reduce overall cardiovascular risk and risk

of stroke. Surgical or endovascular intervention is never indicated on asymptomatic occluded carotid arteries. Current Society for Vascular Surgery guidelines for carotid artery disease surgical treatment (CEA, trans-femoral CAS, or trans-arterial carotid revascularization [TCAR]) include >80% asymptomatic carotid artery stenosis or >50% symptomatic stenosis. Carotid artery stenosis is considered symptomatic if there has been a cerebrovascular event, whether ischemic stroke or transient ischemic attack (TIA), within 6 months of presentation. In this patient, her right carotid stenosis is asymptomatic and was 2 years ago; therefore, the best plan for her is addition of anti-platelet therapy and high-dose statin to her current medical regimen.

2. **D.** This patient is now experiencing Carotid Stump Syndrome, which is the only indication for carotid intervention on the extracranially occluded internal carotid artery. In the setting of left internal carotid artery occlusion, the left cerebral circulation is supplied by the circle of Willis along with collaterals from the external carotid artery on the affected side. This phenomenon is a result of retrograde microembolization from the proximal ICA into the ECA and into the left intracranial circulation via collateral vessels. Treatment of stump syndrome includes common to external carotid endarterectomy, patch angioplasty, and exclusion of the ICA stump to prevent further embolization. Because the right carotid 60% stenosis remains asymptomatic, it does not warrant operative intervention at this time.

3. **C.** While not all carotid surgeons perform completion imaging, it is reasonable to perform either cerebral angiogram or a carotid duplex ultrasound at the conclusion of the case in an effort to ensure adequate revascularization. All patients who undergo carotid revascularization should be awakened in the operating room, and a neurologic examination performed to evaluate for new neurologic deficits. If a new deficit is identified, the wound should be immediately opened and the artery evaluated with Doppler to confirm flow. An artery with flow should be further interrogated with either Duplex ultrasound or cerebral angiography, while a finding of no flow requires arterial re-exploration. Alternatively, if the initial exam has no neurologic deficits but outside of the operating room, the patient develops new deficits, a rapid carotid Duplex ultrasound should

be performed, followed by surgical intervention if an intimal flap or thrombus is noted. If noninvasive studies are negative, head CT scan should be performed to rule out intracranial hemorrhage. If this is negative, cerebral angiogram is warranted to fully evaluate the surgical site as well as the intracranial circulation.

4. **B.** The optimal interval of time between a severe stroke and carotid surgery remains under debate, but most importantly varies from patient to patient based on neurologic deficits. The only immediate action is to administer recombinant tissue plasminogen activator (tPA) if a patient presents within the first 3 hours of symptom onset and meets exclusion and inclusion criteria (additional timing and intracranial intervention recommendations if presenting within 6 hours). Outside this special population, the purpose of extracranial carotid revascularization is to prevent future neurologic events. Endarterectomy should be performed within 2 weeks of the event but after the patient's recovery has plateaued. Patients are at risk for a recurrent neurologic event if endarterectomy is delayed until after 4 to 6 weeks. Asymptomatic severe (>80%) stenosis does not require emergent surgery, and should be addressed only after symptomatic moderate to severe (50% to 99%) stenosis is treated.

5. **C.** The management of patients with concomitant carotid and coronary artery disease is controversial regarding therapy. This patient has symptomatic carotid artery disease and severe asymptomatic coronary disease. If coronary artery stenting is possible, it should be performed prior to the carotid endarterectomy; but this patient needs a 3-vessel CABG, which, by definition, is not amenable to stenting. Patients with severe bilateral asymptomatic carotid stenosis and coronary disease should be considered for CEA before or a concomitant CABG. Patients with symptomatic carotid stenosis and coronary disease not amenable to coronary stenting will benefit from CEA prior to or concomitant with CABG. If a patient undergoes CAS instead of CEA, they should have a delay of at least 2–4 weeks before they undergo CABG due to the dual antiplatelet therapy required for carotid stent placement.

BIBLIOGRAPHY

Arnold M, Perler BA. Carotid Endarterectomy. In: Sidawy AN, Perler BA, eds. *Rutherford's Vascular Surgery and Endovascular Therapy*. 9th ed. Elsevier; 2018:1194–1214.

Bookland M, Loftus CM. 2012 *Surgical Management of Extracranial Carotid Disease. Schmidek and Sweet's Operative Neurosurgical Techniques*. 6th ed. Elsevier; 793–805.

Ricotta, JJ, AbuRahma A, Ascher E, et. al. Updated Society for Vascular Surgery guidelines for management of extracranial carotid disease. *J Vasc Surg*. 2011;54(3):e1–e31.

Ricotta JJ, Ricotta JJ. Cerebrovascular Disease: Decision Making Including Medical Therapy. In: Sidawy AN, Perler BA, eds. *Rutherford's Vascular Surgery and Endovascular Therapy*. 9th ed. Elsevier; 2018:1169–1183.

100

Abdominal Aortic Aneurysm

Dwight C. Kellicut

SCENARIO 1

A 63-year-old male with past medical history significant for well-controlled hypertension, hyperlipidemia, and a remote history of smoking is referred for evaluation of a 5.7 cm infrarenal abdominal aortic aneurysm (AAA) found incidentally on a computerized tomography (CT) scan of the abdomen during a recent emergency room visit for abdominal pain. The patient recently underwent a cardiac stress test by his primary care physician, which was normal and is now being considered for open versus endovascular repair.

1. **Which of the following is considered a major risk factor in the development of AAA?**

    A. Diabetes mellitus
    B. Hypertension
    C. Smoking
    D. Collagen vascular disease
    E. Obesity

2. **For patients with major risk factors, what would be the best method to screen for AAA?**

    A. Physical exam
    B. Abdominal ultrasound
    C. CT scan
    D. MRI
    E. Angiography

3. **Regarding the size of his aneurysm, when should an elective abdominal aortic aneurysm be repaired?**

    A. 4.5 cm
    B. 5 cm

    C. 5.5 cm
    D. 6.0 cm

4. **Regarding survival after endovascular repair (EVAR), compared with open repair, which of the following is true?**

    A. EVAR demonstrates equal survival both in the first 30 days and long term.
    B. EVAR demonstrates better long-term survival and equals 30 days' survival.
    C. EVAR demonstrates better 30 days' survival and no difference in long-term survival.
    D. In patients with minimal, well-controlled comorbidities, EVAR provides the better long-term results.
    E. In patients with poorly controlled co-morbidities, the open repair has a 15% mortality rate.

SCENARIO 2

A 69-year-old male with a history of smoking undergoes screening ultrasound and is diagnosed with a 7.2 cm infrarenal aortic aneurysm. He undergoes preoperative workup and a non-obstructing sigmoid mass is discovered. Staging workup and biopsy reveal a 2-cm adenocarcinoma without metastasis.

5. **What treatment strategy is most appropriate?**

    A. Proceeding with colonic resection and observation of the aneurysm
    B. Open repair of the aortic aneurysm and concomitant neoadjuvant treatment of the cancer with bevacizumab.

C. Endovascular repair of the aneurysm, followed by colon resection.

D. Combined procedure with the colon resection and anastomosis done first.

6. The patient has no prior cardiac history, which is true regarding the patient's pre-operative cardiac evaluation?

A. If he has no history of myocardial infarction and is younger than 70, his cardiac risk is low and no further screening is warranted.

B. If the patient can perform at least four metabolic equivalents (METs), he is low risk for cardiac complications and can proceed with surgery.

C. All patients undergoing major aortic surgery should have a transthoracic echo because of the high rate of LV dysfunction found in patients with vascular disease.

D. A patient with a normal preoperative ECG is low risk for cardiac event and can proceed with surgery.

SCENARIO 3

A 60-year-old male with a known AAA presents in extremis. Just prior to presentation, he had acute onset abdominal pain with syncope. After initial resuscitation in the ED, he was transported to the OR for open AAA repair. In the OR, you find a retroperitoneal rupture of his aortic aneurysm, and an incidental mass that is confined to the left colon. There is no evidence of large bowel obstruction.

7. What is the appropriate management of an incidentally found mass?

A. Proceed with open aneurysm repair and perform a left hemicolectomy, provided the patient remains hemodynamically stable.

B. Proceed with aneurysm repair and perform a limited resection involving only the involved segment without attempting to obtain margins

C. Proceed with aneurysm repair and perform a diverting ostomy to prevent obstruction.

D. Proceed with aneurysm repair without performing a resection.

8. Which of the following is true regarding management of the inferior mesenteric artery during aortic surgery?

A. Evidence of colonic ischemia during open repair is an indication for reimplantation of the Inferior Mesenteric Artery.

B. The colon has sufficient collateral blood supply and as such the IMA can always be ligated.

C. The IMA is always ligated during surgery and if bowel ischemia is noted, a limited resection is performed.

D. The IMA is the sole source of perfusion to the left colon and must be preserved.

ANSWERS

1. C. The major risk factors associated with increased likelihood of aneurysm formation include: age >65, male gender, history of smoking, and family history of AAA in a first-degree relative.

2. B. Abdominal ultrasound has been evaluated in numerous studies and has been found to be available, accurate, and low cost. CT and MRI are excellent modalities for evaluating the aorta regarding accuracy, but fail on cost effectiveness and availability. Angiography actually underestimates the size of an AAA because it only outlines the arterial lumen. It is also not cost-effective as a screening tool.

For patients with major risk factors, the question becomes what is the best methodology to detect aneurysms in regard to screening? In the U.S. Preventative Services Task Force (USPSTF) January 2014 bulletin, the following recommendations were made: the Task Force found that one-time AAA screening can be effective and recommends it for men ages 65 to 75 who have ever smoked. This is a B recommendation. For men ages 65 to 75 who have never smoked, the Task Force recommends that these men talk to their doctor or nurse about whether one-time AAA screening might be right for them based on their health history and the potential benefits and harms of screening.

For women, the Task Force found that the benefits and harms of screening are different. In the draft recommendation statement, the Task Force calls for more research to determine if AAA screening is beneficial for women ages 65 to 75 who smoke or have smoked in the past. Based on the lack of evidence, the Task Force determined it could not recommend for or against screening older female smokers and issued an I statement (issued when evidence is insufficient to fully assess benefits and harms). Research is critically needed in this area to determine if AAA screening could be beneficial for women who smoke or who have ever smoked. Among nonsmoking women, the chance of developing AAA is extremely low (well under 1%), and the Task Force found that AAA screening is very unlikely to benefit these women and may even cause harm. The Task Force recommends against screening for AAA in these women; this is a D recommendation.

Physical examination is highly dependent upon the experience of the examiner and on patient body habitus. As a general rule, patients with a 5.0-cm AAA are palpable 75% of the time and those measuring 3.0 to 3.9 cm are palpable 25% of the time.

3. **C.** The natural history of AAA is such that most aneurysms expand at a rate of 0.3 cm/year. Two randomized, prospective trials have demonstrated that there is no survival benefit to repairing AAA <5.5 cm, even in well-selected patients who are considered to have a favorable operative risk. All aneurysms greater than 4.0 cm should be followed on a yearly basis. For patients who have an aneurysm that measures greater than 4.0 cm, but less than 5.5 cm, their aneurysm should be followed every 6 months as approximately 25% of those aneurysms will expand at a rate greater than or equal to 0.5 cm in 6 months, an indication for repair. Other indications to repair an AAA less than 5.5 cm include embolization, occlusion, symptoms (back/abdominal pain/tenderness on exam), and patients located in a remote area.

4. **C.** As a general rule, patients may be considered for open aortic surgery if they are under the age of 65, provided they are an acceptable surgical risk. EVAR may also be considered, but multiple anatomic considerations must be taken into account to include: neck diameter, neck length, angulation of neck, reverse taper of neck, calcification, thrombus, diameter of common femoral/iliac arteries, distal seal length, iliac tortuosity, and renal/splanchnic blood flow. Given all of the technical considerations associated with EVAR, there are significant immediate and late complications that include device failure, arterial embolization, limb thrombosis, graft migration, graft infection, and endoleaks.

Two trials (EVAR I and DREAM) have compared open aortic surgery versus EVAR in patients considered fit for open surgery. In both studies (EVAR I/DREAM), open surgical repair was found to have increased 30-day mortality (4.7%/4.6% vs. 1.7%/1.2%), increased blood loss, longer operative time, and increased blood transfusion. The long-term

survival between open surgery and EVAR have been shown to be equal. EVAR demonstrates significant graft-related complications (41% vs. 9%) and higher revision rates (20% vs. 6%) making open surgery in this case a better long-term option. The EVAR 2 trial found patients deemed unfit, defined somewhat nebulously, for open surgery had the substantial operative mortality of 7%, indicating that those patients that are high risk will remain high risk regardless of what procedure is chosen. Of note, both EVAR 1 and DREAM excluded emergent cases.

5. **C.** This patient has both an aortic aneurysm that requires intervention, and colon cancer that is resectable. A decision should be made as to which pathology to address first. Aortic aneurysms with a diameter ≥7 cm have up to a 32% chance of rupture within 1 year, and thus should be repaired. Combined procedures, while appealing because it limits the patient to a single anesthesia and avoid delay in treating either problem, is controversial. If it is to be attempted, aortic repair should occur first, and the graft isolated from the field by covering it with remaining aortic sac, retroperitoneal tissue, or omentum to avoid contamination. The discussion of endovascular vs open repair should be individualized to the patient and take into account the risk/benefit to the patient and the technical considerations involved in selecting an adequate repair. In general, EVAR will allow for a shorter delay in surgery, allowing for shorter recovery before colon resection.

6. **B.** All patients undergoing major vascular surgery should be risk stratified based on the guidelines provided by the American College of Cardiology for preoperative risk stratification. A patient with no cardiac history is considered low risk if they can perform >4 METS, roughly equivalent to climbing a flight of stairs or walking 3–4 mph on level ground. Preoperative ECG can provide an important baseline for the patient but are an insufficient screening tool and can easily miss demand related to ischemia. Preoperative echo should not be routinely obtained but are reasonable for symptomatic patients or patients with documented LV dysfunction without a recent study.

7. **D.** This patient presents with incidental abdominal pathology during an emergent surgery for ruptured AAA. When concomitant pathology is discovered during emergent surgery, priority should be given to

whichever pathology presents the greatest risk to the patient. In this question, the patient has a contained rupture, which requires repair. Simultaneous repair is not advised unless the second abdominal process is considered life threatening or extremely urgent. This patient who presents with an incidental finding of a non-obstructing colonic mass can likely be managed by completing the aortic repair, undergo appropriate staging workup, and interval resection after recovery. In the aforementioned scenario, if the patient appeared obstructed, a resection may be necessary.

8. A. Under most conditions, the IMA can be ligated because the colon receives collateral blood supply from the superior mesenteric artery (SMA) and rectal arteries. Preop imaging should be evaluated for significant SMA or hypogastric artery disease, which would suggest poor collateral flow and the need for reimplantation. Other indications for reimplantation include a large IMA suggesting that it provides dominant flow, and poor back bleeding from the IMA.

BIBLIOGRAPHY

Endovascular Aneurysm Trial Participants. Comparison of endovascular aneurysm repair with open repair in patients with abdominal aortic aneurysm (EVAR I trial): randomized controlled trial. *Lancet.* 2004;365:1179.

Endovascular Aneurysm Trial Participants. Endovascular aneurysm repair and outcome in patients unfit for open repair of abdominal aortic aneurysm (EVAR trial 2): randomized controlled trial. *Lancet.* 2005;365:9478.

Fink HA, Lederle FA, Roth CS, et al. The accuracy of physical examination to detect abdominal aortic aneurysm. *Arch Int Med.* 2000;160:833–836.

Fleisher LA, Fleischmann KE, Auerbach AD, et al. 2014 ACC/AHA guideline on perioperative cardiovascular evaluation and management of patients undergoing noncardiac surgery. *J Am Coll Cardiol.* 2014;64(22):e77LP–e77137.

Fleming C, Whitlock EP, Beil T, Lederle FA. Screening for abdominal aortic aneurysm: a systematic review and meta-analysis for the U.S. Preventative Services Task Force. *Ann Intern Med.* 2005;142:203–211.

Kim LG, Scott RAP, Ashton HA, Thompson SG. A sustained mortality benefit from screening for abdominal aortic aneurysm. *Ann Intern Med.* 2007;146(10):699–706.

Lederle FA. Rupture rate of large abdominal aortic aneurysms in patients refusing or unfit for elective repair. *JAMA.* 2002;287(22):2968.

Lederle FA, Johnson GR, Wilson SE, et al. for the Aneurysm Detection and Management (ADAM) Veterans Affairs Cooperative Study Investigators. Relationship of age, gender, race, and body size on infrarenal aortic diameter. *J Vascular Surgery.* 1997;26:595–601.

Lederle FA, Johnson GR, Wilson SE, et al. for the aneurysm detection and management study screening program: validation cohort and final results. *Archives Internal Medicine.* 2000;160:1425–1430.

Lederle FA, Wilson SE, Johnson GR, et al. for the Aneurysm Detection and Management (ADAM) Veterans Affairs Cooperative Study Investigators. Immediate repair compared with surveillance of small abdominal aortic aneurysms. *N. Engl. J. Med.* 2002;346:11437–11444.

Lin PH, Barshes NR, Albo D, et al. Concomitant colorectal cancer and abdominal aortic aneurysm: evolution of treatment paradigm in the endovascular era. *J Am Coll Surg.* 2008;206:1065–1073.

Nevitt MP, Ballard DJ, Hallett JW. Prognosis of abdominal aortic aneurysms: a population based study. *N Engl J Med.* 1989;321:1009–1014.

Prinssen M, Verhoeven ELG, Buth J, et al. A randomized trial comparing conventional and endovascular repair of aortic aneurysms. *N Engl J Med.* 2004;351:1607.

U.K. Small Aneurysm Trial Participants. Mortality results for randomized controlled trial of early elective surgery or ultrasonographic surveillance for small abdominal aortic aneurysms. *Lancet.* 1998;352:1649–1655.

U.S. Preventative Services Task Force. Abdominal aortic aneurysm: screening. http://www.uspreventiveservices-taskforce.org/uspstf14/abdoman/abdomandraftrec

Woo E, Damrauer S. Abdominal aortic aneurysms: open surgical treatment. Cronenwett JL, Johnston KW, eds. *Rutherfords Vascular Surgery.* Vols 1 and 2. Elsevier Saunders; 2014.

Yi J, Ali, Aamna M., Glebova, Natalia Abdominal aortic aneurysm and unexpected abdominal pathology. In: Cameron JL, Cameron AM, eds. *Current Surgical Therapy.* Elsevier; 2017.

Vascular Access

Booker T. King, Steven Vang, and Peter R. Nelson

1. A 40-year-old left-handed female with end-stage renal disease is being evaluated in the clinic for permanent hemodialysis access. Ultrasound venous mapping shows on the left a distal cephalic vein measuring 3.3 mm at the wrist and a basilic vein measuring 3.5 mm in the upper arm, and on the right, a cephalic vein measuring 3.1 mm above the elbow and 1.9 mm at the wrist. The best option for initial long-term hemodialysis access is:

   A. A left radial-cephalic arteriovenous (AV) fistula
   B. A right radial-cephalic AV fistula
   C. A left brachial-basilic AV graft
   D. A right brachial-cephalic AV fistula
   E. A right brachial-cephalic AV graft

2. A 65-year-old male with end-stage renal disease has recently had an autogenous right radial-cephalic AV fistula performed. The patient will require temporary dialysis access until the fistula matures. The best option for temporary access is:

   A. A cuffed, tunneled central venous dialysis catheter in the ipsilateral internal jugular vein
   B. A cuffed, tunneled central venous dialysis catheter in the contralateral subclavian vein
   C. A cuffed, tunneled central venous dialysis catheter in the contralateral internal jugular vein
   D. An uncuffed central venous dialysis catheter in the right femoral vein
   E. An uncuffed central venous dialysis catheter in the contralateral internal jugular vein

3. You are evaluating a patient for an autogenous AV fistula for long-term dialysis access. The patient has an abnormal right arm Allen test, and further workup confirms stenosis of the ulnar artery on that side. The patient has a temporary left subclavian central venous dialysis catheter currently. Vascular evaluation of the left arm and hand was unremarkable. What is the best option for long-term dialysis access in this patient?

   A. Placement of a radial-cephalic AV fistula in the right arm
   B. Placement of a brachial-basilic AV fistula in the right upper arm, as the more proximal location will not be affected by the ulnar artery stenosis
   C. Placement of a long-term central venous dialysis catheter (Permacath)
   D. Placement of a femoral-saphenous AV fistula in the left groin
   E. Change to a cuffed, tunneled central venous catheter in the right internal jugular vein, and proceed with creation of a left arm AV fistula

4. A 67-year-old patient presents in your office as a referral for urgent dialysis access, for immediate use. He was recently diagnosed with Stage IV pancreatic cancer, and was given a life expectancy of 3 to 6 months by his oncologist. Vascular evaluation of his bilateral upper extremities demonstrates adequate vasculature for autogenous access creation. What is the best option for dialysis access in this patient?

   A. Placement of a radial-cephalic AV fistula in his dominant arm
   B. Placement of a radial-cephalic AV fistula in his nondominant arm

C. Placement of an axillary-brachial AV synthetic graft in his dominant arm to prevent steal syndrome

D. Placement of a radial-cephalic AV fistula in his nondominant arm and an uncuffed central venous dialysis catheter in the contralateral side

E. Placement of a cuffed, tunneled central venous dialysis catheter alone

5. **A 50-year-old male presents with fever to 102.5°F, tachycardia, and malaise two months after placement of a prosthetic AV graft in his right forearm. The patient has erythema around the AV graft incision site, and the AV graft is warm and painful upon palpation. Blood cultures were obtained and preliminary gram stain shows a large number of gram positive cocci in clusters. A course of empiric intravenous antimicrobial therapy was started. What is the next step in the management of this patient?**

A. Schedule surgery urgently for the removal of prosthetic material from the right forearm and placement of a temporary dialysis catheter.

B. Continue culture-directed intravenous antibiotics for a 4-week course in an attempt to "sterilize" the AV graft.

C. Inject broad-spectrum antibiotics into the AV graft directly and place a tourniquet above the fistula for 30 minutes.

D. Continue empiric intravenous antimicrobial therapy for 7 days and then repeat blood cultures. No additional therapy is needed if blood cultures are negative.

E. Surgically remove prosthetic material from the right forearm and placement of an autogenous ipsilateral brachial-basilic AV fistula concurrently during this operation.

ANSWERS

1. **D.** The decision of where AV access should be created can be complex and needs to be individualized, but should start with three basic principles: (1) placement in the nondominant arm, (2) creation in most distal position possible, and (3) suitability of the vein conduit. Placement of the AV access in the nondominant arm allows for patients to remain functional and productive during the several hours of hemodialysis treatment. Additionally, the AV fistula is less likely to be unintentionally injured through the use

of the arm in daily activities; and, if there are complications such as steal, then the dominant arm is spared disability. The creation of the AV fistula at the most distal possible location in the arm preserves the more proximal veins of the arm for future access, if needed. Thresholds of a vein diameter of 2.5 mm and an arterial diameter of 2.0 mm have been previously recommended but not validated. However, patients with larger vein diameter have a higher maturation rate and better long-term patency rate compared to those with smaller veins. Arteries and veins smaller than 2.0 mm should undergo careful evaluation for feasibility. Lastly, autologous vein is preferred over grafts due to lower risk of infection, thrombosis, and need for access intervention.

2. **C.** A cuffed, tunneled dialysis catheter can be maintained for 6 weeks or more, while uncuffed catheters will need to be replaced at 3 weeks. An autogenous AV fistula on average will take 6 weeks to mature. Catheters placed in the ipsilateral internal jugular vein or either subclavian vein are associated with higher rates of AV fistula failure due to partial venous outflow obstruction; there is decreased risk of venous outflow obstruction with temporary dialysis catheter placed in the contralateral internal jugular vein. Catheter placement in the femoral vein is not ideal, especially in patients who are ambulatory. Femoral venous catheters have been associated with higher rates of venous thrombosis and bloodstream infections in several reports.

3. **E.** AV fistula placement in the right arm, given the right ulnar artery stenosis and normal vascular exam of the left upper extremity, is not an optimal choice, as either a radial artery- or brachial artery-based fistula places this patient at an increased risk for hemodialysis access-induced distal ischemia (HAIDI), also referred to as steal syndrome. Femoral-saphenous AV fistula is an inferior option due to increased risk of thrombosis and infection in this location. AV fistula placement in the left arm is the best option, and the temporary dialysis should be removed and a cuffed, tunneled catheter placed in the right internal jugular vein to decrease the risk of subclavian venous stenosis and thereby optimize fistula maturation as well as long-term patency.

4. **E.** This patient has a limited life expectancy. An autologous AV fistula usually takes 2 to 3 months

to mature before it can be used for hemodialysis. Alternatively, an AV graft is a looped, plastic tube that reduces the time to use to 2 to 3 weeks, but carries an increased risk of infection and thrombosis compared to an AV fistula. The patient in this question requires immediate use, which would require a temporary dialysis catheter to be placed. A non-cuffed tunneled catheter can be used for emergencies, however, should only be used for short periods (up to 3 weeks). For temporary access, longer than 3 weeks, either as a bridge to AV fistula use or in patients with limited life expectancy, a cuffed tunneled catheter is the ideal access option for hemodialysis.

5. **A.** The patient in this question has an infected AV graft. This patient is bacteremic as result of the graft infection and is at risk to progress to severe systemic sepsis, which can lead to death if not treated appropriately and expeditiously. Antibiotic therapy should be introduced immediately, and empiric broad spectrum antibiotics are advised since the patient has likely been exposed to resistant hospital pathogens. In this case, methicillin-resistant Staphylococcus aureus (MRSA) is the most likely pathogen, and vancomycin provides targeted antimicrobial treatment. The prosthetic material in the graft is the source of the infection and therefore must be removed in its entirety. Any attempt to eradicate the graft infection with antibiotic therapy alone will fail. The placement of a new autogenous AV fistula should be postponed until the infection is adequately treated. A temporary uncuffed central venous dialysis catheter can be utilized during this hospitalization, with transition to a cuffed, tunneled central venous dialysis catheter after the infection is adequately treated and blood cultures are negative.

BIBLIOGRAPHY

Bashar K, Clarke-Moloney M, Burke PE, Kavanagh EG, Walsh SR. The role of venous diameter in predicting arteriovenous fistula maturation: when not to expect an AVF to mature according to pre-operative vein diameter measurements? A best evidence topic. *Int J Surg.* 2015;15: 95–99.

Hall RK, Myers ER, Rosas SE, O'Hare AM, Colón-Emeric CS. Choice of hemodialysis access in older adults: a cost-effectiveness analysis. *Clin J Am Soc Nephrol.* 2017;12(6): 947–954.

Lauvao L, Ihnat D, Goshima K, Chavez L, Gruessner A, Mills J. Vein diameter is the major predictor of fistula maturation. *J Vasc Surg.* 2009;49(6):1499–1504.

Lee T. Fistula first initiative: historical impact on vascular access practice patterns and influence on future vascular access care. *Cardiovasc Eng Technol.* 2017;8(3):244–254.

Pereira K, Osiason A, Salsamendi J. Vascular access for placement of tunneled dialysis catheters for hemodialysis: a systematic approach and clinical practice algorithm. *J Clin Imaging Sci.* 2015;5:31.

Segal M, Qaja E. Types of arteriovenous fistulas. StatPearls [Internet]. https://www.ncbi.nlm.nih.gov/books/NBK493195/

Siddiqui MA, Ashraff S, Carline T. Maturation of arteriovenous fistula: analysis of key factors. *Kidney Res Clin Pract.* 2017;36(4):318–328.

Vascular Access 2006 Work Group. Clinical practice guidelines for vascular access. *Am J Kidney Dis.* 2006;48(Suppl 1): S176–S247.

Whittier WL. Surveillance of hemodialysis vascular access. *Semin Intervent Radiol.* 2009;26(2):130–138.

102

Complications of Hemodialysis

Alexander Malloy, Vernon Horst and Kelly Kempe

1. **A 67-year-old male with end stage renal disease returns to your vascular clinic 2 weeks after he had a left autogenous brachio-basilic AV fistula performed. He complains of intractable pain in his left hand and that hand is colder. He also has dark ulcers of the distal end of fingers 2 to 4 with purulent fluid on digit 3 from the ulcer. His left hand is without radial or ulnar pulses, but he is palpable on the right hand for both. What is the most likely cause of this condition?**

   A. Emboli that have traveled from the brachial artery to the radial artery

   B. Arterial flow is being shunted away from the distal radial and ulnar arteries into the venous outflow of the AV fistula.

   C. An air embolus formed in the radial artery from air trapped in the dialysis circuit that has traveled to the arterial system of the hand.

   D. An unrecognized arterial stenosis in the distal radial artery that has become symptomatic

   E. Intermittent vasospasm of the brachial artery brought on by hemodialysis

2. **For the patient in Question 1, what is the best definitive treatment of his condition?**

   A. Fogarty catheter balloon thromboembolectomy of the brachial, radial, and ulnar arteries

   B. Ligation of the fistula, and placement of a cuffed, tunneled central venous dialysis catheter in the left internal jugular vein and consulting hand surgery

   C. Consulting hand surgery and requesting amputation of the distal phalanges of fingers 2 to 4

   D. Left upper extremity angiogram with balloon angioplasty of a distal radial artery lesion

   E. Topical nitroglycerin paste to the fingers during hemodialysis to improve blood flow via vasodilation

3. **You receive a phone call from an outpatient hemodialysis unit regarding your 57-year-old female patient with end-stage renal disease. The patient undergoes hemodialysis thrice per week via a left arm brachiobasilic fistula that is 12 years old. She last underwent successful hemodialysis 2 days ago; the dialysis staff are unable to access the fistula, and they can no longer hear a thrill or feel a bruit. From prior vein mapping, she is known to have adequate forearm and upper arm vasculature for hemodialysis creation in the right arm. What is the best treatment plan for this patient?**

   A. Placement of an uncuffed central venous dialysis catheter in the left subclavian vein

   B. Urgent thrombectomy, fistulogram, and revision/endovascular therapy of the fistula

   C. Systemic thrombolysis with recombinant tissue plasminogen activator (tPA)

   D. Creation of a right forearm radiocephalic fistula and placement of a cuffed, tunneled central venous dialysis catheter in the right subclavian vein

   E. Creation of a left axillary-brachial arteriovenous fistula using synthetic graft, and placement of a right internal jugular cuffed, tunneled central venous dialysis catheter

4. You are called to the post-anesthesia recovery room to evaluate your patient with left arm pain after you successfully created a left arm brachiobasilic arteriovenous fistula. She is a 64 year-old lady with a medical history of well-controlled diabetes mellitus diagnosed 18 years ago; and chronic kidney disease, stage IV; and left below-knee amputation. She is complaining bitterly of left forearm pain, and she is unable to move her entire left hand. Her fistula has a palpable thrill and an audible bruit with stethoscope evaluation, her bilateral radial pulses are easily palpable, and her hands are warm. What is the best treatment for this patient?

   A. Increase in her narcotic pain regimen
   B. Immediate left brachial-radial bypass graft with reversed greater saphenous vein harvest
   C. Immediate ligation of her arteriovenous fistula.
   D. Outpatient referral to physical therapy for strengthening exercises
   E. Immediate distal revascularization and interval ligation (DRIL) procedure

5. You are called to the emergency department to evaluate a 49-year-old patient with end-stage renal disease on dialysis via a right forearm brachiobasilic fistula that was created 7 years ago. He takes 81 mg of aspirin, but no anticoagulants or other antiplatelet agents. He underwent successful dialysis yesterday, and when he took the bandages off this morning, he had pulsatile bleeding from one of his access sites; direct pressure was applied by the patient until emergency medical services (EMS) arrived, and EMS applied a pressure dressing for transport to the hospital. The patient has stable vital signs, all well within normal limits. On your evaluation, the fistula is pulsatile, with a bruit noted on stethoscope examination; a fresh drop of blood is noted on the skin, and the patient indicates that this is the location that bled this morning. The radial pulse is palpable, and the hand is warm. He has had a similar episode 3 weeks ago. His hemoglobin is similar to that hospital visit. What is the best treatment of this patient's bleeding diathesis?

   A. Pressure dressing until the bleeding stops, then discharge home
   B. Place a purse string suture using dissolvable suture at the bleeding site for hemostasis, and discharge home with follow-up as needed

   C. Schedule for urgent fistulogram
   D. Full biochemical workup to evaluate for medical causes of bleeding
   E. Compress the fistula to cause it to thrombose, and subsequently place a tunneled, cuffed central venous dialysis catheter.

6. A 46-year-old patient who undergoes peritoneal dialysis for end-stage renal disease develops peritonitis. The patient is hemodynamically normal, without volume overload or significant electrolyte abnormality. What is the recommended treatment?

   A. Laparotomy and peritoneal washout
   B. Peritoneal dialysis catheter removal
   C. Empiric gram negative and gram positive coverage with intraperitoneal and oral antibiotics
   D. Empiric gram negative, gram positive, and antifungal intravenous coverage
   E. Emergent temporary uncuffed central venous dialysis catheter placement and initiation of hemodialysis

7. This patient's peritonitis does not improve, and yeast is isolated on the gram stain. What is the recommended management of this patient?

   A. Peritoneal lavage, intraperitoneal fluconazole, and catheter removal
   B. Catheter removal and intravenous fluconazole
   C. Intraperitoneal amphotericin B followed by catheter removal
   D. Peritoneal lavage followed by catheter removal
   E. Catheter removal and immediate hemodialysis

ANSWERS

1. **B.** The arterial insufficiency with new fingertip ulcerations that is seen in this patient is an example of hemodialysis access-induced distal ischemia (HAIDI), also referred to as steal syndrome. Arterial flow is being diverted away from the hand into the venous outflow (in this case, the basilic vein) after fistula creation. This phenomenon occurs in all AV fistulas to some degree, but in some cases, the extent of arterial insufficiency is such that the condition becomes symptomatic. Patients may present with a wide constellation of symptoms, from mild tingling in the fingertips that occurs only during hemodialysis to severe pain in the hand or gangrene, and the severity dictates treatment; left untreated in a severe

form, this can progress to digit loss as well as permanent dysfunction of the hand. The diagnosis can be confirmed by improvement of distal blood flow noted on PPGs or duplex ultrasound with compression of the fistula.

2. **B.** Given the presentation of HAIDI, this patient needs surgical treatment to improve blood flow to the distal extremity. The preferred treatment for HAIDI depends on the severity of the presentation. In patients without tissue loss (dry gangrene, ulcers, or open wounds), decreasing the flow through the fistula may sufficiently treat their symptoms by either plication or banding of the fistula, or revision of the anastomotic revision. However, patients with tissue loss require treatment that is more definitive in order to optimize salvage of the hand and fingers. This usually includes ligation of the fistula to maximize arterial pressure to the digits, and placement of a cuffed, tunneled central venous dialysis catheter in patients already on hemodialysis. Amputation of fingers can be severely disabling, and a digital amputation due to ischemia, without revascularization, would not be expected to heal.

3. **B.** Dialysis access thrombosis is a known complication, which must be treated promptly. Thrombectomy can be done by either percutaneous or open surgical techniques, with some studies suggesting that percutaneous thrombectomy may have more favorable outcomes. Regardless of the technique used, after successful thrombectomy, it is important to evaluate the entire length of the access via a fistulogram, from the arterial anastomsosis to the central veins, for areas of stenosis that may have contributed to the thrombotic event and treat the found cause. Thrombosis of the access causes concern for a failing access, and development of a plan for future access creation is important; however, immediate abandonment of an access due to thrombosis is not the best plan. If the surgeon is unable to successfully perform a thrombectomy, then a tunneled, cuffed central venous dialysis catheter should be placed in the internal jugular vein, contralateral to the next intended access site if possible. Catheter placement within the subclavian veins is known to increase intimal hyperplasia and therefore outflow stenosis, and should be avoided. Use of tissue plasminogen activator (tPA) is common in percutaneous thrombolysis, but this is catheter-directed into the thrombosed access, not administered systemically. Lastly, as this patient has adequate vasculature for autogenous access creation, use of synthetic graft should be avoided.

4. **C.** Ischemic monomelic neuropathy (IMN) is a rare complication of brachial artery fistula creation. Most cases occur in elderly patients with long-standing diabetes and preexisting peripheral neuropathy. Upon emergence from anesthesia, patients will complain of intense arm pain with associated weakness or paralysis. These patients will clinically have excellent distal perfusion, with palpable pulse or strong Doppler signals in the distal radial and ulnar arteries, and a bypass or thrombectomy of the arterial tree will ineffectively treat this pathology. The surgical site must be evaluated for a hematoma, as a brachial sheath hematoma will compress the median nerve; the radial and ulnar nerves, however, would be spared in that scenario. Treatment of IMN incudes immediate ligation of the fistula to optimize arterial flow to the peripheral nerves. Extensive physical therapy will be necessary after ligation of the fistula, in an effort to optimize functional recovery, but therapy alone will be ineffective at treating her injury.

5. **B.** Intimal hyperplasia (IH) is a common issue related to both autologous and synthetic hemodialysis access. IH can occur at any location along the outflow of an autologous access, including in the central venous outflow (axillary, subclavian, and innominate veins), while IH is typically is found at the venous anastomosis in patients with synthetic grafts. This insidious buildup results in stenosis, and this can present as a pulsatile fistula with increased bleeding after decannulation. Therefore, the proper treatment for patients who present with increased access bleeding is a contrast fistulogram, which allows for the diagnosis of stenosis at any location along the outflow as well as treatment of the stenosis. Discharging the patient without addressing the etiology of his bleeding is an unsafe plan. While both medical anticoagulation as well as intrinsic bleeding diatheses can certainly contribute to access bleeding, bleeding due to IH should be evaluated and treated first. Significant effort should be made to preserve dialysis access and to limit catheter reliance.

6. C. Peritonitis is a common complication of peritoneal dialysis and is the primary reason for cessation of peritoneal dialysis with transition to hemodialysis. Peritonitis in patients who undergo peritoneal dialysis has significant morbidity but are managed with empiric outpatient antibiotics in over 75% of cases. Current guidelines state that empiric gram negative and gram positive coverage with antibiotics are indicated. Outpatient antibiotics typically include intraperitoneal and oral administration, such as intraperitoneal cefazolin and oral ciprofloxacin, but inpatient regimens can include intravenous, intraperitoneal, or oral modalities. Monotherapy is also available in intravenous form with imipenem/cilastatin. Empiric antifungal coverage is not recommended due to emerging resistance to antifungals and a large review revealed that only 2% of peritoneal dialysis-associated peritonitis were from fungal elements. Laparotomy would not be recommended even if the patient were hemodynamically unstable, unless there was another precipitating cause of peritonitis such as bowel perforation or hemorrhage. Peritoneal dialysis catheter removal is not a first-line treatment for microbial peritonitis. Indications for catheter removal are relapsing peritonitis, lack of antimicrobial response within 5 days of initiation, or tunnel or insertion sites that involve infection. Placement of a temporary dialysis catheter and initiation of hemodialysis is not indicated in this patient, as he is hemodynamically normal without any gross electrolyte disturbance.

7. A. If fungal elements are isolated on gram stain or culture, prompt removal of the dialysis catheter and administration of intraperitoneal or intravenous antifungals should be initiated. Intraperitoneal amphotericin B is generally not recommended as it causes additional pain to the patient and is known for developing significant intraperitoneal adhesions. Typically, the peritoneal fluid has a grossly cloudy appearance and should be lavaged with normal saline until clear. The patient should undergo hemodialysis in the near future for a minimum of 6 weeks. Immediate hemodialysis is not necessary unless clinically indicated via signs of acidosis, electrolyte imbalance, uremia, or fluid overload. After the 6-week period, a new peritoneal catheter can be placed if the patient desires.

BIBLIOGRAPHY

Harris LM, Rivero M. Hemodialysis access: nonthrombotic complications. In: Sidawy AN, Perler BA, eds. *Rutherford's Vascular Surgery and Endovascular Therapy.* 9th ed. Elsevier; 2019:2335.

Li PK, Szeto CC, Piraino B, et al. Peritoneal dialysis-related infections recommendations: 2010 update. *Perit Dial Int.* 2010;30(4):393.

Meier GH. Hemodialysis access: failing and thrombosed. In: Sidawy AN, Perler BA, eds. *Rutherford's Vascular Surgery and Endovascular Therapy.* 9th ed. Elsevier; 2019:2324–2333.

Port FK, Held PJ, Nolph KD, Turenne MN, Wolfe RA. Risk of peritonitis and technique failure by CAPD connection technique: a national study. *Kidney Int.* 1992;42(4):967.

Sherman RA, Daugirdas JT, Ing TS. Complications during hemodialysis. In: Daugirdas JT, Ing TS, eds. *Handbook of Dialysis.* 4th ed. Lippincott Williams and Wilkins; 2007:170.

Stablein DM, Nolph KD, Lindblad AS. Timing and characteristics of multiple peritonitis episodes: a report of the National CAPD Registry. *Am J Kidney Dis.* 1989;14(1):44.

Wang AY, Yu AW, Li PK, et al. Factors predicting outcome of fungal peritonitis in peritoneal dialysis: analysis of a 9-year experience of fungal peritonitis in a single center. *Am J Kidney Dis.* 2000;36(6):1183.

103

Lymphatic Disease

Hyein Kim

SCENARIO 1

A 65-year-old man presents to your clinic with complaints of increasing right lower extremity "heaviness" and swelling over the last 2 to 3 months. He states his symptoms worsen throughout the day and his shoes feel tight by the time he takes them off at night. He denies any skin changes, wounds, or recent trauma to the area. He also denies any fevers, chills, fatigue, weight loss, or weight gain. His past medical history is significant for hypertension, obesity, and a recent history of melanoma of the right lower extremity for which he underwent resection of the lesion with regional lymph node dissection. His social history and family history are unremarkable and he denies any recent travel.

He has never smoked and denies any alcohol use. He does not exercise regularly and takes an ACE inhibitor and a multivitamin daily. His vital signs are a temperature of 38°C, heart rate of 72 beats per minute, blood pressure of 135/74 mmHg, respiratory rate of 14 breaths per minute, and oxygen saturation of 99% on room air. Physical examination demonstrates diffuse non-painful pitting edema over his right lower extremity that extends over the dorsum of his foot including his toes. There is no evidence of skin discoloration or open wounds. He has easily palpable pulses and good capillary refill. His right lower extremity measures 4 cm greater in circumference than his left lower extremity. There are no palpable masses in his groin. His other extremities are normal in appearance and the rest of his physical exam is unremarkable.

1. **This patient is most likely suffering from which disease process?**

    A. Chronic venous insufficiency

    B. Filariasis

    C. Nephrotic syndrome

    D. Lymphedema

2. **The most common cause of secondary lymphedema worldwide is:**

    A. Malignancy or a result of its treatment

    B. Lymphedema praecox

    C. Wuchereria bancrofti

    D. Lymphedma tarda

3. **The best test for diagnosing this patient with suspected lymphedema is:**

    A. Lymphangiography

    B. Computerized tomography (CT) scan

    C. Magnetic resonance imaging (MRI)

    D. Detailed history and physical exam

    E. Lymphoscintigraphy

4. **The first-line treatment of lymphedema consists of:**

    A. Diuretics

    B. Lymphatic reconstruction or excision of diseased channels

    C. Compressive therapy

    D. Benzopyrones (Coumarin) and long-term antibiotics

5. **You diagnose this patient with lymphedema and start him on the appropriate therapy. He returns to your clinic a few years later with a painful, purplish ulcerating macule on his right lower extremity. This presentation is most concerning for:**

    A. Lymphangitis

    B. Lymphangiosarcoma

C. Hematoma

D. Thrombophlebitis

SCENARIO 2

A 23-year-old female presents with symptoms of unilateral right lower extremity swelling. She complains of "heaviness" as well as concerns for cosmesis. Her swelling started about 6 months ago and has been progressively worse since. She underwent excision of melanoma of the right leg with regional lymph node dissection 1 year ago. She denies any pain or redness of the right leg, shortness of breath, chest pain, fever, chills, weight loss, weight gain, or any other complaints. She has never smoked and denies alcohol use. She denies any family member with similar problem or recent travel. On physical exam, she has non-pitting edema involving right lower calf, ankle, foot, and toes. The skin fold at the base of the second toe is significantly thickened (Stemmer's sign). Prior to today's visit, her primary care provider obtained bilateral lower extremity venous duplex and reflux studies, which were within normal limits.

6. **What is the condition that she is most likely suffering from?**

   A. Acute on chronic deep venous thrombosis

   B. Lipedema

   C. Primary lymphedema

   D. Secondary lymphedema

7. **What is the most appropriate anatomic location for injection of radioactive solution (i.e., Tc-99m sulfur colloid mixed with saline) for lymphoscintigraphy to evaluate lymphedema of the lower extremity?**

   A. Intravascularly, to the posterior tibial artery or vein

   B. Intradermally, between the first and second toe web space

   C. Subcutaneously, on the dorsum of the foot

   D. Intramuscularly, in the calf

ANSWERS

1. **D.** This patient is most likely suffering from lymphedema. He is suffering from unilateral lower extremity edema, which excludes systemic etiologies of his edema, such as nephrotic syndrome, liver disease, and heart failure. Infection is a more common cause of secondary lymphedema worldwide, although this patient denies any travel history. Venous pathology, such as chronic venous insufficiency, is by far the most common cause of unilateral lower extremity edema. Lower extremity edema caused by venous pathology typically presents with pitting edema that spares the feet. Due to the prolonged venous disease, the skin can become atrophic with hemosiderin pigmentation.

   This patient has a history of lower extremity melanoma with regional lymph node dissection, which is a risk factor for developing lymphedema. Other risk factors include increased body mass index, tumor location, postoperative infection or hematoma, and radiation therapy. Additional malignancies that have been associated with the development of lymphedema are sarcomas, gynecologic cancer, genitourinary cancer and head and neck cancer, but the most common malignancy to be associated with the development of lymphedema is breast cancer, with an incidence of 17% among survivors.

2. **C.** The most common cause of secondary lymphedema worldwide is filariasis from infection by the *nematodes Wuchereria bancrofti*. In developed nations, almost all cases of secondary lymphedema are caused by a sequela of malignancy or as a result of its treatment. Lymphedema praecox is the most common form of primary lymphedema and accounts for around 94% of cases. The onset is usually seen in children and teenagers and is predominantly seen in women with a ratio of 10:1 compared to men. Lymphedema tarda is an uncommon cause of primary lymphedema with an age of onset of 35 years old or greater and accounts for less than 10% of cases.

3. **D.** Diagnosis of lymphedema is relatively simple in the second and third stages of the disease. When lymphedema is in the first stage (i.e., pitting, mild, and relieved by elevation), diagnosis can be more difficult. In patients with suspected secondary forms of lymphedema, CT scan and MRI are useful in excluding an underlying malignant etiology. In most patients, the diagnosis of lymphedema can be made based on a thorough history and physical exam alone. Also, patients with previous known lymph node excision, such as the patient in the vignette, do not require additional studies for diagnosis of lymphedema (further imaging is only necessary as

needed for follow-up for each underlying malignancy). In cases where the diagnosis of lymphedema is suspected but the etiology is unclear, lymphoscintigraphy is the diagnostic test of choice.

Lymphoscintigraphy has a sensitivity around 70% to 90% and a specificity of nearly 100%. Lymphangiography provides the best detail of the lymphatic system, but due to complications such as lymphangitis, pulmonary embolism, allergic reaction to the contrast dye, and further damage to the lymphatic vessels, it is reserved for patients being considered for lymphatic reconstruction.

4. C. There is no curative treatment for lymphedema. The goals of treatment are to minimize swelling and prevent infections to the affected limb. Patients are at increased risk of developing recurrent infections such as cellulitis, erysipelas, and lymphangitis. A combination of physical therapies (CPT) is the primary approach to the management of lymphedema. CPT involves good skin care followed by manual lymphatic drainage through massage, bed rest with leg elevation, and application of graded compression stockings and sequential pneumatic compression devices. When worn daily, compression stockings have shown long-term maintenance of reduced limb circumference, and may protect against external trauma and the development of skin and subcutaneous tissue thickening.

No drug therapy for the treatment of lymphedema has been shown to be effective. Diuretics can be useful in an acute exacerbation secondary to infection or if seen with coexisting venous disease, but is not useful for long-term care of lymphedema. Coumarin is still under investigation as a potential treatment for lymphedema, but currently has no role in treatment in the United States.

Although patients with lymphedema are at increased risk of developing recurrent infections, prophylactic use of antibiotics has no role in the treatment. Instead, patients should be prescribed antibiotics that they can keep with them and take at the first signs or symptoms of an infection.

Patients with lymphedema can be managed nonoperatively 95% of the time. Operative intervention may be considered for patients with Stage II or Stage III disease who have severe functional disability.

Stage I: Mild disease, self-limiting symptoms such as edema which often resolves with elevation

Stage II: Moderate disease, non-resolving edema with elevation and fibrosis

Stage III: Severe disease, irreversible edema, fibrosis, and sclerosis of the skin/subcutaneous tissue as well as large deformed limb (lymphostatic elephantiasis)

Surgical intervention is made up of two categories: excisional or reconstructive. Long-term follow-up data for surgical care of lymphedema is not available currently, and is therefore not well accepted as a mainstay of treatment throughout the world.

5. B. This clinical presentation is most concerning for lymphangiosarcoma. Lymphangiosarcoma is a rare malignant tumor that can occur in patients suffering from chronic lymphedema. The tumor originates in vascular endothelial cells and manifests clinically as a reddish-blue or purple skin lesion with a macular shape, an ulcer, a poor healing eschar, or a firm painful nodule.

Lymphangitis is usually caused by group A beta-hemolytic streptococcal or staphylococcal infections and presents in an area of cellulitis. It clinically presents with pain and multiple linear, long, red streaks toward the regional lymph nodes and can even manifest as a systemic response with fevers, chills, sepsis, or death. Treatment consists of warm compresses and intravenous antibiotics.

Thrombophlebitis clinically presents with an erythematous palpable cord along a superficial vein. Causes of thrombophlebitis are from an indwelling catheter, venous stasis, intravenous drug use, or an occult hypercoagulable state. Treatment includes compression stockings and anti-inflammatory medications with surgery being reserved for clusters of varicosities or cases of suppurative septic thrombophlebitis.

6. D. Secondary lymphedema is the most likely diagnosis for this patient as she underwent melanoma excision with reginal lymph node dissection, which put her at high risk of developing lymphedema. Secondary lymphedema is mostly associated with previous surgery, trauma, or infection. Primary lymphedema is associated with unclear ethology. Lipedema is a disorder of adipose tissue and usually presents with swelling of bilateral lower extremities symmetrically without involvement of the feet and toes. Given the normal venous duplex and reflux studies, it is unlikely that this patient is suffering from acute chronic venous thrombosis.

7. B. In most patients, the diagnosis of lymphedema can be made based on obtaining history and physical exam alone. However, in cases where the diagnosis and etiology of lymphedema are unclear, lymphoscintigraphy can be utilized as the diagnostic modality. Lymphoscintigraphy is 70% to 90% sensitive and nearly 100% specific; therefore, it is the primary imaging choice for diagnostic confirmation of lymphedema and to define lymphatic anatomy. This imaging modality uses the transport system of lymphatic and its mobile proteins from the interstitial space into the venous system. Radiolabeled colloids such as sulfur colloid with technetium-99m are injected into intradermal space because of the highest concentration of lymphatics in the dermal layer. Intravascular and intramuscular injections are not utilized for lymphoscintigraphy.

BIBLIOGRAPHY

Browse N, Burnand K, Mortimer P, eds. *Diseases of the Lymphatics*. Arnold (Hodder Headline); 2003.

Burnand KG, McGuinness CL, lagattolla NR, et al. Value of isotope lymphography in the diagnosis of lymphedema of the leg. *BR J Surg*. 2002;89:74–78.

Cambria RA, Gloviczki P, Naessens JM, et al. Noninvasive evaluation of the lymphatic system with lymphoscintigraphy: a prospective semiquantitative analysis in 386 extremities. *J Vasc Surg*. 1993;18:773–782.

Cormier JN, Askew RL, Mungovan KS, et al. Lymphedema beyond breast cancer: a systematic review and metaanalysis of cancer-related secondary lymphedema. *Cancer*. 2010;116:5138.

Disipio T, Rye S, Newman B, Hayes S. Incidence of unilateral arm lymphoedema after breast cancer: a systemic review and meta-analysis. *Lancet Oncol*. 2013;14:500.

Freischlag JA, Heller JA. Venous disease. In: Beauchamp RD, Evers BM, Mattox KL, et al., eds. *Sabiston Textbook of Surgery: The Biological Basis of Modern Surgical Practice*. 19th ed. Elsevier Saunders; 2008:2017.

Gamble F, Cheville A, Strick D. Lymphedema: medical and physical therapy. In: Glovinczki P, ed. *Handbook of Venous Disorders*. 3rd ed. Hodder Arnold; 2008.

Liem TK, Moneta GL. Venous and lymphatic disease. In: Brunicardi FC, Andersen DK, Billiar TR, et al., eds. *Schwartz's Principles of Surgery*. 9th ed. McGraw-Hill Professional; 2009:1–47.

Marotel M, Cluzan R, Ghabboun S, et al. Transaxial computer tomography of lower extremity lymphedema. *Lymphology*. 1998;31:180–185.

Moshiri M, Katz DS, Boris M, et al. Using lymphoscintigraphy to evaluate suspected lymphedema of the extremities. *Am J Roentgenol*. 2002;178(2):405–412.

Pipinos II, Baxter BT. The lymphatics. In: Beauchamp RD, Evers BM, Mattox KL, et al., eds. *Sabiston Textbook of Surgery: The Biological Basis of Modern Surgical Practice*. 19th ed. Elsevier Saunders; 2008:2020–2027.

Rockson SG. Lymphedema. Lymphedema. Current treatment options. *Cardivasc Med*. 2006;8:129–136.

Rooke TW, Felty CL. Lymphedema: pathophysiology, classification, and clinical evaluation. In: Glovinczki P, ed. *Handbook of Venous Disorders*. 3rd ed. Hodder Arnold; 2008.

Tiwari A, Cheng KS, Button M, et al. Differential diagnosis, investigation, a current treatment of lower limb lymphedema. *Arch Surg*. 2003;138:152–161.

Tomita K, Yokogawa A, Oda Y, Terahata S. Lymphangiosarcoma in postmastectomy lymphedema (Stewart-Treves Syndrome): ultrastructural and immunohistologic characteristics. *J Surg Oncol*. 1988;38:275.

Tretbar LL, Morgan CL, Lee BB, et al., eds. *Lymphedema: Diagnosis and Treatment*. Springer-Verlag Limited; 2008:45.

Wakefield TW, Rectenwald JR, Messina LM. Veins and Lymphatics. In: Doherty GM, ed. *Current Diagnosis and Treatment Surgery*. 13th ed. McGraw-Hill Medical; 2009:804.

Warren AG, Brorson H, Borud LJ, Slavin SA. Lymphedema: a comprehensive review. *Ann Plast Surg*. 2007;59(4):464–472.

Weissleder H, Weissleder R. Interstitial lymphangiography: initial clinical experience with a dimeric nonionic contrast agent. *Radiology*. 1989;170:371–374.

Werner GT, Scheck R, Kaiserling E. Magnetic resonance imaging of peripheral lymphedema. *Lymphology*. 1998;31: 34–36.

Yasuhara H, Shigematsu H, Muto T. A study of the advantages of elastic stockings for leg lymphedema. *Int Angiol*. 1996;15:272.

104
Venous Stasis Disease

Hyein Kim

SCENARIO 1

A 48-year-old female presents with a 10-month history of left, lower extremity swelling with worsening swelling and "crampy" pain over the last 2 days. She has a history of hypertension for which she takes hydrochlorothiazide. Her medical history is otherwise unremarkable. She has no family history of thrombophilia. On physical examination, her distal pulses are easily palpable. She is noted to have multiple bilateral lower extremity varicosities as well as a brawny appearing, well-granulated ulcer over the left medial malleolus. The circumference of her left thigh is noted to be 5 cm greater than that of the right thigh and her left calf is 4 cm greater in circumference than that of the right calf. CT scan of the pelvis is consistent with May-Thurner Syndrome (MTS).

1. **Which of the following statements regarding MTS is true?**

   A. MTS-related thrombus accounts for 15% to 20% of all lower extremity deep venous thromboses.

   B. Compression of the right common iliac vein by the left common iliac artery is the most common cause of MTS.

   C. A common cause of MTS-related mortality is acute pulmonary embolism.

   D. Duplex ultrasound is the best imaging modality with which to assess for iliac thrombus.

   E. In the setting of MTS associated thrombosis, anticoagulation alone is the most effective first-line treatment.

2. **Which of the following statements regarding chronic venous insufficiency (CVI) is true?**

   A. Venous stasis ulcers are often located over the lateral malleolus.

   B. Ultrasound is of limited utility in the diagnosis of venous insufficiency.

   C. Distal extremity ulcerations associated with arterial disease are twice as common as venous stasis ulcers.

   D. The Trendelenberg test can be used to distinguish between superficial and deep venous system reflux.

   E. Calf muscle dysfunction plays no role in venous insufficiency.

3. **Which of the following is true regarding the medical management of CVI?**

   A. Systemic antibiotics are recommended as part of the routine treatment of venous stasis ulcers.

   B. Hydrocolloid dressings have not been shown to improve ulcer wound healing over simple non-adherent dressings.

   C. Inelastic compression systems are more effective than multilayer compression systems with an elastic component.

   D. Moderate exercise may limit venous ulcer wound healing.

   E. Intermittent pneumatic compression devices are considered first-line treatment in the majority of patients.

4. **Which of the following is true regarding the surgical management of CVI?**

   A. The risk of greater saphenous nerve injury is increased with greater saphenous vein (GSV) stripping distal to the knee.

B. Radiofrequency ablation of the GSV is not effective at preventing long-term recurrence of venous reflux.

C. Tumescent solution is not commonly used when performing endovenous laser ablation.

D. With regard to endovenous laser ablation, longer laser wavelengths are better absorbed by hemoglobin and therefore exert less of an ablative effect on the vein wall.

E. Allograft placement in conjunction with compression has not been shown to improve wound healing.

5. **Which of the following is true regarding varicose veins?**

A. They are more prevalent in men.

B. Liquid sclerotherapy is superior to foam treatment in the setting of GSV reflux.

C. Ischemic stroke has been reported as a complication of the use of foam sclerotherapy.

D. Varicose veins are rarely painful.

E. The use of compression stockings prevents the progression of uncomplicated varicose veins.

SCENARIO 2

A 67-year-old woman, former smoker, who was recently diagnosed with a metastatic lung cancer, is admitted to the hospital with one-day history of extensive right iliofemoral venous thrombosis. She is retired but used to work as a hairstylist. On physical examination, she has easily palpable femoral, popliteal and pedal pulses, bilaterally. However, she has multiple bilateral lower extremity varicose veins, dark brownish skin discoloration and superficial, well-granulated ulcer over the right medial malleolus. She is scheduled to undergo a surgical resection for her lung cancer within a month. She is very anxious to know about treatment and long-term sequela of the deep vein thrombosis (DVT) as she is very active and athletic and wants to go back to her regular exercise regimen as soon as possible.

6. **Which of the following is true regarding the most common presentation of primary CVI?**

A. Superficial thrombophlebitis is the most common manifestation.

B. Varicose veins are the most commonly presenting symptoms.

C. Unilateral disease is more common than bilateral presentation.

D. More than 90% of patients present for cosmetic reasons.

E. Lateral malleolar venous stasis ulcers and edema are the most frequently presenting symptoms.

7. **As compared to anticoagulation alone, which of the following statements regarding catheter-directed thrombolysis (CDT) for the management of acute iliofemoral deep venous thrombosis (DVT) is true?**

A. Anticoagulation alone is the first-line treatment.

B. CDT is associated with higher mortality.

C. The risk of intracranial hemorrhage is decreased with CDT.

D. CDT decreases the risk of post-thrombotic syndrome (PTS).

E. CDT patients have higher readmission rates.

8. **Which of the following statements is the recommended venous thromboembolism (VTE) prophylaxis in the setting of the surgical resection for a metastatic malignancy?**

A. Sequential compression devices (SCDs) are recommended.

B. Unfractionated heparin (UFH) 5,000 units subcutaneously three times a day while in the hospital and then low-dose warfarin for life.

C. Routine prophylactic inferior vena cava (IVC) filter placement.

D. SCDs and low molecular weight heparin (LMWH) for 4 weeks of LMWH postoperatively.

E. UFH 5,000 units subcutaneously three times a day while in the hospital and then aspirin for life.

ANSWERS

1. C. Causes of mortality in the acute setting include pulmonary embolism and iliac vein rupture resulting in a retroperitoneal hemorrhage. Individuals with chronic MTS may develop chronic left lower extremity edema as well as venous stasis ulcers. MTS-related thrombosis accounts for 2% to 3% of lower extremity DVTs and is most often seen in females 20 to 40 years old. Autopsy studies indicate that anatomic features consistent with MTS are found in 22% to 32% of individuals in the general population.

MTS is most commonly the result of compression of the left common iliac vein by an overlying right common iliac artery, although anatomic variants involving compression of the IVC and right common iliac vein do exist. Over time, chronic compression of the iliac vein leads to endothelial injury and thrombus formation. Acute MTS-related thrombosis is often heralded by the sudden onset of left lower extremity pain and swelling and may be precipitated by pregnancy or recent abdominal surgery.

Duplex ultrasound lacks the sensitivity to detect most cases of ileofemoral thrombus. The preferred imaging modalities in cases of MTS include CT with venous-phase contrast or magnetic resonance (MR) venogram.

Catheter-directed thrombolyses as well as percutaneous mechanical thrombectomy with the addition of endovascular stent placement are the treatments of choice for the management of acute MTS-associated thrombosis. Anticoagulation alone or with mechanical thrombectomy without stent placement results in re-thrombosis rates upward of 70%. Endovascular stent placement is also considered the first-line treatment of MTS without evidence of iliac thrombus.

2. **D.** The Trendelenberg test can be used to distinguish between superficial and deep venous system incompetence. To perform the test, the patient is placed in the supine position and the affected leg is elevated in order to empty the superficial venous system. Either manual compression or a tourniquet is applied proximally and the patient is moved to an upright position. Individuals with deep venous system insufficiency will have rapid filling of the superficial veins, whereas patients with reflux that is limited to the superficial venous system will not have filling for greater than 20 seconds after changing position.

Venous stasis ulcers are often located over the distal-medial aspect of the lower extremities, commonly in the vicinity of the medial malleolus. In contrast, ulcers associated with arterial disease tend to occur over the distal digits or over distal-lateral bony prominences. Both forms of ulceration can be painful. Venous stasis ulcers are typically shallow with irregular boarders and commonly have a granulated or fibrinous base. Venous stasis ulcers are present in around 1% of the population in Westernized countries and account for around 80% of lower extremity ulcers.

Evaluation with duplex ultrasonography is recommended for most patients with a new clinical diagnosis of venous insufficiency. Ultrasound is useful in the assessment of proximal venous compression, deep vein thrombosis, and for determining the direction of venous flow. By using a rapid cuff inflation-deflation maneuver while the patient is upright, the extent of the reversal of venous flow in the superficial system can be determined. Reversal of flow for greater that 0.5 seconds in duration is consistent with incompetent superficial valves, whereas reversal of flow for greater than one second is consistent with reflux originating in the deep venous system.

Normal calf muscle function is thought to improve venous return via a pump-like action during ambulation and lower extremity exercise. Impaired calf muscle function has been shown to positively correlate with the severity of venous insufficiency as well as with the formation of stasis ulcers.

3. **B.** A meta-analysis of 42 randomized trials comparing the use of different dressing types in individuals with venous stasis ulcers demonstrated no significant difference in wound healing rates when using a hydrocolloid dressing verses a simpler, less expensive non-adherent dressing.

Bacterial colonization of stasis ulcers is common. A meta-analysis that reviewed 22 trials involving the use of topical antibiotics, antiseptics, or systemic antibiotics found no clear evidence to support the routine use of systemic antibiotics in individuals with venous stasis ulcers. There was some data to suggest the usefulness of topical cadexomer iodine (not readily available in the United States); however, the authors concluded that more data was needed to determine the efficacy of alternative topical antibiotics/antiseptics such as povidone iodine and mupirocin. Systemic antibiotics are recommended in cases of ulcers with surrounding cellulitis.

A recent Cochrane review found that the use of compressive dressings promotes increased ulcer healing rates when compared to dressings without an element of compression (i.e., Unna boot). Single-layer dressings were less effective than multilayered dressings and multilayered dressings utilizing an elastic component were found to be more effective than those without. Increased calf muscle function as the result of structured exercise is likely to improve venous return and thereby promote ulcer healing.

Intermittent pneumatic compression devices are not considered first-line treatment for most individuals with CVI as they are both expensive and require patient immobilization while in use.

4. A. The classic GSV stripping procedure involves stripping of the vein from the ankle to the groin with high ligation at the sapheno-femoral junction. The greater saphenous nerve, which is a sensory cutaneous branch of the femoral nerve, is at risk of injury as it emerges from the adductor canal (formed by the tendons of the gracilis and sartorius muscles) to run with the GSV just posterior-medial to the tibia. Injury to the nerve results in loss of cutaneous sensation over the medial leg and can be avoided by not stripping the GSV distal to the knee.

Radiofrequency ablation has been shown to result in long-term GSV occlusion with occlusion rates upward of 88% at 4 years in one large trial. Another recent study reports GSV and small saphenous vein occlusion rates of up to 94.6% and 94.5%, respectively, at 14 months after radiofrequency ablation.

Tumescent solution is used in both radiofrequency ablation as well as endovenous laser ablation to anesthetize the tissue surrounding the vein as well as to protect the area from thermal injury.

Shorter laser wavelengths are better absorbed by hemoglobin, whereas longer wavelengths are better absorbed by water allowing them to have greater ablative effects on vein walls. Commonly used endovenous laser wavelengths are between 810 and 1470 nm.

A Cochrane review from 2013 found that allograft when used in conjunction with compression resulted in superior healing of longstanding stasis ulcers when compared to treatment with compression alone. Of note, the authors concluded that current data is insufficient to determine whether the use of autograft or xenograft results in increased rates of healing.

5. C. Although uncommon, ischemic strokes as well as transient ischemic attacks have been reported after foam sclerotherapy. Additional complications include DVT, anaphylactic reactions, and local tissue necrosis.

Varicose veins are approximately twice as common in women with a reported prevalence of 15% to 30.1% in men and 28% to 50.5% in women. Risk factors associated with the formation of varicose veins include prior pregnancy, standing occupations, prior episodes of thrombophlebitis, DVT, family history, and obesity.

Foam sclerotherapy, typically using 1% or 3% polidocanol in a gas to liquid ratio of 4:1, has been found to be superior to liquid polidocanol in the treatment of varicose veins due to GSV reflux. Lower extremity varicosities can be painful with standing. In addition to cosmetic complaints, patients frequently report feelings of heaviness, aching, or itching sensations.

Despite numerous studies and randomized controlled trials, compression stockings have not been clearly shown to halt the progression or slow the recurrence of uncomplicated varicose veins.

6. B. There are many patients who suffer from lower extremity CVI. CVI can be manifested as edema, dark skin discoloration, ulceration, deep venous thrombosis, superficial thrombophlebitis, and so on; but varicosities are the most common presentation of primary CVI. By definition, varicose veins are large and tortuous veins, which are greater than 3 mm in diameter. Bilateral lower extremity varicose veins are present in more than 50% of patients. Symptomatic varicosities are also common in approximately 40% of patients and are associated with the symptoms of venous hypertension such as heaviness, aching, cramping, tingling, and pruritus of the lower extremity. Approximately 25% of patients present with their lower extremity varicose veins for primarily cosmetic reasons. Although patients with chronic venous disease may certainly present with superficial thrombophlebitis, deep venous thrombosis, edema, or ulceration, these are much less frequently presenting symptoms. Additionally, venous stasis ulcers are more often located over the medial malleolus.

7. D. The best management strategy for acute iliofemoral deep venous thrombosis (DVT) is still controversial. However, the setting of an acute iliofemoral DVT, CDT, and anticoagulation together can provide prevention of thrombus propagation, fast removal of the thrombus, and preservation of functional venous valves. According to a study evaluating the Nationwide Inpatient Sample (NIS) data, CDT was not associated with an increased mortality compared to anticoagulation alone. However, CDT was associated with higher risk of intracranial hemorrhage, blood transfusion, and longer length of stay in the hospital. CDT, though, was also associated with a decreased risk of developing PTS and its severity. PTS is the long-term sequela of a DVT, which may present as chronic edema, pain, skin discoloration, paresthesia, pruritus, venous hypertension, difficulty walking, and so on. Acute iliofemoral DVT carries a high risk of PTS that potentially impairs walking in

15% to 40% of patients. According to a randomized controlled trial (CaVenT), there was a 28% absolute risk reduction of PTS with in the CDT group compared to anticoagulation alone. CDT is not associated with higher readmission rate.

8. D. There are many factors that may contribute to an increased risk of perioperative venous thromboembolism (VTE): chronic non-ambulatory status, advanced age, obesity, surgery, genetic predisposition, previous history of VTE, active malignancy, and so on. Among those with the risk factors, the patients with active malignancy are at the highest risk of developing VTE, approximately 15% at 1 year. Therefore, for the patients at higher risk, combination of both mechanical and pharmacological VTE prophylaxis is strongly recommended. Based on current consensus and randomized trial study data, it is recommended for the patients with active malignancy undergoing major surgery to receive pharmacological prophylaxis with LMWH both in hospital and for a month after discharge in addition to the use of SCDs during hospitalization. Subcutaneous UFH or SCDs alone for VTE prophylaxis would not be sufficient for this high-risk patient with metastatic malignancy. Routine IVC filter placement prior to the surgical resection is not recommended.

BIBLIOGRAPHY

Bashir R, Zack C, Zhao H, et al. Comparative outcomes of catheter-directed thrombolysis plus anticoagulation vs anticoagulation alone to treat lower extremity proximal deep vein thrombosis. *JAMA Intern Med.* 2014;174(9):1494–1501.

Bergqvist D, Agnelli G, Cohen AT, et al. ENOXACAN II investigators. Duration of prophylaxis against venous thromboembolism with enoxaparin after surgery for cancer. *N Engl J Med.* 2002;346(13):975–980.

Cavezzi A, Parsi K. Complications of foam sclerotherapy. *Phlebology.* 2012;27(1):46–51.

Choi JH, Park HC, Joh JH. The occlusion rate and patterns of saphenous vein after radiofrequency ablation. *J Korean Surg Soc.* 2013;84(2):107–113.

Coleridge SP. Sclerotherapy and foam sclerotherapy for varicose veins. *Phlebology.* 2009;24(6):260–269.

Criqui MH, Jamosmos M, Fronek A, et al. Chronic venous disease in an ethnically diverse population: the San Diego Population Study. *Am J Epidemiol.* 2003;158(5):448–456.

Delis K, Bountouroglou D, Mansfield A. Venous claudication in iliofemoral thrombosis. *Ann Surg.* 2004;239:118–126.

Evans CJ, Fowkes FG, Ruckley CV, Lee AJ. Prevalence of varicose veins and chronic venous insufficiency in men and women in the general population: Edinburgh vein study. *J Epidemiol Community Health.* March 1999;53(3):149–153.

Fagarasanu A, Alotaibi G, Hrimiuc R, et al. Role of extended thromboprophylaxis after abdominal and pelvic surgery in cancer patients: a systematic review and meta-analysis. *Ann Surg Oncol.* 2016;23(5):1422–1430.

Fernando RR, Koranne KP, Schneider D, Fuentes F. May-Thurner syndrome. *Tex. Heart Inst J.* 2013;40(1):82–87.

Fretz V, Binkert CA. Compression of the inferior vena cava by the right iliac artery: a rare variant of May-Thurner syndrome. *Cardiovasc Intervent Radiol.* 2010;33(5):1060–1063.

Geerts WH, Bergqvist D, Pineo GF, et al. Prevention of venous thromboembolism: American College of Chest Physicians Evidence-Based Clinical Practice Guidelines (8th Edition). *Chest.* 2008;133(6 Suppl):381S–453S.

Gillespie DL, Writing Group III of the Pacific Vascular Symposium 6, Kistner B, et al. Venous ulcer diagnosis, treatment, and prevention of recurrences. *J Vasc Surg.* 2010;52(5):8S–14S.

Haig Y, Enden T, Grotta O, et al. Post-thrombotic syndrome after catheter-directed thrombolysis for deep vein thrombosis (CaVenT): 5-year follow-up results of an open-label, randomized controlled trial. *Lancet Haematology.* 2016;3(2):e64–e71.

Jones JE, Nelson EA, Al-Hity A. Skin grafting for venous leg ulcers. *Cochrane Database Syst Rev.* 2013;1:CD001737.

Kibbe MR, Ujiki M, Goodwin AL, et al. Iliac vein compression in an asymptomatic patient population. *J Vasc Surg.* 2004;39(5):937–943.

Kim JY, Choi D, Guk Ko Y, et al. Percutaneous treatment of deep vein thrombosis in May-Thurner syndrome. *Cardiovasc Intervent Radiol.* 2006;29(4):571–575.

Meissner MH. Pathophysiology of varicose veins and chronic venous insufficiency. In: Hallett JW, Mills JL, Earnshaw J, eds. *Comprehensive Vascular and Endovascular Surgery.* Elsevier Health Sciences; 2009.

Merchant RF, Pichot O, Myers KA. Four-year follow-up on endovascular radiofrequency obliteration of great saphenous reflux. *Dermatol Surg.* 2005;31(2):129–134.

Molloy S, Jacob S, Buckenham T, Khaw KT, Taylor RS. Arterial compression of the right common iliac vein: an unusual anatomical variant. *Cardiovasc Surg.* 2002;10(3):291–292.

Nelson EA, Mani R, Thomas K, Vowden K. Intermittent pneumatic compression for treating venous leg ulcers. *Cochrane Database Syst Rev.* 2011;16(2):CD001899.

O'Meara S, Al-Kurdi D, Ologun Y, et al. Antibiotics and antiseptics for venous leg ulcers. *Cochrane Database Syst Rev.* 2014;10(1):CD003557.

O'Meara S, Cullum N, Nelson EA, Dumville JC. Compression for venous leg ulcers. *Cochrane Database Syst Rev.* 2012;14(11): CD000265.

Osborne NH, Wakefield TW, Henke PK. Venous thromboembolism in cancer patients undergoing major surgery. *Annals Surg Oncol.* 2008;15(12):3567–3578.

O'Sullivan GJ. The role of interventional radiology in the management of deep venous thrombosis: Advanced therapy. *Cardiovasc Intervent Radiol.* 2011;34(3):445–461.

O'Sullivan GJ, Semba CP, Bittner CA, et al. Endovascular management of iliac vein compression (May-Thurner) syndrome. *J Vasc Interv Radiol.* 2000;11(7):823–836.

Padberg FT Jr, Johnston MV, Sisto SA. Structured exercise improves calf muscle pump function in chronic venous insufficiency: a randomized trial. *J Vasc Surg.* 2004;39(1): 79–87.

Palfreyman SJ, Michaels JA. A systematic review of compression hosiery for uncomplicated varicose veins. *Phlebology.* 2009;24(1):13–33.

Palfreyman S, Nelson EA, Michaels JA. Dressings for venous leg ulcers: systematic review and meta-analysis. *BMJ.* 2007;335(7613):244.

Rabe E, Otto J, Schliephake D, Pannier F. Efficacy and safety of great saphenous vein sclerotherapy using standardised polidocanol foam (ESAF): a randomised controlled multicentre clinical trial. *Eur J Vasc Endovasc Surg.* 2008;35(2):238–245.

White-Chu EF, Conner-Kerr TA. Overview of guidelines for the prevention and treatment of venous leg ulcers: a U.S. perspective. *J Multidiscip Healthc.* 2014;11(7): 111–117.

105

Thoracic Outlet Syndrome

Robert McMurray

A 32-year-old right-hand-dominant construction worker presents to the Emergency Department with a 2-day history of worsening swelling and pain in his right arm. He also reports a recent 3-week history of right-arm fatigue and soreness during work. He has no other medical history. On exam, his right arm is diffusely edematous with prominent chest and shoulder varicosities. He has 2+ radial and ulnar pulses. Sensation and motor function are intact.

1. **Which of the following is most likely true regarding the pathophysiology of the condition in this patient?**

   A. Scalene muscle fibrosis is the major causative factor.
   B. It is due to compression from a cervical rib.
   C. It is due to intimal and endothelial injury of the axillary and subclavian veins.
   D. A hypercoaguable state is present, leading to spontaneous subclavian vein thrombosis.

2. **Which of the following is the most common order of anatomic structures in the thoracic outlet, moving from anteromedial to posterolateral?**

   A. Subclavius muscle, subclavian artery, subclavian vein, phrenic nerve, anterior scalene muscle, brachial plexus, middle scalene muscle
   B. Subclavius muscle, subclavian vein, phrenic nerve, anterior scalene muscle, subclavian artery, brachial plexus, middle scalene muscle
   C. Anterior scalene, subclavian vein, subclavius muscle, subclavian artery, brachial plexus, middle scalene muscle, phrenic nerve

   D. Anterior scalene, subclavian vein, subclavius muscle, brachial plexus, subclavian artery, middle scalene muscle, phrenic nerve

3. **Which of the following is true with regard to the diagnosis of thoracic outlet syndrome?**

   A. Electromyography and nerve conduction tests alone exhibit a strong degree of specificity in the diagnosis.
   B. Scalene muscle injection is not helpful in diagnosing neurogenic thoracic outlet syndrome (nTOS) but serves as a useful temporizing measure prior to definitive surgery.
   C. Venography is required for the diagnosis of venous thoracic outlet syndrome (vTOS).
   D. In vTOS, findings on dynamic ultrasound scan include a decrease in venous velocity by 50% with abduction.

4. **The most common site of brachial plexus compression causing neurogenic thoracic outlet syndrome is:**

   A. Costoclavicular space
   B. Pectoralis minor
   C. Scalene triangle
   D. Subclavius muscle

5. **Which of the following is the most common complication of a first-rib resection?**

   A. Lymphatic leakage
   B. Pneumothorax
   C. Intercostal brachial cutaneous nerve injury

D. Long thoracic nerve injury

E. Subclavian vein injury

6. **A woman presents with evidence of acute upper extremity limb ischemia with discoloration of her 4th and 5th digits that are painful to the touch. There is a pulsatile mass appreciated inferior to her clavicle, with no mass on the contralateral side. The condition most likely responsible for this patient's condition is:**

A. Raynaud's disease

B. Subclavian venous occlusion

C. Buerger's disease (thromboangiitis obliterans)

D. Compression of the brachial plexus

E. Embolization from a subclavian artery aneurysm

ANSWERS

1. C. The thoracic outlet is defined as the anatomic area bound by the clavicle superiorly, first rib inferiorly, subclavius muscle anteriorly, and the middle scalene muscle posteriorly. It is through this region that the subclavian artery, vein, and brachial plexus pass as they exit the chest. TOS refers to the compression of one or more of the neurovascular structures as they exit this region, and can be subdivided into three major classes depending upon the structure that is compressed (in order of decreasing incidence): neurogenic, venous, and arterial. nTOS is by far the most common type, comprising greater than 95% of all cases.

Scalene muscle fibrosis as the result of a traumatic event such as an MVC (classically whiplash injury) or engaging in repetitive upper extremity activity is a major causative factor. Occasionally, an anomalous first rib or cervical rib can result in nTOS. The most common presenting symptom is arm paresthesias, present in approximately 90% of patients. Other classical symptoms are pain and weakness in the upper extremity, neck pain, and occipital headaches. Pain and paresthesias are most commonly noted in the C8-T1 (ulnar distribution).

Arterial TOS (aTOS) is the least common variant with an incidence of approximately 1%. Patients typically present with ispilateral hand or digit ischemia from distal embolization of a subclavian artery stenosis or aneurysmal dilation, almost always as a result of extrinsic compression from a cervical or anomalous first rib.

The patient described earlier suffers from vTOS, also known as Paget-Schroetter Syndrome, which is thrombosis or severe narrowing of the subclavian or axillary vein from chronic extrinsic compression at the level of the costoclavicular space. Repetitive injury to the intima and endothelium results in a fibrotic response and loss of normal endothelial function. This damaged endothelium is thought to be a nidus for thrombus formation. vTOS accounts for approximately 2% to 3% of all TOS cases. It is classically seen in young, healthy patients with a history of repetitive motion (swimmers, baseball pitchers, manual laborer, nurse) or those with an active lifestyle. Symptoms include arm swelling (unique to vTOS), cyanosis, pain/aching, and occasionally paresthesias in the fingers or hands (often secondary to hand swelling).

2. B. Moving from anteromedial to posterolateral, the subclavius muscle is the first anatomic structure, which attaches from the first rib to the inferior portion of the clavicle and can be a source of compression of the next structure, which is the subclavian vein. The phrenic nerve usually runs immediately posterior to the subclavian vein along the anterior scalene muscle. However, in approximately 5% to 7% of individuals, it can run anterior to the subclavian vein, and can be a rare cause of subclavian vein compression.

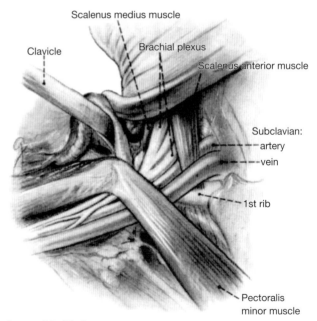

Source: Machleder, 1998.

The subclavian artery is separated from the vein via the anterior scalene muscle. Posterior and lateral to the artery are the brachial plexus and finally the middle scalene muscle.

3. **D.** The diagnosis of nTOS can be challenging but can be made when the patient demonstrates symptoms appropriate to the neurovascular bundle at the thoracic outlet, has physical exam findings that indicate neurovascular compression, and testing that supports the diagnosis of nTOS and a history consistent with the development of nTOS. The single best test to determine whether symptoms are related to the compression of the neurovascular bundle at the thoracic outlet is an EMG-guided scalene muscle stimulation and block test. In one study, 122 patients being evaluated for nTOS underwent anterior scalene block using electrophysiologic guidance. Of the patients who were ultimately diagnosed with a condition other than TOS, only 5% had a positive response to the block, compared to 92% of patients with confirmed TOS. In addition, of the patients who underwent surgical decompression for TOS, 94% with a positive response to scalene muscle block preoperatively had successful surgery, while only 50% of those with negative response preoperatively had good outcomes.

In addition to standard chest radiographs to detect the presence of a cervical or anomalous first rib, dynamic duplex ultrasonography is used to identify axillosubclavian thrombus as well as evaluate for venous compression by having the patient abduct the ipsilateral arm, which should result in a decrease in venous velocity by 50%. Ultrasound is recommended by the American College of Radiology as the best first approach for direct evaluation of arm veins, although venography is still considered the gold standard for making the diagnosis of vTOS (Paget-Schroetter syndrome). The treatment of vTOS includes the administration of anticoagulation once the diagnosis of a DVT is made. If the diagnosis is before 14 days after the onset of symptoms then catheter directed thrombolysis can be considered with reported excellent results, although attempts at thrombolysis after 14 days days have a decreased chance of successful re-establishment of luminal patency. After successful thrombolysis, thoracic outlet decompression should be pursued. However, ultrasound-guided access to the deep system (true brachial veins) at the antecubital fossa or upper arm is needed to obtain optimal visualization and also perform intervention. If the cephalic vein is used for contrast injection, the diagnosis can be missed.

4. **C. Neurologic thoracic outlet syndrome is by far the most common form of TOS, accounting for more than 95% of all cases. vTOS occurs in 2% to 3% of patients and aTOS occurs in less than 1% of all TOS cases.** The brachial plexus arises from nerve roots C5 to T1, and the scalene triangle is the most common site of compression. The compression can occur as the brachial plexus passes over the first rib between the anterior and middle scalene muscles (through the scalene triangle). In the scalene triangle area, the five nerve roots become three trunks. The branches of the brachial plexus lie deep to the pectoralis minor along with the axillary artery and vein. The scalene triangle is made up of anterior scalene muscle, the middle scalene muscle and the first rib. Since outcomes is in large part, based on functional improvements, outcomes in large part depend on the extent of the disability prior to the operation. Unfortunately, there are no well-defined classification algorithms that are in common use by which to stratify patients. Most post-surgical outcomes are divided into the categories of excellent (complete relief of symptoms), good (relief of major symptoms but some symptoms still persist), fair (partial relief of symptoms but some major symptoms still exist), and poor (no relief of symptoms). Also, there is no outcome measures that distinguish between the different operative approaches which further confounds the data. For thoracic outlet decompression using the supraclavicular approach, seven different publications totaling 1222 patients was pooled. Overall, the results listed were good outcomes in 59% to 91% (mean 77%), fair in 5% to 33% (mean 15%), and poor in 3% to 18% (mean 8%) of patients.

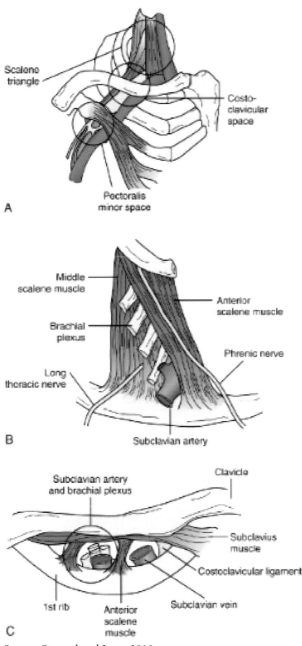

A

B

C

Source: Osgood and Lum, 2019.

5. B. All of the answers have been reported as complications after first-rib resection, with pneumothorax being the most common, occurring in up to 1/3 of patients by some reports.

Entry into the pleural space with resultant pneumothorax or pleural effusion is a known hazard of first-rib resection. At the completion of the procedure, it is generally recommended to instill irrigation into the field and perform a Valsalva maneuver in order to check for pneumothorax. If present, a small chest tube can be placed. In a large retrospective

series of 770 patients who underwent supraclavicular first rib resection and scalenectomy, very few operative complications were noted. Although pneumothorax is a known complication of this procedure, no patients developed postoperative pneumothorax because for the 20% of patients in whom the pleural space was inadvertently entered during the procedure, a closed suction drain was placed to seal the defect. Postoperative causalgia requiring sympathectomy occurred in two patients. One patient experienced lymphatic leak.

In another series examining 334 surgeries for nTOS, 13 complications (3.9%) occurred. The most common was pneumothorax (*n* = 7), for which six patient required chest tubes and one patient required additional surgery. There were five instances of vascular injury (four minor subclavian vein injuries and one transection of the internal mammary artery resulting in a 2 L blood loss). There was also one minor injury to the long thoracic nerve.

The intercostal brachial nerve is encountered during the transaxillary approach as it exists between the 1st and 2nd ribs, and should be preserved if possible. Damage to this nerve would result in loss of sensation over the medial aspect of the arm.

6. E. The patient is presenting with signs of upper extremity ischemia secondary to embolization from a subclavian artery aneurysm. Radiography should be done in cases of upper extremity acute arterial occlusion to look for the presence of a cervical rib. This is due to the high correlation of aTOS with cervical ribs (up to two-thirds of cases). Cervical ribs occur in less than 1% of the population, and most are asymptomatic. There is an anatomic spectrum of cervical ribs, from the presence of a prominent C7 transverse process to a full C7 rib with fusion to the first thoracic rib. Repetitive trauma to the subclavian artery during arm motion can result in aneurysmal degeneration and thrombus formation. It has been reported that aTOS occurs more frequently on the dominant handed side, even in the face of bilateral anatomic abnormalities, due to the more frequent repetitive trauma. First-rib abnormalities occur in 20%, fibrocartilagnious bands in 10%, and both prior clavicular fractures and enlarged C7 transverse processes in less than 5% each. The most symptomatic presentation of aTOS is arterial thromboembolism to the ipsilateral arm, as described in this case. There is no role for conservative treatment with symptomatic arterial TOS. There are 3 main principles to treating aTOS. The first is to relieve the extrinsic compression of the artery, the second is to remove the source of embolus and the third is to restore distal circulation. Relieving arterial compression is performed by removing cervical or first ribs and the anterior scalene, plus any other anomalous anatomy that is causing impingement. Removing the source of embolus involves removing the damaged artery and performing an interposition bypass or by placing a stent graft across the injured arterial segment. Restoring distal cirsulation involving either performing thrombolysis, thromboembolectomy or bypass.

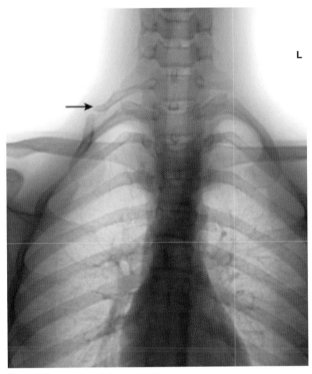

Source: Osgood and Lum, 2019.

BIBLIOGRAPHY

Adelman MA, Stone DH, Riles TS, Lamparello PJ, Giangola G, Rosen RJ. A multidisciplinary approach to the treatment of Paget Schroeter syndrome. *Ann Vasc Surg.* 1997;11:149–154.

Altobelli GG, Kudo T, Ahn SS, et al. Thoracic outlet syndrome: Pattern of clinical success after operative decompression. *J Vasc Surg.* 2005;42:122–128.

Brooke BS, Freischlag JA. Contemporary management of thoracic outlet syndrome. *Curr Opin Cardiol.* 2010;25:535–540.

Chang KZ, Likes K, Davis K, et al. The significance of cervical ribs in thoracic outlet syndrome. *J Vasc Surg.* 2013;57:771–775.

Criado E, Berguer R, Greenfield L. The spectrum of arterial compression of the thoracic outlet. *J Vasc Surg.* 2010;52:406–411.

Desai SS, Toliyat M., Dua A, et al. Outcomes of surgical paraclavicular thoracic outlet decompression. *Ann Vasc Surg.* 2014;28:457–464.

Doyle A, Wolford HY, Davies MG, et al. Management of effort thrombosis of the subclavian vein: today's treatment. *Ann Vasc Surg.* 2007;21:723–729.

Hempel GK, Shutze WP, Anderson JF, Bukhari HI. 770 consecutive supraclavicular first rib resections for thoracic outlet syndrome. *Ann Vasc Surg.* 1996;10:456–463.

Illig KA, Donahue D, Duncan A. Reporting standards of the Society for Vascular Surgery for thoracic outlet syndrome. *J Vasc Surg.* 2016 Sep;64(3):e23–e35.

Illig KA, Doyle AJ. A comprehensive review of Paget-Schroetter syndrome. *J Vasc Surg.* 2010;51:1538–1547.

Jordan SE, Machleder HI. Diagnosis of thoracic outlet syndrome using electrophysiologically guided anterior scalene blocks. *Ann Vasc Surg.* 1998;12:260–264.

Lee JT, Karwowski JK, Olcott C, et al. Long-term thrombotic recurrence after nonoperative management of Paget-Schroetter syndrome. *J Vasc Surg.* 2006;43:1236–1243.

Leffert RD. Complications of surgery for thoracic outlet syndrome. *Hand Clin.* 2004;20:91–98.

Machleder HI, ed. *Vascular Disorders of the Upper Extremity.* 3rd ed. Futura Publishing; 1998.

Meier GH, Pollack JS, Gusberg RJ, et al. Initial experience with venous stents in exertional axillary-subclavian vein thrombosis. *J Vasc Surg.* 1996;24:974–981.

Osgood MJ, Lum YW. Thoracic outlet syndrome pathophysiology and evaluation. In: Sidawy AN, Perler BA, eds. *Rutherford's Vascular Surgery.* 9th ed. Elsevier Saunders; 2019:1607–1618.

Propper BW, Freischlag JA. Thoracic outlet syndromes. In: Cameron JL, Cameron AM, eds. *Current Surgical Therapy.* 11th ed. Elsevier Saunders; 2014:924–927.

Sanders R. Thoracic outlet syndrome: general considerations. In Cronenwett JL, Johnson KW, eds. *Rutherford's Vascular Surgery.* 7th ed. Elsevier Saunders; 2010:1865–1877.

Sanders RJ, Annest SJ. Thoracic outlet and pectoralis minor syndromes. *Semin Vasc Surg.* 2014;27(2):86–117.

Sanders RJ, Hammond SL, Rao NM. Diagnosis of thoracic outlet syndrome. *J Vasc Surg.* 2007;46:601–604.

Schroeder WE, Green FR. Phrenic nerve injuries: report of a case, anatomical and experimental researches, and critical review of the literature. *Am J Med Sci.* 1902;123: 196–220.

Urschel HC, Patel AN. Paget-Schroetter syndrome therapy: failure of intravenous stents. *Ann Thorac Surg.* 2003;75:1693–1696.

Urschel HC, Patel AN. Surgery remains the most effective treatment for Paget-Schroetter Syndrome: 50 years' experience. *Ann Thorac Surg.* 2008;86:254–260.

Urschel HC Jr, Razzuk MA. Paget-Schroetter syndrome: what is the best management? *Ann Thorac Surg.* 2000;69:1663–1668.

Index

Page numbers followed by "f" denote figures; those followed by "t" denote tables.